FIFTH EDITION

Perspectives on Nursing Theory

EDITED BY

Pamela G. Reed, PhD, RN, FAAN
Professor
University of Arizona, College of Nursing
Tucson, Arizona

Nelma B. Crawford Shearer, PhD, RN
Associate Professor
Arizona State University, College of Nursing & Healthcare Innovation
Phoenix, Arizona

 Wolters Kluwer | Lippincott Williams & Wilkins
Health
Philadelphia · Baltimore · New York · London
Buenos Aires · Hong Kong · Sydney · Tokyo

Senior Acquisitions Editor: Margaret Zuccarini
Managing Editor: Michelle Clarke
Editorial Assistant: Season Evans
Production Project Manager: Cynthia Rudy
Director of Nursing Production: Helen Ewan
Senior Managing Editor / Production: Erika Kors
Design Coordinator: Holly Reid McLaughlin
Cover Design: Melissa Walter
Manufacturing Coordinator: Karin Duffield
Production Services / Compositor: Aptara, Inc.

5th edition

9 8 7 6 5 4 3 2 1

Printed in the United States of America

Library of Congress Cataloging-in-Publication Data

Perspectives on nursing theory / edited by Pamela G. Reed, Nelma B. Crawford Shearer. – 5th ed.
      p. ; cm.
   Anthology of previously published articles.
   Includes bibliographical references and index.
   ISBN-13: 978-0-7817-7383-6
   ISBN-10: 0-7817-7383-0
   1. Nursing–Philosophy.   2. Nursing models.   I. Reed, Pamela G., 1952–   II. Shearer, Nelma B. Crawford, 1950–   III. Title: Nursing theory.
   [DNLM: 1. Nursing Theory – Collected Works.   2. Philosophy, Nursing – Collected Works. WY 86 P467 2008]
   RT84.5.P47 2008
   610.7301 – dc22

                                    2007039314

LWW.com

ABOUT THE EDITORS

Pamela G. Reed is Professor at the University of Arizona College of Nursing in Tucson, Arizona, where she also served as Associate Dean for Academic Affairs for seven years. She is a three-time graduate of Wayne State University in Detroit, receiving a BSN in 1974, an MSN in 1976 (with a double major in child-adolescent psychiatric mental health nursing and teaching) and her PhD, with a major in nursing (focused on lifespan development and aging), in 1982. Dr. Reed pioneered research into spirituality and well-being with her doctoral research with terminally ill patients. She also developed a theory of self-transcendence and two widely used research instruments, the *Spiritual Perspective Scale* and the *Self-Transcendence Scale*. Her publications and funded research reflect a dual scholarly focus: Spirituality and other facilitators of well-being and decision-making in end-of-life transitions; nursing metatheory and knowledge development. Dr. Reed also enjoys time with her family, reading, classical music, swimming, and hiking in the mountains and canyons of Arizona.

Nelma B. Crawford Shearer is Associate Professor at Arizona State University College of Nursing & Healthcare Innovation in Phoenix, Arizona. She received her BS in Nursing from South Dakota State University in 1972, an MEd from the University of Missouri–St. Louis in 1977, an MS in Nursing from Southern Illinois University–Edwardsville in 1987, and a PhD with a major in Nursing from the University of Arizona in 2000. Dr. Shearer is an American Nurse Foundation Scholar and a John A. Hartford Foundation Institute of Geriatric Nursing Research Scholar. In 2006 she received the Geriatric Nursing Research award from the Western Institute of Nursing in partnership with the Hartford Institute for Geriatric Nursing. Dr. Shearer conducts research in promoting health empowerment in adults, and is currently funded by NIH/NINR for the study "Health Empowerment Intervention with Homebound Older Adults." In her spare time, Dr. Shearer enjoys her family, entertaining friends, antiquing, gardening, and going for long bike rides.

*W*e dedicate this book to the student and teacher in all of us who, in reading and reflecting on its chapters, may be more informed and inspired to extend nursing knowledge.

Pamela G. Reed
Nelma B. Crawford Shearer

Contributors

Donna L. Algase, PhD, RN, FAAN, FGSA
Professor and Faculty Associate, Institute of Gerontology
Director, Center on Frail and Vulnerable Elders
School of Nursing
University of Michigan
Ann Arbor, Michigan

Joan M. Anderson, RN, PhD
Professor Emerita
School of Nursing
University of British Columbia
Vancouver, British Columbia, Canada

Cynthia Arslanian-Engoren, PhD, APRN, BC, CNS
Assistant Professor
University of Michigan School of Nursing
Ann Arbor, Michigan

Mark Avis, MSc, BA(Hons), RGN, RMN, RNT
Chair in Social Contexts
School of Nursing
University of Nottingham
Nottingham, England, United Kingdom

Alan Gordon Barnard, BA, MA, PhD, RN
Senior Lecturer and
Course Coordinator for the Bachelor of Nursing Program
School of Nursing
Queensland University of Technology
Brisbane, Australia

Elizabeth Ann Manhart Barrett, RN, PhD, FAAN
Professor Emerita of Nursing
Hunter College
City University of New York
New York, New York

Jennifer L. Baumbusch, MSN, RN
Doctoral Candidate at the School of Nursing
University of British Columbia
Vancouver, British Columbia, Canada

Ian Beech, RMN, RGN, BA(Hons), PGCE
Senior Lecturer in Mental Health Nursing
School of Care Sciences
University of Glamorgan
Pontypridd, Wales, United Kingdom

Heather A. Biasio, RN, BSN
Faculty
Camosun College
Victoria, British Columbia, Canada

Anne H. Bishop, EdD
Professor Emerita of Nursing
Lynchburg College
Lynchburg College, Virginia

Kristín Björnsdóttir, RN, EdD
Professor
Faculty of Nursing
University of Iceland
Reykjavik, Iceland

Barbara A. Carper, EdD, RN, FAAN
Professor Emerita
Former Associate Dean for Academic Affairs
University of North Carolina–Charlotte
Charlotte, North Carolina

William K. Cody, RN, PhD, FAAN
Dean
Presbyterian School of Nursing
Queens University of Charlotte
Charlotte, North Carolina

Sheila A. Corcoran-Perry, PhD, RN, FAAN
Professor Emerita
University of Minnesota
Minneapolis, Minnesota

William Richard Cowling, III, RN, PhD, APRN-BC
Professor and Director of PhD Program
School of Nursing
University of North Carolina
Editor, *Journal of Holistic Nursing*
Greensboro, North Carolina

Holly DeGroot, PhD, RN, FAAN
CEO of Catalyst Systems
Novato, California

Freda G. DeKeyser, RN, PhD
Head, Clinical Masters Program and
Coordinator, Nursing Research
Hadassah-Hebrew University School of Nursing
Jerusalem, Israel

James Dickoff, PhD
Professor
Department of Philosophy
Kent State University
Kent, Ohio

Gweneth Hartrick Doane, PhD, RN
Professor
University of Victoria School of Nursing
Victoria, British Columbia, Canada

*****Rosemary Ellis,** PhD, RN
Former Professor
Frances Payne Bolton School of Nursing
Case Western Reserve University
Cleveland, Ohio

Joan Engebretson, DrPH, AHN-BC, RN
Professor, Nursing for Target Populations
School of Nursing
University of Texas Science Center at Houston
Houston, Texas

Jacqueline Fawcett, PhD, FAAN
Professor, College of Nursing and Health Sciences
Director, Office of Urban Family Health
University of Massachusetts–Boston
Boston, Massachusetts

Linda M. Ferguson, RN, BSN, PGD MN, PhD
Professor, College of Nursing
University of Saskatchewan
Saskatoon, Saskatchewan, Canada

Anastasia A. Fisher, RN, DNSc
Associate Professor
School of Nursing and Health Science
University of San Diego
San Diego, California

Joyce J. Fitzpatrick, PhD, MBA, RN, FAAN, FNAP
Elizabeth Brooks Ford Professor of Nursing
Case Western Reserve University
Frances Payne Bolton School of Nursing
Cleveland, Ohio

Dawn Freshwater, PhD, BA(Hons), RGN, RNT, FRCN
Professor and Director, Centre for Applied Research
Institute of Health and Community Studies
Bournemouth University
Bournemouth, Dorset, England, United Kingdom

Sally Gadow, PhD, RN
Professor
School of Nursing
University of Colorado Health Services Center
Denver, Colorado

Denise Gastaldo, BScN, MSc, PhD
Associate Professor
University of Toronto
Lawrence Bloomberg Faculty of Nursing
Toronto, Ontario, Canada

Karen K. Giuliano, RN, PhD, FAAN
Clinical Scientist
Philips Medical Systems
Andover, Massachusetts

Suzanne Gordon, BA
Freelance journalist, author, and lecturer
Visiting Professor
University of Maryland School of Nursing
Baltimore, Maryland
Assistant Adjunct Professor
University of California San Francisco School of Nursing
San Francisco, California

***Susan R. Gortner,** MN, PhD, FAAN
Professor Emerita
School of Nursing
University of California, San Francisco
San Francisco, California

Margaret E. Hardy, PhD, RN, FAAN
Professor of Nursing, Retired
University of Rhode Island College of Nursing
Kingston, Rhode Island
Independent Scholar
Holliston, Massachusetts

Angela Henderson, RN, PhD
Associate Professor and Associate Director of
    Faculty Development
University of British Columbia
School of Nursing
Vancouver, British Columbia, Canada

Frank D. Hicks, PhD, RN
Associate Professor, Adult Health Nursing Director,
    Generalist Education Programs
Rush University College of Nursing
Chicago, Illinois

Patricia A. Higgins, RN, PhD
Associate Professor of Nursing and Researcher
Frances Payne Bolton School of Nursing
Case Western Reserve University
Cleveland, Ohio

Colin Adrian Holmes, BA(Hons), TCert, MPhil, PhD
Adjunct Professor of Nursing
James Cook University
Townsville, Queensland, Australia
Honorary Visiting Professor
University of Central Lancashire
Preston, Lancashire, England

Dave Holmes, RN, BScN, MSc, PhD
Associate Professor
University of Ottawa, Faculty of Health Sciences, School of Nursing
Ottawa, Ontario, Canada

Linda Carol Hughes, PhD, RN
Research Associate Professor
School of Nursing
University of North Carolina at Chapel Hill
Chapel Hill, North Carolina

Judith E. Hupcey, EdD, RN, CRNP
Associate Professor of Nursing, College of Health
    and Human Development
Associate Professor of Humanities, College of Medicine
The Pennsylvania State University
University Park, Pennsylvania

Eun-Ok Im, PhD, MPH, RN, CNS, FAAN
Professor
School of Nursing
The University of Texas at Austin
Austin, Texas

Patricia James, PhD
Professor
Department of Philosophy
Kent State University
Kent, Ohio

Cheryl Bland Jones, PhD, RN
Associate Professor and Health Care Systems Coordinator,
    School of Nursing
Investigator at the Southeast Regional Health Workforce Center
University of North Carolina at Chapel Hill
Chapel Hill, North Carolina

*Deceased

June F. Kikuchi, RN (Retired), BScN, MN, PhD
Professor Emerita
Faculty of Nursing
University of Alberta
Edmonton, Alberta, Canada

Hesook Suzie Kim, PhD, RN
Professor Emerita
College of Nursing
University of Rhode Island
Kingston, Rhode Island

Sheryl Reimer Kirkham, RN, PhD
Associate Professor in the Nursing Department and
Coordinator, Scholarship Initiatives in the Master of Arts
    in Leadership Program
Trinity Western University
Langley, British Columbia, Canada

Gerri C. Lasiuk, RN, BA (Psych), MN
Certified Mental Health/Psychiatric Nurse
Doctoral Candidate
Faculty of Nursing
Women's Health Research Unit
University of Alberta
Edmonton, Alberta, Canada

*Susan K. Leddy, RN, PhD
Professor Emerita
Widener University
School of Nursing
Chester, Pennsylvania

Joan Liaschenko, RN, PhD
Professor
Center for Bioethics
School of Nursing
University of Minnesota
Minneapolis, Minnesota

Patricia Liehr, PhD, RN
Professor
Associate Dean for Nursing Research and Scholarship
Christine E. Lynn College of Nursing
Florida Atlantic University
Boca Raton, Florida

Ruth Palan Lopez, RN, PhD
Assistant Professor and Coordinator of the Gerontological
    Nurse Practitioner Program
Massachusetts General Hospital Institute of Health Professions
Boston, Massachusetts

Lois W. Lowry, RN, DNSc
Professor and Coordinator of the DSN Program
College of Nursing
East Tennessee State University
Johnson City, Tennessee

Kara Lee Schick Makaroff, RN, BScN
Staff Nurse
Vancouver Island Health Authority
Victoria, British Columbia, Canada

Barbara A. Mark, PhD, RN, FAAN
Sarah Frances Russell Distinguished Professor in Nursing Systems
University of North Carolina at Chapel Hill
Chapel Hill, North Carolina

Jo-Ann Marrs, BS, MS, MSN, EdD
Associate Dean of Academic Programs and Student Services
East Tennessee State University
Johnson City, Tennessee

Joan McCarthy, MA, PhD
Lecturer, Healthcare Ethics
School of Nursing and Midwifery
Brookfield Health Sciences Complex
University College Cork
Cork, Ireland

Gladys McPherson, BScN, PhD
Independent Researcher
Tsawwassen, British Columbia, Canada

Barbara Medoff-Cooper, PhD, RN, CRNP, FAAN
Ruth M. Colket Professor in Pediatric Nursing and
Director of the Center for Biobehavioral Research
School of Nursing
University of Pennsylvania
Philadelphia, Pennsylvania

Afaf I. Meleis, PhD, DrPS(Hons), FAAN
Margaret Bond Simon Dean of Nursing
University of Pennsylvania
Philadelphia, Pennsylvania

*Deceased

Shirley M. Moore, PhD, RN, FAAN
The Edward J. and Louise Mellen Professor of Nursing and
Associate Dean for Research
Frances Payne Bolton School of Nursing
Case Western Reserve University
Cleveland, Ohio

Sioban Nelson, RN, BA(Hons), PhD
Professor and Dean of the Faculty of Nursing
University of Toronto
Toronto, Ontario, Canada
Editor-in-Chief of *Nursing Inquiry*
Co-editor of the Culture and Politics of Healthcare Work List for
    Cornell University Press

Betty M. Neuman, PhD, RN, FAAN
Independent International Consultant
Watertown, Ohio

Margaret A. Newman, RN, PhD, FAAN
Professor Emerita
University of Minnesota
Minneapolis, Minnesota

Deborah Thoun Northrup, RN, PhD
Associate Professor
University of Victoria
Victoria, British Columbia, Canada

Joanne K. Olson, RN, PhD
Professor and Associate Dean
Undergraduate Programs
Faculty of Nursing
University of Alberta
Edmonton, Alberta, Canada

Valeria G. Olynyk, RN, BSN
Staff Nurse
Vancouver Island Health Authority
Nanaimo, British Columbia, Canada

Kader Parahoo, PhD, RN
Professor and Director of Research
University of Ulster
Coleraine, Northern Ireland

Rosemarie Rizzo Parse, PhD, FAAN
Distinguished Professor Emeritus
Loyola University Chicago
Chicago, Illinois
Visiting Scholar, New York University
Founder and Editor of *Nursing Science Quarterly*
President, Discovery International

Janice Penrod, PhD, RN
Associate Professor of Nursing, College of Health and
    Human Development
Associate Professor of Humanities, College of Medicine
Professor in Charge of Graduate Programs, School of Nursing
The Pennsylvania State University
University Park, Pennsylvania

Barbara K. Pesut, PhD, RN
Assistant Professor of Nursing
University of British Columbia
Kelowna, British Columbia, Canada

Mary E. Purkis, RN, PhD
Dean of the Faculty of Human and Social Development
University of Victoria
Victoria, British Columbia, Canada

Pamela G. Reed, PhD, RN, FAAN
Professor
University of Arizona
College of Nursing
Tucson, Arizona

*Martha E. Rogers, RN, ScD, FAAN
Professor Emerita
New York University
New York, New York

Gary Rolfe, PhD, MA, BSc, RMN, PGCEA
Professor of Nursing
Swansea University
Swansea, Wales, United Kingdom

Daniel Rothbart, PhD
Associate Professor of Conflict Resolution and Philosophy
George Mason University
Institute for Conflict Analysis and Resolution
Fairfax, Virginia

*Deceased

Carole A. Schroeder, RN, PhD
Associate Professor
Psychosocial and Community Health
School of Nursing
University of Washington
Seattle, Washington

Annette S. H. Schultz, PhD, RN
Postdoctoral position
University of Manitoba, Faculty of Nursing
Winnipeg, Manitoba, Canada

Phyllis R. Schultz, PhD, FAAN
Associate Professor Emerita
School of Nursing
University of Washington
Seattle, Washington

John R. Scudder, Jr., EdD
Professor of Philosophy, Emeritus
Lynchburg College
Lynchburg, Virginia

Nelma B. Crawford Shearer, PhD, RN
Associate Professor
College of Nursing & Healthcare Innovation
Arizona State University
Phoenix, Arizona

Mary Cipriano Silva, PhD, RN, FAAN
Professor Emerita of Nursing
George Mason University
Fairfax, Virginia

A. Marilyn Sime, PhD
Professor Emerita
University of Minnesota
Minneapolis, Minnesota

Marlene Sinclair, PhD, MEd, DASE, BSc, RNT, RM, RN,
    Cert Neurosurgical / Neuromedical Nursing
Chair in Nursing Research and
Professor of Midwifery Research, Institute of Nursing Research
University of Ulster
Jordanstown, Northern Ireland

Mary Jane Smith, PhD, RN
Associate Dean and Professor
School of Nursing
West Virginia University
Morgantown, West Virginia

Chris Stevenson, RMN, BA(Hons), MSc(Dist), PhD
Chair in Mental Health Nursing
Dublin City University
Dublin, Ireland

Joanna Szabo, RN, BN
Sessional Instructor
Camosun College
Victoria, British Columbia, Canada

Denise S. Tarlier, PhD, MSN, FNP-C, RN
Assistant Professor, School of Nursing
Thompson Rivers University
Kamloops, British Columbia, Canada

Sally E. Thorne, RN, BSN, MSN, PhD
Professor and Director of British Columbia School of Nursing
University of British Columbia
Vancouver, British Columbia, Canada

Coby L. Tschanz, RN, BN
Sessional Instructor
University of Victoria and Camosun College
Victoria, British Columbia, Canada

Lynda A. Tyer-Viola, RNC, PhD
Clinical Nurse Specialist
Massachusetts General Hospital
Boston, Massachusetts

Colleen Varcoe, PhD, RN
Associate Professor
University of British Columbia School of Nursing
Vancouver, British Columbia, Canada

Deborah Lowe Volker, RN, PhD
Associate Professor and Division Chair of the Holistic
    Adult Health Faculty
University of Texas at Austin
School of Nursing
Austin, Texas

Patricia Hinton Walker, PhD, RN, FAAN
Professor
Graduate School of Nursing
Uniformed Services University of Health Sciences
Bethesda, Maryland

Philip John Warelow, RPN, RN, PhD
School of Nursing and Midwifery
Deakin University
Geelong, Victoria, Australia

Catherine A. Warms, PhD, RN
Biobehavioral Nursing and Health Care Systems
School of Nursing
University of Washington
Seattle, Washington

Jean Watson, RN, PhD, FAAN, HNC
Distinguished Professor and Murchinson-Scolville Chair in
    Caring Science
University of Colorado Health Sciences Center School of Nursing
Denver, Colorado

Kathryn Weaver, RN, PhD
Assistant Professor Faculty of Nursing
University of New Brunswick
New Brunswick, Canada
AHFMR Postdoctoral Fellow
Faculty of Nursing, University of Alberta
Edmonton, Alberta, Canada

Ann L. Whall, PhD, RN, FAAN, FGSA
Professor
University of Michigan School of Nursing
Associate Director of University of Michigan Geriatric Center
Ann Arbor, Michigan
Distinguished Visiting Professor
The Allesee Endowed Chair in Gerontological Nursing
Oakland University School of Nursing
Rochester Hills, Michigan

Jill White, RN, RM, MEd, PhD
Professor of Nursing and Midwifery
Dean of Nursing, Midwifery and Health
University of Technology
Sydney, Australia

Michael Yeo, PhD
Associate Professor
Department of Philosophy and M.A.
Laurentian University
Sudbury, Ontario, Canada

Reviewers

Linda Carman Copel, PhD, RN, CS, DAPA
Associate Professor
Villanova University
Villanova, Pennsylvania

Rose Ann DiMaria, PhD, RN, CNSN
Associate Professor
West Virginia University School of Nursing–
   Charleston Division
Charleston, West Virginia

Eleanor Donnelly, PhD, RN
Associate Professor
Indiana University School of Nursing
Indianapolis, Indiana

Barbara H. Fleming, BSN, MN
Associate Professor of Nursing (Retired)
California State University, Bakersfield
Bakersfield, California

Angela Gillis, PhD, RN
Professor
Saint Francis Xavier University
Antigonish, Nova Scotia, Canada

Teresa M. O'Neill, APRNC, PhD
Associate Professor of Nursing
Our Lady of Holy Cross College
New Orleans, Louisiana

Donna Romyn, PhD, RN, BScN, MN
Director, Centre for Nursing and Health Studies
Athabasca University
Athabasca, Alberta, Canada

Karen Moore Schaefer, DNSc, RN
Assistant Professor
Director, Undergraduate Program
Temple University College of Health Professions, Department of Nursing
Philadelphia, Pennsylvania

Lee Schmidt, PhD, RN
Assistant Professor
University of Miami School of Nursing
Coral Gables, Florida

Teresa Walsh, PhD, RN, NC
Assistant Professor
Texas Woman's University College of Nursing
Houston, Texas

Preface

Theory is a tool for knowledge development that enhances the effectiveness and status of a discipline. The term "theory" holds special meanings across disciplines, from the humanities to the sciences. In nursing, the term may have one of several meanings: A well-known conceptual model of nursing; a middle range theory newly proposed by a doctoral student; the unobserved and conceptual as distinguished from the observed and clinical; and the metatheoretical and philosophical dimensions of knowledge development in the discipline. This fifth edition of *Perspectives on Nursing Theory* embraces all of these perspectives and some new perspectives that will challenge basic assumptions as well as clarify thinking about theory.

This book is an anthology of classic and contemporary nursing articles that address various theoretical and philosophical perspectives on the nature of theory and knowledge development. It is designed to provide a comprehensive overview of the important discussions taking place regarding the structures and processes of knowledge building in nursing. A sampling of the articles within this book may be considered prerequisite or co-requisite knowledge for graduate level nurses, students, and faculty who, as part of their teaching, research, and practice, inevitably will philosophize, theorize, and contribute to nursing knowledge.

As many of you know, this book has an important history. It began in 1985 with Leslie Nicoll as the founding editor, and continued through two additional editions at six-year intervals, in 1991 and 1997. Dr. Nicoll selected articles that captured 40 years of significant theoretical thinking in nursing. She included biographical information and original commentary by the authors. Pertinent articles were added in each new edition, with her 3rd edition comprising 80 articles.

The 4th edition, published in 2004 with Reed and Shearer as the new editors, maintained elements of previous editions that reviewers found valuable, but it also marked a departure from the first three editions: The *fin-de-siècle* was accompanied by new and revisioned perspectives on nursing theory, which necessitated the addition of many new articles and a reconceptualization of the framework for the book. The revised 4th edition featured 41 new articles and was trimmed down to 62 articles, replacing redundancies with substantive additions of cutting-edge and sometimes controversial ideas on nursing theory that included international perspectives.

This 5th edition continues in the same spirit, revising the framework and refreshing the text with 31 new articles that reflect the changes in theoretical thinking in nursing that have occurred since the 2004 edition, and are occurring as we move deeper into the new millennium. Forty-one articles—indisputable classics in nursing theory and their authors a who's who in theoretical nursing—were retained from the 4th edition. Biographical information and personal commentaries by each author extend readers' insight into the authors' theoretical ideas and encourage their own reflection on the readings. Together, the 72 articles orient readers to

21st century thought while maintaining a vital connection to the history of nursing theory.

The 72 articles comprise the chapters of the book. The chapters are organized topically into eleven units that represent important domains of nursing metatheory and tools for knowledge development:

- Unit One: Structures of Nursing Knowledge
- Unit Two: Historical Contexts of Nursing Knowledge Development
- Unit Three: Theoretical Thinking in Practice
- Unit Four: Nursing Philosophies and Paradigms
- Unit Five: Philosophies of Science and Knowledge Development
- Unit Six: Epistemologies, Evidence, and Practice
- Unit Seven: Tools for Theory Development
- Unit Eight: Characteristics and Criteria of Nursing Theories
- Unit Nine: Ethics Inquiry
- Unit Ten: Philosophic Views on Nursing and Its Practice
- Unit Eleven: Future Directions for Nursing Theory

The units are not mutually exclusive, but they represent clusters of articles that present key ideas for each metatheoretical domain. For example, the topics in Units Four and Five are placed sequentially because each focuses on philosophies of science, originating in nursing and in philosophy or other disciplines, respectively. Units Three and Six were developed to convey the importance of theory-based evidence and to show how theoretical thinking and knowledge development occur in practice. The intent in part was to demonstrate that philosophical thinking and knowledge development are the purview of all nurses—in academia and in clinical settings.

The transformation of knowledge into nursing knowledge through theory development requires active participation of nurses with practice doctorates as well as research doctorates, and of nurses with advanced practice degrees as well as the BSN. This new edition is intended to not only inform scholars and future scholars of nursing, but to serve as a catalyst to facilitate continued thought and discussion among students and teachers, researchers, and practitioners about the development of nursing knowledge. A diversity of philosophic views is presented, from Rogerian to Foucauldian, as relevant to nursing. May these chapters be read more than once for the dialogue and enthusiasm they can generate about nursing knowledge and one's role in its evolution.

Pamela G. Reed
Nelma B. C. Shearer

Acknowledgments

Many people have contributed to making this book a success for nursing. We first thank the contributors whose timeless ideas and insights about nursing are recorded between the covers of this book. Their articles comprise the substance of the book and, together, provide conceptual perspectives about our discipline that are relevant to nursing theorizing.

We thank our students—past, present, and future—who helped inspire the selection of these chapters. It is our hope that the chapters will further students' learning about the metatheoretical foundations of the discipline.

We appreciate everyone at Lippincott Williams & Wilkins for their careful, expert work in transforming ideas about nursing metatheory into this portable package. We especially thank Michelle L. Clarke, Managing Editor at Lippincott Williams & Wilkins, for her expertise in managing the myriad details while maintaining the big picture of this project. She was an invaluable guide and support to us. We also acknowledge and thank Stephanie Lentz, Project Manager, Aptara, Inc. for her dedication to authors and her expertise in pulling everything together.

Contents

UNIT **THREE**
Theoretical Thinking in Practice

UNIT **FOUR**
Nursing Philosophies and Paradigms

UNIT **SEVEN**
Tools for Theory Development

UNIT **EIGHT**
**Characteristics and Criteria of
Nursing Theories**

Structures of Nursing Knowledge

This section is designed to ease the reader into the realm of metatheory, with its special vocabulary and philosophic dimensions of knowledge production and application. The reader is the first to appreciate the place of metatheoretical thinking, and then able to consider through various dimensions of nursing knowledge. Metatheory is important in referring to philosophical differences among philosophic systems and theory. The metatheory level is another vocabulary relevant to building knowledge. Metatheoretical helps is often understanding in terms of level of abstraction, from concrete to the various levels of theory.

This unit considers essential overview of key elements of nursing knowledge and how to view each element, along with the relationships among these elements and the different ways to frame or structure nursing knowledge. The reader is introduced to important elements in the structure of nursing knowledge that are views between philosophy and science.

Questions for Discussion

- Is nursing knowledge scientific knowledge?

- How do nursing's various patterns of knowing (addressed in Unit Six) fit within the structure of knowledge presented in this unit?

- How is the practice dimension (addressed more in-depth in Unit Three) related to the elements identified in these structures of nursing knowledge?

CHAPTER 1

Nursing Theory and Practice: Connecting the Dots

Jo-Ann Marrs
Lois W. Lowry

The authors propose connecting the dots among theory, practice, and research by adopting an expanded conceptual-theoretical-empirical structure of nursing knowledge and matrix process to guide the placement of nursing knowledge in a contextual whole. An overview of the theoretical journey of nursing knowledge development is contrasted with the journey from practice resulting in a theory-practice disconnect. Both approaches are united to present an integrated view of the dimensions of the knowledge development of nursing as a professional discipline.

Much as a young child struggles to connect the dots on a picture in an activity book, nursing has been trying to connect the dots between nursing theory, research, and practice. It is the hypothesis of the authors that *the picture* is about to be completed, but that the pattern of the dots has been somewhat divergent and scattered among nurse theorists, researchers, and practitioners as they have each taken different approaches in completing the holistic picture of nursing knowledge. Some have traveled inductively and others, deductively. Both are about to meet in the middle in order to *connect the dots* for a holistic view of nursing. The journey to completion will focus on a matrix that can provide a logical process for practitioners and theoreticians to access the state of the nursing knowledge development.

We propose an approach that combines an expanded conceptual-theoretical-empirical (CTE) structure of knowledge development and a process for adding

About the Authors

Jo-Ann Marrs was born in Linz, Austria. She graduated from St. Mary's School of Nursing in Knoxville, TN, with a diploma in nursing. She received a BS, an MS in education, an MSN in nursing, and her EdD from the University of Tennessee. She received a post master's certificate in Family Nurse Practitioner from Pittsburg State University in Pittsburg, KS. Dr. Marrs also holds a Legal Nurse Consultant Certificate. She led a national effort to implement background checks for nursing programs, and has written articles and spoken on the subject. She is interested in educational research and in obesity in children. As an administrator, she has developed numerous degree programs and has taught nursing since 1972. She is presently the Associate Dean of Academic Programs and Student Services at East Tennessee State University. She likes to do arts and crafts and garden.

Lois W. Lowry received her BSN degree from Cornell University-New York Hospital School of Nursing in 1955, achieved her MN from the University of Florida in 1977 with a double major in maternal–infant health and psychiatric/mental health, and earned her DNS in educational administration from the University of Pennsylvania in 1987. Dr. Lowry is currently Professor and Coordinator of the DSN program in the College of Nursing at East Tennessee State University. Her research areas include studies in patient satisfaction with prenatal care, spirituality and aging, and the development of critical thinking in baccalaureate nursing students. Dr. Lowry's interest in nursing theory began with her first course in her doctoral program, taught by Dr. Jacqueline Fawcett, who sparked her desire to contribute to theoretical knowledge development. She is a charter member of Neuman Systems Model (NSM) Trustees, Inc., and continues to write, consult, and lecture about the NSM in practice, education, and research. Dr. Lowry is married to Dr. Robert L. Lowry, a Presbyterian minister, and has 5 children and 12 grandchildren. Her hobbies are hiking, camping, swimming, and singing.

to, revising, and moving about within the field of nursing knowledge. Fawcett's (2000) five-level hierarchical structure of nursing knowledge, now referred to as a holarchy (Fawcett, 2005) provides the *what* of nursing knowledge to be included within the field. We propose that practice theory be explicitly added to the present structure. The essence of practice theory is a focus on a limited number of variables, a desired goal, and specific actions necessary to achieve the goal. At present, practice theories are included in the level of mid-range theory at a low middle-range level. This is confusing and does not add clarity to the CTE structure. In our proposal, theories that meet the criteria of practice theory will be explicitly designated in the CTE structure.

The *how* of adding to, refining, or revising the CTE structure is an adaptation of a matrix process used to promote learning and change within organizations (Shibley, 2001). The five-step matrix proposed here guides the process for considering contributions to the hierarchy of nursing knowledge. Setting forth a vision is the first step. Our vision is to establish a clearinghouse in which all contributions to nursing knowledge will be registered and analyzed. The second step is the development of a cognitive infrastructure or mental model to guide placement of nursing knowledge within the clearinghouse in a way that connections between theories and action can be demonstrated. The third step in the process, the systemic structure, is the plan for operationalization. The fourth and fifth steps are key to success of the matrix process, that is, the identification of events and an analysis of patterns among the contributions to new nursing knowledge so that theoretical linkages are identified.

Prior to a detailed discussion of the expanded CTE structure and the matrix process, a brief historical overview of the development of nursing knowledge through deductive and inductive means is provided as the backdrop for understanding the respective contributions to nursing knowledge of each type of thinking. We will begin our discussion through the theoretical lens.

Theoretical Overview

Our theoretical journey has taken the discipline of nursing through various stages and milestones. In the beginning, Florence Nightingale focused on patient care and hygiene to enhance healing, which gave nursing its mission and focus. Throughout the first half of the 20th century nursing practice was based on principles and traditions through an apprenticeship form of education. By mid-century the emphasis was that of nursing as a service requiring a strong scientific base that was acquired within university settings. As our nurse leaders shared their ideas about the essences and empirics of nursing, they spoke out about the need for theory to guide the practice of nursing. They reminded us that theory is the goal of scientific work and is essential to the development of any profession (Chinn & Kramer, 1999; Meleis, 1997). Thus, through the second half of the 20th century, nursing made rapid progress toward the development of theoretical knowledge; first, through the application of theories borrowed from other disciplines, followed by the creation of grand theories and conceptual models. Much of the early theory development was based on the ideal of nursing, or what ought-to-be nursing practice (Barnum, 1990). However, the conceptual models for education and practice contributed to defining a unique nursing perspective that was useful in practice settings. Each model's description of the nursing process encouraged reflective problem-solving and showed nurses the connection between nursing models and practice (Chinn & Kramer, 1999). In addition, the identification of the dominant phenomena within the field of nursing knowledge, the metaparadigm, asserted the distinct domain of the discipline of nursing (Fawcett, 1996).

At one time, nursing was greatly influenced by the writings of Dickoff and James (1968) who advocated a model of *practice-oriented theory* including four levels of theorizing: factor-isolating, factor-relating, situation-relating, and situation-producing. Since nursing is a practice discipline, it is logical that situation-producing theory be given the greatest consideration because it will guide actions that have an impact on reality (Walker & Avant, 2005). Other pioneers of nursing theory supported the necessity of building theoretical knowledge from the study of nursing actions for the goal of providing better nursing care (Ellis, 1968; Jacox, 1974; McCarthy, 1972).

Given the importance of practice theory, it is interesting that there was little growth of this level of theory. A reason posited for the lack of growth was its practical nature, thus, it was not very exciting (Walker & Avant, 2005). It may be thought of as *common sense* or too time and place bound to be considered theory. Practitioners may not be aware that the assessing, planning, prioritizing, and decision-making that engages them while caring for their clients reflects processes necessary in theoretical thinking. Practice theory is based on the assumption that the practitioner has the cognitive skills necessary to be able to discriminate among several patients with the same symptoms, and would take the action that is most effective in each case. With a thorough education in nursing theory, and the opportunity to engage in theory-based practice over time, practitioners can be expected to contribute to nursing theory development. Nurses learn to practice nursing very well by studying nursing theories intensely. Problem-solving at the midrange and practice levels must be aligned with the whole gestalt of philosophy, theory, and method in order to advance the body of knowledge which is nursing (Cody, 2003). Practitioners' attention to and appreciation of theory is more likely to be caught when theoretical knowledge focuses on specific nursing phenomena from practice.

However, the abstract nature of theory has created a schism between nurse theorists, nurse scientists, and practitioners. Nurse theorists emphasize the *knowing* that is based on philosophies and theories of nursing. On the other hand, practicing nurses focus on the *doing* and often deny that theories are useful to them in their everyday work. Yet all professional nurses are urged to build bridges between knowing and doing.

The complexity of nursing practice requires the efforts of practitioners who encounter phenomena and theorists/ researchers who discover new relationships among concepts. It is the position of the writers that the advancement of nursing knowledge only occurs when discipline-specific research is conducted. If practice theory is to gain acceptance, it must demonstrate the hierarchical connection between midrange and grand theories; which in turn, stem from the philosophy of nursing science, paradigms, and worldviews of nursing. Often, the knowledge and skill sought at the practice level follows the requirements for licensure and expectations of corporate employers or are just practical solutions to nursing problems (Cody, 2003).

Utilizing a multitude of methods for knowledge development, including inductive approaches, could enhance the progress of nursing knowledge development as long as connections to theoretical knowledge are made explicit. Other disciplines, such as sociology and psychology, have developed theory from observing reality. What has been the pathway of practitioners in nursing who have attempted to connect the dots inductively?

Practice Overview

From the practitioner's point of view, the development of nursing knowledge has somewhat mirrored that of the development of medicine. This is particularly noticeable when one examines the inductive development of practice theory with the development of medicine. In ancient Greece the Hippocratic School of ancient Greece classified disease using the concept of *humors* rather than supernatural or magical forces. By 1893, the International Classification of Diseases and Causes of Death was being used by medicine to categorize illness. Other nomenclature systems used in medicine include the Standard Diagnostic and Statistical Manual of Mental Disorders; International Classification of Injuries, Disabilities, and Handicaps; Standard Nomenclature of Disease and Operations; Systematized Nomenclature of Pathology; and Systematized Nomenclature of Medicine (Gordon, 1998).

Historically, nursing also used these medical classifications to organize its knowledge, since these were the only concepts available to use until the mid-20th century. As nursing research increased, there was an interest in classification systems for coding studies. The best known system is that of the North American Nursing Diagnosis Association (NANDA; Gordon, 1998). NANDA is recognized as one of the pioneer organizations in the development of a classification system for nursing practice. Several nurse theorists, including Roy, King, Newman, and others, joined their efforts and presented an organizing framework for nursing diagnoses called Patterns of Unitary Man (Humans) to the NANDA and Taxonomy Committee in 1977. While there was much controversy over this as a framework, and some theorists (Roy, Parse, and others) disagreed with the paniculate nature of the diagnostic system, in 1984, this framework was renamed Human Response Patterns and was accepted in 1986. This consists of the patterns of choosing, communicating, exchanging, feeling, knowing, moving, perceiving, relating, and valuing. The nursing diagnoses were intended to provide a conceptual model for interpreting a set of observations which would be firmly grounded in studies of the phenomenon. An inductive approach was used initially by NANDA to identify these concepts within the medical model frame of reference. Up to this point, research was minimal and literature about the concepts negligible. With an inductive methodology that NANDA leaders used, diagnostic concepts were formed from a set of empirical indicators (signs/symptoms), arising from practice observations. Further studies led to the identification of contributing factors that came to be the focus of nursing interventions. NANDA's (2001) latest work, *Nursing Diagnoses: Definitions and Classifications (2001-2002)*, features a new multiaxial framework that organizes the diagnoses into domains according to Gordon's functional health patterns (NANDA, 2001). These formulations, however, were not connected to existing theories and models. Likewise, as nursing followed medicine in developing nursing diagnoses, nurses used medical treatments and the patient's ability to carry out physicians' orders as a high priority in the traditional typology of nursing interventions. Eventually, following the format of nursing diagnoses, and nursing clinical judgment development, nurses began to name nurse-initiated interventions in textbooks.

Since 1987, research to develop a vocabulary and nursing intervention classification system (NIC) has been conducted at the University of Iowa by Bulechek and McCloskey (1992). The nursing intervention classification (NIC) research team identified a set of nursing intervention concepts through content analysis of the literature and linked them to NANDA diagnoses and to nursing outcomes classification (NOC). The research team identified three types of interventions. They are defined as "any direct care treatment that a nurse performs on behalf of a client. These treatments include nurse-initiated treatments resulting from nursing diagnoses, physician-initiated treatments resulting from medical diagnoses, and performance of the daily essential functions for the client [who] cannot do these" (Bulechek & McCloskey, 1992, p. 21).

Since 1998, there have been biennial NANDA-NIC-NOC conferences to help to link these three systems. Outcomes are linked to the problem (nursing diagnosis) in a diagnostic statement. Interventions are linked to the related or contributing factors. Diagnosis-intervention linkages (McCloskey & Bulechek, 1996) assume that a nursing diagnosis is being used as a contributing factor for another nursing diagnosis and that the classification is similar to a dictionary of terms. These three taxonomies are becoming the standard for nursing practice because they provide the content focus for nursing process and serve to identify and communicate the unique function of nursing. Thus the taxonomies provide a standardized vocabulary to clarify nursing's role to other healthcare professionals and patients. A caution is in order, however, for taxonomies represent the realities of nurses who developed them, but not necessarily the majority of nurses who care for patients (Meleis, 1997). More important, the nursing process and classification systems are not based on theoretical underpinnings and do not allow nurses to connect the dots in the CTE structural hierarchy without further research.

The current emphasis on evidence or outcomes-based practice in nursing is another example of the tendency to follow the lead of medicine. Evidence-based medical practice originated as the gold standard for integrating individual clinical expertise with the best available clinical evidence from clinical research studies, particularly clinical trials. It has been suggested that the roots of evidence-based practice can be traced as far back as the 3rd century B.C. Whatever the origin, it appears that nursing has once again adopted a process utilized by medicine to guide nursing practice, rather than building upon our unique nursing knowledge. The trend toward evidence-based practice and its focus on outcomes as the end results of care, linked to diagnoses and interventions, does not support a theoretical link. Rather this approach is fostered by institutions and typically reinforces and supports the medical model, without concern for connections to the structural hierarchy of nursing knowledge.

Conceptual-Theoretical-Empirical Structures

Whereas the historical developments have claimed to further the advancement of nursing knowledge, there continues to be a *disconnect* among the works of theorists, researchers, and practitioners. Is there a way to unite the approaches in thinking so that theorists, researchers, and practitioners can embrace an integrated view of the dimensions of our professional discipline and the activities associated with those dimensions? These authors believe that this is possible through enhancing the development of our existing CTE systems of knowledge. Fawcett (2000) posited a five-level hierarchical structure of nursing knowledge based upon levels of abstraction. This heuristic device places the metaparadigm of nursing at the highest level of abstraction, the philosophies of nursing science just below the metaparadigm, and the conceptual models of nursing at the third level. Below the conceptual models are theories and the lowest level of abstraction is represented by empirical indicators. Each of these levels is well-defined and described in the literature (Fawcett), so will not be further explicated here.

Table 1-1
Expanded Hierarchy of Nursing Knowledge

Components	Level of Abstraction
Metaparadigm	Most abstract
Philosophies	
Conceptual models	
Grand theories	
Middle-range theories	
Practice theories (situation-producing, situation-relating, factor-relating, factor-isolating)	
Empirical indicators (standards for practice, assessment formats, classification taxonomies, intervention protocols, evaluation criteria)	Most concrete

These authors propose that the CTE hierarchy be expanded to explicitly place additional elements into the structure that have guided scholars in their thinking and practitioners in their practice as the discipline has expanded its roles. Table 1-1 displays the proposed hierarchy. Table 1-2 provides the definitions for each component in the hierarchy. Note that grand theories are placed just below conceptual models, indicating that they are derived from conceptual models, such as Newman's (1994) theory of health as expanding consciousness and Parse's (1998) human becoming theory, both of which were sparked by Rogers' (1970) science of unitary human beings. Middle-range theories are located somewhat below grand theories on the hierarchy because they are made up of fewer concepts and propositions. These theories are written at a more concrete level of abstraction so that they can assist in interpreting behaviors, situations, and events. They can be applied to practice situations and can be tested through research methodologies. Some midrange theories are derived from nursing conceptual models, such as Orem's (2001) theories of self-care, self-care deficit, and nursing systems, and Neuman's (2002) theory of prevention as intervention. Other midrange theories

identify other disciplines as their source, such as social support (Norbeck, 1981); or nursing observations and taxonomies as sources of their generation, like the Omaha Classification System for community health nursing (Martin & Scheet, 1992). The literature has indicated that the level of abstraction attributed to mid-range theories is quite broad. Thus, Liehr and Smith (1999) have categorized midrange to include high-middle, middle and low middle, depending on scope and level of abstraction. Their categorization tends to add confusion rather than clarity to the CTE hierarchy. Rather, we suggest explicit placement of practice theory below the midrange level to include those theories that focus on a narrow view of reality and may be considered as low middle-range; for example, the theory of balance between analgesia and side effects (Good & Moore, 1996) and the theory of acute pain management in infants and children (Huth & Moore, 1998).

Practice theories may be as simple as a single concept that is operationalized, and may be linked to a special population or situation. Practice theories can evolve deductively from a midrange or grand theory (Newman, 1994), or may be inductively formulated from a specific situation, as demonstrated by Im and Meleis (1999) who brought theoretical understanding to a delimited clinical situation. It is important, however, that practice theories be aligned with the whole gestalt of philosophy of nursing science, theory, and method in order to advance the body of knowledge of nursing (Cody, 2003). Within our expanded CTE structure, the four levels of theory proposed by Dickoff and James (1968) are situated below practice theory. Finally, at the lowest and most concrete level of the hierarchy are the empirical indicators. Empirical indicators are directly connected to midrange and/or practice theories by means of operational definitions for each theory concept that is being generated or tested. Empirical indicators are the tools, instruments, and procedures that the researcher uses to test midrange or practice theories. Likewise, empirical indicators can be the protocols or clinical procedures that a practitioner will use to direct nursing actions in a precise manner (Fawcett, 2000). In our hierarchy, standards for practice, assessment formats, classification

Table 1-2
Definitions of Conceptual-Theoretical-Empirical Components

Component	Definition	Example
Metaparadigm	Global concepts that identify the phenomena of the discipline	Person, environment, health, nursing
Philosophies	Ontological and epistemological claims about values and beliefs of the discipline	Totality and simultaneity paradigms
Conceptual models	Set of abstract concepts and their propositional statements that address the metaparadigm concepts	Neuman systems model, Orem's self-care framework, Rogers' science of unitary human beings
Grand theories	Set of fewer abstract concepts and propositional statements that are broad in scope and derived from conceptual models	Newman's theory of health as expanding consciousness, Parse's theory of human becoming, Watson's theory of human caring
Middle-range theories	Limited number of concepts and propositions written at a more specific level	Mishel's uncertainty in illness, Norbeck's model for social support, Swanson's theory of caring
Practice theories (practice-oriented focus, predictive focus)	One or two variables and their propositional connection stated in prescriptive terms or predictive terms and related to a specific situation	Huth and Moore's theory of acute pain management
Empirical indicators	Real world proxy for midrange or practice theory concept	Instruments, protocols

taxonomies, intervention protocols, and evaluation criteria are given as examples of empirical indicators from the practice arena. Each of these must be connected to the more abstract elements of the hierarchical structure (philosophies, conceptual models, or grand theories) to be considered as contributions to the development of nursing knowledge. A caution is in order here. Many protocols, taxonomies, critical pathways, and other such systems are created and required by corporate employers with no intent to develop nursing knowledge. This has contributed to confusion for practicing nurses, and the opinion that theory is unnecessary for practice.

Strategies for Implementation

A matrix provides a logical map to guide the process for connecting the dots. The matrix includes five 5 parts: vision, a mental model, systemic structures, patterns, and events. The matrix process (Figure 1-1) illustrates the interaction among the parts. *Vision* suggests the creation of a clearinghouse that contains the field of nursing knowledge. This clearinghouse will be centrally

located so that there will be global access at all times. Contributors to nursing knowledge can go to the clearinghouse to explore the state of the science in nursing at any hour of the day or night, for the purpose of finding gaps and areas for further study. For example, an online site could be created or incorporated into an existing site, such as the Sigma Theta Tau International online library, and will contain references to theories and research studies that currently represent the field of knowledge in nursing.

The *mental model* that stems from the vision can be illustrated as a sea of dots within a frame. Each dot represents a separate piece of nursing research or theoretical knowledge. The expanded CTE hierarchy (Table 1-1) adds the basic structure to guide placement of a new dot. Further delineation within the structure will be necessary to complete the picture of the connected dots. For example, major categories will be identified, such as focus areas in practice, education, and administration. Each major category will be further subdivided by more defining attributes; for example, the practice focus may include adult issues, women's health issues, children's health, and

Gordon, M. (1998, September 30). Nursing nomenclature and classification system development. *Online Journal of Issues in Nursing, 3*(2). Retrieved October 15, 2005, from http://www.nursing-world .org/ojin/tpc7/tpc7_1.htm

Huth, M. M., & Moore, S. M. (1998). Prescriptive theory of acute pain management in infants and children. *Journal of Society of Pediatric Nurses, 3,* 23–32.

Im, E., & Meleis, A. I. (1999). Situation-specific theories: Philosophical roots, properties, and approach. *Advances in Nursing Science, 22*(2), 11–24.

Jacox, A. K. (1974). Theory construction in nursing: An overview. *Nursing Research, 23*(1), 4–13.

Liehr, P., & Smith, M. J. (1999). Middle range theory: Spinning research and practice to create knowledge for the new millennium. *Advances in Nursing Science, 21*(4), 81–91.

Martin, L. S., & Scheet, N. J. (1992). *The Omaha system: Applications for community health nursing.* Philadelphia: Saunders.

McCarthy, R. T. (1972). A practice theory of nursing care. *Nursing Research, 21,* 406–410.

McCloskey, J. C., & Bulechek, G. M. (1996). *Nursing intervention classification (NIC)* (2nd ed.). St. Louis, MO: Mosby.

Meleis, A. I. (1997). *Theoretical nursing: Development and progress* (3rd ed.). Philadelphia: Lippincott.

North American Nursing Diagnosis Association. (2001). *Nursing diagnosis: Definitions and classification, 2001–2002.* Philadelphia: Author.

Neuman, B., & Fawcett, J. (2002). *The Neuman systems model* (4th ed.). Upper Saddle River, NJ: Prentice Hall.

Newman, M. A. (1994). *Health as expanding consciousness* (2nd ed.). New York: National League for Nursing.

Norbeck. J. S. (1981). Social support: A model for clinical research and application. *Advances in Nursing Science, 3*(4), 43–59.

Orem, D. E. (2001). *Nursing: Concepts of practice* (6th ed.). St. Louis, MO: Mosby.

Parse, R. R. (1998). *The human becoming school of thought: A perspective for nurses and other health professionals.* Thousand Oaks, CA: Sage.

Rogers, M. E. (1970). An *introduction to the theoretical basis of nursing.* Philadelphia: F. A. Davis.

Shibley, J. J. (2001). *A primer on systems thinking and organizational learning.* Portland, OR: Portland Learning Organization Group.

Walker, L. O., & Avant, K. C. (2005). *Strategies for theory construction in nursing* (4th ed.). Upper Saddle River, NJ: Pearson Prentice Hall.

The Authors Comment

Nursing Theory and Practice: Connecting the Dots

This work arose from our concern about the disconnect between theory and practice. Theoreticians develop their thinking deductively, whereas practitioners use an inductive approach. We hope to integrate both approaches into a meaningful whole that will advance the development of nursing knowledge. Our idea combines the structure of nursing knowledge with a process for adding to, revising, and identifying new contributions to knowledge in a uniform way. We invite readers to respond to our proposal.

—Jo-Ann Marrs
—Lois W. Lowry

Philosophy, Science, Theory: Interrelationships and Implications for Nursing Research

Mary C. Silva

If nurse researchers are to study the structure of nursing knowledge, they must first understand the relationships among philosophy, science, and theory. Although many articles have spoken to the nature of theory or science in nursing (Andreoli & Thompson, 1977; Hardy, 1974; Jacox, 1974; Leininger, 1968; Walker, 1971), few have examined the links between them and fewer yet have examined the role of philosophy in the deriving of nursing knowledge. To bridge this gap, I would like to present an overview of the relationships among philosophy, science, and theory, and then describe some implications for the conduct of nursing research.

Relationships Between Philosophy and Science

Although in western civilization the precise origin of what we call pure knowledge is difficult to trace, most scholars agree that significant advancements occurred during the great Age of Greece (500 B.C. to 300 B.C.). During this time those ideals commonly associated with western civilization—freedom, optimism, secularism, rationalism, and high regard for the dignity and worth of the individual—were developed (Burns, 1955).

Greek learning formed a single entry called philosophy and, even into the nineteenth century, this term was

From M. C. Silva, Philosophy, science, theory: Interrelationships and implications for nursing research, Journal of Nursing Scholarship *1977, 9(3), 59–63. Copyright 1977 by Blackwell. Reprinted with permission by Blackwell Publishing.*

About the Author

MARY CIPRIANO SILVA was born and raised in the small town of Ravenna, OH. She earned a BSN and an MS from Ohio State University and a PhD from the University of Maryland. She also undertook postdoctoral study at Georgetown University in health care ethics. The focus of her scholarship and key contributions to nursing has been in philosophy, metatheory, and health care ethics. She is a Professor Emerita, at George Mason University, Fairfax, VA. When not working, she attends foreign films, the Shakespeare Theatre, and fine and performing arts events.

used to designate man's total knowledge. To designate all knowledge as philosophy was possible because our body of knowledge was relatively small and no real distinctions were made between different kinds of knowledge.

The Industrial Revolution, however, dramatically altered man's perception about the structuring of knowledge. The Darwinian hypothesis of natural selection, cell and germ theories, revolutionary discoveries about energy and matter, and the advent of psychoanalysis were but a few contributors to the knowledge explosion. No longer was philosophy considered adequate to answer questions about natural phenomena, and science divorced itself from it. New disciplines were formed—embryology, cytology, immunology, anesthesiology, to name a few—each asking their own questions and seeking their own answers.

This specialization, however, created a new problem: Although each discipline revealed unique and enlightening aspects of man, the ultimate questions about his nature and purpose went unanswered. Science had taken man apart but had not put him back together. Once again philosophy was sought out—this time to unify scientific findings so that man as a holistic being might emerge. This is in keeping with Kneller's (1971) view of the philosopher as one whose work begins before and after the scientist has done his job.

The philosopher is concerned with such matters as the purpose of human life, the nature of being and reality, and the theory and limits of knowledge. Questions the philosopher might ask are "Is man inherently good or evil?", "Is truth absolute or relative?", "What does 'knowing' mean?". His approach to understanding reality is characterized by formulating sets of assumptions and beliefs derived from his own personal experience and his contemplation of it in relation to the studied experiences of others (Association for Supervision and Curriculum Development [ASCD] Commission on Instructional Theory, 1968). Intuition, introspection, and reasoning are some of his methodologies.

The scientist, on the other hand, is primarily concerned with causality. Cause and effect, in one way or another, are central to his goal of deriving scientific laws (Labovitz and Hagedorn, 1976). Questions the scientist might ask are "Does treatment X, and only treatment X, cause Y?", or "What is the relationship between X and Y?" His approach to understanding reality is characterized by tentativeness, verifiability, observation, and experience. Reality becomes interpretable to him through such mechanisms as hypothesis-testing, operational definitions, and experiments. The scientists' position is summarized by Kerlinger (1973): "If an explanation cannot be formulated in the form of a testable hypothesis, then it can be considered to be a metaphysical explanation and thus not amenable to scientific investigation. As such, it is dismissed by the scientist as being of no interest" (p. 25).

However, despite different focuses and methodologies, the philosopher and scientist share the common goal of increasing mankind's knowledge.

Relationships Between Science and Theory

Before analyzing the relationships between science and theory, let us first briefly review some characteristics of science as a system, based on principles of Van Laer (1963, pp. 8–19):

1. **Science must show a certain coherence.** Science must constitute a coherent whole of interrelated facts, principles, laws, and theories which are appropriately ordered. An explication of unrelated data, no matter how valuable, does not constitute a science.

2. **Science is concerned with definite fields of knowledge.** Man is no longer able to know all things. Consequently, he must specialize so that he might know one field, or an aspect of it, well.

3. **Science is preferably expressed in universal statements.** Science ultimately is concerned with commonalities of properties that transcend the specific; science seeks to discover the universal characteristics of phenomena under investigation. Its goal is to reduce data to their most fundamental common denominator.

4. **The statements of science must be true or probably true.** What constitutes truth is a vexing epistemological question. One may suggest, however, that scientific statements are true if they express the nature of things as they are. But man, being finite, frequently does not know the true nature of things. And so it is to the scientist we often turn to help us find reality in a systematic, scholarly, and trustworthy way. His job, according to Scheffler, is "not to judge the truth infallibly, but to estimate the truth responsibly" (Scheffler, 1965, p. 54).

5. **The statements of science must be logically ordered.** One does not draw conclusions before stating hypotheses. Science is usually best served through careful observance of scientific methods such as the deductive-inductive or analytic-synthetic method.

6. **Science must explain its investigations and arguments.** Scientists have a responsibility not only to report their research findings, but as importantly, to explain the arguments and demonstrations which led them to their conclusions.

The above six principles certainly are not the exclusive domain of science. Many of them apply equally as well to philosophy or theory, once again underscoring the ebb and flow of relationships among philosophy, science, and theory.

We again see these relationships when we ask the question, "What is the aim of science? "Typical responses are that science aims to describe, understand, predict, control, or explain phenomena. But Kerlinger offers a different perspective: "The basic aim of science is theory" (Kerlinger, 1973, p. 8).

But what are the components of theory and how do they relate to science? There is no easy answer, no one correct response. Basic philosophical differences exist among scientists regarding the constructional processes composing science and theory. These differences stem from varying philosophical orientations—realism, idealism, pragmatism, and others—each with its own interpretation of reality.

To complicate the situation further, the many terms used to define theory can be bewildering. For example, words such as propositions, assertions, axioms, postulates and maxims, to name a few, are sometimes used interchangeably, at other times with different meanings. When one looks carefully, however, some common denominators of theory emerge. They are set, postulates, definitions, and hypotheses. Let us now briefly examine how each contributes to theory, and consequently, to science.

1. **Set.** Set is a well-defined collection of objects or elements. Facts, principles, and laws do not, in and of themselves, constitute theory. However, when a scientist selects particular facts, principles and laws from the universal set (i.e., from the set of all elements under discussion) because of their interrelationships and relevance to the problem under investigation, he fulfills the requirements of set needed for theory development.

2. **Postulates.** The central core of a theory consists of its postulates. These are statements of general truth that serve as essential premises for whatever is being investigated. Postulates are usually stated as generalizations which are consistent with scientific evidence related to one's research problem. They form the essential presuppositions from which hypotheses are deduced and tested. Rogers (1970), for example, in developing her theoretical basis of nursing, identified four essential postulates about man. These

postulates speak to man's wholeness, fluidity, sense of pattern and organization, and sentence.

3. **Definitions.** Definitions of terms are important for communication among scholars. Terms can be defined as primitive, theoretical, and key (ASCD Commission on Instructional Theory, 1968). Primitive terms are those which cannot be defined by specifying operations or by referring to other operationally defined terms. They represent entities which one can only intuitively experience. Purpose and need are examples of primitive terms. Theoretical terms are those which cannot be defined by pointing to particular operations, but which can be defined by their relationship to other terms which are operationally defined. Motivation is an example of a theoretical term. Key terms are those which can and must be operationally defined so that hypotheses under study can be tested. Learning is an example of a key term when it is essential to a hypothesis and can be operationally defined by use of valid and reliable instruments. Key terms are essential for replication research and theory verification.

4. **Hypotheses.** Hypotheses are predictions which have been deduced from a set of postulates and which state the relationship between two or more variables. They imply that the relationship between these variables can be observed and tested. This is no small matter, but one that is crucial in bridging theory and science. For if we cannot observe what we study, we cannot measure it. If we cannot measure it, we do not know whether or not it contributes to theory. If we do not know its impact on theory, we cannot know its potential contribution to science. Nurses are becoming more aware of these relationships. In a study of priorities in clinical nursing research, the highest priority in regard to "impact upon patient welfare" was given to items concerned with determining reliable and valid indicators of quality nursing care (Lindeman, 1975).

Because well stated hypotheses are based on observation of fact which permit them to be "proven" or "disproven," they are powerful instruments of science.

Through systematic and rigorous testing of hypotheses, phenomena are explained and, depending on the amount of verifiable evidence, these phenomena have predictive ability, first as theory, then principles and laws (Weinland, 1975). Through the power of hypotheses, mankind's knowledge is increased, or at the very least in the case of disproven hypotheses, his ignorance is reduced.

If we now synthesize the above four common denominators of theory, we arrive at a workable definition: Theory refers to a set of related statements (most commonly, **postulates** and **definitions**) which have been derived from scientific data and from which plausible **hypotheses** can be deduced, tested, and verified. If verified, theory becomes part of the body of science from which other sets of postulates can be derived. The process of theory building, therefore, involves the formulation and testing of hypotheses which have been deduced from a set of statements derived from scientific knowledge and philosophical beliefs.

Implications for Nursing Research

When the research process is examined by studying the relationships among philosophy, science, and theory, one arrives at perspectives different from traditional viewpoints about the derivation and significance of nursing knowledge. These perspectives are discussed below:

1. **Ultimately, all nursing theory and research is derived from or leads to philosophy.** Traditionally, one is led to believe that nursing research begins with theory. I believe it begins and ends with philosophy and this awareness enhances one's perspective about the research process.

   If one examines the four main branches of philosophy—logic, epistemology, metaphysics, and ethics—one begins to see the links between them and the process of nursing research. Through logic, researchers are able to establish the validity of various thoughts and the correctness of their reasoning. Germane to the research process is the ability to establish logical relationships between theory selection and problem identification, problem identification and hypothesis testing, hypothesis testing and derivation of valid conclusions.

Epistemology, the study of the theory of knowledge, is also crucial to the process of nursing research. For is not the aim of research to discover, expand, or reaffirm knowledge? Yet, what constitutes knowledge is no simple matter. Inherent in the concept of knowledge are conditions of truth, secure belief, and evidence (Scheffler, 1965). The truth condition claims that if one "knows" something to be true, he must be judged not to be in error. The belief condition stipulates if one "knows" something to be true, he also believes it to be true. The evidence condition states that one evaluates knowledge against all adequate standards of evidence at a particular time. Although nurse researchers have recognized the evidence condition of knowledge, they seemingly have paid less attention to the truth and belief conditions. By identifying and applying the contributions of epistemology to nursing, nurse researchers can gain further insights into the research process.

Metaphysics studies the most general concepts used in ordinary life and science by examining the internal structure of the language used in various disciplines (Harré, 1972). Of particular interest to the nurse researcher is an examination of the concept of causality. Questions the researcher might ask include: Is causality a necessary condition of objective experience? Can causality be demonstrated empirically? What are acceptable scientific criteria for the establishment of causality?

Finally, the study of ethics comes to grips with moral principles and values. Although all researchers are, I hope, familiar with the ethical requirements of informed consent and protection of the rights of human subjects, some, perhaps, have not considered other pertinent concepts. For example, what are ethical implications inherent in the nature of the research problem? What ethical considerations do advancements in science and technology present? What are the ethics involved in collaborative research and the reporting of research?

To whom are researchers ultimately accountable? Although the "pure" scientist may argue that the use to which knowledge is put is not his business, I believe research cannot be conceived apart from its moral implications.

2. **Philosophical introspection and intuition are legitimate methods of scientific inquiry.** Historically and traditionally, nurses have been indoctrinated into a singular approach to the derivation of nursing knowledge—the scientific method. As early as the 1930s, scientific criteria were used to evaluate procedural demonstrations (Gortner & Nahm, 1977). In the 1960s, McCain (1965) stressed nursing by assessment, not intuition. This stress on the scientific method continues strongly today. For example, Riehl and Roy (1974), among others, express disapproval about nursing actions based on intuition. Gortner (1974) suggests that the logic of science is closed to intuition. In addition, many graduate nursing students have been indoctrinated into a methodology of nursing research which excludes anything but strict adherence to the scientific method.

The time has come to question this singular approach to the study of nursing knowledge. The time has come to value truths arrived at by intuition and introspection as much as those arrived at by scientific experimentation. For, in fact, the scientist has no greater claim to truth than does the theoretician or the philosopher. Yet, nurse scholars seem hesitant to acknowledge intuition and introspection as valid methods of acquiring knowledge.

However, what we scorn, others praise. Burner (1977), for example, tells us that the development of intuitive thinking is an objective of many highly regarded teachers and is considered to be a valuable asset in science. Intuition is not knowledge arrived at out of nothing; rather, it is knowledge arrived at by a deep grasp of a subject, although one may not be able to articulate the process by which a conclusion is reached. The derived knowledge may not always be correct, but neither is knowledge arrived at with all the advantages of the scientific method. The large numbers of unsubstantiated hypotheses support this assertion.

In addition, knowledge gained through introspection cannot be overlooked as it constitutes one of the major approaches to the derivation of knowledge—rationalism. The prime example, of course, is mathematics where truth is deduced from reasoning and not contingent on observation or experience. According to Scheffler, mathematicians conduct no experiments, surveys, or statistics, yet "they arrive at the firmest of all truths, incapable of being overthrown by experience" (Scheffler, 1965, p. 3).

The point to be made here is that we must keep our minds open to all potential avenues which lead to advancement of nursing knowledge. We must be careful not to impose our value judgments about the research process on others if, in the end, we narrow their thinking and undermine their creativity. For example, during the conduct of my dissertation, although never explicitly stated, it was inferred time and again that the experimental research design with its emphasis on causality is superior to all other types of research. Descriptive, historical, and other valuable types of research were quietly but steadfastly refuted.

3. **Nursing knowledge arrived at by the scientific method too often sacrifices meaningfulness for rigor.** Although rigorous research designs are praiseworthy, if not used judiciously, they can impede rather than enhance the research process. Too much rigor can (and often does) lead to trivial research problems with the logical outcome of trivial research results. The same is true of definition of terms and statistics. One can meticulously operationally define the independent and dependent variables in one's hypotheses, but if these definitions are so narrow that they have little or no meaning for nursing practice, what is the point? In terms of statistics, one can find statistically significant differences among groups (if they exist) if a large enough sample is used. However, for practical purposes, the differences may be so small as to be negligible. Such statistics can be impeccably and rigorously applied, yet offer little to the advancement of nursing knowledge and, at best, be misleading.

Although one expects sufficient rigorism of design so that there is confidence in the results, the pursuit and worship of rigorism and experimentation for their own sake—as at times seems the case—needs questioning. Cook and LaFleur (1975) maintain that experimentation (with its implications for rigorism) as an exclusive method of obtaining knowledge is becoming a dead end as too little meaningful behavior can be understood by this method alone.

How can this situation be improved? As previously noted, researchers can begin to examine other ways to derive nursing knowledge. This does not necessarily mean that we give up a method we believe in, only that we open our minds to other approaches. Most of us, for example, have traditionally considered probability theory as the basis for accepting or rejecting hypotheses. Yet, Frank (1957) discusses another option: logical probability. Instead of reducing probability statements to statements about relative frequencies, one uses inductive logic to arrive at the probable truth or falsity of the data. The statements of inductive logic are purely logical and say nothing about physical facts; that is, they are not statements that are derived from observations. The basic premise is as follows: The inductive probability of a hypothesis h on the basis of a certain evidence e is high; or stated in another way, the evidence e confirms to a high degree the hypothesis h. Although the precise logical formulations derived to arrive at the above premise are beyond the scope of this paper, the possibilities of validating hypotheses in nontraditional ways are interesting to ponder.

In summary, when nurse researchers examine the total philosophy-science-theory triad, they develop a more holistic and less traditional approach to the possibilities of deriving nursing knowledge. They are more open to contributions of other disciplines and less likely to see the research process as though through a glass darkly.

REFERENCES

Andreoli, K. G., & Thompson, C. E. (1977). The nature of science in nursing. *Image, 9,* 32–37.

Association for Supervision and Curriculum Development Commission on Instructional Theory (ASCD). (1968). *Criteria for theories of instruction.* Washington, DC: National Education Association.

Bruner, J. (1977). *The process of education*. London: Harvard University Press (Originally published 1960).

Burns, E. M. (1955). *Western civilization: Their history and their culture* (4th ed.). New York: W. W. Norton.

Cook, D. R., & LaFleur, N. K. (1975). *A guide to educational research* (2nd ed.). Boston: Allyn and Bacon.

Frank, P. (1957). *Philosophy of science: The link between science and philosophy*. Englewood Cliffs, NJ: Prentice-Hall.

Gortner, S. R. (1974). Scientific accountability in nursing. *Nursing Outlook, 22,* 764–768.

Gortner, S. R., & Nahm, H. (1977). An overview of nursing research in the United States. *Nursing Research, 26,* 10–33.

Hardy, M. E. (1974). Theories: Components, development, evaluation. *Nursing Research, 23,* 100–107.

Harré, R. (1972). *The philosophies of science: An introductory survey*. London: Oxford University Press.

Jacox, A. (1974). Theory construction in nursing: An overview. *Nursing Research, 23,* 4–13.

Kerlinger, F. N. (1973). *Foundations of behavioral research* (2nd ed.). New York: Holt, Rinehart, and Winston.

Kneller, G. F. (1971). *Introduction to the philosophy of education* (2nd ed.). New York: John Wiley & Sons.

Labovitz, S., & Hagedorn, R. (1976). *Introduction to social research* (2nd ed.). New York: McGraw-Hill.

Leininger, M. (1968). Conference on the nature of science and nursing: Introductory comments. *Nursing Research, 17,* 484–486.

Lindeman, C. A. (1975). Delphi survey of priorities in clinical nursing research. *Nursing Research, 24,* 434–441.

McCain, R. F. (1965). Nursing by assessment—not intuition. *American Journal of Nursing, 65,* 82–84.

Riehl, J. P., & Roy, C. (1974). *Conceptual models for nursing practice*. New York: Appleton-Century-Crofts.

Rogers, M. E. (1970). *An introduction to the theoretical basis of nursing*. Philadelphia: F. A. Davis.

Scheffler, I. (1965). *Conditions of knowledge: An introduction to epistemology and education*. Glenview, IL: Scott, Foresman.

Van Laer, P. H. (1963). *Philosophy of science: An introduction to some general aspects of science* (2nd ed.). Pittsburgh: Duquesne University Press.

Walker, L. O. (1971). Toward a clearer understanding of the concept of nursing theory. *Nursing Research, 20,* 428–435.

Weinland, J. D. (1975). *How to think straight*. Totowa, NJ: Littlefield, Adams (Originally published 1963).

The Author Comments

Philosophy, Science, Theory: Interrelationships and Implications for Nursing Research

My inspiration for this article came from a long-standing interest in philosophy and the need I saw to bridge the gap between philosophy, science, and theory. In addition, when this article was written, the strong emphasis on empirical research offended my integrative and intuitive nature. The three implications for nursing research contained in this article continue to be important to the development, testing, and evaluation of nursing theory in the 21st century.

—MARY CIPRIANO SILVA

CHAPTER 3

Nursing Questions
That Science Cannot Answer

June F. Kikuchi

Science—what nursing questions can it answer? What nursing questions can it *not* answer? Indeed, are there *any* nursing questions that science, as a mode of inquiry, cannot answer? Certainly, given the tremendous success of science to date and the omnipresence of science, it is easy to be lured into thinking that we not only can, but must, turn to science for answers to all of our questions. That we have been so lured is clear: Science reigns supreme in the world of nursing research.

That science dominates nursing research is not problematic—in fact, because nursing as a discipline is a science, it is to be expected. What *is* of concern is that nurses are erroneously subjecting to scientific study nursing questions that are nonscientific—beyond the scope of science to answer. This misuse of science is clearly evident in the scientific studies being conducted using the grounded theory method (à la Glaser and Strauss) to answer philosophical nursing questions such as "What is the nature of nursing?" and "What is the nature of the nurse-client relationship?" Adequate answers to such questions will not be forthcoming until they are recognized as philosophical in nature and are pursued philosophically, not scientifically.

It is my contention that the present misuse of science by nurses, and its attendant consequences, will persist unless and until philosophy, as a mode of inquiry, is allowed to take its rightful place in the nurse's world, for it is only by philosophizing that we can ascertain the kind of nursing question that is (and those that are not) amenable to scientific study. In this essay, with the hope of goading us into philosophizing about those nursing questions that

About the Author

JUNE F. KIKUCHI was born on the west coast of Canada in 1939 and, being of Japanese ancestry, she spent some of her early years in an internment camp in the interior of British Columbia during World War II. She received her BScN degree in 1962 from the University of Toronto and her MN and PhD degrees in the nursing care of children in 1969 and 1979, respectively, from the University of Pittsburgh. Postdoctorally, she studied philosophy at the University of Toronto. She has held various nursing positions, including staff nurse, instructor, head nurse, clinical nurse specialist, clinical nurse researcher, and, most recently, professor. With Dr. Helen Simmons, she cofounded the Institute for Philosophical Nursing Research at the University of Alberta in 1988 and served as its director until 1997, when she retired early to engage leisurely in philosophic nursing inquiry, gardening, and volunteer work with hospitalized children. The aim of her scholarly work continues to be raising nurses' awareness of the need to think philosophically about their world.

science cannot answer, I present a position that is grounded in the *moderate realist* view of reality—a view that in my estimation is the most tenable and that nurses must adopt if nursing is to have a future as a learned profession (i.e., as a societal institution with an organized body of knowledge and with activities of its own, which exists to serve a practical end, a "particular human good" (Maritain, 1930, p. 111). I say this because in this view the existence of reality independent of the mind is supposed: objective reality with natural forms, boundaries, and orders, against which the truth of propositions can be tested, making possible the attainment of knowledge (in the form of probable truth) of reality. The importance of this supposition becomes evident as this essay unfolds.

In putting forward my position, given the time constraint and the theme of the conference, I have decided to focus on only one kind of nursing question that science cannot answer: the philosophical. Let me begin by defining three key terms: nursing question, science, and philosophy. Other key terms will be defined as they arise.

What is a nursing question? An answer to this philosophical nursing question presupposes an answer to another philosophical nursing question: What is the nature of nursing? As we all know, in searching for an adequate definition of nursing, we have hit dangerous potholes and landmines. Given that we are without adequate answers to both of these questions and that in this essay I do not intend to seek such answers, in order that I might proceed,

permit the term *nursing question* to be incompletely defined as follows: questions that are controlled by the end or goal of nursing practice. To define it in terms of the end or goal of nursing practice seems proper because, as Wallace (1977) correctly states, "That which is final in the place of action is the cause of all the activity leading to it" (p. 157). I acknowledge that for many purposes this definition would not be useful, in that it includes the undefined term *nursing;* however, it is adequate to the task at hand.

Because of the various ways in which the terms *science* and *philosophy* are used, it is problematic, especially in epistemological treatises, if these terms are left undefined. Unless otherwise specified, in speaking of science and philosophy, I am referring to specific modes of inquiry, the aim of which is to attain knowledge, in the form of probable truth, about reality—a world of real existences that exists outside and independent of our minds (Adler, 1965). As a mode of inquiry, science inquires into the phenomenal aspects of reality, philosophy into those aspects that transcend the phenomenal (Maritain, 1930). An elaboration of this distinction follows in the next section.

In agreement with Adler (1965), I am taking probable truths to be truths that are "(1) testable by reference to evidence, (2) subject to rational criticism, and either (3) corrigible and rectifiable or (4) falsifiable" (p. 28). Such truths are distinctively different from necessary truths, which are characterized by certainty and finality, such as self-evident truths; and from statements we make from time to time about our own subjective experiences, such as "I feel ill," which unless we are prevaricating also have certitude and finality for us when we make them (p. 26). Furthermore, probable truths are not to be confused with mere opinion, which is "irresponsible, unreliable, unfounded, unreasonable" (p. 29).

Having defined some key terms, let me now present my position. I will proceed by first establishing the essential distinction between scientific and philosophical questions. Then I will consider the kinds of questions that constitute the realm of philosophical nursing questions—a realm beyond science's investigative power.

Scientific and Philosophical Questions

Why is it that science cannot answer philosophical questions? Is it merely that science does not yet have the means to do so? What if we devised additional scientific methods? It is my contention that no scientific method would help us here. Philosophical questions are questions regarding aspects of reality that are not amenable to scientific study in that they transcend the material. Being metaphysical, they lie outside science's realm— the realm of the phenomenal (Maritain, 1930). Scientific questions, then, are questions regarding the phenomenal (material) aspects of reality. Let me try to make this distinction between philosophical and scientific questions clear, by calling upon the work of Aristotle (as interpreted by Wallace, 1977) concerning the matter of change.

In grappling with the perplexing philosophical problem of change (how it is that things change and yet remain the same), Aristotle reasoned that two coexisting intrinsic principles were operative in every change: (a) *form*, the principle that actuates matter (i.e., that makes a thing be what it is); and (b) *matter*, the principle that receives the actuation (i.e., that of which a thing is made). Now, there are (a) two kinds of form: substantial and accidental, and (b) two kinds of matter: primary

and secondary. *Substantial form* actuates *primary matter* (or what may be thought of as undifferentiated protomatter) making it *be* a thing of a specific kind or essence (such as "a dog" or "a human"), or what is called *secondary matter.* Operating on this secondary matter (i.e., the actuated primary matter), *accidental forms* qualify it to be this way or that in certain respects (such as its color and size), resulting in, for example, "a large, brown dog."

According to Aristotle, *substantial change* entails a change of substantial form; in such a change, a thing wholly becomes a thing of another kind, such as takes place at death. *Accidental change* entails a change of accidental form(s); in this kind of change, a thing changes in one or more respects while retaining its substantial form, such as takes place when a baby grows. To illustrate, as a baby grows, it changes only in an accidental way. For example, it becomes larger in size, and its hair color and tone of voice may change; however, throughout such changes, the baby does not change substantially—it retains the human form or essence that it had at conception (albeit in potency) and will retain until death.

Now—relating Aristotle's work to the matter at hand—science concerns itself with the accidental or phenomenal; philosophy with the substantial or nonphenomenal. Science has the power to answer questions regarding the accidental aspects of things (e.g., questions about how babies change as they grow); however, it has no power to answer questions regarding the substantial aspect of things (the essence of things, such as the babies' humanness). Questions about essences or forms per se, the metaphysical aspects of things, lie in the metaphysical realm, a realm addressed by philosophy.

When we are faced with philosophical questions (speculative questions regarding metaphysical aspects of reality and the normative questions grounded in them), science's investigative observational and measurement tools are useless. We have no recourse but to use that wonderful power that we possess—reason— which, unfortunately, seems to be taking a backseat to feelings lately. Moderate realism, a common-sense philosophy, holds that by reflecting on and discursively analyzing our common-sense knowledge (that which we know, not through investigation, but by common sense in light of common experience available to all of us by virtue of being awake), answers to philosophical questions can be attained that are empirically grounded and, furthermore, do not conflict with our common-sense knowledge (Adler, 1965). If you will recall, I have grounded my position on the matter of nursing questions that science cannot answer in moderate realist thought. Therefore, all of its tenets are presupposed, the most important being that philosophy can attain probable truths about reality through the use of reason.

Having made the essential distinction between philosophical and scientific questions, let us turn to the nurse's world and consider the structure of the realm of philosophical nursing questions: philosophical questions controlled by the end or goal of nursing practice.

Philosophical Nursing Questions

An examination of the contemporary nursing literature (apart from an examination of the reported methods used by nurse researchers) might lead one to conclude that philosophical nursing questions are of two kinds: ethical and epistemological. Would we be correct in so concluding? To answer this question, it may be fruitful to look first at ethical nursing questions: There seems to be little dispute within nursing that these questions are philosophical in nature.

Ethical Nursing Questions

In the last decade, numerous publications have appeared in which the term *nursing ethics* has been used, leading one to conclude that the realm of philosophical nursing questions includes, at minimum, ethical nursing questions. In point of fact, ethical nursing knowledge is the only kind of philosophical nursing knowledge identified by Carper (1975), Jacobs-Kramer and Chinn (1988), Schlotfeldt (1988), and Walker (1971) in their conceptualizations of nursing knowledge. Furthermore, it is equated by the latter two authors with "nursing philosophy" and "philosophy of nursing," respectively. However,

as a recent issue of *Advances in Nursing Science* devoted to ethical issues (Chinn, 1989) indicates, a point yet to be resolved is whether or not there are, indeed, ethical nursing questions—whether or not the ethical principles that guide nursing activities are attained by nursing ethics or by ethics proper.

It would seem that because ethics proper addresses questions about what is good to do and to seek, specifically as human, in order to attain a good human life, nursing ethics would be required to address questions about what is good to do and to seek, specifically as nurses, in order to attain the end or goal of nursing practice—in short, to answer ethical nursing questions. It would also seem that given the nature of ethics proper and of nursing ethics, the latter derives ethical nursing principles from principles that the former has worked out. If so, nursing ethics, as knowledge, would not (as the previously mentioned nurse scholars claim) consist of ethical theories or professional codes of behavior: the former would be presupposed and the latter derived from nursing ethics (ethical nursing principles).

Let me hasten to add that nursing politics would also be required to address questions about what nursing, as a political institution, ought to do and to seek in order to meet its social mission—to answer political nursing questions. As is the case for nursing ethics, answers to political nursing questions, it would seem, are derived from principles that politics proper (i.e., political philosophy) has worked out.

Moving along to epistemological questions, let us consider the existence of epistemological nursing questions.

Epistemological Nursing Questions

As is the case for nursing ethics, it would seem that because epistemology proper addresses questions regarding human knowledge in general (its nature, scope, and object), nursing epistemology would be required to address questions regarding nursing knowledge (its nature, scope, and object)—epistemological nursing questions. That these questions do exist and have been addressed by nurse scholars with increasing frequency is evident, for example, in the compilation of papers published in *Perspectives on Nursing Theory* by Nicoll (1986).

Again, it would seem that, as is the case for nursing ethics and nursing politics, answers to epistemological nursing questions are derived from principles that epistemology proper has worked out. It is important to note that this would only be the case if epistemology were conceived as giving us new knowledge. It would not be the case if the position taken up by some contemporary philosophers, such as Adler (1965), were adopted: the position that epistemology "gives us no new knowledge, it serves only to clarify what we already know . . . [it gives us] only a better understanding of the facts already known by other disciplines" (Adler, 1965, p. 47).[1]

In adhering to the positive position—that epistemology proper and nursing epistemology give us new knowledge—it then becomes possible to raise epistemological nursing questions with a future, the asking and answering of which will bring us ever closer to identifying and developing the body of nursing knowledge required for attaining the end of nursing practice. What are these questions? Because the focus of the conference is epistemological in nature, it may be helpful to identify some of these questions and also concerns related to them.

Some critical questions come immediately to mind: Is there such an entity as nursing knowledge? If so, what is its nature? What are its parameters? What is its object? There are those who have dismissed these questions, saying that it is pointless to ask them because there are no genuine boundaries to knowledge of any sort. Others who have tried to answer them, but without success, have dismissed them, saying that it is a waste of time and energy to continue to struggle with them because the answers are too elusive. Still others, myself included, contend that these questions are not so easily dismissed. They continually crop up in our interactions with other disciplines, funding agencies, the public, the media, health care institutions, and so forth. I submit that we must *not* try to escape asking and answering these questions but

rather face them squarely. Only by so doing can we attain the knowledge that will ensure that the research endeavors of nurses directly and essentially serve the end or goal of nursing.

In addressing the aforementioned epistemological nursing questions, three epistemological distinctions must be made. It is of concern that these distinctions are not being made in the nursing literature. If made, the confusion that currently pervades our thinking stands to be replaced by clarity.

First, a distinction must be made between (a) the knowledge nurses use in order to nurse, and (b) the knowledge that comprises the body of nursing knowledge. Are these synonymous? Some nurses certainly seem to be treating them as such. I contend that they are not synonymous and that the latter is part of the former—the knowledge that comprises the body of nursing knowledge is only one kind of knowledge that nurses use in order to nurse. Furthermore, it is only the body of nursing knowledge that nursing is responsible for developing. Nursing is not responsible for developing the other kinds of knowledge nurses use, such as the preclinical and personal knowledge nurses use to do their work. By *preclinical knowledge* I mean that knowledge that nurses use or take on as assumption, which lies outside their discipline; by *personal knowledge* I mean that knowledge described by Carper (1975) as subjective, incommunicable, publicly unverifiable, and therefore not possessed by anyone other than the one whose direct knowledge it is. Indeed, how could nursing be held responsible for developing such private knowledge?

Another distinction requiring our attention is the difference between (a) private ways of knowing, such as intuiting, that may contribute to the development of nursing's body of knowledge but *only* indirectly; and (b) public ways of knowing, such as scientizing and philosophizing, that stand to contribute directly. Private ways of knowing serve only as possible means to public ways of knowing—ways that possess the power to make available, for public examination and testing, their methods and resultant evidence and, thereby, directly serve the development of knowledge. How can intuition be other than an indirect contributor, given that it is a private experience?

The failure to make these two distinctions may be a result, in part, of the failure to make a third distinction: the difference between (a) that which is private, and (b) that which is public. According to Adler (1985), that which is private "belongs to one individual alone and cannot possibly be shared directly by anyone else" (p. 10); and that which is public is "common to two or more individuals" (p. 10). Private ways of knowing and knowledge, then, are subjective: "differ[ent] from one person to another and . . . exclusively the possession of one individual and no one else" (p. 9). They are incommunicable and publicly unverifiable. Public ways of knowing and knowledge, on the other hand, are objective: "the same for me, for you, and for anyone else" (p. 9). They are communicable and publicly verifiable.

Of late, nurses (e.g., Carper, 1975; Jacobs-Kramer & Chinn, 1988; Kidd & Morrison, 1988; Schultz & Meleis, 1988) seem not to be paying heed to these three distinctions in setting down their conceptualizations of nursing knowledge. Consequently, when a reference is made to nursing knowledge, at times it is impossible to determine if the referent is (a) the knowledge that nurses possess and/or use, or (b) the knowledge that lies within the body of nursing knowledge. Perhaps the failure to make these distinctions is intentional in that it is being presupposed that there are no differences in kind (i.e., no natural forms and boundaries) in reality, only differences in degree. Such a presupposition would explain nurses' growing reluctance to differentiate between (a) nursing's body of knowledge and (b) those of other disciplines; and between (a) ways of knowing and knowledge that are public and objective and (b) those that are private and subjective. It seems likely that this presupposition may be operative, because questions about whether or not nursing knowledge is borrowed or unique seem to have disappeared from the nursing literature and to have been replaced with questions about the knowledge that nurses possess and use.

Let me move on now to another kind of philosophical nursing question, a kind that is, unfortunately, neglected in the nursing epistemological literature: the ontological.

Ontological Nursing Questions

It is problematic that in contemporary conceptualizations of nursing knowledge, for the most part, no reference is made to ontological nursing knowledge: knowledge about nursing as a *being*. Are we to take, from this absence, that it is being presupposed, as identified earlier, that there are no differences of kind in reality, only differences of degree? I suspect this may be so because, if such were the case, no ontological nursing questions regarding the nature, scope, and object of nursing would be asked. However, we do ask such questions. How would those who deny the existence of ontological and ontological nursing questions account for the occurrence of such questions? I suspect that they would identify them as scientific, in which case they would also claim that answers to such questions would be found in the science of nursing, both of which are errors.

I submit that if ontological nursing questions are treated as scientific and "answered" scientifically, then we will attain merely knowledge of nursing as it exists phenomenally or accidentally and as it appears to us. But then, if it is being presupposed that there are no natural forms and boundaries in reality, this is the end of the line. To acknowledge the existence of ontological nursing questions and the possibility of attaining philosophical knowledge of nursing as it exists substantially, as a being, would require our holding the presupposition that natural forms and boundaries, differences of kind, do exist in reality. In my estimation, to do otherwise is suicidal. If only differences of degree exist, then we are left with no universal natural truths or order and with having to impose meaning and order on the world. This bodes ill in terms of knowledge development, because all we can possibly attain in that case is a plurality of mere opinions, which may be upheld by consensus or by what can be referred to as "might makes right."

The Author Comments

Nursing Questions That Science Cannot Answer

My doctoral nursing studies in the 1970s focused only on the scientific mode of inquiry, and I graduated thinking that science was the only road to knowledge. A few years later, I discovered to my amazement that the question "What is nursing?" is a philosophic question to be answered philosophically. I then realized that I was ignorant about philosophic inquiry, and, as they say, the rest is history. Nursing Questions That Science Cannot Answer is one of the first papers I wrote after my life-changing discovery. The sound development of nursing theory in the 21st century depends, in part, on our seeking answers to the types of philosophic nursing questions identified in that paper, particularly those of an ontologic nature about the nature, scope, and object of nursing.

—June F. Kikuchi

CHAPTER 4

The Relationship Between Theory and Research: A Double Helix

Jacqueline Fawcett

Both theory development and research, when isolated endeavors, are excursions into the trivial. What could be less important than a theory about sweet peas or research that involved mating the peas? Yet Mendel combined these seemingly trivial activities and formulated classic genetic theory (Gardner, 1968). And what could be less meaningful than trying to interpret x-rays of sugars and proteins, drawing pictures of protein pairs and tinkering with cardboard and tin replicas of the substances? Yet from these activities emerged an understanding of the double helix structure of DNA (Watson, 1968). Thus only when theory and research are integrated do both become non-trivial; and only then can they contribute to the advancement of science.

The relationship between theory and research may be thought of as a double helix, much like DNA. Theory is one helix from the conception of an idea through modifications and extensions to eventual confirmation or refutation. Research is the second helix, spiralling from identification of research questions through data collection and analysis to interpretation of findings and recommendations for further study. The core of the double helix is the pairing of theory development with the research process. In the core, theory directs research and research findings shape the development of theory. It is this core that avoids the potential triviality of the separate helices.

The Theory Helix

The primary function of the theory helix is the development of theory. It is also concerned with such philosophic issues

About the Author

JACQUELINE FAWCETT received her Bachelor of Science degree from Boston University in 1964, her master's in Parent–Child Nursing from New York University in 1970, and her PhD in Nursing, also from New York University, in 1976. Dr. Fawcett currently is Professor, College of Nursing and Health Sciences, University of Massachusetts-Boston. She is Professor Emerita at the University of Pennsylvania. Starting with her dissertation, Dr. Fawcett conducted a program of research dealing with wives' and husbands' pregnancy-related experiences that was derived from Martha Rogers' conceptual system. Subsequently, she undertook a program of research dealing with responses to Cesarean birth derived from the Roy Adaptation Model of Nursing. A third program of research, also derived from the Roy Adaptation Model, focuses on function during normal life transitions and serious illness. Dr. Fawcett is perhaps best known for her meta-theoretical work, including many journal articles and several books. Since 1996, Dr. Fawcett has lived in the mid-coast region of Maine with her husband John and a now-tame feral cat, Lydia Dasher. She and her husband own Fawcett's Art, Antiques, and Toy Museum. She swims laps and walks on a treadmill at a fitness center for exercise and relaxation and sails on a windjammer off the Maine coast during the summer.

as "truth, the nature of reality, the processes of knowing, and the logic of meaning statements" (Dubin, 1978, p. 17).

A theory is defined as "a set of interrelated [concepts], definitions, and propositions that present a systematic view of phenomena by specifying relations among variables" (Kerlinger, 1973, p. 9). An empirically testable theory is composed of concepts that are narrowly bounded, specific and explicitly interrelated.

Content and Structure of Theory

As noted, a theory comprises concepts, definitions and propositions. A concept is an abstract idea expressed in words, a generalization from observed events which may range from a single word to several sentences to entire paragraphs. Concepts enable scientists to categorize, interpret and structure events and objects, helping them to make some sense of their world. Concepts refer to properties of things, not to the things themselves. Usually, they represent phenomena that vary in some manner and are thus referred to as variables (Burr, 1973; Dubin, 1978).

Concepts are the basic building blocks of theories and must therefore be precisely and explicitly defined to enable scientists to distinguish between the meanings of one concept and another. Concepts are defined constitutively and operationally. The constitutive definition, also referred to as the rational approach or the nominal definition, provides meaning for a concept by defining it in terms of the other concepts; it is a circular definition. The operational definition, in contrast, gives concepts empirical utility by linking them with the real world. These definitions, also called real definitions, rules of correspondence or rules of interpretation, define concepts in terms of observable data; i.e., the activities necessary to measure the concept or manipulate it.

Constitutive definitions facilitate communication about the meaning of concepts. Without them, as circular and imprecise as they are, it would not be possible to construct meaningful, logical theories. A theory composed of undefined concepts would be unintelligible, while one composed of only operationally defined concepts would probably be so complex that it too would be unintelligible. While all concepts in a theory should be defined constitutively, such a theory can be evaluated only on logical grounds and cannot be considered scientific. Therefore, for a theory to be empirically testable, operational definitions are required of at least some of its concepts. The operationally defined terms are called empirical indicators. Each is fully specified in terms of its measurement and is therefore clearly differentiated from others. It is important to point out that while constitutive definitions are a distinct part of a theory, operational definitions may be thought of as standing just outside the theory, serving as a link between it and research (Burr, 1973; Hempel, 1952; Torgerson, 1958).

Concepts are connected in a theory by verbal or mathematical statements called propositions. Propositions described the theoretical linkages between concepts. Two types of propositions are generally found in a theory. Axioms, or initial propositions, are the starting points for derivations; they are not to be tested, but rather are taken as givens in the theory. In contrast, postulates, also called deduced propositions or theorems, are statements of supposition regarding the type of relation between the concepts of the theory. A theory's explanatory power is found in its postulates (Burr, 1973; Skidmore, 1975).

The hypothesis is a postulate containing operationally defined terms. It is a descriptive, predictive or prescriptive statement about the presumed relations between the values of two or more empirical indicators. Like the operational definitions they contain, hypotheses are not part of a theory, but are derived from it. The theory is the explanation of relations between concepts; this explanation is tested through the tests of hypotheses (Dubin, 1978).

Theory-Building Strategies

Knowing what the elements of theory are does not, by itself, ensure adequate theory construction. For theory does not emerge out of a random selection and combination of concepts, definitions and propositions; it must be carefully constructed according to a defensible plan. Burr (1973) identified a taxonomy of theory building which includes strategies to assist the scientist to create, extend, integrate or modify theories.

Inductive strategies of theory building use relatively specific, concrete ideas to generate more general, abstract ideas. One such strategy is Glaser and Strauss's (1967) grounded theory, which requires scientists to immerse themselves, without preconceived ideas, in the data (preferably qualitative) of a research project in an attempt to generate new theoretical notions.

Merton (1957) describes another inductive strategy, codification; this is the process of systematizing apparently different empirical generalizations and using them as the basis for inducing new propositions. A third inductive approach is Zetterberg's (1965) definitional reduction in which several variables are redefined, or "collapsed," into a single variable. Thus a new theoretical formulation, more general than the original notions, is suggested.

A fourth theory-building strategy is Zetterberg's (1965) propositional reduction. This approach requires the scientist to select some of the original propositions as general axioms and then to derive other statements of relationships in a logical manner. This strategy qualifies as an inductive one because some propositions are taken to be more general than others.

Deductive strategies of theory building involve starting with relatively abstract, general propositions as the basis for logically deducing new theories that are more specific. One such strategy involves borrowing propositions from one discipline and applying them in another. However, this approach is appropriate only when the initial propositions are rather general and logically congruent with other knowledge in the discipline (Aldous, 1970; Jacox, 1969).

Another deductive strategy is the process of constructing a new theory by deductively extending an already established one. Zetterberg (1965) alludes to this approach, but it is not fully described in the literature.

Other theory-building strategies are not clearly classifiable as either inductive or deductive. The retroductive strategy, described by Hanson (1958), combines the two methods for the purpose of expanding theory. This approach requires the scientist to identify many specific propositions and then induce a more general proposition from which new, specific ones are deduced. Gibson's (1960) factor strategy is similar to induction and generates new theories by examining the interactions and contingencies of various independent variables and their influence on one or more dependent variables.

The final strategy in Burr's taxonomy is theory reworking, or the modification of a theory in light of new methodological tools, new conceptualization, new insights or new empirical data. Burr commented that while this strategy may not increase the amount of theory, "it can build theory in the sense of improving such things as the clarity, testability, communicability, parsimony, and heuristic value" (Burr, 1973, p. 281).

Burr (1973) also identified other activities that are indispensable to theory building. These include development of conceptual models; gathering of empirical data to generate, test of modify theory; improvement of data retrieval systems; and improvement of measurement instruments. However, the discussion of these techniques is beyond the scope of this article.

The ultimate purpose of theory is to order and systematize empirical observations. The scientist desires theory that is highly predictive and thus narrowly bounded; at the same time, he seeks theory that is highly explanatory and thus broad in scope. Since it is not possible to have both at once, decisions must be made as to which type of theory is most needed at any given time in the evolution of a science.

Merton's is perhaps the most popular solution for this paradox. He urged construction of "theories of the middle range" (Merton, 1957, p. 9)—that is, theories that focus on and are applicable to somewhat limited ranges of data. Such theories have some explanatory power and some predictive precision. Moreover, they are more readily testable than either grand theories that are initially too abstract for empirical testing, or partial theories that lack sufficient specification for empirical testing.

If scientists follow the procedures outlined above, they will produce theories that will probably have a degree of esthetic appeal. However, such theories could still be trivial. The theory helix becomes nontrivial only when theory is tested in the real world and modified accordingly.

The Research Helix

The primary function of the research helix is the development of prescriptions for empirical investigations. Its foci are measurement issues, translation of propositions into testable hypotheses and reliability of empirical indicators (Dubin, 1978).

Kerlinger defined scientific research as the "systematic, controlled, empirical, and critical investigation of hypothetical propositions about the presumed relations among natural phenomena" (Kerlinger, 1973, p. 11). Scientific research is systematic and controlled in that observations are sufficiently disciplined so that the investigator has confidence in the research outcomes. Systematization and control come from application of the "max-con-min principle" by which the investigator maximizes the variance of the variables of the research hypothesis, controls the variance of extraneous variables, and minimizes the error variance (Kerlinger, 1973, p. 306).

The empirical and critical nature of scientific research requires scientists to compare subjective belief against objective reality. They must continually subject their ideas to empirical inquiry and view their own and others' findings hypercritically.

Scientific research is a multiphase process which proceeds through several well-known stages: (a) formulation of a research issue, (b) identification of a specific research problem, (c) development of an appropriate research design, (d) selection of research instruments, (e) sampling of units of interest, (f) collection and analysis of data, (g) interpretation of findings and (h) dissemination of results.

Formulating Research Issues and Problems

The choice of research issues is typically based on scientists' current interests and their perceptions of what the crucial questions are in their discipline. Webb (1961) pointed out that scientists commonly base studies on: (a) their interest in the issues, (b) their belief that the answers to the problems inherent in the issues are available, (c) their compassion for society, (d) their belief that these issues will lead to expensive (and therefore important) studies, (e) their belief that the research will yield substantial personal rewards, (f) and their knowledge that everyone else is doing similar work. He noted that while each of these reasons may result in investigations of significant issues in the discipline, more often they result in delineation of pedestrian problems and trivial results.

Research Design and Instruments

The empirical expressions of research issues are the specific research problems, which state the relation between two or more variables. These statements should clearly indicate the scope of the research and should imply possibilities of empirical testing. Research design is the translation of research issues and derived problems into action. As noted above, scientific research attempts to deal with all sources of variance. The "max-con-min principle" is the basis of Campbell and Stanley's classic monograph comparing various research designs with regard to their likelihood of yielding valid inferences. Their work provides specific guidelines for research free from threats to internal and external validity (Campbell & Stanley, 1963).

The instruments selected for a particular study obviously should measure the variables identified in the problem statements. A major concern at this stage of the research process is the evaluation of instrument validity and reliability—their sensitivity in detecting significant differences or relations; their applicability to and appropriateness for the population of interest; and their objectivity. (Fox, 1976).

Sampling

Sampling techniques allow scientists to select for study groups of subjects that permit generalizations to the population of interest. While random samples are traditionally the most valued, they are not the ones that are most precise and they cannot be used under some circumstances. It is therefore not surprising to find an increased interest in sampling methods that are more generally applicable and which yield more precise estimates of the population (Kish, 1965). Sample size must also be considered. Various techniques exist for the determination of optimum sample size and are documented in the literature (Cohen, 1969).

Data Collection and Analysis

Data collection, of course, directly depends on the research problems and instruments. However, it is not unusual in the course of a study for the scientist to collect data that are only indirectly related to specific study problems. As will be seen later, often these additional data ultimately prove more valuable in terms of the overall research issue.

Data analysis is a focal point of contemporary research. As more sophisticated and complex analyses are facilitated by the use of computers, it becomes increasingly possible for scientists to examine more sources of variance among study variables. However, it is important that they not be so seduced by advanced analytical methods as to lose sight of the original study issues and problems.

Interpretation and Dissemination of Findings

Interpretation of research findings follows the rules of logic explicit in the statistical procedures used in the investigation. Objectivity is a key component of this stage of the research process. While statistical significance of findings is almost always reported, few scientists consider the strength of association between variables, despite repeated urging by experts to do so (Dunnette, 1966).

The scientist has not completed the research helix until findings are reported to peers. The purpose of the research report is to communicate as precisely, concisely and clearly as possible "what was done, why it was done, the outcome of the doing, and the investigator's conclusions" (Kerlinger, 1973, p. 694). The readers must then make their own judgments regarding the adequacy and validity of the study.

Relating Research to Theory

If scientists apply the research process carefully, it is likely they will conduct sophisticated investigations free from methodological flaws. However, it is quite possible the studies will be irrelevant, for, just as the theory helix is trivial in isolation, so is the research helix. Knowledge of research methodology, no matter how extensive, is meaningless unless it can be utilized in the design and conduct of investigations that are grounded in theory.

The ultimate purpose of a research study, according to Popper (1965), is to refute the theory on which the study is based. The Popperian stance focuses on improving rather than proving a theory. This approach allows all data collected during an investigation to be used, giving "particular attention to deviant cases and nonfitting data that feed back immediately into the theory-building process by resulting in theory modifications" (Dubin, 1978, p. 232). From this perspective, it is impossible to discuss research without discussing theory.

The Core of the Double Helix

The double helix has as its core the interrelation between theory and research. As in DNA, the core is essential for structure and function. Merton emphasized this point by noting, "It is commonplace that continuity, rather than dispersion, can be achieved only if empirical studies are theory-oriented and if theory is empirically confirmable" (Merton, 1957, p. 100). Thus the body of knowledge of a science must rely on the repeated investigation of theoretically based problems that are redefined as research results accumulate. Theory should guide all phases of the research process, from choice of research issue to dissemination of results. All research, in turn, should be directed to one of two goals—theory building or theory testing.

Types of Theory-Related Research

Theory-building research has as its primary purpose the discovery of relations between variables on the basis of empirical observations. Once observations are made, they are analyzed and examined for generalizations that might lead to formulation of concepts and propositions. Traditionally, these activities have been labeled theoretical, descriptive, inductive or hypothesis-generating research. This type of research stems mainly from and relies heavily on inductive strategies of theory building to create new theories or to modify existing ones.

Theory-testing research, on the other hand, seeks to confirm or refute previously postulated relations between variables. Its major function is to determine the degree of correspondence between predicted and observed relations. These activities are usually labeled empirical, deductive or hypothesis-testing research. Predominantly through deductive theory-building strategies, hypotheses are formulated and tested in the real world (Dubin, 1978).

It should be clear that the two types of research are inextricably bound to theory and are differentiated only by the direction of movement between observation and theory within the double helix. It should also be obvious that all phases of the research process should be based on theory. Of course, research can be conducted without an explicit theoretical base. However, according to Popper (1965), even the most creative induction is based on observations made within some theoretical frame of reference.

Designing and Implementing Theory-Related Research

Since there is some evidence that scientists are not highly successful in uniting theory and research in their work, and since few research or theory construction texts consider this in any detail, the content of the double helix core needs to be examined.

The formulation of a research issue may justifiably stem from either theoretical or pragmatic concerns of the scientist. If theoretical interest is the point of departure, the research may lead to theory building or theory testing, depending on the state of theory in the discipline. Pragmatic concern, on the other hand, often leads initially to theory-building research, since frequently there is no prior theory bearing on this issue available for testing.

Many failures to integrate theory and research occur when the research impetus is pragmatic and the scientist "does not bother" to develop a theory to explain results. Such research may be very important in practical terms, but it is likely to be sterile and not advance the discipline. However, a theoretical interest can also get in the way of integration when scientists put all their energies into constructing elegant theoretical edifices which they do not trouble to test, or which, even worse, may be untestable.

Once the research issue has been identified, specific research problems must be outlined. The relation between theory and research is perhaps more clearly illustrated at this point than at any other in the double helix core. The specific problems ultimately derive from theory and prior research. Scientists should take care at this stage to explicitly relate the present study to the larger body of knowledge in the discipline. Furthermore, they should take care to either state the propositions of the theory being tested and to clearly derive hypotheses from them, or to identify specific observations expected to lead to propositions of the theory being built. The expression of the research problem is the culmination of the theoretical process, "the final step in the unfolding of the logic that provides the foundation for the empirical phase of research" (Batey, 1977, p. 329).

The specific research problems will suggest the research design to be used in conducting the investigation. The level of knowledge from which the research problem is derived is even more influential in selecting the design. For instance, if a review of the literature reveals no previous study of the relations between variables of interest, an exploratory theory-building study might be undertaken. Such a study enables the investigator to collect preliminary data which can then be used to formulate specific concepts and propositions using inductive theory-building strategies. However, if the literature indicates a well-developed body of theory, the research might focus on derivation of hypotheses using deductive strategies and empirical testing of hypothesized relations.

The choice of research instruments should also be guided by the study's theoretical base. Extreme care must be taken to select tools that are valid and reliable empirical indicators of the relevant concepts. It is important to recognize that the tools of a research project are the links between "a theoretically formulated research problem and the data to be gathered from observations" (Lin, 1976, p. 10).

Sampling, too, is based on the theory underlying the investigation. The majority of theories should be limited to certain populations. The scientist who wishes to build or test a theory must therefore be explicit about its boundaries. Furthermore, if the research is designed to extend a theory, the scientist must be certain it has been confirmed in one population before testing it in another.

The data analysis stage links research problem and the raw data. The form of analysis is also dictated by the theoretical base of the study. The statistics used in the analysis should come as no surprise to the reader, since the hypotheses should reveal these, at least in the broad categories of analysis of relations or of difference. Once data analysis is completed, the task is to interpret the findings. Theory serves to order the findings and to place them in context. Research findings should be clearly and explicitly related to the theory being built or tested.

Interpreting Theory-Related Research

The results of research lead directly to confirmation or rejection of hypotheses. If they are confirmed, the scientist should plan even more stringent tests of the theory or studies which will continue to build it. If, on the other hand, the hypotheses are rejected and the scientist is convinced the study was a legitimate test of the theory, it is probable the theory requires modification and subsequent rigorous testing.

Regardless of the outcomes of the study and of the care taken to integrate theory and research, several additional should be considered at this point in the research process. Those relating mainly to the theory include reexamination of the causal structure and of variables identified as causes and effects. (Although the scientist may not have considered his theory as causal, these factors require examination because causal thinking and theory cannot be separated.) Factors relating primarily to reexamination of the data include scale of measurement assumed, coding procedures used and validity of the data as empirical indicators of the concepts (Smelser & Warner, 1976). The conclusions which may be reached from such a critical review include: (a) the data are faulty and cannot be relied on; (b) the theory is faulty and should be discarded; (c) the data are accurate and the theory requires modification; and (d) the data are accurate but have no relevance to the theory (Downs, 1973).

Ultimately, a theory can never be confirmed or refuted. Since hypotheses are tested in a probabilistic manner, and since the probability of error in inference is normally never zero or one, it is always possible that replications of a study will yield different results. Moreover, there is always the possibility of other logical explanations why the data of one study provided or failed to provide support for the hypotheses. Any theory can therefore be considered no more than an approximation of the real world or a plausible explanation of events. As Selltiz and her associates commented:

> . . . the most plausible theory is the one for which we have the strongest evidential support. And it is this theory that is to be provisionally "believed" or "accepted" until another theory gains superior evidential support. Scientific knowledge is knowledge under conditions of uncertainty (Selltiz, Wrightsman, & Cook, 1976, pp. 47-48).

Theory and Research in Nursing Science

Nursing Theory

Nursing theory is not trivial; it is practically nonexistent. The nursing literature yield little evidence of formulations that might be considered nursing theory, that is, "a set of interrelated propositions and definitions which present a systematic view of one or more of the essential [concepts] of nursing—person, environment, health, nursing—by specifying relations among relevant variables" (Fawcett, 1978, p. 26).

Currently, nursing science has not progressed much beyond a knowledge base composed of conceptual models. A conceptual model is a highly abstract umbrella of related multidimensional concepts that provide a broad perspective for scientists, telling them what to look at (Reilly, 1975). The conceptual models of nursing certainly are not trivial, since they have a demonstrated usefulness in guiding nursing practice, research and education (Riehl & Roy, 1974). However, they cannot be empirically tested because of the abstract nature of their concepts. Nursing science thus

remains essentially devoid of any substantive nursing theories that could be related to nursing research.

Nursing's theory helix has received considerable attention over the past several years. Nurse scholars have offered definitions of nursing theories and urged their construction; they have described techniques of theory formalization and construction; and they have cited the advantages and disadvantages of theory-building strategies using borrowed theories (Cleland, 1967; Hardy, 1974; Jacox, 1974; Silva, 1977). More recently, it has been advocated that nursing theories be derived from the conceptual models of nursing and that theory construction follow the master plan offered by Dickoff and James' (1968) four levels of theory (Fawcett, 1978; Menke, 1978).

Nursing scholars are essentially in agreement on the need for nursing theory and the strategies for its construction. They even seem to agree that nursing knowledge may be a synthesis of theory borrowed from other disciplines. What, then, has been the payoff for the theory helix of nursing science? Apparently, it has been almost nil. As Menke stated:

> Thus far there has been a dearth of theory developed for nursing. Efforts have not been organized in any specific manner. The theory that has been developed has followed a laissez-faire route or has not necessarily been focused in any specific direction (Menke, 1978, p. 218).

It may be concluded then that while knowledge of the content of the theory helix exists in nursing science, the application of that knowledge is not evident.

Nursing Research

The content of the research helix of nursing science is better developed. Even a cursory review of nursing research publications and presentations reveals increasing attention to the cornerstones of scientific research, i.e., systematization, control, empiricism and critical review. Despite this, given the preceding discussion, it should be clear that most nursing research must be trivial, since it is not connected to theory in any discernible way. This assertion is supported by Batey's (1977) review of 25 years of research published in

Nursing Research, which discovered few explicit theoretical bases for the research. Batey's findings suggest that while nurse researchers may know that theory and research should be interrelated, they apparently do not comprehend this, or do not accept it, or do not know how to apply this knowledge.

The Theory-Research Core

It should by now be apparent that the double helix core is essentially nonexistent in nursing science. While this situation is not unique to nursing, as pointed out earlier, it is important that some rapid progress be made if nursing is to retain and increase its respectability as a science.

The underdevelopment of the theory helix of nursing science is obviously the main factor impeding the development of the double helix core. For without nursing theory, it is rather difficult, if not impossible, to design theoretically based nursing research. A review of the literature has identified several other factors retarding the development of the double helix core of nursing science.

First, nursing has no scientific heritage. There is no comprehensive body of knowledge or research tradition on which to construct a core of unified theory and research (Johnson, 1974). Second, although the derivation of research problems from the conceptual frameworks of nursing has been advocated (Schlotfeldt, 1975), there is little evidence that nurse researchers have adopted this strategy, perhaps because of the effort required to deduce a theory and relevant empirically testable problems from these highly abstract models.

Third, the favoring of experimental research as the best way to test theories and of research with direct clinical practice implications has led away from basic descriptive studies that might provide the baseline data crucial for theory building. These research biases have, unfortunately, encouraged nurses to conduct "more sophisticated" studies that lack a firm theoretical foundation.

Fourth, the value placed on creativity, together with a "do your own thing" orientation in nursing, has inhibited study replication research that might provide empirical data needed for modification, extension or refutation of theories.

Fifth, since nurses are oriented to doing, it is evidently difficult for them to value "the time-consuming analysis and testing demanded by research before action is initiated" (Martinson, 1978, p. 159).

Sixth, as long as editorial reviews of research reports are less rigorous regarding theory helix content than for research helix content, it is doubtful that nurse researchers will be motivated to carefully delineate the type of research (theory building or theory testing) they are conducting or to explicitly integrate theory with research (Batey, 1977).

Finally, as long as published research is not related to theory, an implicit message of "why bother" is given to those who might otherwise attempt to relate theory to research and research to theory. Or, even worse, the effective message may be that this is not necessary.

Many other sciences have gone through a similar phase before the double helix core has come into being. For instance, only in the past decade has the literature of many of the behavioral sciences revealed integration of theory and research. It should not be surprising then that such integration has not yet occurred in the embryonic science of nursing. And it is probable that nursing's current preoccupation with this lack is the result of its quest for recognition as a distinct science, particularly in academe, but also in hallways of practice settings.

REFERENCES

Aldous, J. (1970). Strategies for developing family theory. *Marriage and the Family, 32*(2), 250–257.

Batey, M. V. (1971). Conceptualization: Knowledge and logic guiding empirical research. *Nursing Research, 26*(5), 324–329.

Burr, W. R. (1973). *Theory construction and the sociology of the family.* New York: John Wiley & Sons.

Campbell, D. T., & Stanley, J. C. (1963). *Experimental and quasi-experimental designs for research.* Chicago: Rand McNally.

Cleland, V. S. (1967). The use of existing theories. *Nursing Research, 16*(2), 118–121.

Cohen, J. (1969). *Statistical power analysis for the behavioral sciences.* New York: Academic Press.

Dickoff, J., & James P. (1968). A theory of theories: A position paper. *Nursing Research, 17,* 197–203.

Downs, F. S. (1973). Elements of a research critique. In F. S. Downs & M. A. Newman (Eds.), *A source book of nursing research.* Philadelphia: F. A. Davis.

Dubin, R. (1978). *Theory building* (rev. ed.). New York: Free Press.

Dunnette, M. D. (1966). Fads, fashions, and folderol in psychology. *American Psychologist, 21*(4), 343–352.

Fawcett, J. (1978). The 'what' of theory development. In *Theory development: What, why, how?* New York: National League for Nursing.

Fox, D. J. (1976). *Fundamentals of research in nursing* (3rd ed.). New York: Appleton-Century-Crofts.

Gardner, E. J. (1968). *Principles of genetics* (3rd ed.). New York: John Wiley & Sons.

Gibson, Q. (1970). *The logic of social enquiry.* New York: Humanities Press.

Glaser, B. G., & Strauss, A. L. (1967). *The discovery of grounded theory: Strategies for qualitative research.* Chicago: Aldine.

Hanson, N. R. (1958). *Patterns of discovery.* New York: Cambridge University Press.

Hardy, M. (1974). Theories: Components, development, evaluation. *Nursing Research, 23*(2), 100–107.

Hempel, C. G. (1952). *Fundamentals of concept formation in empirical science.* Chicago: University of Chicago Press.

Jacox, A. (1969). Issues in construction of nursing theory. In C. M. Norris (Ed.), *Proceedings, First Nursing Theory Conference.* Kansas City: University of Kansas Medical Center Department of Nursing Education.

Jacox, A. (1974). Theory construction in nursing. An overview. *Nursing Research, 23*(1), 4–13.

Johnson, D. E. (1974). Development of theory: A requisite for nursing as a primary health profession. *Nursing Research, 23*(5), 372–377.

Kerlinger, F. N. (1973). *Foundations of behavioral research* (2nd ed.). New York: Holt, Rinehart and Winston.

Kish, L. (1965). *Survey sampling.* New York: John Wiley & Sons.

Lin, N. (1976). *Foundations of social research.* New York: McGraw-Hill.

Martinson, I. (1978). Why research in nursing? In N. L. Chaska (Ed.), *The nursing profession: Views through the mist.* New York: McGraw-Hill.

Menke, E. M. (1978). Theory development: A challenge for nursing. In N. L. Chaska (Ed.), *The nursing profession: Views through the mist.* New York: McGraw-Hill.

Merton, R. F. (1957). *Social theory and social structure* (rev. ed.). New York: Free Press.

Popper, K. R. (1965). *Conjectures and refutations: The growth of scientific knowledge.* New York: Harper and Row.

Reilly, D. E. (1975). Why a conceptual framework? *Nursing Outlook, 23*(8), 566–569.

Riehl, J. P., & Roy, C. *Conceptual models for nursing practice.* New York: Appleton-Century-Crofts.

Schlotfeldt, R. M. (1975). The need for a conceptual framework. In P. J. Verhonick (Ed.), *Nursing Research, Vol 1.* (pp. 3–24). Boston: Little, Brown.

Selltiz, C., Wrightsman, L. S., & Cook, S. W. (1976). *Research methods in social relations* (3rd ed.). New York: Holt, Rinehart and Winston.

Silva, M. C. (1977). Philosophy, science, theory: Interrelationships and implications in nursing research. *Image, 9*(3), 59–63.

Skidmore, W. (1975). *Theoretical thinking in sociology.* New York: Cambridge University Press.

Smelser, N. J., & Warner, R. S. (1976): *Sociological theory: Historical and formal.* Morristown, NJ: General Learning Press.

Torgerson, W. S. (1958). *Theory and methods of scaling.* New York: John Wiley & Sons.

Watson, J. D. (1968). *The double helix.* New York: New American library.

Webb, W. B. (1961). The choice of the problem. *American Psychologist, 16*, 223–227.

Zetterberg, H. L. (1965). *On theory and verification in sociology* (3rd ed.). Totowa, NJ: Bedminster Press.

CHAPTER 5

Theoretical Thinking in Nursing: Problems and Prospects

Hesook Suzie Kim

The development of nursing's knowledge-base for its practice has exercised the minds of nursing scholars in recent years as evidenced in the literature. Many of the nursing theories and conceptual frameworks initially proposed in the 1970s have gone through several revisions and testing by nursing scientists. There are some evidences that nursing's theoretical frameworks are producing an array of explanatory knowledge and some predictive or prescriptive notions about human phenomena and nursing practice. Many doctoral programs in nursing which have been implemented during the past 5 years to a total of more than 40 in the United States have also been instrumental in forcing nursing scientists to seek theoretical bases of their own research and of their students within the nursing perspective.

However, such culmination has received very little systematic scrutiny in the literature as to how far and to what extent the nursing's theoretical development has progressed. Nursing scientists in general are either interested in or pressured into 'testing' theories empirically rather than 'evaluating' or 'reflecting' on what theories are being produced or how they are being produced. Of course this is not to say that there have not been any critical analyses of nursing theories. Summaries and critiques of nursing theories and conceptual frameworks have been published in recent years as evidenced in such books as Chinn and Jacobs (1983), Fitzpatrick and Whall (1983), Fawcett (1984), and Meleis (1985). However, much of these analyses were limited to evaluation of the contents of theories and conceptual frameworks which I consider to be only one level of analysis.

Inherent in this state of affairs is a lack of systematic framework upon which various levels of questions related

Reprinted from Recent Advances in Nursing, *24, H. S. Kim, Theoretical thinking in nursing: Problems and prospects, 106–122.*
Copyright © 1989 with permission from Elsevier Ltd.

About the Author

HESOOK SUZIE KIM was born in Korea and came to the United States as an undergraduate student at Indiana University. She received a BS in nursing and an MS in nursing education from Indiana University and an MA and a PhD in sociology from Brown University. She has been in Rhode Island since 1964 and was a faculty member at the University of Rhode Island College of Nursing since 1973, and is now Professor Emerita there. Her scholarly work has focused on metatheoretical questions in nursing, and she considers her two books, *The Nature of Theoretical Thinking in Nursing* (2nd edition published in 2000) and *Nursing Theories: Conceptual and Philosophical Foundations* (edited with Ingrid Kollak, published in 1999), to be her major contributions to the discipline. Her empirical research has been on nursing practice issues from the cross-national perspective, including research on collaboration, pain assessment, clinical decision making, and the nature of nursing practice carried out in Finland, Japan, Korea, Norway, the United States, and Sweden. She reads (Günter Grass is her favorite author), listens to jazz, plays golf, and skis for sheer enjoyment and relaxation.

to knowledge generation can be posed for the discipline of nursing. In general, questions related to how theories should be developed and what theories should be like are left to scholars in the philosophy of science to grapple with while very little systematic attention is paid to such questions by nursing scholars. In nursing, the products of theoretical work are evaluated only with respect to their contents and forms. My view is that this approach is limiting. A comprehensive system of theory evaluation that poses questions beyond those related to theory's content and form is needed to assess the broader questions of epistemological orientations as well as content adequacy.

This paper attempts to integrate several levels of analysis to examine the nature of theoretical thinking in nursing, beginning with the questions at the level of the philosophy of science and moving to the examination of the contents of theories being developed in nursing. The major assumption underlying this form of analysis is in the belief that the nature of scientific products is influenced by the scientists' views regarding the methods of knowledge generation, the definitions of knowledge structure, and the aims of disciplines as well as the focus of scientific attention.

A Framework for Examining the Nature of Theoretical Thinking

Whether or not a scientist is aware of the connections among his/her theory or research piece and the beliefs about what a theory should be like or what the content of a theory should be and the contributions of the work on the discipline is irrelevant. This is because the articulation between what Popper (1972) calls World 2, a 'subjective' world, and World 3, 'an objective' world occurs in scientific activities regardless of such awareness. What cannot be ignored is the idea that a scientist who is working within the frame of his/her own World 2 (a personal data system) is engaged in creating and adding to a World 3, the objective world of ideas, knowledge, and understanding which becomes interwoven with that particular scientist's perspectives about the world and science.

While it is apparent that most scientists go about with their work, i.e. their scientific activities, paying very little attention to fundamental questions related to the nature of science and scientific methodologies, cumulatively their work results in forming prevailing patterns and forms in the discipline's scientific development. Hence the nature of theoretical thinking or theorizing in nursing has to be examined by looking not only into the contents of theories being developed or the products of theory testing but more importantly into the various levels of philosophical and perspective based orientations from which the scientist's work is being developed. From this assumption, I propose a five-level analysis framework for reviewing and evaluating theoretical work in nursing, articulating the following questions. These questions are similar to the ones discussed by Turner (1986) for sociological theorizing.

- What is the kind of knowledge possible for nursing? And, what kinds of theories are possible for nursing?
- What procedures are appropriate for developing this knowledge for nursing? And, what are the appropriate ways to develop nursing theories?
- What is it that nursing should try to develop knowledge about?
- What should nursing theories be concerned with? And, how can we decide what are important questions for nursing science?
- What are the ultimate goals of nursing knowledge being generated?
- What qualifies a given nursing theory to be scientifically sound?

These questions within the five-level framework are shown within the Figure 5-1, indicating the increasing specificity with which descending level influences theorizing and theoretical products in nursing. The five levels are thus specified as (1) the philosophy of science level, (2) the metaparadigm level, (3) the nursing philosophy level, (4) the paradigm level, and (5) the theory level.

The philosophy of science level is concerned with questions related to a scientist's positions regarding the nature of nursing as a science and the nature of scientific theory and theorizing. Analyses at this level will reveal the foundations upon which theories take their form and theorizing progresses. The second level focuses on a scientist's definitions regarding the essential phenomena of nursing requiring scientific attention and the selection of subject matters with which a given nursing theory is concerned. This level of analysis can be examined within a metaparadigmatic structure for nursing science as developed by Kim (1983, 1987). What the analysis at this level can reveal is the boundary within which nursing theories are being developed and how such a boundary changes over time within the discipline's revisions regarding the 'critical problems' for scientific attention. While the first level (the philosophy of science level) is concerned with the fundamental positions regarding scientific methodologies for theory development and theory testing, the second level (the metaparadigm level) allows examinations of the 'content' choices which are made for the science.

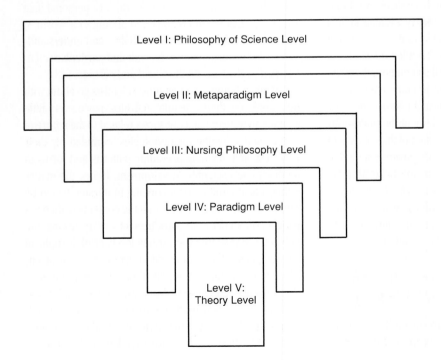

Figure 5-1 *Framework for analysis of theoretical thinking in nursing.*

The third level concerned with nursing philosophy is essential to the extent that a given nursing philosophy directs the development of nursing theories in their orientations for understanding, explanation, prediction, and prescription. Therefore, this level articulates closely with the philosophy of science level by directing the nature of nursing theory being developed in a methodological sense.

The fourth level is concerned with paradigmatic orientations and perspectives from which the actual theorizing is carried out. The term paradigms is used to mean general scientific perspectives and traditions in this discussion, not used in the strict sense with which Kuhn (1962, 1970) described paradigms for the natural sciences. The concept of paradigm for this level is appropriate for our analysis because nursing science is being developed from various scientific traditions, maybe because it is paradigmatic as Kuhn might argue, and furthermore because the critical scientific problems of the discipline seem to require various perspectives for understanding.

The fifth level is concerned with theories themselves. Analyses at this level will reveal the content of a theory with respect to its scope, logic and preciseness (i.e. form) of theoretical statements, testability and use. While there have been many nursing theoreticians who proposed different criteria for theory analysis and evaluation, for example, Stevens (1984), Hardy (1974) and Meleis (1985) among many, these four criteria have been adopted to be critical for the analysis of the contents of theory for nursing within this proposed framework. These four criteria have linkages to the preceding four levels of analysis, in that the questions of scope and use have direct relevance to the metaparadigm and nursing philosophy levels while the questions of form and testability are related to the philosophy of science and paradigm levels.

For the present exposition, this framework is used to scan the status of nursing's theoretical development and point up the areas in which gaps and deficiencies are apparent with respect to our efforts in nursing science. However, many fundamental questions related to the nature of nursing knowledge and scientising of nursing vis-à-vis nursing practice are lurking unresolved behind the scene of fervour with which scientific knowledge is being produced within nursing. Such questions are most troublesome, for example, as we encounter a nurse at a patient's bedside who is grappling with a decision to apply or not to apply a bed restraint.

Theoretical Development in Nursing: Status, Problems and Prospects

Level I: Philosophy of Science Questions

Nursing within the last three decades in its attempt to be treated as a legitimate knowledge discipline has embraced the belief that its knowledge has to be scientific and that scientific theories are the foundations upon which knowledge about nursing phenomena may be accumulated. There are three basic questions which have constantly been circumvented by nursing scientists in their quests for nursing knowledge:

1. Is the primary goal of nursing science in understanding or in control?
2. What kinds of knowledge are appropriate for nursing discipline and nursing science?
3. What is (are) the appropriate form(s) of theorizing in nursing?

While it appears that modern nursing is comfortable with the notion that the best way to accumulate knowledge relevant to nursing and nursing practice is through scientific methods, we continue to argue regarding the extent to which the science of nursing should control nursing practice. In addition, dichotomising the science and art of nursing as separate entities requiring some form of integration has been one of the major struggles articulated by many nursing scholars including Florence Nightingale, Henderson, and more recently Carper (1978) and Watson (1981). On the one hand is the belief that nursing practice encompassing the art of nursing goes beyond the scope of nursing science, while the counter argument goes with the belief that nursing practice has to be based on scientific knowledge and the science of nursing. This argument, in a sense, is more fundamentally embedded in the question regarding the nature of nursing science rather than the seeming dichotomy of the science and art. The fundamental question therefore is whether the nursing science is concerned with 'what is' or 'what should be.'

Since all prescriptive theories must be based on the notion of what is the right thing to do, they are based on value premises. The proposal for situation-producing theories as the ultimate goal of nursing in the early years of nursing theory development (Dickoff, James & Wiedenbach, 1968a) had set the stage for nursing science to be normative science for many nursing theorists. Donaldson and Crowley (1978) also argue for the development of prescriptive theories which can govern the clinical practice of nursing. They view 'the syntax of nursing as value systems (both of science and professional ethics) . . . ' (p 119), and suggest that this syntax influences theory generation in nursing by providing a context from which judgments regarding the appropriateness, reliability and validity of knowledge being developed are made.

Suppe and Jacox (1985) also argue that since situation-producing theories presume goal states as the starting points, they are normative although satisfying as a species of teleological theory within the semantic concept of theories, and indicate that goal selection or the justification of selection are based on nonscientific normative or ethical assumptions requiring extra scientific procedures for analysis.

To the extent that prescriptive theories presume to differentiate what should be desired or preferred from what should not be, they are ideological and normative in nature. However, the procedures followed by developing prescriptive theories in nursing have not incorporated the procedures which are necessary in developing ideological knowledge. One form of argument has been advanced by Beckstrand (1978a, 1978b, 1980) in arguing against practice theories and by proposing that 'the goal of modern 'scientific' practice is to bring about changes in entities through scientific and moral means so that a good is acknowledged and defined within the ethical theory of value is realized or becomes increasingly capable of being realized' (Beckstrand, 1978a, p. 136). Beckstrand thus believes that scientific theory as value-forming knowledge may be developed separately, requiring juxtapositioning of two bodies of knowledge at the instances of practice.

It appears then that there are at least two schools of thought regarding the nursing science as value-free or value laden. Nursing scientists who believe in the notion that science is 'value-free' will have to be interested in understanding the nature of nursing phenomena as the basic goal of nursing's scientific enterprise, while prescriptive theorists' goal of nursing science is in controlling nursing phenomena in selected contexts of goal attainment. This differentiation certainly will result in different types of nursing theories advanced and different methodologies used to develop such theories. Whether or not nursing scientists in general are aware of this differentiation in orientation is highly questionable in the light of the paucity of literature available on the subject.

Somewhat related to the above problem but related to the maturing of nursing as a scientific discipline is the current awareness among the nursing scholars of the role that various philosophies of science have played in influencing the kinds of nursing knowledge being developed. It appears that the debates in the philosophy of science have finally filtered onto nursing scientists, raising sensitivities and questions about the nursing's scientific enterprise as well as their own work in terms of methodologies and contents. This awareness may have been stimulated in recent years by the necessity to delve into the developments in philosophy of science by faculty members in the many newly created doctoral programs in nursing. Hence, we are recently engaged in debating about the nature of nursing science in terms of form and procedures of development (Watson, 1981; Webster, Jacox, & Baldwin, 1981; Hardy, 1983; Gortner, 1983). Uys (1987) even suggests that many of the so-called nursing theories are pretheoretical and may be considered as foundational studies that try to answer such questions as foundationalism, development of language system, and philosophical analysis regarding the discipline of nursing science.

Nevertheless, the literature indicates that during the past 30 years many nursing scientists who had been trained in the tradition of the received view of science, with or without realizing their commitment to it, led the development of nursing science to the path that emphasized essentialism (Silva, 1977; Jacox, 1974), deductive theory building and formalization (Hardy, 1974; Chinn & Jacobs, 1983; Walker & Avant, 1983), operationalization and empirical testing (Fawcett & Downs, 1986) and the rules of confirmation and verification (Silva, 1977; Gortner, 1980).

However, sensitizing to the new developments in the philosophy of science with the exposures to and assimilation of the works by Hanson (1958), Popper (1968), Kuhn (1962, 1970), Lakatos and Musgrave (1970), Suppe (1977), Laundan (1978), and Feyreabend (1978) has created a great deal of confusion and uncertainties among nursing scientists in recent years (see Silva & Rothbart, 1984; Suppe & Jacox, 1985). Thus, many theoretical writings by metatheorists and theorists in nursing (e.g., Fawcett, 1980; Stevens, 1984; Meleis, 1985; Rogers, 1983; King, 1981) seem to have embraced selected views regarding the nature and form of nursing science. Some are holdovers from the Received View tradition, while others are encompassing of the new ideas suggestive of the perspective view of Hanson, the semantic conception of theories espoused by Suppe, and the historicism of Kuhn, Laudan, and Shapere, henceforth creating muddiness in the position taken by them regarding the nature and form of nursing theories and theory development. Whether or not this is only transitional and should eventually fall into distinct positions and schools of thought regarding the nature of nursing science has to be borne out by the history, it seems.

Attempts deviating from the earlier efforts in nursing theory development and methodologies for theory testing have become more varied and aggressive in recent years. Phenomenological theories (Parse, 1981; Paterson & Zderad, 1976), inductive theorizing (Benoliel, 1977, 1983; Norris, 1982), use of qualitative methodologies (Munhall, 1982; Watson, 1985), and hermeneutics (Benner, 1983) have been proposed as appropriate or better ways of developing nursing knowledge.

Level II: Metaparadigm Questions

A metaparadigm refers to a boundary structure which consists of items or phenomena for investigation for a given disciplinary perspective. Thus a nursing metaparadigm provides a structure from which the subject matters for nursing may be described and/or selected for scientific attention. Fawcett (1980) uses four essential concepts: person, environment, health, and nursing (Yura & Torres, 1975) as those encompassing the phenomena of

interest to nursing science, and suggests these concepts as the components of a metaparadigm for nursing. Meleis (1985) expands this list in what she terms 'domain concepts' for a metaparadigm of nursing theories, and includes nursing client, transitions, interaction, nursing process, environment, nursing therapeutics, and health. Both authors use these metaparadigm concepts to indicate the extensiveness of a given nursing theory in its scope, and suggest that theories describing or dealing with any one of the major concepts are nursing theories—although Fawcett (1984) considers that the most sophisticated nursing theory would encompass all four of the essential concepts. With a view that these metaparadigms are limited in the specification for the purpose of subject matter selection and of considering what would constitute critical scientific problems, a more comprehensive metaparadigm was proposed for consideration (Kim, 1983, 1987).

A metaparadigm topology of four subdomains for structuring nursing knowledge proposed in my earlier work (Kim, 1987) provides a freedom with which nursing theorists and scientists can select out phenomena of concern for theoretical or empirical attention within the nursing perspective at various levels of scope. This metaparadigm containing four subdomains (the client domain, the client-nurse domain, the practice domain, and the environmental domain) is based on the assumption that the goal of nursing science is to gain knowledge about the nature of human phenomena in the context of nursing practice. With such knowledge, it is possible to understand, explain, or predict human phenomena requiring nursing attention with respect to other human phenomena, environment, client-nurse interaction, or practice. Further, it is also possible to understand the nature of nursing therapeutics and interpret or predict outcomes of nursing practice. Table 5-1 shows a matrix based on this metaparadigm useful in examining the concept selections within nursing theories. It can be used to analyze theories in terms of in what domain the concepts requiring explanation reside and from what domain or domains the concepts providing explanation are selected.

Obviously, the domain of environment does not qualify to be the major domain of interest for explanation in the nursing perspective and is only appropriate in providing the focus of explanation. The matrix therefore can point up within-domain theories and across-domain theories at various degree of scope.

What has been found in our analyses of nursing theories so far is that the general theoretical frameworks, such as Rogers's unitary man model, Orem's self-care model, Roy's adaptation model, and Parse's man-health-living model deal with the client domain concepts in either nonselective or holistic manners, in the form of what Turner (1986) calls 'analytical schemes' rather than as theories containing a network of well developed propositions. Hence, these models may be considered theoretical to the extent that they try to order human phenomena in specific schemata with given orientations for the client domain.

In contrast, many middle range theories being developed and tested in nursing are more specific in the selection of metaparadigm concepts. For example, Johnson's theoretical and empirical work on a theory of self-regulation (1983) is concerned with the concept of identity development, both of them with the metaparadigm orientation in the client domain.

Interests in concepts of the client-nurse domain among nursing scholars are longstanding. Peplau (1962), Orlando (1961), Wiedenbach (1963), and King (1981) have taken concepts from the client-nurse domain for explanation of client phenomena or nursing practice. As it is true of the client domain theories, nursing theories dealing with the client-nurse domain tend to focus on global concepts of interaction and communication rather than on delineated aspects of client-nurse phenomena such as conflict, collaboration, competition, frequency, or quality of interaction.

What is important at this level of analysis is the identification of metaparadigmatic focus with the ultimate purpose of assessing whether or not nursing's theoretical work is adequately and sufficiently dealing with critical problems of the discipline. As one fills the matrix with nursing theories in the process of analysis, it is possible to identify the gaps in theoretical development in nursing. We have thus far limited theoretical advances in making specific connections between concepts from the client domain and the environment domain and between those from the client domain and the practice domain. Hence, the metaparadigm level questions permit us to examine to what extent a given theory or a collection of theoretical work handle the critical problems or subject matters of interest to the discipline of nursing.

Level III: Nursing Philosophy Questions

As debated by Walker (1971), the term "philosophy of nursing" has been used in several senses in the literature. The specific sense it is adopted for this level of analysis refers to one's beliefs about the nature of humanity and what nursing "should" do about this humanity. These are preparadigmatic choices one has to be committed to in order to streamline one's theoretical thinking, and are closely related to the kinds of philosophic choices one makes in terms of the nature of science and scientific theories. This notion of choice in philosophies of nursing is not universally accepted.

Table 5-1
Nursing Domain in Matrix for Identification of Metaparadigm Focus of Theories

Domain of Focus Providing Explanation	Domain of Focus for Theory		
	Client Domain	Client-Nurse Domain	Practice Domain
Client domain	*		
Client-nurse domain		*	
Practice domain			*
Environment domain			

*Within domain theories.

Munhall (1982) treats as given that there is an adherence to "a basic philosophy" of individuality and advocacy in nursing. Sarter (1988) points out common philosophical views as well as some divergent ones in her analysis of four nursing theorists' work, and suggests dangerously that the commonly shared philosophical views among the four theories may form "an appropriate philosophical foundation for the discipline." Sarter's conclusion thus is derived with the assumption that nursing science requires a single metaparadigm based on an appropriate philosophical foundation. Sarter therefore equates a common metaparadigm of nursing with a world view, a philosophical foundation for the discipline of nursing. This notion is contrary to the position expressed in this paper, calling for multiple philosophies of nursing as appropriate.

While it is possible that there can be a prevailing philosophy of nursing at a given time, it does not mean that multiplicity in philosophies of nursing is impossible or inappropriate insisting on a unified philosophy of nursing is pigeon-holing the development of theoretical thinking in nursing to only one direction and one paradigm. Certainly for an essentialist who believes in one and only one truth, this view would be appropriate. However, philosophy is an intellectual choice and commitment one makes regarding metaphysics which becomes integrated into the lower level theoretical thinking.

My review, contrary to Sarter's analysis, indicates divergent nursing philosophies with orientations in such positions as rationalism, existentialism, causal determinism, instrumentalism, humanism, and pragmatism. As stated by Bernstein (1986), intellectual currents of a given period may have common philosophical concerns, but philosophical positions culminate into diverse idea systems according to the way the problems of humanity are analyzed. For nursing, this diversity in philosophical orientations will eventually influence the types of praxiology (theories of practice) that get developed.

What is usually portrayed in the nursing literature is a separate treatment of nursing philosophy without integrating it into theoretical positions. Hence, it is often that we encounter a theorist who advocates free will and

individualism but whose theory is based on the assumption of normative determinism or behaviouristic holism. It appears that nursing scholars in general take the position that there is a unified nursing philosophy upheld by the nursing community, national or international, and that its significance to theory development is rudimentary at best. My view is contrary to this in that nursing philosophy having a close linkage to the philosophy of science has to be articulated into theory so that the whole network of theoretical thinking that goes into theory building maintains internal consistency and is based on a compatible thread of idea-system.

Level IV: Paradigm Choices

Paradigm choices in theory development refer to choices related to theoretical tradition and perspective as discussed earlier. A given theoretical tradition for nursing holds specific assumptions about the nature of human phenomena or nursing. A theoretical perspective also advocates specific ideas about theory building and theory testing, thus guides theoretical activities in dealing with selected metaparadigm concepts. The most prevailing paradigm choices which seem to have guided and continue to guide the theoretical work in nursing are:

1. General systems perspective in the tradition of von Bertalanffy's work
2. Behavioral perspective inclusive of all varieties of stimulus-response and adaptation/coping frameworks
3. Phenomenological perspective
4. Functional perspective
5. Sensory/cognitive perspective
6. Interaction perspective.

Although these seem to be the major paradigms, theories are more often based not on a single perspective but on two or more perspectives combined to guide the work.

At the same time, nursing scholars are beginning to pay attention to nontraditional theoretical perspectives such as Habermas' critical theory (Holter, 1988) and hermeneutics and interpretive perspective (Benner, 1984). It appears that as we become increasingly sophisticated and diversified in asking questions about the nature of critical nursing problems, we seek out alternative explanations based on different theoretical perspectives rather than holding onto those which have offered unsatisfactory answers in the past. This diverse approach to theory building in nursing may eventually fall into major paradigms for the three domains of nursing, as theorists and researchers working independently with concepts from different domains but from similar theoretical perspective begin to realize integration into major theoretical themes.

Level V: Aspects of Theory

This level of analysis is concerned with the content of a theory in terms of key concepts and propositions. Questions of "form" and "testability" refer to the internal structure of a theory, while the questions of "scope" and "use" refer to the degree with which a theory contributes to the development of nursing science. These four are considered to be the elementary, fundamental criteria to evaluate the content of a theory partly in line with Reynolds (1971), Hardy (1978), Stevens (1984), and Meleis (1985).

Form as the criterion of evaluation deals with:

1. The clarity, abstractness and consistency with which key concepts in a theory are specified and derived, and
2. Identification of the types, network and internal structure of propositions and theoretical statements contained within a theory.

An evaluation of a theory with respect to form will reveal the degree of completeness in the development of conceptual system in terms of logic, clarity, and abstractness. On the other hand, testability as the criterion of evaluation deals with the degree with which a theory can be translated for empirical testing. Hence, the more abstract a theory is the more deductive or interpretive steps it would require for empirical testing.

The questions of scope and use have been well articulated by Stevens (1984), and refer to degrees with which a given theory provides explanations for various subject matters in nursing and suggests usefulness in providing the types of knowledge for application. While middle range theories tend to be narrower in scope but are more useful in providing both explanatory and predictive knowledge, grand theories of nursing tend to be broader in scope but very troublesome in terms of utility.

Summary

The foregoing exposition suggests a global approach to evaluate theoretical thinking in nursing. Several issues have come to light in examining the current status of nursing's theoretical work within the proposed framework.

In most of the theoretical pieces of work in nursing, major threads of theoretical thinking are difficult to identify. It seems that even if it were to be an after-thought, any major theoretical work should be committed to certain positions at the four higher levels so that it becomes obvious for the kind of theory that gets developed.

As has been stated by many nursing scholars, the so-called grand nursing theories or conceptual frameworks require further specification to be called theories. There seems to be two ways these frameworks could be developed further:

1. They may be developed into paradigms of nursing by specifying advocated assumptions about the nature of human beings and nursing, theory-building strategy or strategies assumed to be appropriate for the perspective, an image of nursing practice the perspective holds, and types of theoretical statements that are possible within the perspective; or
2. They may be developed as bona-fide theories by rigorously following the criteria at the fifth level.

It seems that the time is ripe for nursing scholars working within similar theoretical perspective to come together in order to formulate integrative nursing theories covering concepts from different domains of nursing.

For example, much work in nursing within the symbolic interactionist tradition may be ready to be assimilated into a nursing theory of "self-identity."

Similarly, much of the theoretical and empirical work dealing with how people develop competence in living with chronic illness (for example, cancer) can also be integrated into one nursing theory for further testing.

The community of nursing scholars at large has not dealt with the meaning of prescriptive theories for nursing science and nursing practice. There should be more rigorous debates regarding the normative nature of prescriptive theories and their effects on the development of nursing science and application to nursing practice in the context of scientific philosophy, nursing philosophy, and praxiology. The beliefs that praxiology follows naturally from prescriptive theories and that prescriptive theories are naturally the goal of nursing science are both naive and dangerous.

Certainly, we are becoming increasingly sensitive and competent to carve out those requiring scientific explanation in the nursing perspective. And in doing so, we have created world views of nursing that seem both socially and epistemologically relevant to pursue. However, theoretical thinking in nursing will require a greater degree of specificity in terms of process and products if we are to move away from the intellectual infancy on which we have been comfortably resting. This attempt will require not only a greater degree of specificity, but also a more rigorous self-criticism.

REFERENCES

Beckstrand, J. (1978a). The notion of a practice theory and the relationship of scientific and ethical knowledge to practice. *Research in Nursing and Health, 1,* 131–136.

Beckstrand, J. (1978b). The need for a practice theory as indicated by the knowledge used in the conduct of practice. *Research in Nursing and Health, 1,* 175–179.

Beckstrand, J. (1980). A critique of several conceptions of practice theory in nursing. *Research in Nursing and Health, 3,* 69–79.

Benner, P. (1983). Uncovering the knowledge embedded in clinical practice. *Image, 15,* 41.

Benner, P. (1984). *From novice to expert: Excellence and power in clinical nursing practice.* Menlo Park, CA: Addison-Wesley.

Benoliel, J. (1977). The role of the family in managing the young diabetic. *The Diabetic Educator, 3,* 5–8.

Benoliel, J. (1983). Grounded theory and qualitative data: The socializing influences of life threatening disease on identity development. In P. J. Wooldridge, M. H. Schmitt, J. K. Skipper Jr., & R. C. Leonard (Eds.). *Behavioral science and nursing theory* (pp. 141–187). St. Louis: C. V. Mosby.

Bernstein, R. J. (1986). *Philosophical profiles: Essays in a pragmatic mode.* Cambridge: Polity Press.

Carper, B. A. (1978). Fundamental patterns of knowing in nursing. *Advances in Nursing Science, 1,* 12–23.

Dickoff, J., James, P., & Wiedenbach, E. (1968a). Theory in a practice discipline: Part I, Practice-oriented theory. *Nursing Research, 17,* 415–435.

Dickoff, J., James, P., & Wiedenbach, E. (1968b). Theory in a practice discipline: Part II, Practice-oriented theory. *Nursing Research, 17,* 545–554.

Donaldson, S. K., & Crowley, D. M. (1978). The discipline of nursing. *Nursing Outlook, 26,* 113–120.

Fawcett, J. (1980). A framework for analysis and evaluation of conceptual models of nursing. *Nurse Educator, 5,* 10–14.

Fawcett, J. (1984). *Analysis and evaluation of conceptual models in nursing.* Philadelphia: F. A. Davis.

Fawcett, J., & Downs, F. S. (1986). *The relationship of theory and research.* Norwalk, CT: Appleton-Century-Crofts.

Feyerabend, P. (1978). *Against method.* London: Verso.

Fitzpatrick, J. J., & Whall, A. L. (1983). *Conceptual models of nursing: Analysis and application.* Bowie, MD: Brady.

Gortner, S. R. (1980). Nursing science in transition. *Nursing Research, 29,* 180–183.

Gortner, S. R. (1983). The history and philosophy of nursing science and research. *Advances in Nursing Science, 5,* 1–8.

Hanson, N. R. (1958). *Patterns of discovery.* Cambridge, England: Cambridge University Press.

Hardy, M. E. (1974). Theories: Components, development, evaluation. *Nursing Research, 23,* 100–107.

Hardy, M. E. (1978). Perspectives on nursing theory. *Advances in Nursing Science, 1,* 27–48.

Hardy, M. E. (1983). Metaparadigms and theory development. In N. L. Chaska (Ed.). *The nursing profession: A time to speak* (pp. 427–437). New York: McGraw-Hill.

Holter, I. M. (1988). Critical theory: A foundation for the development of nursing theories. *Scholarly Inquiry for Nursing Practice, 2,* 223–232.

Jacox, A. (1974). Theory construction in nursing: An overview. *Nursing Research, 23,* 4–13.

Kim, H. S. (1983). *The nature of theoretical thinking in nursing.* Norwalk, CT: Appleton-Century-Crofts.

Kim, H. S. (1987). Structuring the nursing knowledge system: A topology of four domains. *Scholarly Inquiry for Nursing Practice, 1,* 99–110.

King, I. M. (1981). *A theory for nursing: Systems, concepts, process.* New York: John Wiley & Sons.

Kuhn, T. S. (1962). *The structure of scientific revolutions.* Chicago: University of Chicago Press.

Kuhn, T. S. (1970). *The structure of scientific revolutions* (2nd ed.). Chicago: University of Chicago Press.

Lakatos, I., & Musgrave, A. (Eds.) (1970). *Criticism and the growth of scientific knowledge.* Cambridge, England: Cambridge University Press.

Laudan, L. (1978). *Progress and its problems: Toward a theory of scientific growth.* Berkeley, CA: University of California Press.

Leventhal, H., & Johnson, J. E. (1983). Laboratory and field experimentation: Development of a theory of self-regulation. In P. J. Wooldridge, M. H. Schmitt, J. K. Skipper Jr., &

R. C. Leonard (Eds.). *Behavioral science and nursing theory* (p. 262). St. Louis: C. V. Mosby.

Meleis, A. I. (1985). *Theoretical nursing: Development and progress.* Philadelphia: J. B. Lippincott.

Munhall, P. L. (1982). Nursing philosophy and nursing research: In apposition or opposition? *Nursing Research, 31,* 176–181.

Norris, C. M. (1982). *Concept clarification in nursing.* Rockville, MD: Aspen.

Orlando, I. (1961). *The dynamic nurse-patient relationship.* New York: J. P. Putnam's Sons.

Parse, R. R. (1981). *Man-living health: A theory of nursing.* New York: John Wiley & Sons.

Paterson, J. G., & Zderad, L. T. (1976). *Humanistic nursing.* New York: John Wiley & Sons.

Peplau, H. (1962). Interpersonal techniques: The crux of psychiatric nursing. *The American Journal of Nursing, 62,* 50–54.

Popper, K. R. (1972). *Objective knowledge.* Oxford, England: Clarendon Press.

Reynolds, P. D. (1971). *A primer in theory construction.* Indianapolis, IN: Bobbs-Merrill.

Rogers, M. E. (1983). Science of unitary human being: A paradigm for nursing. In I. W. Clements & F. B. Roberts (Eds.). *Family health: A theoretical approach to nursing.* New York: John Wiley & Sons.

Sarter, B. (1988). Philosophical sources of nursing theory. *Nursing Science Quarterly, 1,* 52–59.

Silva, M. C. (1977). Philosophy, science, theory: Interrelationships and implications for nursing research. *Image, 9,* 59–63.

Silva, M., & Rothbart, D. (1984). An analysis of changing trends in philosophy of science on nursing theory development and testing. *Advances in Nursing Science, 6,* 1–13.

Stevens, B. J. (1984). *Nursing theory: Analysis, application, evaluation* (2nd ed.) Boston: Little, Brown.

Suppe, F. (Ed.) (1977). *The structure of scientific theories* (2nd ed.). Urbana, IL: University of Illinois Press.

Suppe, F., & Jacox, A. K. (1985). Philosophy of science and the development of nursing theory. In H. H. Werley & J. J. Fitzpatrick (Eds.). *Annual review of nursing research: Vol. 3* (p. 267). New York: Springer.

Turner, J. H. (1986). *The structure of sociological theory* (4th ed.). Chicago: Dorsey Press.

Uys, L. R. (1987). Foundational studies in nursing. *Journal of Advanced Nursing, 12,* 275–280.

Walker, L. O. (1971). Toward a clearer understanding of the concept of nursing theory. *Nursing Research, 20,* 428–435.

Walker, L. O., & Avant, K. C. (1983). *Strategies for theory construction in nursing.* Norwalk, CT: Appleton-Century-Crofts.

Watson, J. (1981). Nursing's scientific quest. *Nursing Outlook, 29,* 413–416.

Watson, J. (1985). *Nursing: Human science and human care.* Norwalk, CT: Appleton-Century-Crofts.

Webster, G., Jacox, A., & Baldwin, B. (1981). Nursing theory and the ghost of the received view. In J. C. McCloskey & H. K. Grace (Eds.). *Current issues in nursing* (pp. 26–35). Boston: Blackwell.

Wiedenbach, E. (1963). The helping art of nursing. *American Journal of Nursing, 63,* 54–57.

Yura, H., & Torres, G. (1975). Today's conceptual frameworks within baccalaureate nursing programs. In National League for Nursing. *Faculty, curriculum development. Part 3: Conceptual framework: its meaning and function* (pp. 17–25). New York: Author.

The Author Comments

Theoretical Thinking in Nursing: Problems and Prospects

This article was written to address my concerns regarding the one-dimensional approach to analysis and evaluation of nursing theories espoused by many authors who are mostly concerned with the structure and meaning of theories rather than with the fundamental epistemologic roots from which nursing theories emerged. I found that when master's and doctoral students relied on such sources to understand nursing theories, they often became dogmatic, procedural, and superficial. I believe that nursing theories, as any other theories, emerge from and are rooted in various sorts of epistemologic assumptions. To understand theories more comprehensively, it is necessary to engage in analyzing and evaluating their epistemologic foundations before addressing theory structure and contents. My doctoral students have been engaged in the framework I proposed in this article to study nursing theories, as well as other theories they encounter, and their work has shown this approach to be valuable and enriching. My hope is that any nursing scholar who engages in theory building would consider the epistemologic questions I address in this article as the starting points for theory development.

—HESOOK SUZIE KIM

CHAPTER 6

Levels of Theoretical Thinking in Nursing

Patricia A. Higgins
Shirley M. Moore

Development of a knowledge base is an iterative and ongoing process that requires periodic analysis and synthesis of an entire body of work. This article examines 4 related levels of theoretical thinking that are currently used in developing knowledge for nursing practice, education, and science: meta-theory, grand theory, middle-range theory, and micro-range theory. Each level of theory is discussed according to typology, scope, and generalizability, level of abstraction, and role. Suggestions are made for clarification of terminology, and examples are provided for each level of theoretical thinking. Evidence associated with the 4 levels of theoretical thinking is discussed, and applications for use of the levels of theoretical thinking to meet future challenges in nursing's knowledge development are offered.

In an effort to build a knowledge base for the clinical, educational, and scientific endeavors of the discipline, nursing theory has undergone several phases of development. In the earliest period, scholars focused their attention on building grand theory and debating the structure and methods for developing nursing theory. More recently, there has been a call for the development of middle-range theory. Thus theory in nursing has been conceptualized as existing on several levels although there are wide differences in the definitions and terminology associated with the levels of theoretical thinking and the classification of theoretical products. This lack of clarity impedes our use of theoretical thinking to extend and communicate our nursing knowledge. Therefore, the purpose of this article is to present an examination of levels of theoretical thinking in nursing and provide

Reprinted from Nursing Outlook, *48(4), P. A. Higgins & S. M. Moore, Levels of theoretical thinking, 179–183.*

About the Authors

PATRICIA HIGGINS is an Associate Professor of Nursing, Case Western Reserve University (CWRU). Her first nursing diploma was from Henry Ford Hospital (1970) and her second from Akron University (BSN, 1986). These were followed by graduate degrees from CWRU (MSN, 1989; PhD, 1996). Her teaching concentrates on theory and philosophy of science, and her program of research focuses on understanding and improving the health of adults who live with chronic conditions. In her time off, Dr. Higgins enjoys her family, gardening, and reading.

SHIRLEY MOORE is the Edward J. & Louise Mellen Professor of Nursing and Associate Dean for Research and Associate Professor of Nursing at Case Western Reserve University (CWRU), Cleveland, OH. Born at the beginning of the baby boom, she began her nursing career during a shift in nursing education from hospital training programs to more academic-focused programs, and she considers herself a product of both. Dr. Moore received her diploma of nursing from the Youngstown Hospital Association School of Nursing (1969) and her bachelor's degree in nursing from Kent State University (1974). At CWRU, she earned a master's degree in nursing-psychiatric mental health nursing (1990) and a PhD in nursing science (1993). Dr. Moore has taught nursing theory and nursing science to all levels of nursing students and has a program of research and theory development that addresses recovery after acute cardiac events. Her hobbies include traveling with her family, reading, and music.

examples of how several existing nursing theories can be classified within the theoretical levels. Applications of levels of theoretical thinking to meet challenges in knowledge development in nursing are suggested.

A theory in its simplest view is the creation of relationships among two or more concepts to form a specific view of a phenomenon. As constructions of our mind, theories provide explanations about our experiences of phenomena in the world.[1] The understanding provided by theories is of two types: explanatory (describing concepts and understanding interactions among concepts) or predictive (anticipating a particular set of outcomes).[2] Theories consist of the following components: (1) concepts that are identified and defined, (2) assumptions that clarify the basic underlying truths from which and within which theoretical reasoning proceeds, (3) context within which the theory is placed, and (4) identified relationships between and among the concepts.[3]

The terms theory, theoretical (or conceptual) model, theoretical framework, and theoretical system are often used to distinguish different types of theory. This practice has created confusion among scholars and practitioners, and we believe a more useful approach to understanding theory is to consider all of the aforementioned terms as parallel synonyms. Each can be used interchangeably, but each term also requires further specification through an adjective modifier, such as "grand" or "middle range," that describes its fit with other theoretical work. Thus the notion of different levels of theoretical thinking can be a more useful way to develop, disseminate, and use knowledge in nursing. We use the word "level" to imply a relative degree of relationship rather than a ranking or a distinct advantage. Each level of theoretical thinking has defining characteristics and purposes that are specific to that level. The scope or breadth of the concepts and goals of a theoretical system determine its use for research and practice. Therefore, theoretical thinking in nursing uses concepts and their relationships to organize and critique existing knowledge and guide new discoveries to advance practice. Its development and use is not limited to particular venues, time frames, or formats, and although *all* nurses may not use theoretical thinking *at all times,* its actual use is more frequent than some nurses may acknowledge. For instance, theoretical thinking regarding a family's psychologic well being can be briefly and automatically accessed as part of the gestalt of clinical practice or formally developed into a more permanent, written framework. Both types of theoretical thinking are crucial for practice, and either may be critiqued, modified, and tested.

Linkages between the theoretical world and the empirical world to which it applies are made through the formulation and testing of hypotheses. Both scientists and practitioners use this process to make the empirical world and the theoretical world as congruent as possible. It is important to distinguish an empirical system from a theoretical system. An empirical system is what we apprehend, through senses, in the environment. A theoretical system is what we construct in our mind's eye to model the empirical system.[1] Nurse scientists and practitioners focus on understanding the variables of a particular practice situation. To better understand a specific event, they formulate working definitions and associations among variables (hypotheses)

and either develop a new theoretical system or link them to existing organizing frameworks. The theoretical system then serves as guidance about how to proceed, and as long as the abstraction of a theory can be represented with empiric indicators, hypotheses can be generated and empirically tested.[2]

Levels of Theoretical Thinking

Theory in the human sciences has been used to delineate and legitimate the emerging disciplines and substantiate knowledge development.[4] There are 4 levels of theoretical thinking in nursing: meta-theory, grand theory, middle-range theory, and micro-range theory.[5] Each level of theory will be discussed according to level of abstraction and scope, generalizability, typology, and role. Figure 6-1

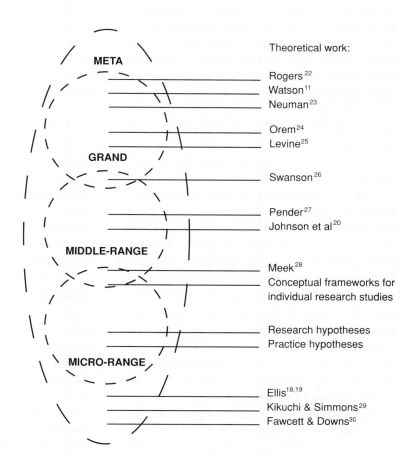

Figure 6-1 *Levels of theoretical thinking.*

describes the relationships among the 4 levels and provides examples of theoretical thinking for each level.

Meta-theory

Meta-theory, the most abstract and universal of the 4 levels of theoretical thinking, addresses issues related to the conduct of inquiry. Therefore, it is the theory of inquiry. Meta-theory or philosophic inquiry uses logic and analytic reasoning to examine the direction, methods, and standards of inquiry and thus it differs from the other levels of theory as its product is primarily knowledge-about-knowledge (second-order knowledge), rather than specific theoretical frameworks that explain the empirical world (first-order knowledge). Meta-theoretical inquiry related to scientific issues is known as philosophy of science, and it focuses on a critical examination of science, its processes, and products. Used by both scientists and practitioners, meta-theoretical inquiry also addresses questions that science cannot answer. For example, in the study of death and dying, scientific inquiry seeks to answer questions about the physiologic changes leading to death. However, philosophic inquiry is needed to address the question, "Is death best understood as a process or a product?" Therefore, an understanding of meta-theoretical thinking is central to both the research and practice of nursing.

As the most well established of the 4 levels, the significance and role of meta-theoretical knowledge in nursing is revealed through a partial list of issues addressed through this mode of inquiry: (1) clarification of the relationship between nursing science and practice, (2) definition, development, and testing of nursing theory, (3) establishment of the academic discipline of nursing, and (4) examination and interpretation of fundamental philosophic perspectives and their connection to nursing science. The long list of exemplary scholarship that represents these 4 categories of philosophic inquiry in nursing is well represented in anthologies such as the one by Nicoll,[6] but one example also illustrates the value of the discipline's meta-theoretical thinking. In 1978 when Carper[7] published her influential article on the fundamental patterns of knowing in nursing, she initiated a spirited dialogue that continues to this day—in print, classrooms, and practice arenas throughout the world.

Grand Theory

Nursing grand theories are the global paradigms of nursing science.[8] They are formal, highly abstract theoretical systems that frame our disciplinary knowledge within the principles of nursing, and their concepts and propositions transcend specific events and patient populations. The substantial body of analytic and philosophic reasoning that has emerged from grand theory provides evidence of scholarship that distinguishes nursing from other closely related disciplines and legitimizes its existence among academic disciplines.[9] Thus grand theory's most significant contribution to nursing is the establishment and substantiation of the discipline's identity and boundaries.

Given their abstract nature, grand theories provide universal explanations and an understanding of nursing, but not the particulars that are necessary for empirical testing. As a result, they have little predictive capability. Some grand theories also use language that is difficult for the beginning student and unfamiliar to many potential users. Nevertheless, they have significantly influenced knowledge development within the discipline and there are numerous examples of their use in guiding nursing research, practice, and education. Grand theories also contribute to the historical perspective of nursing, reflecting the time and context in which the authors developed their theories, as well as their philosophic underpinnings and their educational and practice perspectives. In charting the growth of the discipline, Nightingale[10] can be considered the first grand theorist and *Notes on Nursing,* the original paradigm of contemporary nursing.

There is debate about what constitutes a grand theory and thus, which nursing scholars' work should be classified as grand theory. For example, is Jean Watson's[11] *Philosophy and Science of Caring* more accurately categorized as a "philosophy" or "grand theory" of nursing? Further, should Madeleine Leininger's[12] conceptual model, *Culture Care: Diversity and Universality Theory,* be classified as a grand or middle-range theory? Our view is that this type of debate reflects the growth of nursing's disciplinary knowledge. Although we may never have a consensus of answers for such questions, it also indicates that we have sufficiently established our external boundaries, and we can now redirect our energy to further distinguish the internal substance and structure of our knowledge through the construction of middle-range theories.

Middle-range Theory

In terms of historical development, middle-range theory is the relative newcomer to nursing science. Similar to grand theory, middle-range theory explains the empirical world of nursing, but it is more specific and less formal. For example, the philosophic underpinnings and assumptions of the middle-range theorist may be more implicit than explicit. As indicated by its name, any explanation of middle-range theory requires discussing "what it is" and "what comes before and after in its range." Suppe[4] was one of the first to clarify and define middle-range theory for nursing science. By using Merton's examination of sociologic theory,[13] Suppe[4] provided 3 criteria for delimiting middle-range theory from grand theory and the next lower level, micro-range theory. These 3 criteria, scope, level of abstraction, and testability are widely accepted.[14,15]

In terms of scope and level of abstraction, Lenz et al[15] stated that "middle-range theories (are those) that are sufficiently specific to guide research and practice, yet sufficiently general to cross multiple clinical populations and to encompass similar phenomena." In the quote from Lenz et al,[15] the guidance for research and practice is much more direct than is that offered by grand theory; therefore, middle-range theory can be tested in the empirical world. The concepts or phenomena of interest can be coded objectively (by using either qualitative or quantitative methods) and it has the potential to postulate measurable relationships between the phenomena; thus it has a "time-relativistic distinction."[4] The generalizability of middle-range theory is further defined by boundaries that limit measurement of the person-environment interaction. Although testable across several different patient populations and environments, a particular middle-range theory does *not* address *all* patients in *all* environments. For example, Good and Moore's[14] theory on pain management applies only to adults who experience acute surgical pain and is appropriately tested only during the immediate postoperative period. Because of the aforementioned characteristics, middle-range theory is not as limited as grand theory in its typology and can be classified as either explanatory or predictive. A major role of middle-range theory is to define or refine the substantive content of nursing science and practice, and it should be an important focus of both nurse scholars and practitioners as we continue to build knowledge for the discipline.

Micro-range Theory

Micro-range theory is the least formal and most tentative of the theoretical levels discussed in this article. It also is the most restrictive in terms of time and scope or application. However, its particularistic approach is invaluable for scientists and practitioners as they work to describe, organize, and test their ideas. We propose 2 levels of micro-range theory. At the higher level, micro-range theory is closely related to middle-range theory but is comprised of 1 or 2 major concepts, and its application frequently is limited to a particular event; for example, theories related to decubitus or catheter care.[16]

At the lower level, micro-range theory is defined as a set of working hypotheses or propositions.[17] Scientists and practitioners use these working propositions to tentatively categorize, explain, or test health-related person-environment interactions. As such, they are not coded and entered into a formal theoretical system, but two examples serve to illustrate their invaluable contribution to science and practice. In the first example, scientists interested in developing and testing larger theoretical frameworks isolate and organize proposed conceptual relationships into propositions. The scientific literature is then used to investigate the relationships of the propositions and, if there is evidence for the truth of the relationships, to determine conceptual-empirical correspondence. In the second example, the clinician also uses propositions to identify, describe, and organize the working conceptual relationships in practice. The investigation, although identical in process to the scientist's, differs in terms of its scope and its generalizability; that is, the practitioner investigates more particular and immediate relationships in a smaller group of persons; or frequently, a single person. For instance, a nurse working on a general medical unit is assigned to admit an elderly patient with the medical diagnosis of chronic obstructive pulmonary disease. Before meeting the patient, and in attempt to organize knowledge, the nurse hypothesizes several possible conceptual relationships; for example, the patient's age and medical diagnosis limit the patient's functional status. The nurse then tests the working hypothesis through assessment and works to directly change the concepts' relationships through manipulation of the person-environment interaction.

Any discussion of micro-range theory must consider the term "practice theory." We jump into the debate on what constitutes practice theory with the realization that numerous definitions exist and many authors consider micro-theory, as the most concrete and applicable of all theoretical levels, to be an equivalent term for practice theory.[5,16] We believe this categorization limits the understanding of theoretical thinking in nursing and a broader definition of practice theory is more useful. Based on Ellis,[18,19] who stated that *all* nursing knowledge ultimately is developed for practice, we maintain that all nursing theory, regardless of level, is practice theory.

Evidence and Levels of Theoretical Thinking

Regardless of the method used to create the theory or whether the theory is explanatory or predictive, the amount of evidence accrued to support it promotes confidence in its use by practitioners and scientists. In addition to the previously cited examples, varying degrees of evidence exist among the different types and levels of theoretical thinking.

On the meta-theoretical level, the accrual of bodies of research findings (evidence) demonstrates our ability to produce and critique our knowledge. Our progress is measured by the usefulness of the knowledge that is accrued, the explanatory and predictive theories that are created and tested, and the articulation of philosophic perspectives that are connected to nursing science and practice.

At the grand theory level, evidence is represented by practitioners' and scientists' use of the philosophic approaches presented in the theories. As we have sought to build an academic discipline, grand theories have assisted in legitimizing the emerging discipline by providing broad guidelines about the focus of the discipline. There are varying degrees of evidence about the usefulness of existing nursing grand theories. Their frequent use by schools of nursing, care institutions, and practitioners, and their use in guiding research initiatives are examples of their value.

Middle-range theories often have evidence that is acquired by using many repetitions under controlled conditions (scientific method). An example is Johnson's[20,21] self-regulation theory that addresses the use of preparatory information to assist persons in coping with threatening illness situations. Middle-range theoretical frameworks provide some evidence to support the relationships posed. However, to date no nursing theories have sufficient evidence to be considered "laws," which is not unexpected, given that nursing is a newly established discipline and our phenomena of interest are highly complex.

In micro-range theory, relationships exist among a limited number of concepts that characterize a specific situation. The working hypothesis (of either the practitioner or the scientist) has the least amount of evidence behind it. The evidence behind this kind of theoretical thinking is not usually accrued by planned repetitions under controlled situations, but instead it is built from a limited number of repetitions and observations. For example, the best way to approach first-time ambulation for surgical patients may be hypothesized by a nurse as the result of providing postoperative care to a series of patients. The theoretical-empirical congruence of this hypothesis is then tested in subsequent surgical patients.

Use of Levels of Theoretical Thinking to Enhance Knowledge Development in Nursing

Several challenges prevail in the development of nursing knowledge. Conceptualizing theory at different levels of theory may assist us to address some of these challenges. For example, one challenge is to determine how different levels of theory relate to each other. How can one level of theory be used to develop related theories at another level? As we analyze and generate theory, we often use traditional methods of theory construction and substruction. The appropriate use of inductive and deductive approaches to develop nursing knowledge may be improved by the consideration of the relationships among levels of theories. Conceptualizing levels of theories also provides a beginning tool to assess whether the philosophic roots of our grand theories are reflected in our middle-range and micro-range theories. Such analyses can potentially enhance the consistency and logic in our decision making about care issues and the theoretical design of future research.

As a discipline, we also are looking for ways to integrate related theories that have arisen from the multiple ways of building knowledge. For instance, how does the theory about stages of behavior change, developed from grounded theory methods, relate to theories of self-efficacy for health behaviors that were developed by using hypothesis-testing methods? Similarly, we are searching for ways to integrate related theories from different disciplines. For example, how do middle-range theories of health promotion in psychology relate to those in sociology and nursing? The analysis and integration of related theories may be facilitated by comparison of related theories at the same theoretical level across disciplines and arising from multiple methodologic approaches.

Another challenge in the discipline's knowledge development is understanding the mechanisms needed to enhance articulation of the knowledge produced by practitioners and researchers. Regardless of whether the methods used to develop theory are inductive or deductive, and originate from a philosophic, practice, or research perspective, multiple levels of theoretical thinking exist. Although practitioners and researchers may use divergent methods, each uses theoretical thinking for the generation of knowledge. Recognition and discussion about the levels of theoretical thinking can serve as a vehicle for increased communication between practitioners and scientists about the knowledge each is developing.

Conclusion

Knowledge development in any discipline is a dynamic process that pursues probable truths about reality. It begins with creative approaches from multiple perspectives and continues by testing the knowledge according to appropriate truth criteria. In nursing, our "reality" is clinical practice, and we construct theories about probable truths related to the experience of health in the person-environment interaction. Development of a knowledge base is an iterative and ongoing process that requires periodic analysis and synthesis of an entire body of work. In an attempt to further the understanding of the current status of nursing theory, we provided an examination of the different levels of theory currently being used to develop nursing knowledge. This meta-theoretical discussion of theory is not meant to create artificial domains; rather, it is an attempt to understand the current status of nursing theory through clarification of the terminology and a discussion of the related categories of theoretical thinking. Perhaps more important, the final purpose of this article is to recognize the strength of our disciplinary knowledge base and generate public discussion about the future of theory development and testing.

REFERENCES

1. Stevens BJ. Nursing theory, analysis, application, evaluation. 2nd ed. Boston: Little Brown & Co Inc; 1984.
2. Dubin R. Theory building. 2nd ed. New York: Free Press; 1978.
3. Chinn PL, Kramer MK. Theory and nursing. 5th ed. St. Louis: Mosby; 1999.
4. Suppe F. Middle range theories: what they are and why nursing science needs them. Proceedings of the ANA/Council of Nurse Researchers Symposium; 1993 Nov 15.
5. Walker LO, Avant KC. Strategies for theory construction in nursing. 3rd ed. Norwalk (CT): Appleton & Lange; 1995.
6. Nicoll LH. Perspectives on nursing theory. 3rd ed. Philadelphia (PA): Lippincott-Raven; 1997.
7. Carper BA. Fundamental patterns of knowing in nursing. Adv Nurs Sci 1978;1:13–23.
8. Whall AL. Current debates and issues critical to the discipline of nursing. In: Fitzpatrick JJ, Whall AL. Conceptual modes of nursing. 3rd ed. Stamford (CT): Appleton & Lange; 1996. p. 1–12.

9. Fawcett J. Analysis and evaluation of conceptual models of nursing. 3rd ed. Philadelphia (PA): FA Davis Co; 1995.

10. Nightingale F. Notes on nursing. New York: Churchill Livingstone; 1859.

11. Watson J. Nursing: the philosophy and science of caring. Boston: Little Brown & Co Inc; 1979.

12. Leininger M. Transcultural nursing: concepts, theories, and practices. New York: Wiley; 1978.

13. Merton RK. On sociological theories of the middle range. In: Merton RK. Social theory and social structure. New York: Free Press; 1968. p. 39–72.

14. Good M, Moore SM. Clinical Practice guidelines as a new source of middle-range theory: focus on acute pain. Nurs Outlook 1996;44:74–9.

15. Lenz ER, Suppe F, Gift AG, Pugh LC, Milligan RA. Collaborative development of middle-range nursing theories: toward a theory of unpleasant symptoms. Adv Nurs Sci 1995;17(3): 1–13.

16. Whall AL. The structure of nursing knowledge: analysis and evaluation of practice, middle-range, and grand theory. In: Fitzpatrick JJ, Whall AL. Conceptual modes of nursing. 3rd ed. Stamford (CT): Appleton & Lange; 1996. p. 13–25.

17. Kim HS. The nature of theoretical thinking in nursing. East Norwalk (CT): Appleton-Century-Crofts; 1983.

18. Ellis R. The practitioner as theorist. Am J Nurs 1969;69:428–35.

19. Ellis R. Values and vicissitudes of the scientist nurse. Nurs Res 1970;19:440–5.

20. Johnson JE, Fieler VK, Jones LS, Wlasowicz GS, Mitchell ML. Self-regulation theory: applying theory to your practice. Pittsburgh (PA): Oncology Nursing Press; 1997.

21. Leventhal H, Johnson JE. Laboratory and field experimentation: development of a theory of self-regulation. In: Wooldridge PJ, Schmitt MH, Skipper JK, Leonard RC, editors. Behavioral science and nursing theory. St Louis: Mosby; 1983, p. 189–262.

22. Rogers ME. An introduction to the theoretical basis of nursing. Philadelphia (PA): F. A. Davis Company; 1970.

23. Neuman B. The Neuman systems model: application to nursing education and practice. New York: Appleton-Century-Crofts; 1982.

24. Orem DE. Nursing: concepts of practice. New York: McGraw Hill; 1971.

25. Levine ME. The four conservation principles of nursing. Nurs Forum 1967;6:45–59.

26. Swanson KM. Empirical development of a middle range theory of caring. Nurs Res 1991;40(3): 161–6.

27. Pender NJ. Health Promotion in nursing practice. New York: Appleton-Century-Crofts; 1982.

28. Meek SS. Effects of slow stroke back massage on relaxation in hospice clients. IMAGE J Nurs Sch 1993;25:17–20.

29. Kikuchi JF, Simmons H, editors. Philosophic inquiry in nursing. Newbury Park (CA): Sage Publications; 1992.

30. Fawcett J, Downs FS. The relationship of theory and research. 2nd ed. Philadelphia (PA): FA Davis Co; 1992.

The Authors Comment

Levels of Theoretical Thinking in Nursing

We wrote this article in response to our need to understand and explain middle-range theory to our students. As the discipline's understanding of theoretic thinking evolved, we were asked for detailed definitions of theory and how to distinguish the meaning and application of the different types. Because we both also have programs of research, we're pragmatists when it comes to theoretic thinking. Therefore, using "levels" of theory was a natural approach for categorizing and explaining the range of theoretic thinking used by all nurse theorists, from practitioners to scientists to philosophers. The article is dedicated to all our students. Thank you for your questions, skepticism, and willingness to take on the adventure of understanding human health and illness.

—PATRICIA HIGGINS
—SHIRLEY MOORE

Historical Contexts of Nursing Knowledge Development

The chapters in this unit provide an overview of the history and trends in nursing theory. Practice and education are addressed in their critical roles in knowledge development. The distinction between borrowed and unique theories in nursing as first put forth by Dorothy Johnson in the 1960s re-emerges as an issue of the 1990s and as a non-issue in the new millennium. Authors propose other positions and issues that have become integral to understanding the history and possible future of nursing theory.

The chapters span a century of ideas about nursing as they relate to nursing knowledge, and conclude with a call for a nursing reformation.

Questions for Discussion

- How would you characterize the history of nursing theory—as a change of ideas or a progress in ideas?
- Are there foundational views about nursing knowledge that remain more or less constant over time?
- What philosophic views best characterize the context of nursing knowledge development?
- Is there any need for a nursing reformation in our theoretical thinking?

CHAPTER 7

A Non-Theorist's Perspective on Nursing Theory: Issues of the 1990s

Freda G. DeKeyser
Barbara Medoff-Cooper

The basis of all nursing endeavors, including practice and research, lies in theory. While nursing theorists are postulating and debating, practicing nurses are continuing with their daily routines and are often unaware that the world of nursing theory is changing. It is important, however, for all nurses to keep abreast of the latest developments in nursing theory. This article discusses some of the key developments within nursing theory based on a review of the nursing literature from 1990 through 1999.

The basis of all nursing endeavors, including practice and research, lies in theory. While nursing theorists are postulating and debating, practicing nurses are continuing with their daily routines and are often unaware that the world of nursing theory is changing. It is important for all nurses to keep abreast of the latest developments in nursing theory. As Fawcett (1999) points out, "Many disciplines exist to generate, test and apply theories that will improve the quality of people's lives. Every such theory-development effort is based on a particular frame of ref-

erence that provides an intellectual and socio-historical context for theoretical thinking, for research, and ultimately, for practice" (p. 1). Theory development is then seen as a basis for the advancement of research as well as practice. Few studies have investigated attitudes of practicing nurses toward nursing theory. A study conducted in 1991 (Laschinger) found that 367 Canadian staff nurses considered nursing theory development and its use important to the advancement of the nursing profession. While this study is rather old, no other study was

From Scholarly Inquiry for Nursing Practice: An International Journal, *15(4). DeKeyser, F. G. & Medoff-Cooper, B. A non-theorist's perspective on nursing theory: Issues of the 1990s, 329–341. Copyright © 2001, Springer Publishing Company. Used with permission.*

About the Authors

FREDA DEKEYSER was born in New York. She received her BSN from New York University, MA and PhD from the University of Maryland at Baltimore, and a Postdoctoral Fellowship from Johns Hopkins University. Dr. DeKeyser's clinical area is critical care. Her research also focuses on critical care, as well as psychoneuroimmunology. Several years ago, Dr. DeKeyser moved with her family to Jerusalem, Israel, where she was appointed coordinator of nursing research of a new clinical master's program, the first one in Israel. She has actively worked toward advancing the academic level of research among nurses, as well as advancing the awareness of nurses and fellow health care practitioners toward nursing research, especially clinically based research.

BARBARA MEDOFF-COOPER was born in Philadelphia at the Hospital of the University of Pennsylvania. Her education includes a BSN from the College of New Jersey, an MS in pediatric nursing from the University of Maryland, and a PhD in educational psychology/child development research from Temple University. Dr. Medoff-Cooper was a Robert Wood Johnson Clinical Nurse Scholar at the University of Pennsylvania and then joined the faculty as an assistant professor. Currently, she is the Ruth M. Colket Professor in Pediatric Nursing & Director of the Center of Biobehavioural Research in the School of Nursing, University of Pennsylvania. Her program of research has focused on the neurobehavioral development of high-risk infants, which has included both feeding behaviors and infant temperament. Dr. Medoff-Cooper's two key contributions to the discipline are the Early Infancy Temperament Questionnaire and the development of feeding norms for both high-risk and healthy neonates.

found which asked staff nurses their attitudes toward nursing theory. Laschinger concludes that the cadre of nurses familiar with theory-based nursing practice will only increase due to the increased numbers of nursing programs including nursing theory in their curriculum. This reported increase in exposure to nursing theory is even more appropriate today, more than 10 years later.

The purpose of this article is not to teach or review nursing theory. It is assumed that the reader has some general knowledge of nursing theory and its importance to nursing. Instead this discussion is aimed at exposing the reader to some, not all, of the issues which concerned authors who wrote about nursing theory over the previous decade. This article addresses some of the key developments within nursing theory based on a review of the nursing literature from 1990 through 1999. The authors are not nurse theorists themselves but rather nurses who base their practice and research on contemporary nursing theory. Therefore, it is anticipated that this discussion will be useful and accessible to a wide range of nurses.

A Medline and CINAHL search was performed on articles published between January 1990 and December 1999 which referred to nursing theory. Many issues related to nursing theory were presented in the literature. It is beyond the scope of this article to review all of the literature published during the 1990's dealing with nursing theory. Topics which were more commonly discussed and/or had relevance to practicing nurses were chosen for review and discussion. Some of the issues discussed are controversies that have been debated for several decades; others are new areas of discussion. The controversial areas discussed are: is nursing theory dead?; unique as opposed to borrowed theory in nursing; and the theory-practice gap. Newer issues discussed are the use of philosophy as opposed to theory; types of knowing; and changes in the meta-paradigm of nursing.

Continuing Controversies

Is Nursing Theory Dead?

Over the decade of the '90s nursing theory seemed to take an increasingly smaller role in the content of nursing schools' curricula and in the literature. It seemed that nursing theory was "out" and possibly even dead.

Theories that are dead are those that lie on a shelf somewhere, in some journal or book, without being used or applied. Several reasons cited in an article by Nolan, Lundh, and Tishman (1998) for the disenchantment with nursing theory are: that theories were considered too abstract and general; grand theories attempted to explain everything while explaining nothing; and there was little empirical evidence to back theories up. Most nurses had exposure to such nursing theory in their undergraduate courses and were expected to uncritically accept theories that did not necessarily agree with traditional nursing values such as holism and attention to cultural needs (Whall, 1993).

According to Fawcett (1999), nursing models and theories are by definition abstract and general and, therefore, cannot meet clinicians' expectations for concrete prescriptions directed toward the solution of problems. Grand nursing theories were developed thoughtfully, using creative intellectual leaps in order to go beyond existing knowledge. They were not based on empirical research (Fawcett, 1999). Consequently, many nurses became disappointed by the grand theories.

Due to these arguments, many abandoned the use of grand theory or conceptual models and a movement began which stressed the intuitive side of nursing, a "know how" rather than a "know that" approach. This movement is reflected in the development of theories such as that of Benner (1984) that led to a more practice-based approach rather than a purely theoretical one (Nolan, Lundh, & Tishelman, 1998). Theory derived from practice is based on the Heidegerrian view that actions are more basic than thinking. This approach reflects the presence of embodied intelligence; people learn at an unconscious level by doing instead of at a conscious level by thinking. This view is in contrast to that of Descartes, who claimed that we know the world through observation and that we consciously place these observations into mental representations by thinking (Ward, 1993). This new approach is philosophically different from that of the traditional nursing theories. Previous nursing theorists observed their nursing world and then designed their theories based on their use of reason. For example, Betty Neuman logically derived her Health Care Systems Model (1972) from her observations as a nurse and nurse educator. These new approaches, similar to that of Benner, do not focus on conclusions based on reasoning alone but on the experience itself.

Another response to the grand theories or conceptual models was the introduction and incorporation of middle-range theories. Middle-range theories are made up of a limited number of concepts and are written at a relatively concrete and specific level. Unlike grand theories, middle-range theories are generated and tested by means of empirical research (Fawcett, 1999). These types of theories are thought to be more useful in everyday practice (Nolan, Lundh, & Tishelman, 1998), possibly due to their lower level of abstraction and greater substance (Lenz, Pugh, Milligan, Gift & Suppe, 1997). Cody (1997a) categorizes middle-range theories as incipient nursing theories. Others (e.g., Liehr & Smith, 1999) state that middle-range theories are extremely appropriate for the current historical context that calls for the development of a knowledge base supported by art and science as well as by practice and research. An example of a middle-range theory in nursing is the theory of unpleasant symptoms (Lenz, Pugh, Milligan, Gift, & Suppe, 1997).

While it is possible to conclude that nursing as a discipline has moved away from the use of grand theories or conceptual models, there are some who carry on the work of individual grand theorists such as Rogers or Orem. Some claim that middle-range theories can be developed from these grand theories thereby making the grand theories more "user friendly" (Fawcett, 1999). Others see grand theories or conceptual models as the means by which practitioners can develop systematic reasoning and as a tool to develop a sense of collective self for the discipline of nursing (Kozol-McLain & Maeve, 1993). Grand theory has been described as a method to help nurses find the trees, while middle-range and other less abstract theories are used to describe more details such as the reason the leaves grow in a certain pattern (Oberst, 1995). Finally, some are concerned with the rapidity with which nursing has adapted to changes in the economic market place versus the extremely slow adaptation of the field to changes in theory and philosophy (Cody, 1997b).

In summary, while the majority of articles reviewed tended to devalue the use of grand theories at this time, there are still major supporters of such theories. In addition, middle-range theories and other less abstract schools of thought have revitalized the development of nursing theory. In the long run, the issue of whether nursing theory is dead or alive is less important than whether nurses can incorporate theory into their daily lives. This is possible whether the theory is at the grand or middle-range levels. Many nurses, usually as students, learn, think about, and eventually internalize conceptual models and nursing grand theories. These thoughts get filtered and modified through the prism of experience. Nurses in clinical practice may find themselves in a specific situation and reflect that the situation reminds them of a nursing theory or conceptual model. For example, a pediatric nurse might find him- or herself confronting issues related to control with a 2-year-old and with a 15-year-old. The 2-year-old might want to play with a specific toy only when the toy is unavailable. The 2-year-old wants to control the environment and be able to play with the desired toy when she wants to play with it. A 15-year-old might want to smoke cigarettes in his room despite rules against it. He wants to control his actions and be able to do what he wants to do where he wants to do it. While these two behavioral issues look similar, they are actually quite different. Martha Rogers (1970) describes such situations within the concept of helicy. Certain situations may appear to be the same with similar characteristics but because space-time moves forward and there is no going back, these situations are inherently different. Therefore, specific clinical situations can shed light on the most abstract concepts and theories. Middle-range theories are used often as the theoretical basis for many research studies. For example, the middle-range theory of Psychoneuroimmunology has been used by one of the authors in her research (DeKeyser, Wainstock, Rose, Converse, & Dooley, 1998). Psychoneuroimmunology theory describes interactions between psychosocial factors and the neurological and immune systems. This theory has direct bearing on the nature of the author's research. For example, Psychoneuroimmunology theory suggests that stress and anxiety impact on immune function. Several research studies were conducted by the author which attempted to evaluate this interaction. Therefore, we personally find that while grand theories and conceptual models influence our way of thinking about nursing in general, middle-range theories can be more easily applied to our work on a day-to-day basis.

Unique Versus Borrowed Theory

There is an ongoing debate as to whether nurses should use only theories that are developed by nurses or whether it is of value to borrow theories from other disciplines and adapt these theories to nursing. An example of a borrowed theory is the use of Self-Efficacy Theory to describe many nursing-related phenomena. For example, Chever and Hardin (1998) evaluated the effects of traumatic events, social support and self-efficacy on adolescents' self-health assessments. Self-Efficacy Theory, however, though widely used in nursing research, was developed by Bandura (1977), a psychologist.

Those who take the more conservative approach, refusing to accept external theories, cite several reasons for their stand. One argument is that only nursing science can describe the phenomena of nursing (Phillips, 1996). Also, non-critical acceptance of theories from other disciplines has led to the potential for overlooking the cultural needs of clients as well as the acceptance of values which may be contrary to nursing (Whall, 1993). Cody (1996a) adds that theories from varying sources do not necessarily coincide with one another. Northrup (1992) states that nursing theories need to be placed within a larger context that is consistent with the values of knowing nursing. The use of borrowed theory makes the foundation of nursing into a grab bag where nurses have minor knowledge of many theories but have in-depth knowledge of none, thus making nurses into the Jack or Jill of all trades and master of none (Cody, 1996a). Some maintain that the empirical gains won, such as advances in clinical practice, are offset by the conceptual losses brought about by compromise (Northrup, 1992). One author commented how ironic it is that many disciplines have called for interdisciplinary theory and research yet only nursing is willing to leave its roots to accomplish this (Cody, 1997a). Practically speaking, when nurses are constantly borrowing from other disciplines they have less energy to devote to sustaining, growing and developing their own (Cody, 1996a).

While still in its early stages, nursing needed to establish itself as a unique discipline, separate from others such as medicine and to develop its unique knowledge base in order to achieve academic and professional status (Cody, 1996a; Nolan, Lundh, & Tishelman, 1998). Nurses were trained to do (i.e., to practice nursing) and not to know. What nurses needed to know they learned from other disciplines and so became more familiar with these (Cody, 1996a). Northrup (1992) suggests that when nursing began to develop as a discipline it borrowed from others; however, she states that with continuing research nursing will develop to be unique. One example of this development is cited by Cody (1997b) who stated that theory-based guides for practice have been created over the previous decades that are unique to nursing science and distinct from other sciences. These purists, therefore, believe that while initially nursing theorists were forced to borrow from other fields, with time nursing theory will develop without the influence of other disciplines.

On the other hand, other authors claim that nursing cannot develop independently and use only its unique theory due to historical as well as practical reasons. The original nurse scientists received their academic training in fields other than nursing. They learned the tools necessary to build theory and research in those other fields. These tools were those of the home discipline (Cody, 1996a; Monti & Tingen, 1999). Nurse educators have handed down these tools to subsequent generations of nurse scientists. As a result, many nurse scientists have been trained to borrow and incorporate theories from other fields.

Another view is that nursing cannot develop its own theory because nursing deals with the complexity of humans. This wish for a unique theory can be called "physics envy." In physics, a pure basic science, it is possible to develop theories unique to the discipline. Theories dealing with the complexity and variability of humans, however, must draw upon more than one discipline (Levine, 1995).

Finally, others state that theories are relevant to nursing if they relate to nursing and the source of the theory is irrelevant. Oberst (1995) contends that as long as a theory helps nurses solve nursing problems, the theory is applicable and useful and thereby helps the discipline progress. Its origin is of little consequence. Nursing can be viewed as unique if it uses knowledge in a unique manner (Nolan, Lundh, & Tishelman, 1998). Booth, Kenrick and Woods (1997) strongly adhere to the conception of knowledge as a "web of belief" as described by Quine. According to this view, knowledge consists of various elements interconnected like a spider's web. The web is anchored where reality converges with beliefs through experiences. Experience is seen as the testing ground for knowledge. Therefore, the knowledge and experiences of other disciplines which are associated with nursing could be accommodated within the 'web' of nursing knowledge without compromising the core of nursing.

We agree with the position of Sims as cited by Timpson (1996) that knowledge gained from borrowed theories is changed once used within the context of the nursing discipline. The borrowed knowledge can eventually emerge as nursing theory because it is used in a way unique to nursing. Both of the present authors have used borrowed theories as the basis for their research (for example, Medoff-Cooper, McGrath, & Bilker, 2000). In both our cases theories from other disciplines, biology and psychology, have added to the richness of the theoretical underpinnings of our programs of research and allowed for a more operational/direct use of theory. As researchers and practitioners, we agree with the position that knowledge cannot be owned by one discipline or another. What makes a discipline unique is not only what problems it addresses but how it addresses, as well as solves, those problems with the knowledge it has.

Theory Practice Gap

During the 1990s and for many years before that, there was a heightened awareness in the nursing literature of the gap between nursing theory and practice. Differences between the language used to describe practice as opposed to the language of theory have been one major cause noted for this gap (Levine, 1995; Tolley, 1995). Another reason cited is that the people who develop theories have for the most part not been practitioners. Clinical nurses have not historically developed nursing theory and that trend continues to this day (Tolley, 1995). In a call for increased attention to nursing science in advanced practice graduate curricula, Huch (1995) states that students need more than one theory course to be able to apply theory to practice. Levine (1995) states that many practicing nurses were trained by those who believed that there was a chasm between practice and theory. Therefore curricula were developed such that theory and clinical practice were taught in courses independent of one another.

Engebretson (1997) adds that an understanding of the theory-practice gap can be informed by the dichotomy between medicine and nursing. Nursing theory has traditionally been developed within nursing academia, while nursing practice has dwelled within the medical model. These conflicting world views have contributed to the gap.

Some authors caution the developers of nursing diagnoses. They predict a similar progression to the one that occurred in the development of nursing theory. Many theorists designed their own language or words to describe nursing when developing their nursing theories, thereby making theory inaccessible to many. While there is a need to establish the uniqueness of nursing, at the same time these theorists may be isolating nursing by creating a language that is idiosyncratic (Nolan, Lundh, & Tishelman, 1998). In addition, practicing nurses utilize diagnoses, interventions and outcome classification systems. They deal with the specific details or "the parts." The concept of holism, however, is very prevalent among nurse theorists. Therefore, according to this view many clinical practices are incongruent with theoretical holism (Engebretson, 1997).

Some disagree with the usefulness of practice theory in general (Koziol-McLain & Maeve, 1993). They state that a theory that defines or delineates practice is by its very nature a prescriptive theory. These types of theories are problematic because the clinical environment is constantly changing. By accepting a theory, one has, in essence, accepted a stable structure that does not exist in a realistic setting.

A recent development associated with the theory-practice gap is the inclusion of action research in nursing. Action research is thought to be a means of narrowing the theory-practice gap by researching clinical problems and introducing improvements based on the research into practice (Clark, 2000). It involves four major characteristics; collaboration between researchers and practitioners, a solution of practical problems, change in practice and the development of theory. It contains three major phases, the first being a fact-finding phase where a goal or action intention is defined. This phase also includes observations to discover the true theoretical nature of the situation. The second, or action, phase, involves an action or intervention where data are collected to help achieve the designated goal. Each action taken is part of a larger plan to bring about a specific change. Activities can be either practical or theoretical. The third phase is that of evaluation. Action research simultaneously attempts to implement a practical change while generating an action theory (Greenwood, 1994). An action theory is then developed that is prescriptive and situation specific. Therefore, action research is both practical and theoretical. It attempts to solve clinical problems and then develops theories based on an evaluation of the problem and the attempts at solving it.

Theory by its very nature is abstract. Practice by its very nature is not. Therefore, an inherent gap must exist between theory and practice. Perhaps, then, the problem is not that there is a gap between theory and practice but our expectations of what theory can do for us as practitioners. Perhaps we as practitioners should see theory as a guide and not as a prescription. Theory cannot tell us what to do in a specific situation but it can be used in clinical practice as a general guide to help us channel our thinking. In turn, clinicians should learn to abstract the lessons they have learned from their practice. Here is the opportunity for clinicians to translate lessons learned from practice into theory and thereby contribute to the discipline of nursing as well as to nursing theory development.

New Issues

The phrase, "There is nothing new under the sun," can certainly be applied to the discussions of nurse theorists. While controversy around the issues related above has been prominent in the nursing literature for a while, there are several issues which while not new, have gained increased attention during the 1990s.

Nursing Philosophy Versus Theory

An interesting shift in thought is the movement from discussions about theories of nursing to more recent discussions about the philosophy of nursing. Brunk (1995) describes theory development in nursing as progressing through several stages. The first involved defining the domain of nursing. The second and third phases were the mechanical aspects and conceptual development of nursing phenomena. More recently, philosophical discussions about the nature of nursing have been published. Edwards (1997) states that philosophy of nursing contains three components:

1. Conceptual clarification and assessment of arguments;
2. Consideration of traditional philosophical problems which have relevance to nursing theory and practice; and,
3. A focus on the framework of propositions which constitute nursing discourse and on the concepts from which those propositions are comprised.

Northrup (1992) has suggested that the nursing literature has blurred the distinction between philosophy and theory. Philosophy is concerned with inquiries into the nature of reality, what nursing should be (Northrup, 1992). Philosophical issues are related to a perspective on life. Such perspectives sometimes resemble those of the grand theories such as those of Rogers (1970). Theory, on the other hand, clarifies a domain of a discipline while describing, explaining, predicting or controlling. It has been recommended that future knowledge development in nursing concentrate on philosophies of nursing as opposed to theories of nursing (Koziol-McLean & Maeve, 1993).

Uys and Smit (1994) caution nurses against confusing two different concepts related to philosophy and nursing. They discriminate between "a philosophy of nursing" and "philosophy of nursing." "A philosophy of nursing" refers to a set of beliefs, principles and values which can direct practice while "philosophy of nursing" is a theoretical analysis. The "philosophy of nursing" endeavor is used to define the object of study within the discipline and limit it, analyze basic questions and concepts, and criticize its ideology. "A philosophy of nursing" can, and perhaps should, be held and elucidated by every individual nurse as something personal. "Philosophy of nursing" is not personal but rather is an "objective" evaluation of the discipline of nursing as a source of knowledge.

This more recent trend in theoretical writing has great promise for nurse theoreticians, practitioners and researchers. It is not our view that further development of nursing theories should be stopped. We have a sense, however, that a common philosophy, as opposed to a theory of nursing, might be more accepted and reach a more common consensus among nurses. It seems that nurses can agree, more or less, as to what nursing should contain. Perhaps a further delineation of not only the philosophy of nursing but also of a philosophy of nursing would be of use.

Types of Knowing

Another recent development is the movement from purely abstract theories to those with greater direct clinical relevance. A re-emphasis on a classic article by Carper (1978) has emerged (for example, as described in Cody, 1996b; Koziol-McLain, & Maev, 1993; Nolan, Lundh, & Tishelman, 1998; Rose & Parker, 1994; Tolley, 1995). In her article, Carper describes four ways of knowing related to clinical knowledge. The four ways include: empirics, esthetics, personal knowledge, and moral knowledge. Empirics deal with the science, while esthetics focuses on the art of nursing. Esthetics can only be expressed. It cannot be published or written down and only the client receiving nursing care can observe this form of knowledge. Personal knowledge involves knowledge of the self. This is tacit knowledge that is difficult to teach but is basic to nursing practice. This type of knowledge is the basis of interactions with clients and makes these interactions more reciprocal in nature. Personal knowledge cannot be described. It can only be actualized. Moral knowledge is concerned with the ethics of nursing. The legitimization of all types of knowledge and the attempt to set them on an equal level with empirical knowledge was the theoretical basis for movements such as practice-based theories and action theories.

Cody (1996b) claims that the major impact of Carper's work was to stress that knowledge in nursing can be gained from sources other than those that are empirical or scientific. Cody also suggests that a major aspect of Carper's work is that these sources of knowledge are interrelated and dynamic.

Nolan, Lundh, and Tishelman (1998) cite the increasing popularity of Carper's theory as evidence of the widening gap between theory and practice. They state that nurses have used the theory to advance the importance of the "art" of nursing, or nursing practice, over the "science" of nursing or nursing theory.

As practitioners and researchers, we have experienced these types of knowing and agree with their importance to nursing. We hope, however, that these categories will lead to the advancement of nursing knowledge and not become a weapon to be used by one side in a theoretical debate.

Changes in the Meta-Paradigm of Nursing

The meta-paradigm of nursing has also shifted over the past decade. While each theorist can be associated with a specific interpretation of the four main concepts of the field—person, health, environment and nursing—new aspects related to these concepts have emerged. A summary of these changes is provided by Thorne and colleagues, (1998). These authors point out that for much of nursing's history the patient's body was the primary focus. In the 1970s the holistic movement impacted nursing such that a more holistic view of the person was more accepted. Other more recent theorists, however, de-emphasized the physical body and felt that the entire energy field or lived experience was more important.

Another concept shift is related to the increased emphasis on health promotion and illness prevention. This perspective includes illness as a personal experience.

While health is still considered within nursing theories to be the intended outcome of nursing actions, other nursing outcomes have emerged, such as quality of life. The authors of this review also point to the surroundings between different conceptualizations of health. Some view health as an aspect or dimension of a person which is a normative state or process. Others view health as a reflection of the whole person and not just one aspect. Health has also been viewed from a social critical theory standpoint. According to this approach, nurses must take into account the unique criteria by which people evaluate their own lives and circumstances. What might be considered healthy for one person might be sick for another. What might be considered as a health care decision born of free will for one might be considered forced or denied by another.

While most nursing theories have stated that the environment is important, in fact many deal only with the person and not the society. In keeping with more modern views, it was suggested that the nursing environment should be defined as a multi-layered construct. Two conceptualizations of the environment were also summarized. The environment can be seen as contiguous and inseparable from the person. The other view is that the environment is the surroundings or circumstances of the individual to which the person must adapt. In the first case the person and the environment are essentially one, while in the second, they are connected yet separate.

Finally, the view of the role of the nurse has come into question. The movement to formalize nursing diagnoses, as well as the traditional role of the nurse, has defined the nurse as an expert who helps clients achieve optimal health care. This view is in contrast to the consumer movement that has empowered clients to become experts themselves using media such as the internet. There also exists a conflict between the social mandate of the nurse which is "to do" as opposed to the role of the nurse as viewed by others, to simply "be there." This last conflict relates to whether nurses should be active caregivers or be more passive and allow clients to take the active role in their health care.

It has been suggested (Thorne et al., 1998) that caring be added to "the big four" concepts of nursing. The concept of caring is an attempt to define nursing's unique place in the health care world. This attempt also helps to decrease the theory-practice gap by making theory more meaningful to those practitioners who do their caring in a very technological environment. While the concept of caring is important to nursing, disagreements have arisen as to its place within nursing. Is caring nurse-centered? Patient-centered? Or both? Others stated that the caring debate was distracting nurses from finding the real boundaries of nursing. Caring is the domain of many roles and is not unique to nursing. Therefore why should nursing take on this concept as its own? The last argument against emphasizing the concept of caring in nursing is a political one. In a society that does not value caring, and in fact devalues it because of its association with gender, it is not wise for nurses to position themselves as the primary providers of caring. The role of caring within the framework of nursing remains rather controversial.

Summary

Many of the issues discussed over the past decade related to nursing theory are a continuation of those addressed previously while several have begun to cover new ground. It is safe to say that nursing theory is not dead. It remains an essential component of research and practice. As the discipline has matured, the focus of theory development has changed to more realistically reflect the practice and research environment. There is a place within the discipline of nursing for borrowed theory that can be adapted to our profession. There is no doubt, however, that theory unique to nursing provides the perspective necessary for nursing inquiry and practice. Theory is becoming more integrated into practice in many environments but there is much work to be done to narrow the theory-practice gap.

New ways of exploring old issues within the discipline have been advanced, such as action research and

the various ways of knowing. More recent approaches to the meta-paradigm of nursing have moved from the more abstract to realistically reflect issues such as health promotion and disease prevention as well as the political reality. In conclusion, can theorists and non-theorists talk to one another? We believe that they can and that doing so will advance the art and science of nursing.

REFERENCES

Bandura, A. (1977). Self-efficacy: Toward a unifying theory of behavioral change. *Psychological Review, 84,* 1911–1215.

Benner, P. (1984). *From novice to expert: Excellence and power in clinical nursing practice.* Menlo Park, CA: Addison-Wessley.

Booth, K., Kenrick, M., & Woods, S. (1997). Nursing knowledge, theory and method revisited. *Journal of Advanced Nursing, 26,* 804–811.

Brunk, Q. (1995). Setting the stage for the 21st century. *Clinical Nurse Specialist, 9,* 317.

Carper, B. (1978). Fundamental patterns of knowing in nursing. *Advances in Nursing Science, 1,* 13–23.

Cheever, K., & Hardin, S. (1998). Effects of traumatic events, social support, and self-efficacy on adolescents' self-health assessments. *Western Journal of Nursing Research, 21,* 673–684.

Clark, J. E. (2000). Action research. In D. Cormak (Ed.), *The research process in nursing* (4th ed., pp. 183–198). Oxford, UK: Blackwell Science Ltd.

Cody, W. K. (1996a). Drowning in eclecticism. *Nursing Science Quarterly, 9,* 86–87.

Cody, W. K. (1996b). Occult reductionism in the discourse of theory development. *Nursing Science Quarterly, 9,* 140–142.

Cody, W. K. (1997a). Of tombstones, milestones, and gemstones: A retrospective and prospective on nursing theory. *Nursing Science Quarterly, 10,* 3–5.

Cody, W. K. (1997b). The many faces of change: discomfort with the new. *Nursing Science Quarterly, 10,* 65–66.

DeKeyser, F. G., Wainstock, J. M., Rose, L., Converse, P. J., & Dooley, W. (1998). Distress, symptom distress and immune function in women with suspected breast cancer. *Oncology Nursing Forum, 25,* 1415–1426.

Edwards, S. D. (1997). What is philosophy of nursing? *Journal of Advanced Nursing, 25,* 1089–1093.

Engebretson, J. (1997). A multiparadigm approach to nursing. *Advances in Nursing Science, 20,* 21–33.

Fawcett, J. (1999). *The relationship of theory and research.* Philadelphia: F. A. Davis Company.

Greenwood, J. (1994). Action research: A few details, a caution and something new. *Journal of Advanced Nursing, 20,* 13–18.

Huch, M. H. (1995). Nursing science as a basis for advanced practice. *Nursing Science Quarterly, 8,* 6–7.

Koziol-McLain, J., & Maeve, M. K. (1993). Nursing theory in perspective. *Nursing Outlook, 41,* 79–81.

Laschinger, H. S. (1991). Nurses' attitudes about nursing models in practice. *Journal of Nursing Administration, 21,* 12, 15, 18.

Lenz, E. R., Pugh, L. C., Milligan, R. A., Gift, A., & Suppe, F. (1997). The middle-range theory of unpleasant symptoms: An update. *Advances in Nursing Science, 19,* 14–19.

Levine, M. E. (1995). The rhetoric of nursing theory. *Image, 27,* 11–14.

Liehr, P., & Smith, M. J. (1999). Middle-range theory: Spinning research and practice to create knowledge for the new millenium. *Advances in Nursing Science, 21,* 81–91.

Medoff-Cooper, B., McGrath, J., & Bilker, W. (2000). Nutritive sucking and neurobehavioral development in infants from 34 weeks PCA to term. *Maternal Child Nursing, 25,* 64–70.

Monti, E. J., & Tingen, M. S. (1999). Multiple paradigms of nursing science. *Advances in Nursing Science, 21,* 64–80.

Neuman, B. (1972). The Betty Neuman model: A total person approach to viewing patient problems. *Nursing Research, 21,* 264–269.

Nolan, M., Lundh, U., & Tishelman, C. (1998). Nursing's knowledge base: Does it have to be unique? *British Journal of Nursing, 7,* 271–276.

Northrup, D. T. (1992). Disciplinary perspective: Unified or diverse? *Nursing Science Quarterly, 5,* 154–155.

Oberst, M. T. (1995). To what end theory? *Nursing in Research and Health, 18,* 83–84.

Phillips, J. R. (1996). What constitutes nursing science? *Nursing Science Quarterly, 9,* 48–49.

Rogers, M. E. (1970). *An introduction to the theoretical basis of nursing.* Philadelphia: F. A. Davis Company.

Rose, P., & Parker, D. (1994). Nursing: An integration of art and science within the experience of the practitioner. *Journal of Advanced Nursing, 20,* 1004–1010.

Thorne, S., Canam, C., Dahinten, S., Hall, W., Henderson, A., & Kirkham, S. R. (1998). Nursing's metaparadigm concepts: disimpacting the debates. *Journal of Advanced Nursing, 27,* 1257–1268.

Timpson, J. (1996). Nursing theory: Everything the artist spits is art? *Journal of Advanced Nursing, 23,* 1030–1036.

Tolley, K. A. (1995). Theory from practice for practice: Is this a reality? *Journal of Advanced Nursing, 21,* 184–190.

Uys, L. H., & Smit, L. H. (1994). Writing a philosophy of nursing? *Journal of Advanced Nursing, 20,* 239–244.

Ward, R. (1993). The search for meanings in nursing: Could facet theory be a way forward? *Journal of Advanced Nursing, 18,* 549–557.

Whall, A. L. (1993). Let's get rid of all nursing theory. *Nursing Science Quarterly, 6,* 164–165.

The Authors Comment

A Non-Theorist's Perspective on Nursing Theory: Issues of the 1990s

As the person responsible for continuing education at a school of nursing, I searched for a seminar topic that was general enough to be of interest to all faculty members. Most nurses who received a master's degree have taken at least one course in nursing theory. However, few, if any, return to the subject once they have graduated, nor do they attempt to see how theory relates to their practice. I began to search the literature and found little that summarized what was new in nursing theory or how these advances were related to practice. I asked Dr. Medoff-Cooper to help me prepare and present this seminar. On one of her visits to the Hadassah-Hebrew University School of Nursing as a visiting professor, we jointly presented the material as a seminar to the faculty. The presentation and the ensuring conversation with the faculty made us believe that perhaps the content was part of a bigger discussion. From this came the impetus for the article.

—FREDA DEKEYSER
—BARBARA MEDOFF-COOPER

CHAPTER 8

The Rhetoric of Rupture: Nursing as a Practice With a History?

Sioban Nelson
Suzanne Gordon

In this paper we argue that nursing is consistently presented as a practice without a history, constantly reinventing itself within new professional and technical realms. This rupture with and repudiation of a past deemed to be pejorative, coupled with a rebirth in a "preferred present," raises recurrent problems in the construction of nursing's contemporary professional identity and search for social legitimacy. Furthermore, constituting new nursing knowledge and practice as discontinuous with the past produces a sense of historical dislocation of that nursing knowledge and practice that, in turn, reproduces the need for relocation through reinvention. This phenomenon, which we term the "rhetoric of rupture," in our view, arises from nursing's frustrated attempts to gain social status and legitimacy. Paradoxically, this constant reinvention in fact hampers nurses' attempts to gain that status and legitimacy.

This paper examines one aspect of the troubled history of nursing's search for social legitimacy. Over the past 150 years, nurses have worked to extend and develop the professional image and practice base of nursing. This endeavor has produced training schools, the legal regulation of practice, clinical specializations, university education, a growing body of research on clinical prac-

tice, and the nurse practitioner and advanced practice movement. Despite these achievements, nursing lags well behind other professions in both social status and financial remuneration. There is still no standard entry to practice in the United States or throughout Canada—the word "nurse" applies equally to people with only 1 year of post high school education as well as to those

Reprinted from Nursing Outlook, *52, Nelson, S. & Gordon, S., The rhetoric of rupture: Nursing as a practice with a history?, 255–261.*
Copyright © 2004 with permission from Elsevier Ltd.

increasingly investigator. Yale's School of Nursing is helping to redefine the profession.[8]

In a major report, designed to frame deliberations about how the largest and most influential health care foundation responded to the latest American nursing shortage, authors described nurses' historical role thusly, "In spite of an overwhelming commitment to serve, there was little nurses could provide through the first half of the twentieth century outside of comfort and cleanliness."[9]

In a 1997 article in the *New York Times* describing nurse practitioners' role in primary care, nurse practitioners were described as "the elite of the profession," having "much more responsibility" (as opposed to authority) than other nurses— "the foot-soldiers of the healthcare industry"—whose role is to "carry out doctor's orders and to alert doctor to any changes in the patient condition."[10] According to one nurse practitioner, a new NP-controlled primary care practice described in the article was "moving nurses into the twenty-first century." In discussing a recent nurse practitioner conference, one New York State NP differentiated "advanced practice clinicians" from "nurses," explaining, "We have a nursing background, but do *not* function as *nurses*"[10] (emphasis added).

Two consistent themes emerge in these examples: nursing is new, its practices and knowledge are hot off the press. Nursing is not what you expect, not practiced in the places you expect it to be, and not practiced with the patients and colleagues you expect it to be practiced with. It is young, dynamic, expanding.

In many publications and in discussions about differentiation of practice, the technical skills of these "old-style nurses" are disparaged because they are mere "tasks" that "anyone," "even a trained monkey" could be taught to perform.[11] In arguing for "differentiated practice," deans and professors of nursing commonly make the distinction between technical and professional nursing, describing nurses with less than a 4-year degree as mere "informed hands and feet," or "worker bees" who can't make critical decisions and judgments, and who are "easily controlled by hospitals," and lack "critical thinking skills" and "ability for leadership."[11]

In her examination of the relationship between nursing and technology, Margarete Sandelowski argues that one consequence of this downplaying of nursing skill and technical knowledge has been an intellectual division of labor between nursing and medicine. In the case of the emergence of diagnostic technology in the early part of the twentieth century, Sandelowski claims that,

> The effect of this division and denial of the labor of diagnosis [the labor performed by nurses] was to downplay the technical, interpersonal, and body-tending expertise of nurses and their frequently greater skill in these components of the application of the new diagnostic technology to the patient.[12]

Sandelowski's observations also hold in the examples of distancing presented above. In these quotes from the profession one hears echoes of this denigration of the nursing skills and activities performed in the past— and by many in the present. These views depict nursing as a pyramid, not a spectrum, and create rupture between the new advanced practitioner and the "common" nurse. These examples state or imply that only the "new" or advanced practice nurses are *capable* of interpretation and decision making (diagnosing and treating problems), solving problems and working with the latest scientific knowledge and technology. In so doing, they deny the part that the so-called technical nurses play in those decisions. Moreover, this rhetoric of rupture seems to assign blame for the failures that new nurses remedy on the individual nurses themselves and not on a medical or hospital system that has devalued nurses.

The Historical Record

The lauding of the new or advanced practitioner and the dismissal of the old nurse is based on an inaccurate view of past nursing practice that consistently underestimates what nurses did/do and what they knew/know. Nurses have, historically, made use of the latest medical science and technology and based their practice not only on the latest scientific and technical knowledge but also on cumulative wisdom.

In France, a community of nursing sisters, the Daughters of Charity, began running clean, efficient hospitals under contract to municipal authorities in the seventeenth century when the order was first formed. This community of women "opened their arms" to the young Florence Nightingale when she considered converting to Catholicism to follow her call from God to care for the sick.[13] As part of routine training, a Daughter of Charity was taught to care for the sick in the community's own infirmary (for sick sisters), shown how to grow medicinal herbs, trained in apothecary and how to perform minor surgery as well as to apply leeches—the medical treatments of the era.[14] On completion of her preparation, the Daughter of Charity was contracted to a hospital in the provinces and left Paris equipped with "three boxes of lancets and ligatures plus a case of surgical instruments."[15]

While it is difficult to account for seventeenth-century "clinical skill" in contemporary terms, the attendance upon the sick of reliable, committed women with knowledge of herbs and medicines, minor surgery, dietary regimen, and the domestic management skills to run a clean and economical hospital would surely have produced as good an outcome as any medical attention available at the time.[16] In fact, Colin Jones' study of the Daughters of Charity in Montpellier in the seventeenth century reveals efficient clinical institutions with a high turnover of patients and low death rate—nothing like the death traps of Paris' massive Hotel Dieu, or the similar charitable institutions across the Channel in Britain.[14]

Florence Nightingale's vision for nursing reform also adhered closely to the dominant scientific framework of the mid-nineteenth century—sanitarianism and the miasma theory. For Nightingale, health was the product of moral reform and cleanliness, clean air, rest and moral rectitude.

Indeed, Nightingale succeeded in many of her reform efforts, in part because she borrowed from the clinical knowledge and organizational skill of the Anglican sisterhoods in Britain. British historian Anne Summers argues that it was in fact these Anglican sisters, as the most experienced and best-trained nurses in the country, who raised the standard of care and

organization in London teaching hospitals.[17] Their clinical competence developed from their private work with leading surgeons, whose innovative techniques were carried into the homes of wealthy private patients and whose operative successes depended upon their skilled aftercare.[17] Rather than being acknowledged for their contribution to the development of professional secular nursing, religious nurses, like the Sarah Gamps of Charles Dickens, were also vilified as "old" nurses with the arrival of the Nightingale nurse.

Postoperative care, then and now, has involved the critical management of unstable patients. Janet McCalman's landmark history of the Women's Hospital in Melbourne, Australia charts the intensive nursing required for women undergoing innovative procedures for vaginal repair in the 1860s.[18] After years of pain, debility, and infection, these women were admitted weeks ahead of the scheduled surgery to be rested, nourished, and then prepared. Ulcerated and inflamed perineal tissue was assisted to heal with irrigations, dressings and scrupulous hygiene. The operation was performed on the women while they were fully conscious and tied into a flexed position. Postoperatively the women were also nursed in this position, their bowels kept confined and sedated with opium, regularly catherized with glass catheters (by medical officers), and the vagina irrigated with tepid water after each catheterization. The avoidance of infection was critical to recovery. After several weeks they were weaned off the opium and assisted to manage their own elimination. This was demanding and difficult nursing as the women were frequently (and understandably!) uncooperative and fractious.[18]

Another example of the complex skill and knowledge nurses mobilized to care for patients can be found in Karen Buhler-Wilkerson's history of public health nursing.[19] For the typhoid nurse in the late nineteenth century, the "intelligent understanding of the nature and progress of this 'great' fever was essential."[19] Among the many things the typhoid nurse did was utilize antiseptic mixtures, which she mixed herself, "to treat the effects of typhoid on the tongue or mouth." Special methods of bathing were utilized to "quiet delirium,

In fact, the very leadership and management model upon which the lady nurses, like Nightingale, based their effort to recreate nursing as a respectable career for gentlewomen was adapted from the religious nurses. Nightingale borrowed from Sisters of Mercy (particularly Mother Mary Moore who had been a stalwart friend and mentor of Nightingale in Crimea and for many years after) and Sister Mary Jones of St John's House. Mary Jones was a frequent, privileged visitor to Nightingale, and provided her with copies of St John's House rules for nurses, hospital contracts and other material upon which Nightingale built her "system" for St Thomas' Hospital and the famed Nightingale School.[34]

Although this disparaging view of the "old nurse" was accepted as nursing gospel for decades, the works of Abel-Smith and Christopher Maggs have clearly documented that the "new" Nightingale nurses were in fact the same women who nursed of old. The so-called Sarah Gamps or pre-Nightingale nurses, in fact, included nurses of great experience and skill.[35–37] What Nightingale and her reformers did do was to provide these old nurses with a new leadership.

Like any innovator, Nightingale freely borrowed ideas from experiments that were being conducted around her. She creatively packaged these ideas and innovations into the "new nursing," which was effective in mobilizing political support for nursing and hospital reform. This was a social and political strategy, not a clinical one. Into the twentieth century the pattern continued. Education reformer Isabel Stewart pushed the barrel of nursing as a "science" and an end to "empiric" nursing, arguing "the scientific content of nursing is little more than a thin veneer covering a larger body of traditional material and practice gained largely through experience."[38] In fact, in every period one may chose to examine, whether the post-World War II attempt to increase government investment in nursing education, or the 1970s move to tertiary education for nurses, to the nurse practitioner and advanced practice movement, this reformulation of the "new nurse," at the expense of the old, has been an irresistible political stratagem for the nursing leadership.

A political and public relations strategy that targets the past, however, can have serious consequences for the present. In nursing, the profession and its elites have a well articulated history, but nursing practice does not. If a commonly accepted discourse is blind to the skill and competence of ordinary nurses in the past, it risks denying the skill and competence of ordinary nurses in the present. One cannot help but wonder about the impact of such a strategy on contemporary bedside nurses. If their practice is not anchored to an internally articulated history of that practice within that profession, will they not feel that their own practice is ephemeral, that it too will be denigrated and disappear in a newly written history?

Conclusion

What we call the rhetoric of rupture raises a number of serious problems. The devaluation of nursing skill and competence that takes place within nursing has led to a flight from the "tasks" of nursing and a denigration of technical competence as mindless, mechanical work. It perpetuates the notion that practical knowledge is not knowledge and that the clinical dexterity and acumen does not involve critical thinking or decision making. This, in turn, demeans the skill and knowledge of those nurses who are left out of current reformulations of "advanced" nursing and wipes out the very significant contributions nurses have made over 150 years to the health care system, medical science, and medical and nursing practice.

By constantly repeating the notion, among themselves, in the media, in promotional material, that ordinary, basic nursing practice has been and still is performed by people who lacked and still lack responsibility, the ability to think critically, to make decisions and display leadership, nurses themselves inadvertently reinforce the traditional view that most bedside nursing and clinical skills are by-products of medical knowledge and judgement.

This rhetoric of rupture nursing reproduces, within itself, the oppressive relationship between nursing and medicine that has simultaneously denied and appropriated the contributions, insights and knowledge of nurses. The only way for nursing to achieve social legitimacy is to educate contemporary practitioners to the practice of the past. Simply because earlier nurses may not have been formally educated to the level of contemporary nurses does not mean they did not practice skillfully, solve problems, think critically, and make decisions that significantly improved the care of patients.

To reverse this tendency, nursing could take some lessons from the feminists. Feminists debunked the oppressive stereotyping of female roles by documenting the important roles ordinary women played in their societies and examining the contributions they made; nursing historians, too, are taking up the challenge of rethinking the myths and stereotypes of yesterday's nurses. Nursing students need to be educated in the skill and intelligence required of early surgical nurses, of fever nurses and obstetric nurses. The management of "the sick and helpless,"[31] as Virginia Dunbar called it in her 1946 preface to the revised American edition of *Notes on Nursing*, was and is highly skilled technical work. More nursing leaders, however, need to develop an understanding of the importance of everyday nursing practice and to respect the achievement, skill and competence of the women on whose shoulders this practice stands. Arguments for the advancement of the profession have to be based on this understanding and respect for nursing as a practice with a history.

REFERENCES

1. Thompson EP. *The making of the English working class*, Harmondsworth: Penguin. 1963, p. 13.
2. Buresh B, Gordon S. *From silence to voice*, Ithaca: Cornell University Press; 2000.
3. Gordon S, Nelson S. An end to angels and hearts. Moving beyond the virtue script to a knowledge-based identity for nurses. *Amer J Nurs* (in press).
4. Freidson E. *The profession of medicine: A study of the sociology of applied knowledge*, Chicago; University of Chicago Press; 1988. p. 13.
5. Lown B. *The lost art of healing*. Ballantine Books; 1999, p. xvii.
6. Office of Admissions, University of Pennsylvania School of Nursing. *People shaping the professional*. University of Pennsylvania School of Nursing undergraduate overview 2001.
7. MetroWest Community Health Care Foundation. *Nurse power. Framingham: MetroWest Community Health Care Foundation;* 2003. Available at; www.nursepower.net.
8. Branch MA. *The New Nurses Special Issue*. Graduate and Professional Edition. Yale School Nurs. Alumni Mag 1999. p. 48–51.
9. Kimball B. O'Neill E. *Healthcare human crisis: The American nursing shortage*. A study commissioned by the Robert Wood Johnson Foundation, 2001.
10. Freudenheim M. *As nurses take on primary care, physicians are sounding alarms*. The New York Times. 1997; September 30: Al, D4.
11. Gordon S. S. *Gordon interviews with US nursing leadership* 2000–1.
12. Sandelowksi M. *Devices and desires: Gender and technology in American nursing*. Chapel Hill: University of North Carolina Press; 2000; p. 90.
13. Nightingale to Henry Manning, July 1852, BL Add. MSS. 9095/10, British Library.
14. Jones C. *The charitable imperative: Hospital and nursing in Ancien Regime and Revolutionary France*. London: Routledge, 1989.
15. Jones C. *The construction of the hospital patient in early modern France*. In: Finzsch N. Jutte R, eds. Institutions of confinement. Cambridge University Press. 1996. p. 55–74.
16. Nelson S. Entering the professional domain, the making of the modern nurse in 17th century France. *Nurs Hist Review 1999*; 7:171–88.
17. Summers A. *The cost and benefits of caring: Nursing charities, c. 1830-1860*. In: Berry J, Jones C, eds. Medicine and charity before the welfare state. London: Routledge; 1991. p. 133-48.
18. McCalman J. *Sickness and suffering*. Melbourne: Melbourne University Press; 1998. p. 43–5.
19. Buhler-Wilkerson K. *No place like home; a history of nursing and home care in the United States*. Baltimore: Johns Hopkins Press; 200. p. 129, 131.
20. Doherty MK. *The life and times of Royal Prince Alfred Hospital*. Sydney, Australia; Russell RL, ed. Glebe: New South Wales College of Nursing; 1996. p. 123, 124.
21. Fairman J. Lynaugh J. *Critical care nursing: a history*. Philadelphia; University of Pennsylvania Press; 1998.
22. Risse G. Mending bodies, saving souls: *A history of hospitals*. Oxford: Oxford University Press; 1998.
23. Gordon S. *Life support; Three nurses on the front lines*, Boston: Little, Brown and Co.; 1996.
24. Lynaugh J. Brush B. *American nursing; From hospitals to health systems*. Malden; Blackwell; 1996.
25. Dickens C. *The life and adventures of Martin Chuzzlewit*. Harmondsworth; Penguin; 1968.
26. Summers A. *The mysterious demise of Sarah Gamp: The domiciliary nurse and her detractors, c. 1830–1860*. Victorian Studies 1989; Spring: 365–86.

About the Lead Author

DEBORAH THOUN NORTHRUP was born in Montreal, Quebec, Canada, where she began her lifelong passion for nursing at the age of 6 by holding clinics for the neighborhood children; taking temperatures with popsicle sticks, and offering cough drops. She earned undergraduate and graduate degrees in Nursing from Dalhousie University in Halifax, Nova Scotia, and a PhD in nursing from The University of Texas at Austin. Reading and theatre are her favorite hobbies. She has been employed by the University of Victoria since 1996. Her key contributions to the discipline lie in the focus of her scholarship, which is the advancement of nursing as a scientific discipline, the development of nurse scholars, and the practice of nursing from a human science perspective. The co-authors were graduate students with Dr. Northrup at the University of Victoria.

baccalaureate education" (CNA, 2002, ¶7). The CNA contends further that, "The goal of having a baccalaureate requirement for entry into nursing has been adopted throughout Canada by all provincial and territorial nurses' associations. The decision was taken based on trends affecting health care in Canada and the changing role of the nurse" (¶7). Nevertheless, explicit endorsement of this position in two Canadian provinces (Alberta and Quebec) and three territories (Yukon, Northwest Territories, Nunavet) remains elusive and optional (diploma programs for nursing education remain open), and in some cases quite perplexing (British Columbia) as the inception of college-based applied degrees takes place. The Registered Nurses Association of British Columbia (RNABC) (2003) "believes the competencies required for future nurses are most effectively and economically achieved through baccalaureate nursing education" (¶2) yet, no reference to university level education can be found and neither endorsement nor identification of a plan to sanction university-based baccalaureate education alone for entry into nursing has taken place.

Currently, the education debate in nursing and resulting position statements on appropriate educational requirements and qualifications for entry into nursing appear to support academic preparation for nurses. At the heart of this implied preference however, are recurring themes and core narratives regarding efficiency, economy, shifting trends, and/or changing roles. Indeed, the exclusion of all reference to intellectual inquiry from a disciplinary perspective, conceptions of nursing science,

and issues of theory, practice, and values in nursing in this debate is disconcerting, worrisome, and far from the goal of academic nursing scholarship and practice. Without doubt, time and economic commitments as well as changing health trends and roles have huge implications for students and educational institutions and must be considered in any discussion of access to education and recruitment within the field of nursing. These issues however, lack relevance for nursing qua nursing as a field of study, research, and practice. Moreover, failure to mandate a basic academic qualification for entry into nursing opens the door for differing educational institutions to offer diverse qualifications for the preparation of new graduates, compounding the struggle of eliminating multiple levels of entry into nursing. Furthermore, there can be little doubt that reducing arguments for appropriate and adequate education in nursing to social conditions provides the impetus for that education to be determined and imposed by governments, health and/or education administrators, as well as an array of professionals educated in other disciplines. All too frequently, proposed changes to nursing education are set out as quick-fix solutions to the fiscal and economic woes of healthcare. A perusal of related editorial features and letters in our newspapers from lay persons and other professionals–most notably physicians, various union representatives, and some administrators–demonstrates clearly that people outside the discipline believe they have the right and requisite knowledge of nursing to determine educational preparation for nurses.

Understanding Ourselves as a Profession

In our own experiences as nurse teachers, students, researchers, and practitioners, we have come to understand nursing as a practice profession and academic discipline. In order to substantiate this claim, we would like to unpack the language embedded in this statement and examine the notions of profession and discipline respectively. To begin, we submit that many people confuse the terms profession and discipline and use them interchangeably. There are however, numerous authors in nursing who stress the importance of understanding and considering the differences between and relationships among these concepts in shaping the evolution of nursing (Cody, 1997; Donaldson & Crowley, 1978; Parse, 1999, 2001b; Schlotfeldt, 1989).

A brief review of the literature aimed at locating the origins of professions revealed considerable information related to the Flexner Report. First published in 1910, the Flexner Report (Flexner, 1915) was designed to secure the dominance of allopathic practitioners who were prepared within university-based programs of education and guided by natural science research. Pursuant to his report, Flexner identified several criteria he believed were required for the establishment and legitimation of a profession. These were:

> Professions involve essentially intellectual operations; they derive their raw materials from science and learning; this material they work up into a practical and definite end; they possess an educationally communicable technique; they tend to self-organization; they are becoming increasingly altruistic in motivation, (p. 904)

Although concerned with universally acknowledged professions in the late 19th and early 20th centuries, specifically law, medicine, and the clergy, Flexner's characterization of professions has contributed greatly to contemporary views. For example, *The New Fontana Dictionary of Modern Thought* (Bullock & Trombley, 2000) tells us that,

> One of the key features of 'modern society' . . . is the transformation of many occupations into pro-

fessions. This process involves the development of formal entry qualifications based upon education and examinations, the emergence of regulatory bodies with powers to admit and discipline members, and some degree of state-guaranteed monopoly rights, (p. 689)

When considering the notions of advanced learning, public service and safety, regulation, and rules of membership embedded in the above description, readers may note that these criteria confer professional status on numerous occupations of diverse standing in contemporary society, including the medical profession, the military profession, and groups of persons such as carpenters, golfers, or actors by profession (Bisset, 2000). In British Columbia, the RNABC (1998) assigned a number of similar attributes that serve to legitimate nursing as a practice profession. These include:

> Professionals are responsible and accountable to the public for their work.
> Professional practice is based on a specialized body of knowledge.
> Professionals are bound by a code of ethics.
> A profession provides a service to the public.
> A profession is self-regulating. (p. 5)

Chronicling Nursing's Disciplinary Evolution

When considering nursing as a discipline, it is noteworthy that until an emphasis on development of a specialized body of knowledge engendered nursing's move into the academy, which began in earnest in the early 1950's (Kalish & Kalish, 1995), nursing's evolutionary path was signposted by its transition from vocation to profession; the emergence of diploma granting hospital schools of nursing; a decided focus on what nurses *do* aimed at mastery of technique, and; the valuing of curricula framed predominantly within bio-medical knowledge. While this period did much to sever nursing's link with domestic labor and establish standards of paid work, the appropriation of an apprenticeship model of education to *train* nurses also entrenched the domination of nurses by physicians and hospital administrators. By the 1960's, a heightened awareness and growing need to establish a distinctive science of nursing propelled nursing education into four year university-based programs offering baccalaureate degrees and heralding the inception of nursing as a discipline or branch of knowledge (Bisset, 2000, p. 269). At the same time in the United States, the proliferation of associate degree (A.D.) programs based in community colleges emerged as a substitute for diploma programs. The A.D. programs differed from hospital programs only in the way the programs were administered and the length of the programs, that is, two academic years with practice experiences located in affiliated community health agencies versus three years of bedside instruction.

According to Kozier and DuGas (1967), graduates from diploma or A.D. programs were referred to as *technical nurses* who were prepared to execute technical skills most often guided by a set of rules, routines, and techniques, in the performance of service. Conversely, university-based baccalaureate programs were mandated to prepare *professional nurses* whose broader scope of practice was guided by theoretical knowledge of the biological, physical, and social sciences, as well as the humanities. Such preparation was considered essential to one's "ability to make wise nursing judgments . . . to guide other personnel in their activities," and to pursue graduate education (Kozier & DuGas, 1967, p. 7). Although cursory, this summary sheds light on the ground that has served to shape and foster nursing's rich and dynamic evolution. Sadly, the differing educational preparation and purposes, and divisive character of debate advanced over five decades ago forged an enduring class system in nursing that continues to inform and shape nursing to this very day.

Drawing from the descriptions presented above and a review of related literature it appears that the profession/discipline distinction rests predominantly on the generation and appropriation of a "specialized body of knowledge" (RNABC, 1998, p. 5) related to an associated realm of practice. Accordingly, numerous authors contend that a discipline is known by the knowledge base that embodies its distinctive perspectives, theories, methods, worldviews, and phenomena of concern (Donaldson & Crowley, 1978; Fawcett, 1992; Oldnall, 1995; Parse, 1987, 1999, 2001b). In other words, the discipline of nursing is given structure and form by the nature of its distinct knowledge base, not by the varied and sundry activities in which nurses engage, that is, not by what nurses do. We are not suggesting here that a discipline is limited to its science base, but rather that the relevance of its science is located within its practice. To be sure, the discipline of nursing is broader than its science, and must encompass "all that nursing is and all that nurses do" (Cody, as cited in Daly et al., 1997, p. 12), including nursing philosophy, nursing history, nursing education, and other areas (Donaldson & Crowley, 1978; Schlotfeldt, 1989). Hence, the discipline of nursing can claim nurse philosophers, nurse historians, nurse educators, nurse scientists, nurse practitioners, and others of this genre. Knowledge *about* nursing's history or philosophy however, does not constitute the specialized body of knowledge or science required to inform and guide practice.

Nursing Knowledge: Organizing Frameworks, Structure, and Influences

Continued confusion related to nursing's disciplinary status revolves around differing assertions that nursing is a professional *or* academic discipline. Similar to the profession/discipline distinction, the difference between an academic or professional discipline of nursing rests on the articulation of nursing's "specialized body of knowledge" (RNABC, 1998, p. 5) to guide nursing practice. If nothing else, the proliferation of views on nursing's specialized body of knowledge over the last century attests to the dynamic nature of disciplines in general and nursing in particular. Indeed, the very structuring of human knowledge evolves as disciplines emerge, expand, are revised, fuse, and become extinct relative to changes in the nature of their conceptual bases (Donaldson & Crowley, 1978). And, just as expressions and meanings of nursing as domestic work-vocation-occupation-profession have evolved with the dawning of generative ideas, so too must we acknowledge shifting views in nursing's disciplinary standing. Therefore, as we proceed, we ask that you suspend favored precepts, remain open to new ways of thinking, and take note of language or vocabulary that may hold nursing in controlled patterns of meaning that perpetuate convention, old habits, stereotypes, and subservience.

Understanding Nursing as a Professional Discipline

The notion of nursing as a professional discipline emerged within the strong impetus to establish a specialized knowledge base for professional practice. Hence, the professional discipline classification arose to distinguish nursing from accepted academic disciplines and to connote the practical aims of the discipline. In retrospect, this appears particularly reasonable as nursing, unlike academic disciplines of the day, did not have a specialized knowledge base to articulate. Further, nursing as an emerging discipline, was devoid of all characteristics specific to academic disciplines, such as an "impressive body of enduring works, suitable techniques [or methods], concerns which are significant and relevant to humans, unifying and inspiring traditions, and considerable scholarly achievements" (Shermis, as cited in Donaldson & Crowley, 1978, p. 115). Moreover, nursing's search for its substantive body of knowledge emerged prior to articulation of the nature of nursing knowledge to be developed. Alligood (1997) contended that this void gave rise to the "early valuing of nursing content specific to nursing action" (p. 5) as well as numerous and varied foci for knowledge development which she historically situates and fittingly refers to as the curriculum, research, graduate education, and theory "eras of nursing knowledge" (p. 4). The disparate and unspecified content basis for practice generated throughout these eras, along with nursing's fledgling and limited tenure as a discipline, make it easy to understand why nursing would organize around its practical aims rather than its academic or scientific ones. Interestingly, Meleis (1985) claimed that

it wasn't until the identification of a knowledge structure for nursing, that is, its metaparadigm, and the phenomenal growth of nursing theory during the 1980's, that the foundation for the development of the discipline of nursing was achieved.

Many people argue that the inextricable link between the discipline (branch of knowledge) and the profession (people educated in nursing) implies that persons who practice nursing are best served by a professional discipline. This argument however, rests on historical events (for example, nursing's early search for and articulation of its disciplinary purpose and specialized body of knowledge driven by its move into the academy) and semantics alone, not issues of relevance to nursing as an evolving discipline or science. Furthermore, all disciplines have a related realm of practice (Donaldson & Crowley, 1978). For example archaeologists who choose to work and practice in the field, are challenged to be proficient in many skills, techniques, and approaches related to finding, caring for, and preserving artifacts and archaeological sites. However, archaeology as a discipline seeks to generate a science or specialized body of knowledge related to study of the material remains of humans' past (Bullock & Trombley, 2000). The science and practice of archaeology are inextricably linked. Whether or not archaeology assumes professional status however, is reliant on archaeologists as a group, to acquire and/or conform to attributes that satisfy contemporary notions of a profession. Clearly, not all professions are disciplines and not all disciplines are professions. And indeed, the regulatory purview of our professional body does not extend to the discipline as a branch of knowledge.

The location of nursing within a professional discipline orientation is often supported by opponents of neat disciplinary boxes of scholarship and/or by proponents of inter- or trans-disciplinarity who hold a wide range of related disciplinary perspectives. All too often, these scholars predicate their programs of research on the knowledge base of those other disciplinary boxes, most notably sociology, psychology, and the natural sciences, or argue for an eclectic approach to knowledge development *for* nursing aimed at breaking down professional dominance of one group over another and/or enhancing communication among disciplines. Both approaches toward knowledge development however, are reminiscent of the diverse knowledge forms and practice directions characterized by "eras of nursing knowledge" (Alligood, 1997, p. 4) and, contrary to contemporary arguments, further entrench the subordination of practicing nurses to physicians and/or more recently, social scientists. Additionally, premature movement toward or adoption of nursing as an interdisciplinary endeavor ensures the invisibility of nursing's distinct disciplinary knowledge and places nursing at risk of disappearing in the medicalization of healthcare (Barrett, 2002) and/or of being swallowed by the global hegemony of population health (Hamilton & Bhatti, 1996; Health Canada, 1998).

Interestingly and sadly, knowledge generated within a host of disciplinary perspectives is often named and appropriated uncritically as *new* nursing knowledge, perpetuating an illusory notion of nursing science and multiple understandings of nursing practice. Clearly, this is similar to saying that clinical drug trials, when conducted by nurses, generate knowledge that can be identified as nursing knowledge simply because the person carrying out the study holds professional membership in nursing. Moreover, we believe that when nursing's knowledge base is limited to borrowed knowledge from other disciplines, it announces that nursing science, that is, our specialized body of knowledge, is considered scientifically unimportant.

Our accounting of nursing as a professional discipline and directed focus on nursing's specialized body of knowledge are not intended to narrow nursing's scope of practice, to dismiss practice as the central focus for the discipline of nursing, or to negate the broad range of other disciplinary knowledge needed for safe and appropriate practice. Indeed, preliminary education in nursing like most other disciplinary fields requires a broad base of knowledge from several disciplines. Rather, the position advanced here is intended to clarify the need for specificity related to our specialized body of knowledge and to compel nurse scientists to generate a distinct knowledge base *of* nursing to guide

and enhance professional practice that will, in turn, elucidate and account for the purposes, goals, and values specific to that practice.

Understanding Nursing as an Academic Discipline

When we classify nursing as an academic discipline, nursing is defined accordingly, as a science. Within this classification, the aim of the discipline is to know or understand. In nursing, the focus of our knowing or understanding is structured by our metaparadigm or organizing conceptual framework, commonly identified as our phenomena of concern, that is, person, environment, health. This metaparadigm has given rise to nursing's divergent paradigms and philosophical perspectives, numerous theoretical perspectives and creative conceptualizations, as well as a number of research methodologies. The conceptualizations of science within this disciplinary model are generally referred to as applied or basic science. For some people, this distinction further categorizes academic disciplines into applied or basic disciplines.

Applied sciences or applied branches of academic disciplines aim to answer "questions related to the applicability of basic theories in practical situations" (Donaldson & Crowley, 1978, p. 115). In other words, the practical limits of basic theories are described, explained, or tested in research. Study findings are used to inform practice in ways that are consistent with the nature (ontology and epistemology) of the science. Nursing's recognition as an applied science has rested predominantly on the development of practical knowledge based in or drawn from other disciplines (Benner, 1984). Research studies in this realm are conducted to answer questions related to *best practice* such as tube placement, frequency of catheter changes, skin cleansing, prevention of decubitus ulcers, and others. Similarly, research studies framed within the conceptual basis of a social model of health promotion direct nurses to *take collective action* on the broad social, ecological, political, psychological, or economic determinants/conditions/contexts of health that drive health and social reform (MacDonald, 2002). Processes of monitoring, assessing, risk profiling, and/or measuring the health status of populations engender population-based interventions often targeting aspects of everyday life (Health Canada, 1998; Lupton, 1995) or loftier notions of social justice (Hamilton & Bhatti, 1996). Language appropriated to describe such activities is coined foremost as *health promotion practice* rather than nursing practice. The theoretic knowledge underpinning such applied research is predominantly and variously pulled from a range of natural (biology, chemistry, physics, and others) and social sciences (sociology, psychology, ecology, economics, anthropology, epidemiology, and others). This *means to an end* conceptualization of nursing science has resulted in narrowly defining nursing within a set of skills, strategies, activities, and the like, albeit the research/evidence-based, intent on improving health. Interestingly, the pervasiveness of research-based or evidence-based discourses in the nursing literature, wittingly or unwittingly obscures the conceptual bases of nursing practice by frequently cloaking within objective calculating devices such as scales, indices, and surveillance tools, and fails to address the deterministic view of health held within this stance.

Within contemporary nursing thought, a very large and growing group of nurse scholars claims that research that borrows or uses the theory base of other disciplines and sciences, advances the knowledge base of that discipline and not nursing's (Fawcett, 1992; Johnson, 1991; Parse, 2001a, 2001b). Moreover, Mitchell (2001) asserted, "borrowed theories can leave theoretical residue that also contribute to moral distress and compromise" (p. 112) for nurses. Johnson (1991) contended further that borrowing theories from other disciplines not only places nursing in the hands of other disciplines, but the development of so called nursing knowledge is then "driven by the advancements of other disciplines" (p. 13), not the concerns of nursing. Similarly, when shifts in policy focus by governments or other organizations provide the foremost impetus and direction for knowledge generation in nursing, such knowledge reflects a government or institutionally driven agenda for the governance of health that may or may not be consistent with nursing's values or goals. Indeed, practitioners may become experts in the interests of government, participating in the creation and delivery of nationally organized and politically-directed programs of healthcare and delivery. Elucidating nursing's distinct contribution to humankind in light of such shifts can only occur within nursing's disciplinary frame of reference. Clearly, the requisite body of "specialized nursing knowledge" (RNABC, 1998, p. 5) or theoretically-driven interpretations that are central to the development of a distinct nursing science are conspicuously absent within an applied disciplinary view of nursing. Furthermore, many would argue that advancement of research/evidence-based practice rather than nursing theory-guided practice, is precisely what accounts for nursing's placement within the professional discipline realm.

Memory and Commitment

Advances in nursing science over the past thirty years continue to evolve our specialized body of knowledge and disciplinary footing. The development of our meta-paradigm, identifiable philosophical perspectives, a growing number of nursing theories and frameworks specific to guiding, informing, and enhancing practice, the development of congruent research methods, and a body of impressive and enduring scholarly works have laid the ground for the establishment and recognition of nursing as a basic academic discipline and science (Barrett, 2002; Newman, 1994; Parse, 1987; Phillips, 1996). Such disciplinary standing implies the existence of boundaries that differentiate nursing science from other sciences. Once differentiated as a distinct domain of knowledge, ultimate responsibility for expanding the conceptual basis of nursing science; for explicating the inextricable link between our theories, practice, and research; for articulating and extending nursing's contribution to healthcare, and; for elucidating the difference we make to the people we serve, rests within nursing and not with other disciplines.

A current snapshot of our discipline reveals two major perspectives or paradigms that reflect distinct worldviews about nursing's phenomena of concern or focus of inquiry. These perspectives, posited as the *totality* and *simultaneity* paradigms (Parse, 1987) situate nursing within the natural and human science traditions respectively. As such, each paradigmatic perspective houses a multitude of differing theories nourished by innumerable creative conceptualizations relevant to nursing; diverse nursing practice methodologies, and; various research methods that are congruent with the identified philosophy and framework. Knowledge development within a basic discipline of nursing includes concept development, basic research aimed at expanding nursing science, and applied research aimed at evaluating the usefulness of our theories for practice and healthcare (Barrett, 2002; Donaldson & Crowley, 1978; Parse, 1987; Phillips, 1996; Schlotfeldt, 1989).

Today, political and economic realities are fueling a number of changes in healthcare as well as education. Current conditions within the commodity economy of healthcare find nurses scrambling to provide *evidence* for healthcare decision makers regarding the effects of nursing care on the health of the population. As discussed previously, such evidence is generated predominantly within bio-medical and social science-driven research that gives rise to a set of skills, techniques, and interventions summarily labeled as best practices. When used as the basis for healthcare decisions, the ultimate aim of such evidence is reduction of healthcare costs related to a host of material as well as human resources (Purkis, 1997). At the same time, the government of British Columbia in Canada has proposed an expansion of education mandates that paves the way for applied baccalaureate and applied masters degrees to be offered at public community colleges and university colleges/provincial institutes, respectively. Driven by "labour market need" the focus of the applied degree is on "employment related skills" in business and technical fields, aimed at addressing "pending skill shortages in existing and emerging occupations" (Applied Degrees Advisory Committee, 2002, p. 4). Likewise, the applied focus of the masters degree aims to ensure "an **advanced** level of . . . practice . . . expertise" (Applied Degrees Advisory Committee, p. 5) in response to industry needs. Not surprisingly, much of nursing sees a fit

between the practical aims of evidence-based practice and the focus of an applied degree. Sadly however, the shortsightedness of this view sustains nursing in conventional patterns of meaning, maintains the majority of nurses in roles that are informed by and subordinated to other disciplines, and lays the foundation for advanced technical "training" in "applied fields" (Applied Degrees Advisory Committee, p. 4), in effect, driving us back to the 19th century! An intriguing question for us at this juncture is, *If the interdisciplinary nature of applied degrees is so attractive, why are the disciplines of sociology, psychology, and other health-related disciplines not exploring a move to a college-based applied baccalaureate degree?* Further, and most perplexing, *Why is medicine, the quintessential applied science, not scurrying to establish itself in our community colleges?*

Possibility and Necessity

As discussed, the decisions that are made in relation to entry level education for nursing are far from inconsequential. It seems clear that discerning our disciplinary status, and thus an appropriate education arrangement, is centrally concerned with distinguishing the illusion or pretense of nursing science located within the meaningless sea of interdisciplinary research studies and discourses from the synthesis of thought and distinction of subjects that are solidly anchored in nursing. Indeed, the central conception that addresses the discrepancies of our earlier eras as well as the plurality of motives imposed on nursing practice from myriad perspectives is the development of conceptual language in which *nursing* has primary authority, that is, a nursing science founded on the study of phenomena of concern that are distinguishable from, complementary to, and in some respects conflicting with other disciplines. As soon as we accept this possibility, the necessity of education that is not subordinated to the authority of other disciplines becomes imperative. Without doubt, such education belongs properly only to venues that can play a central role in opening new domains of abstract thought that do not compromise the specific practice and science of nursing. Once accomplished, nursing can enjoy building alliances within multidisciplinary teams that honor its unique life form and its distinct contribution to human health service and multidisciplinary endeavors. Indeed, our ability to communicate with other sciences and even with one another is enhanced greatly when we have something to communicate, something other than the reiteration of teachings from other disciplines. Hence, our ability to communicate demands that we are in the possession of language, self-awareness, subject matter, and foresightedness that taken together can create a true science of nursing. What however, can be done to stem the tide of those who contort themselves and thus nursing to look interesting and credible to other members of healthcare, research funding bodies, and organizations of healthcare delivery?

While governmental influences, that is, policy, economic constraints, and recruitment and retention issues, are cited as major challenges to academic degree preparation for nurses, the greatest obstacle to the establishment of academic disciplinary status for nursing, the development of nursing science, and the establishment of appropriate nursing education rests with nurses themselves. Academic careers built on the subject matter of other disciplines and professional indifference or a *just get on with it* attitude abound in nursing. To be sure, disciplinary expertise that is internal to the discipline is neither valued nor sought. And clearly, organizations are not structured to make advanced nursing practice that claims coherence, economically viable. In short, only medically-driven nursing practice serves the economic purposes of mainstream healthcare.

If nursing is to find full expression within mainstream healthcare, nurses must set the stage for a fuller exploration of their difference, their defining qualities, their unique talents, their distinct purposes, and their revolutionary spirit. Such expression requires a combination of exceptional knowledge in nursing, technical skill, sensitivity, originality, ambition, drive, and self-respect. When connected and reinforced with education, a universe of seemingly infinite possibilities arise for nursing. But not all possibilities are equally alike. And without doubt, our choice of educational path reveals much about who we are and who we value, what we attach importance to, what we wish to build, and what we wish to pass on to the next generation. Clearly, nursing requires careful nurture and progress that will grow works of enduring value that do not debase or demean the intelligence of nurses, that do not rely on the authority of others, that do not diminish the integrity of human wholeness, that do not change our path of service, wisdom, tenderness, or rectitude. We cannot build a discipline that must collapse because its foundations are wrong. Certainly, once we trust and respect ourselves, and once we have faith and confidence in our own innovation, learning, and choice, we will be in a position to demand no less from others.

Conclusion

In British Columbia, the attention generated by the shifting agendas of educational institutions is triggering an interesting and most important debate in nursing familiar to many nurses around the world. Questions raised in this debate are giving rise to choices and decisions that cut to the heart of nursing's position as a scholarly academic discipline and subsequently, the adequacy and appropriateness of education for nurses. Consequently, we might also ask, *Could this ultimately be a global pattern?*

Considering the disciplinary expressions and related arguments presented above, it appears that there are a number of ways of looking at and growing nursing that ultimately constitute and construct our contribution to healthcare, to the people we serve, and to ourselves. Accordingly, we must examine and carefully consider the ramifications and associated implications of each in light of our commitment to the advancement of nursing as a discipline and the fulfillment of professional desires and aspirations. Taking the long view, we recommend strongly, that preparation for entry into nursing as well as the foundations for graduate study in nursing must be located within *nursing science* programs of academic education.

REFERENCES

Alligood, M. R. (1997). The nature of knowledge needed for nursing practice. In M. R. Alligood & A. Marriner-Tomey (Eds.), *Nursing theory: Utilization & application* (pp. 3–13). St Louis: Mosby.

Applied Degrees Advisory Committee. (2002, March). *Applied degrees policy framework* [Draft], Victoria, BC: British Columbia Ministry of Advanced Education, Public Institutions Branch.

Barrett, E. A. M. (2002). What is nursing science? *Nursing Science Quarterly, 15,* 51–60.

Benner, P. (1984). *From novice to expert: Excellence and power in clinical nursing.* Menlo Park, CA: Addison-Wesley.

Bisset, A. (Ed.). (2000). *The Canadian Oxford paperback dictionary.* Don Mills, Ontario: Oxford University Press.

Bullock, A., & Trombley, S. (Eds.). (2000). *The new Fontana dictionary of modern thought* (4th ed.). Hammersmith, London: Harper Collins.

Canadian Nurses Association. (2002). *Education: Requirements for a degree.* Retrieved May 22, 2002, from http:// www.cna-nurses.ca/pages/education/ educationframe.html

Cody, W. K. (1997). Of tombstones, milestones, and gemstones: A retrospective and prospective on nursing theory, c. 1997. *Nursing Science Quarterly, 10,* 3–5.

Daly, J., Mitchell, G. J., Toikkanen, T, Millar, B., Zanotti, R., Takahashi, T, et al. (1997). What is nursing science? An international dialogue. *Nursing Science Quarterly, 10,* 10–13.

Donaldson, S. K., & Crowley, D. M. (1978). The discipline of nursing. *Nursing Outlook, 26,* 113–120.

Fawcett, J. (1992). Conceptual models and nursing practice: The reciprocal relationship. *Journal of Advanced Nursing, 17,* 224–228.

Flexner, A. (1915). Is social work a profession? *School Soc, 1,* 901–911.

Hamilton, N., & Bhatti, T. (1996). *Population health promotion: An integrated model of population health and health promotion.* Ottawa: Health Canada, Health Promotion and Development Division.

Health Canada. (1998). *Taking action on population health.* Ottawa: Author, Population Health Development Division.

Johnson, J. (1991). Nursing science: Basic, applied, or practical? Implications for the art of nursing. *Advances in Nursing Science, 14,* 7–16.

Kalish, P. A., & Kalish, B. J. (1995). *The advance of American nursing* (3rd ed). Philadelphia: J. B. Lippincott.

Kozier, B. B, & DuGas, B. W. (1967). *Fundamentals of patient care: A comprehensive approach to patient care.* Philadelphia, PA: W. B. Saunders.

Lupton, D. (1995). *The imperative of health: Public health and the regulated body.* London: Sage.

MacDonald, M. (2002). Health promotion: Historical, philosophical, and theoretical perspectives. In L. E. Young & V. Hayes (Eds.), *Transforming health promotion practice: Concepts, issues, and applications* (pp. 22–45). Philadelphia, PA: F. A. Davis.

Meleis, A. (1985). *Theoretical nursing: Development and progress.* Philadelphia, PA: J. B. Lippincott.

Mitchell, G. J. (2001). Policy, procedure, and routine: Matters of moral influence. *Nursing Science Quarterly, 14,*109–114.

Newman, M. (1994). *Health as expanding consciousness* (2nd ed.). New York: National League for Nursing.

Oldnall, A. S. (1995). Nursing as an emerging academic discipline. *Journal of Advanced Nursing, 21,* 605–612.

Parse, R. R. (1987). *Nursing science: Major paradigms, theories, and critiques.* Philadelphia, PA: W. B. Saunders.

Parse, R. R. (1999). Nursing: The discipline and the profession. *Nursing Science Quarterly, 12,* 275.

Parse, R. R. (200la). Language and the sow-reap rhythm. *Nursing Science Quarterly, 14,* 273.

Parse, R. R. (2001b). *Qualitative inquiry: The path of sciencing.* Sudbury, MA: Jones and Bartlett.

Phillips, J. R. (1996). What constitutes nursing science? *Nursing Science Quarterly, 9,* 48–49.

Purkis, M. E. (1997). The "social determinants" of practice? A critical analysis of health promoting discourse. *Canadian Journal of Nursing Research, 29,* 47–62.

Registered Nurses Association of British Columbia. (1998, March). *Standards for nursing practice in British Columbia* (Pub. No. 128). Vancouver, BC: Author.

Registered Nurses Association of British Columbia. (2003, September). *Education requirements for entry level registered nurses.* Retrieved September 11, 2003, from http://www.rnabc.bc.ca/pdf/347.pdf

Schlotfeldt, R. M. (1989). Structuring nursing knowledge: A priority for creating nursing's future. *Nursing Science Quarterly, 2,* 14–18.

The Author Comments

Nursing: Whose Discipline Is It Anyway?

This article was inspired by my passion for nursing as a scientific discipline and my commitment to creating opportunities for students to advance as nurse scholars. My coauthors participated in creating this article during their time as graduate students with me at the University of Victoria. I believe that such opportunities help students to create new understandings and to choose from among options as they confront the familiar and unfamiliar and strive to achieve their goals. It is a testament to their courage and integrity. This article contributes to nursing theory in the 21st century through them and all those who wish to examine what has value and importance for them, their discipline, and their profession.

—Deborah Thoun Northrup

An Analysis of Changing Trends in Philosophies of Science on Nursing Theory Development and Testing

Mary C. Silva
Daniel Rothbart

The effects of changing trends in philosophies of science on nursing theory development and testing are analyzed. Two philosophies of science—logical empiricism and historicism—are compared for four variables: (a) components of science, (b) conception of science, (c) assessment of scientific progress, and (d) goal of philosophy of science. These factors serve as the basis for assessing trends in the development and testing of nursing theory from 1964 to the present. The analysis shows a beginning philosophic shift within nursing theory from logical empiricism to historicism and addresses implications and recommendations for future nursing theory development and testing.

Both philosophy of science and nursing theory are in a state of transition. At times this transition is characterized by contradictory, divergent, and confusing points of view that lead to probing questions about the nature of science in general and nursing theory and science in particular. What are the goals and components of science? How should science be conceptualized and scientific knowledge assessed? Have nursing theory development and testing kept pace with changing trends in philosophies of science?

The goal of this analysis is to show the influences of changing trends in philosophies of science on nursing theory development and testing and to encourage dialogue among nurses about the future directions of nursing theory.

Philosophies of Science

Since the 1940s, two major schools of philosophical thought have influenced philosophy of science: logical

traditions, as illustrated by the nursing research traditions of holism and particularism. According to Laudan (1977), three specific components make up a research tradition: (a) specific theories, (b) ontological commitments, and (c) methodological commitments. Some of the specific theories within a given research tradition are new and others are modified versions of older theories that "fit" within the tradition. The function of any theory is to solve scientific problems within the discipline, from the perspective of the research tradition's, ontological commitments. If, for example, one ontological commitment of a research tradition is holism, various theories within this research tradition might address the problem of how to view the person as a holistic being without looking at parts.

In addition to specific theories and ontological commitments, the third component, methodological commitments, is also essential for a research tradition. Methodological commitments define the legitimate methods of inquiry and experimental procedures that are inseparably linked to a research tradition's ontology. To follow the logic of the above example, would not the case study method of inquiry better preserve the ontological commitment to holism than the elemental design method of inquiry with its built-in reductionism?

The components of a scientific system, according to historicists like Laudan, are multiple research traditions, each containing theories that produce a set of ontological viewpoints and methods of inquiry that are not only essentially compatible with the research tradition but also capable of solving problems within it.

Conception of Science

Based on this comparison of the components of science for logical empiricism and historicism, it is apparent that the two schools assume very different views about what science means. Logical empiricists do not understand science in terms of the human activities of working scientists (e.g., experimenting and compiling data). Instead, they conceive of science only in terms of the results of these activities. The term *science* refers only to a product; i.e., a set of statements that purportedly constitute the body of scientific knowledge. The product includes scientific terminology and definitions, propositions, hypotheses,

theories, and laws. This conception of science as product rests on the philosophical goal of articulating the logical foundations of scientific knowledge (Rudner, 1966). Within this viewpoint, it is important to recognize that logical empiricists are not interested in how scientific hypotheses are conceived but rather in how they can be sufficiently supported by empirical evidence. Their emphasis is one of theory validation, not theory discovery (Rudner, 1966).

In contrast, historicists understand science as a process of human behavior and thought exhibited by practicing scientists. Historicists would be interested in different questions. What reasoning patterns do practicing scientists use to accept or reject a theory? To what extent are scientists influenced by the theory's empirical findings in contrast to the theory's logical elegance in such a decision? How do external factors such as religious convictions influence the scientist's decision-making judgments? To the historicist, every facet of the scientific process is subject to philosophical examination, including the process of explaining how fruitful theories are conceived by practicing scientists. With greater understanding of this process, historicists hope to develop models for future theory construction. Within this scientific viewpoint, valid data for theory construction include:

- The psychological factors of individual scientists
- The social forces on the community of scientists at a particular time
- The overall historical environment, especially the "nonscientific" influences on scientists.

Assessment of Scientific Progress

The assessment of scientific progress within the logical empiricist tradition rests on the ability to justify a scientific theory by examining the requirements for the theory's truth and the conditions of its falsehood. If a scientist can demonstrate the truth of a theory, the scientist has acquired scientific knowledge.

Certain criteria identify theory as false or true. Generally, if a theory's predictions are repeatedly disconfirmed, the logic of testing requires a rejection of the problematic dimensions of the theory, assuming that the observations are correct (Hempel, 1966). But logical empiricists have more difficulty explaining the method of proving that a theory is true. According to the logic of theory testing, no finite number of experiments can conclusively prove that a theory is true. If a theory passes many severe tests, it is only empirically confirmed; that is, the theory's probability of truth has increased. Therefore, to logical empiricists, scientific progress is assessed by the degree of probability that the theory is true, based on the number and severity of empirical tests it passes.

In addition, logical empiricists consider theoretical reduction an important scientific goal. In theoretical reduction, one theory can be absorbed by or reduced to some other inclusive theory. The philosophical advantage of reduction lies not only with the simplicity of fewer theoretical concepts and laws but also with the insight into the ultimate character of reality (Nagel, 1961).

For historicists, the question of whether philosophy of science should try to explain when, if ever, a theory is true or false is the subject of considerable debate. Many agree with Laudan (1977), who argues that philosophy should not search for distinguishing characteristics of true theories, primarily because practicing scientists rarely evaluate theories in terms of truth or falsity. The history of science includes many instances in which a theory was accepted even though it contained scientific anomalies or produced false experimental predictions. Conversely, some theories have been rejected even though they received the most empirical confirmation. Thus, Laudan argues that questions about truth are essentially irrelevant to scientific progress. The relevant element is the theory's problem-solving effectiveness; a theory's progress is defined by the degree to which it solves more scientific problems than its rivals. As stated by Laudan, "*the solved problem—empirical or conceptual—is the basic unit of scientific progress*" (Laudan, 1977, p. 66).

Historicists such as Laudan find reductionism counterproductive to the goal of solving scientific problems. Research traditions should not be seen as competitors trying to mutually undermine each other rather as collaborators toward the goal of solving scientific problems. This process of synthesizing

research traditions, thus expanding them, is called the "integration of research traditions," according to Laudan (1977). Two ways in which this integration may occur are described:

1. One research tradition can be grafted onto another without any major modifications in the components of either.
2. Two or more research traditions may each sacrifice fundamental elements that have been refuted while combining their remaining elements in a new way.

An important scientific motivation for integrating research traditions is the goal of explaining different dimensions of the same phenomena under study. For example, in nursing, the integration of divergent research traditions from biology, psychology, and sociology can account for the ontological perspective that individuals are bio-psychosocial beings, which is common in nursing. This pattern of conjoining fundamental perspectives from different traditions is common when scientists develop new interdisciplinary fields of study to account for previously unexplained scientific problems. The integration of research traditions and corresponding theories is shown in Figure 10-1.

Laudan's analysis of integration departs significantly from the logical empiricist contention that science progresses through the elimination of theories by reduction.

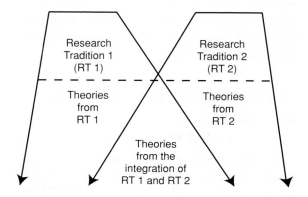

Figure 10-1 *A conceptualization of the integration of research traditions and corresponding theories within historicism.*

But the process of integration does not involve elimination by reducing one tradition to another, because both traditions retain their identity. Integration aims at extracting the progressive components of each tradition in a way that produces solutions to previously unsolved problems.

Goal of Philosophy of Science

According to logical empiricists, the ultimate goal of philosophy of science is to present a formalized account of the nature of scientific knowledge. This includes an application of logical principles to questions about the nature of science, since logic provides the eternal principles for relationships between scientific statements. By examining these relationships, the foundation of science is intended to systematically reveal the logical requirements for all scientific knowledge.

Historicists share with logical empiricists the belief that the philosopher's task is to construct a general account of the nature of scientific knowledge. But for historicists like Laudan, such a task must conform to the human elements of scientific evolution and growth. To meet this goal, historicists engage in studies of the actual activities, behavior patterns, and reasoning processes of working scientists. The belief is that philosophy of science must show how science, as it is actually practiced, can yield knowledge about the world. Such examination of the actual practice of scientists is used by historicists as evidence against logical empiricism, because the growth of scientific knowledge seems at times to be aided by illogical and nonrational decision making. It is believed that illogical processes can contribute to create growth of knowledge within a discipline.

Nursing Theory Development and Testing

Since 1964, nurse scholars have become more aware of the influences of philosophy—in particular philosophy of science—on the development of nursing theory. A review of significant and representative nursing theory literature within three time periods shows the status of nursing theory in regard to logical empiricist and historicist trends in philosophy of science.

1964 to 1969

An important influence on nursing theory development during the 1960s was support given by the Division of Nursing of the U.S. Department of Health, Education, and Welfare (now the Department of Health and Human Services) to nursing schools to sponsor programs on the nature and development of nursing science. An analysis of metatheoretical papers from the proceedings of two such conferences—the Symposium on Theory Development in Nursing held at Case Western Reserve University in 1968 and the Conference on the Nature of Science in Nursing held at the University of Colorado in 1969—gives insight into how nurse scholars and others during the late 1960s conceptualized the derivation of nursing knowledge.

In 1968, Dickoff and James presented a version of their position paper on a theory of theories, introducing the idea that significant nursing theory must be situation producing. Although they modified the orthodox view about the purpose of theory—that is, they postulated that theory could be capable of both more than and less than prediction—they, nevertheless, explicitly stated their faithfulness to the logical empiricist tradition. They forthrightly spoke of their work as a broader interpretation of the writings of such philosophers as Nagel (1961) and Hempel (1965, 1966). The language they used to describe theory supports logical empiricism. They spoke of concepts, propositions, set; they assessed scientific progress in terms of truth; and they insisted on a product orientation to science (i.e., production of desired situations).

In 1969, Abdellah discussed the nature of nursing science. Although no mention was made per se of the writings of philosophers who supported logical empiricism, Abdellah's views of what constitutes a scientific theory were nevertheless consistent with their writings; that is, terms must be operationally defined and preferably observable and quantifiable. Postulates are validated by testing deductions, which either helps to confirm the theory or leads to modifications of the postulates. Abdellah concludes that the reward of nurse scientists for their efforts is the discovery and affirmation of truth. Thus, as with Dickoff and James (1968), the criterion for the assessment of scientific progress is an increase in scientific truths.

Other writings (Dickoff, James, & Widenbach, 1968a, 1968b) related to nursing theory development and testing during the late 1960s all tended to have a logical empiricist perspective, with the exception of Leininger's (1969) introductory comments to the Conference on the Nature of Science in Nursing, which offered an ethnoscience research methodology to the discovery of scientific knowledge. This approach stresses the viewing of behavior from the subject's perspective rather than the researcher's. This accommodation to subjectivism is more compatible with historicism than with the objectivism of logical empiricism.

1970 to 1975

In the first half of the 1970s, two major trends in nursing theory occurred:

1. Metatheoretical formulations relevant to nursing theory and testing within the logical empiricist tradition were developed to a high degree by such investigators as Jacox (1974) and Hardy (1974).
2. A number of conceptual frameworks for nursing were published; for example, the work of Rogers (1970), King (1971), Orem (1971), and Roy (1974).

According to Jacox (1974), the goal of science is the discovery of truths, and the purpose of scientific theory is description, explanation, and prediction of part of our empirical world. In discussing theory construction, Jacox uses the language of the logical empiricists, including concepts, propositions, axioms, and theorems. Hardy (1974) is even more oriented to the formal logic underlying logical empiricism, discussing nine possible relationships that can exist between concepts and presenting a diagrammatic and matrix presentation of a situation that shows (a) the concepts, (b) the sign of the relationship between concepts, and (c) the nature of the relationships between concepts.

These two articles represented a culmination of the metatheoretical notions about logical empiricism in nursing theory. The irony, of course, is that at the time these and similar reports were making a profound impact on the derivation of theory in nursing, the logical

empiricist view-points espoused in them were being strongly repudiated by a growing number of philosophers of science. In other words, nursing's theoretical link to philosophy of science was, from the historicist perspective, about a decade behind the times.

The irony continues in regard to the second trend—the publication of a number of important conceptual frameworks for nursing. Several conceptual frameworks published in the early 1970s were essentially devoid of any explicit linkage to philosophy of science (King, 1971; Orem, 1971). This is in no way meant to diminish the quality or significance of these seminal works but only to point out that a situation existed in which the most influential nursing literature on theory construction and testing followed rather than preceded the derivation of the conceptual frameworks, apparently because the metatheoretical movement in nursing was, for the most part, a separate movement from the conceptual framework movement.

1976 to Present

Since 1976, the following trends have occurred:

1. A continued and relatively stable commitment to logical empiricism, although a beginning trend toward historicism is apparent;
2. A revision of several conceptual frameworks for nursing and the introduction of some new frameworks; and
3. A questioning of the adequacy of strictly quantitative research methods to test nursing theory deductions.

The relatively stable commitment to logical empiricism is reflected in the current writings of several nurse authors (Chinn & Jacobs, 1983; Fawcett, 1983; Menke, 1983; Walker & Avant, 1983). However, there are some new trends. For example, in 1979 when Newman introduced a new theory of health, the viewpoint was one of logical empiricism. However, in a recent work (1983), a shift in her thinking is evident. Reflecting the thoughts of Kuhn (a historicist), Newman defines science as "a process of knowing, a process of challenging, and a continuing revolution" (Newman, 1983, p. 387). This emphasis on process (not product) and revolution (not logic) is a noticeable shift in viewpoint from logical empiricism to historicism.

In a recent publication, Hardy (1983) also extensively cited Kuhn in discussing nursing theory. The primary emphasis is on metaparadigms; however, Hardy also seems to agree, at least implicitly, with Kuhn's definition of the development of scientific knowledge as both nonrational and noncumulative. This represents a marked shift in viewpoint from the 1974 Hardy article, which, of all the metatheoretical articles, represented the most rigorous and logically structured formulations in support of logical empiricism. These contradictions in the works of Hardy and other metatheorists are indicative of the pull between orthodox and new ideas in philosophy of science and in nursing theory development and testing.

Although several other nurse authors (Carper, 1978; MacPherson, 1983; Meleis, 1983; Menke, 1983; Munhall, 1982) briefly address Kuhn's *The Structure of Scientific Revolutions,* with the exception of Meleis (1983) they do not discuss Kuhn's more recent writings or mention Laudan's work, which represents the forefront of philosophy of science today. However, Laudan's work is briefly mentioned in an article by Watson (1981) and cited in the bibliographies of books by Parse (1981) and Chinn and Jacobs (1983). Although this attention to the work of Laudan is scant, it is encouraging because it begins to bring the development of nursing theory knowledge in line with current trends in philosophy of science.

The second trend occurring between 1976 and the present is the expansion and revision of the works of those nurse authors who in the early 1970s had developed conceptual frameworks for nursing. For example, first editions of books and other publications were rewritten, expanded, or revised by Orem (1980), King (1981), Roy (1981), Roy and Roberts (1981), and Rogers (1980). Several of these nurse theorists, in an attempt to bring their works more in line with what the nurse metatheorists of the mid-1970s were espousing—logical empiricism—revised their works to explicitly identify such elements as concepts and propositions that are inherent in the orthodox viewpoint.

Thus, an interesting situation has been created: While these nurse theorists have been updating trends in philosophy of science as espoused in the nursing literature of the mid-1970s, those who espoused these views have begun to question them and some no longer espouse them. This is not to say that individuals should not alter their viewpoints but to point out again the seeming separateness of the metatheoretical and conceptual framework movement in nursing and the effect of this separateness on perpetuating traditional or singular viewpoints about philosophy of science.

Two other conceptual frameworks were developed in books published in 1976 by Paterson and Zderad and in 1981 by Parse. Neither book has received much attention in the nursing literature, although there is some evidence that this is changing (Chinn & Jacobs, 1983; King 1981). Could it be that both of these books have a strong existential-phenomenological perspective that, until recently, was out of the mainstream of the thinking of orthodox nurse scientists about philosophy of science? The underlying assumptions these three authors hold about the nature of science are much more in keeping with nontraditional views about philosophy of science than with traditional views. In particular, they see science as process; they envision a strong link between the theory's ontological commitment and its methodological commitment; and they place little emphasis on precise, logical formulations.

The third trend is a shift in emphasis from quantitative to qualitative research methods to test nursing theory deduction. In the late 1970s, nurse scholars (Silva, 1977) began to question the limits of quantitative research methods because they too often sacrificed meaningfulness for rigor. Out of this questioning, articles suggesting alternative approaches to logical empiricism began to appear in the nursing literature (Munhall, 1982; Oiler, 1982; Omery, 1983; Swanson & Chenitz, 1982; Tinkle & Beaton, 1983; Watson, 1981). These approaches were sought because of the inadequacy of logical empiricism to deal with certain phenomena in nursing, in particular, those phenomena dealing with humanism and holism. By exploring alternative philosophies of science and research methodologies that are compatible, it seems possible to study these phenomena in a more meaningful and creative way and, in so doing, to help bridge the gaps among philosophies of science, nursing theory, and nursing research. Historicism is one of the alternative philosophies that holds promise in helping to bridge these gaps.

Implications and Recommendations for the Future

Since every scientific theory is tied to some philosophical framework as the basis for understanding and assessing theory, it is important for the theorists within a given discipline to be aware of the discipline's philosophical orientation. Therefore, nursing theorists should continue to explore the philosophical underpinnings of their discipline in order to integrate the latest advances in nursing theory development and testing with a coherent philosophical foundation.

This review of the trends in nursing theory from 1964 to the present shows not only that nursing theory is presently in a state of transition, but also that many of the changes in nursing theory reflect a reorientation of the underlying philosophy of the discipline. This is evident in the beginning metatheoretical shift away from a strongly empirical and logical orientation to theory construction reminiscent of logical empiricism and toward a more holistic and humanist approach more in line with historicism. There are several implications for nursing theory development and testing:

- Laudan dismisses as counterproductive the logical empirical goal of reducing one theory to another. Rather than trying to restrict the range of possible theories, Laudan encourages theory expansion through a process of integrating components from different research traditions, which results in a multidimensional understanding of the phenomena. Based on this historicist orientation, there should not be a single, conceptual framework for nursing. This orientation suggests, rather, the expansion of nursing theory through the integration of progressive components of the various existing nursing conceptual frameworks, which results in multiple frameworks. This process should be a cooperative endeavor and, if adhered to, should encourage a cooperative rather than a competitive attitude among nurse scholars. In the future some of the conceptual frameworks for nursing may be integrated so that the unimportant elements are sacrificed and the important elements are combined in a new way.

- The historicist's conception of science as a human process, rather than a product of some endeavor, suggests that nursing theory should always be understood as a stage in its evolution and growth. Although nursing theory is experiencing shifts in its evolution, the result of the transition will not be some final and static body of knowledge. Like any scientific discipline, nursing theory construction will never culminate in some static set of eternal truths but will represent one episode in its evolving history.

- Historicism strongly encourages a careful study of the actual practices, belief systems, and external factors influencing a community of scientists within a given discipline. This has a direct bearing on the type of data relevant for any theory construction. Thus, data for nursing theory development and testing will include the common practices of nurse clinicians, the social and psychological factors affecting the profession of nursing, the widely held beliefs of the community of nurses, and the reasoning patterns of individual nurse theorists. A result of integrating these data will be a nursing theory that more explicitly addresses the human dimensions of nursing and the practitioners of nursing.

- Scientific progress for Laudan reduces to the number of solved problems within a discipline. Therefore, the assessment of progress in nursing theory development and testing will be less rigid and more practical than suggested by a logical empiricist orientation. That is, there will be less emphasis on truth and error as the criteria for assessing scientific progress and more emphasis on the actual solution to nursing care problems. This shift should help to bridge the gap between those persons who are primarily nurse scholars and those who are primarily

CHAPTER 11

Nursing Reformation: Historical Reflections and Philosophic Foundations

Pamela G. Reed

Nursing is in the throes of reform. We are speaking more openly about graduate education as the level of entry for practice, more boldly about the art and spiritual dimensions of nursing care, more matter-of-factly about the necessity of science-based practice, and more creatively about nursing's philosophy and unique methods of building knowledge. Reform means to amend or improve by change of form or removal of faults or abuses (Webster's New Collegiate Dictionary, 1993). But will the changes be radical enough to make a positive difference for those within the discipline, those contemplating a career choice, and those who work and are served within healthcare systems?

When we contemplate the roots of professional nursing in reference to contemporary nursing, it is evident that we have not yet mined the full implications of nursing initiated by Nightingale (1859/1969) in the 19th century and carried forward by other visionaries during the 20th century. Nursing has evolved into a disintegrated profession, due largely to factions of variously educated nurses. The purpose of this dialogue is to propose ideas for clarifying philosophic foundations for reforming nursing in the 21st century.

Historical Reflections

There is a need to revive the roots of professional nursing's existence. These roots are found in Nightingale's (1895/1969) emancipatory spirit for nursing and for her

About the Author

PAMELA G. REED is Professor at the University of Arizona College of Nursing in Tucson, Arizona, where she also served as Associate Dean for Academic Affairs for 7 years. She is a three-time graduate of Wayne State University in Detroit, receiving a BSN in 1974, an MSN in 1976 (with a double major in child–adolescent psychiatric mental health nursing and teaching), and her PhD (with a major in nursing, focused on life-span development and aging) in 1982. Dr. Reed pioneered research into spirituality and well-being with her doctoral research with terminally ill patients. She also developed a theory of self-transcendence and two widely used research instruments, the *Spiritual Perspective Scale* and the *Self-Transcendence Scale*. Her publications and funded research reflect a dual scholarly focus: Spirituality and other facilitators of well-being and decisions in end-of-life transitions: nursing metatheory and knowledge development. Dr. Reed also enjoys time with her family, reading, classical music, swimming, and hiking in the mountains and canyons of Arizona.

patients to not only be well, but to use well every power they have; her spiritual commitment concerning the role of nursing; her clarity of a philosophy for nursing that was both scientific and caring; her revolutionary ideas about formally educating nurses, distinct from other healthcare providers; her pragmatism in addressing the health needs of society; and her vision for nursing as a profession. Despite nurse leaders' revolutionary ideas about health reform, university-based education, theory development, and research during the past 100 years, nursing's roots have not developed the discipline as fully as desired.

Service needs of hospitals and physicians have exploited the nursing vision, twisted its roots and choked potential growth that could have been realized in great part through higher education. There is still a proliferation of technical "nursing" training fostered by political interests and profit-driven employers who quell nursing shortages, and the viability of professional nursing, with employment of nonprofessional "nurses." State boards of nursing, with one exception, maintain an outdated, unenlightened, and dispiriting system of nurse licensure. Furthermore, what occupies too much of state boards' time is implementing disciplinary action against nurses whose most common error, amid all that they do, is the implementation of physicians' (medication) orders. The relentless, dependent activity of passing medications, as well as transcribing, filling, and requesting other orders,

sustains the need for undereducated "nurses" and erodes the creativity and autonomy that could be nursing.

Professional nurses, by definition, are morally obligated to work within their field and to have a knowledge base adequate for ordering their own actions, especially for direct patient care, whether ambulating patients, talking with a grieving family, or distributing medications. And physicians must take the responsibility for fulfilling their own orders. Nurses who identify with the oppressor by integrating if not embracing medical practice across nursing roles, whether advanced, basic, or technical, rob from the potential to advance nursing care. So do nurses, as CEOs and directors, academic administrators, and teachers, who have the leadership but lack the vision and expertise to implement nursing models of care in their systems, and who lack the courage to speak the language of nursing in their daily work.

The tangled roots of nursing are due also in part to the entry-into-practice debacle from the 1960s and the so-called diversity in educational offerings. Well-meaning and not-so-well-meaning officials are trying to reframe the diverse and disintegrated condition of nursing preparation today with euphemisms that speak of promoting a continuum of practice and therefore a continuum of education, as though something less than a baccalaureate degree provides a foundation for professional nursing education. This continuum may better serve the hospitals than the science.

such that qualifying words are often needed to explain holism. For some, holism conjures up vague and sometimes unattainable expectations and stifles attempts to conjecture about nursing phenomena.

It is not inaccurate to describe nursing as a holistic discipline. However, if holism is applicable to only a certain part of the nursing community, as the qualifier in the term holistic nursing implies, then holism is not useful in conveying an integrative perspective for nursing. Alternatively, if the essence of nursing is holism, then use of the term holistic nursing is redundant; the term *nursing* should stand alone. It is more productive to spend our efforts identifying terms that clarify the substance of nursing rather than the substance of holism. These terms will better serve our research and practice endeavors to unite nurses in a deeper understanding of what their discipline is all about.

Thesis 3: Embodiment Is a Core Concept in Understanding Health Experiences

The linguistic focus of postmodernism has emphasized the role of language and discourse in building knowledge. The social, cultural, and political dimensions have garnered recognition of their roles in scientific inquiry. Terms like spiritual, self-transcendence, perception, and consciousness, which tend to emphasize mind over body, have gained increased attention. Nevertheless, embodiment remains a critical context for nursing inquiry into health experiences (Wilde, 1999).

Dewey (1929) addressed the dichotomy in knowledge development found between discursive and nondiscursive experiences, mind and body. He, along with other pragmatists, argued for the importance of nondiscursive experience and he, in fact, posited that nondiscursive experience is foundational to all thinking. Shusterman (1997) extended Dewey's views in a more integrative manner by arguing the need for philosophy to value the somatic as well as the linguistic and rational experience. This was justified, he said, given philosophy's pragmatic goal of not only grounding knowledge but producing a better experience. He proposed, radically, that somatics should be integrated into the discursive practices of philosophy, and in the practices of other disciplines interested in promoting transformation and betterment of life. Similarly, Schneider (1998) called for a revival of romanticism in science and advocated for a more balanced approach to post-modern inquiry that included exploration of peoples' felt impressions, bodily sensations, and existential awareness.

The integration of somatic experience into nursing inquiry helps bridge the gap between the worlds of the patient, the practitioner, and the researcher. The body is an important manifestation of the human being, around which much in nursing revolves. As Gadow (1980) explained, the self is inseparable from the body, and nursing philosophy cannot address human health experiences in abstraction from the existential ground, the body. The quest for nursing knowledge, then, occurs not only through the discursive modes of philosophic inquiry and the research process, but also by attending to the embodiment of health processes and practices.

Thesis 4: Scientific Knowledge Is Transformed Into Nursing Knowledge Through Contexts of Nursing Practice

This fourth thesis moves us beyond traditional and disintegrative pathways of developing and distributing knowledge, that is, moving from the top down, from theorist and researcher to practitioner. Putnam (1988), a contemporary philosopher who espouses a pragmatic approach to philosophy, explained that the traditional pathway to epistemologic justification, from the theoretical to the more observable concepts, was only one approach to knowledge development. He proposed that theory development proceed in all directions, in any direction that may be handy. Philosopher Nancy Cartwright (1988) elaborated on this idea in explaining that it is not enough to know a given law of nature and deduce other occurrences from that law, as one would using Hempel's (1966) covering law. That is to say that nature is not so well-regulated and independent of context that events can be determined from a given law. Science, she explained, cannot shut down once a law is put forward. Rather, explanations entail ongoing consideration of data from an integration of various ways of knowing, of which we have identified many in nursing: empiric, personal, ethical, aesthetic, unknowing, and intuition, to mention some. Similarly, philosopher Susan Haack (1996) argued against the received (realist) view of truth and the perceived (relativist) view of truth as being the only options for selecting an approach to developing knowledge in a discipline. Instead, she proposed a new term that represented a synthesis of the two dichotomous views, foundationalism and coherence, which she called "foundherentism." Foundherentism was a better justified and more practical approach to building knowledge, in which both experience and beliefs provided an epistemologic basis.

In realizing the meaning of Carper's (1978) nursing epistemology and other postmodern perspectives, nursing began reforming its traditional top-down approach to building knowledge. More nurses are using approaches that privilege the experiences and beliefs of multiple individuals, including researcher, practitioner, and patient.

Professional nurses are people who, in their practice, ethically and skillfully engage patients and themselves in application and testing of knowledge. This engagement transforms scientific knowledge into nursing knowledge (Reed, 1996). The mutual process between nurses and patients or, more broadly, between persons and their environments provides contexts for both the discovery and confirmation of knowledge.

Thesis 5: Nursing Is a Spiritual Discipline

Spiritual is defined as existing in an intentional community with others where otherness is an unreduced intrusion into the experience of each person (S. G. Smith, 1988). While intentions are shared across the community, the individuals are neither diminished nor supplanted by the community. In applying this interpretation of spirituality in nursing, it can be said that the nurse participates with the patient, sharing intentions about health through the intimacy and skill of touch and talk. Intentions are spiritual, focused on health as experienced wholeness.

A spiritual discipline is distinguished from the psychosocial sciences in that it is not merely descriptive of behaviors but rather poses a normative and pragmatic call to action, which is freely chosen. A spiritual person is said to be "called" or "launched outward to others to inhabit a world that transcends one's own world" (S. G. Smith, 1988, p. 62). The spiritual is directed toward "enabling, supporting, growing, loving, respecting, and appreciating" (Lane, 1988, p. 335). A spiritual person, like a poet, discovers new things and ideas from "beyond the horizon of the self" (S. G. Smith, 1988, p. 71) for the benefit and transformation of others.

Regarding a profession as spiritual enhances the meaning of a profession. It is more than compassion; it requires a sense of self-transcendence, connectedness to others, a desire to promote life, and a sense of freedom in choosing these things (Lane, 1988). This perspective nourishes the aesthetic as well as other ways of knowing required within a discipline.

The spiritual, then, is a philosophic basis for praxis, uniting values and knowledge with actions in accord with patients' needs for healthcare. In so doing, the spiritual is integrative and promotes unity within a discipline.

Toward Scholarship and Praxis in Nursing

Paradoxically, postmodernism has provided us with an awareness of our freedom to turn toward philosophic foundations to create a possibility for unity within a complex discipline characterized by much diversity. We have come to understand that there is no dichotomy between the theoretical and observable. Kant (1781/1964), Popper (1965), and contemporary philosophers of science have argued convincingly that there is no observation in the absence of theory and values. In nursing, this epistemologic view translates into the realization that some of the distinctions drawn between practitioner and researcher may be reformed in an integrative way to enhance development of nursing knowledge and patient care. This was not so 30 years ago, when Ellis' (1969) idea of practitioner as theorist was dismissed by modernist nurses who regarded science as an endeavor separate from art, values, and practices of nursing.

Contemporary pragmatic approaches to knowledge development diminish the dichotomy between the theoretical and the observable, theory and practice, beliefs and experience. The theses presented here have posited a nursing ontology based upon a relational, embodied, and processual view of health. This view necessitates an epistemology that involves both the scientist's and the practitioner's expertise within what Lerner (1995) called the natural laboratory of the world. Scientific knowledge, which is generated outside of this natural laboratory, is transformed into nursing knowledge by its integration within contexts of nursing practice.

A nursing reformation that derives from an integrated philosophy of nursing is not likely to end in revolt and further divisions. But successful reform will require a type of symbolic home where a diversity of theories and ideas can flourish within a spiritual community of shared values and beliefs. Trainor (1998) distinguished this home from the unshakable foundation of modernism. He described it instead as a home that offers a foundational faith in the connectedness of our ideas to the world and to each other. Nursing reformation will require the participation of theorists, scientists, and practitioners in a shared vision of nursing and of the education needed for nurses to participate in integrated methods of knowledge development. Within this perspective, a reformation may remove faults that divide nurses and may restore the scholarship and praxis to nursing that Nightingale envisioned.

REFERENCES

American Nurses' Association. (1995). *Nursing: A social policy statement* (Rev. ed.). Washington, DC: Author.

Bishop, A. H., & Scudder, J. R. (1999). A philosophical interpretation of nursing. *Scholarly Inquiry for Nursing Practice, 13,* 17–27.

Carper, B. (1978). Fundamental patterns of knowing in nursing. *Advances in Nursing Science, 1,* 13–23.

Cartwright, N. (1988). The truth doesn't explain much. In E. D. Klemke, R. Hollinger, & A. D. Kline (Eds.), *Philosophy of science* (Rev. ed., pp. 129–136). New York: Prometheus.

Dewey, J. (1929). *Experience and nature* (Rev. ed.). Carbondale: Southern Illinois University Press.

Dolan, J. A. (1968). *History of nursing* (12th ed.). Philadelphia: W. B. Saunders.

Ellis, R. (1969). The practitioner as theorist. *American Journal of Nursing, 69,* 1434–1438.

Gadow, S. (1980). Body and self: A dialectic. In S. Specker & S. Gadow (Eds.), *Existential advocacy: Philosophical foundations of nursing* (pp. 86–100). New York: Springer.

Haack, S. (1996). Evidence and inquiry: Towards reconstruction in epistemology. In M. Warnock (Ed.), *Women philosophers* (pp. 273–299), London: J. M. Dent.

Hempel, C. G. (1966). *Philosophy of natural sciences.* Englewood Cliffs, NJ: Prentice-Hall.

Johnson, M. B. (1990). The holistic paradigm in nursing: The diffusion of an innovation. *Research in Nursing & Health, 13,* 129–139.

Kant I. (1964). *Critique of pure reason* (N. Kemp Smith, Trans). New York: Macmillan. (Original work published in 1781).

Kolcaba, R. (1997). The primary holisms in nursing. *Journal of Advanced Nursing, 25,* 290–296.

Lane, J. A. (1988). The care of the human spirit. *Journal of Professional Nursing, 36,* 332–337.

Lerner, R. M. (1995). The integrations of levels and human development: A developmental contextual view of the synthesis of science and outreach in the enhancement of human lives. In K. E. Hood, G. Greenberg, & E. Tobah (Eds.), *Behavioral development* (pp. 421–455). New York: Garland.

Newman, M. (1995). *Health as expanding consciousness* (2nd ed.). New York: NLN.

Nightingale, F. (1859/1969). *Notes on nursing: What it is and what it is not.* New York: Dover.

Owen, M. J., & Holmes, C. A. (1993). "Holism" in the discourse of nursing. *Journal of Advanced Nursing, 18,* 1688–1695.

Parse, R. R. (1995). *Illuminations: The human becoming theory in practice and research.* New York: NLN.

Peplau, H. (1992). Interpersonal relations: A theoretical framework for application in nursing practice. *Nursing Science Quarterly, 5,* 13–18.

Popper, K. R. (1965). *Conjectures and refutations: The growth of scientific knowledge.* New York: Harper.

Putnam, H. (1988). What theories are not. In E. D. Klemke, R. Holllinger, & A. D. Kline (Eds.), *Philosophy of science* (Rev. ed., pp. 178–183). New York: Prometheus.

Reed, P. G. (1996). Transforming knowledge into nursing knowledge: A revisionist analysis of Peplau. *Image: The Journal of Nursing Scholarship 28,* 29–33.

Reed, P. G. (1997). Nursing: The ontology of the discipline. *Nursing Science Quarterly, 10,* 76–79.

Rogers, M. (1990). Nursing: Science of unitary, irreducible human beings: Update 1990. In E. Barrett (Ed.), *Visions of Rogers' science-based nursing* (pp. 5–12). New York: NLN.

Roy, C. (1997). Future of the Roy model: Challenge to redefine adaptation. *Nursing Science Quarterly, 10,* 49–52.

Schlotfeldt, R. M. (1987). Defining nursing: A historic controversy. *Nursing Research, 36,* 64–65.

Schneider, K. J. (1998). Toward a science of the heart. *American Psychologist, 53,* 277–289.

Shusterman, R. (1997). *Practicing philosophy: Pragmatism and the philosophical life.* New York: Routledge.

Smith, M. J. (1988). Perspectives in nursing science. *Nursing Science Quarterly, 1,* 80–85.

Smith, S. G. (1988). *The concept of the spiritual: An essay in first philosophy.* Philadelphia: Temple University Press.

Trainor, B. (1998). The origin and end of modernity. *Journal of Applied Philosophy, 15,* 133–144.

Watson, J. (1997). The theory of human caring: Retrospective and prospective. *Nursing Science Quarterly 10,* 49–52.

Webster's new collegiate dictionary. (1993). Springfield, MA: Merriam-Webster.

Wilde, M. H. (1999). Why embodiment now? *Advances in Nursing Science, 22,* 25–38.

The Author Comments

Nursing Reformation: Historical Reflections and Philosophic Foundations

The impetus for this article came from a contributing editor of *Nursing Science Quarterly,* Dr. Marilyn Rawnsley, who provided me the wonderful opportunity to write about what I believed was significant as nursing moved into the 21st century. As an educator, an administrator, and a nurse, I was frustrated with the state of nursing practice education, which in its diverse forms was incongruous with visions of the kind of education professional nursing requires, nursing shortages notwithstanding. I grounded my ideas in historical visions of nursing, still unrealized, in terms of a truly independently functioning profession. I wanted to expose some key philosophic issues (presented as my "theses") in reforming nursing from within the discipline to put forth a philosophic basis for professional nursing.

—PAMELA G. REED

CHAPTER 12

Theoretical Thinking in Practice

This unit was designed to increase awareness about the theoretical thinking that occurs in nursing practice. The ideas of two noted theorists in nursing history, Rosemary Ellis and Hildegard Peplau, are anchors for this unit. They put forth their progressive philosophy about the dynamic link between practice and theory long before it was fashionable in nursing. Contemporary thought in other articles reveals that nursing is beginning to embrace their vision; practice is no longer the passive recipient of theory. Rather, practice and theory form a reciprocal process in the development of knowledge. The movement toward advanced practice nursing and the practice doctorate will help resurrect this idea and provide the human capital to enact it.

Philosophies and theories of knowledge (epistemology) both within nursing and in other disciplines are presented in his unit as well as in Units Four, Five, and Six. These ideas have stimulated new insights about theoretical thinking—who does it and how it is done.

The chapters in this unit demonstrate some of the approaches to foster links between theory and practice, using practice as inquiry for theory building as well as theory application. Whether we speak of nursing theory-guided practice or practice-guided theory, a key to developing nursing knowledge is built upon the conception of an inseparability of theory and practice.

Questions for Discussion

- Should theory arise out of extant practice or from visions of what practice should or could be?
- Do practitioners have time to theorize?
- Is theorizing inherent to practice?
- What role do patients play in nursing theorizing?
- Does the knowledge that nurses use in practice differ from the knowledge put forth in researchers' theories?

About the Authors

GWENETH HARTRICK DOANE was born in Regina, Saskatchewan. Her educational background includes a diploma and baccalaureate degree in nursing, a master's in counseling psychology, and an interdisciplinary PhD (nursing/psychology). She is currently a professor in the School of Nursing and Associate Dean in the Faculty of Graduate Studies at the University of Victoria in British Columbia. Her scholarly work has focused on relational practice and epistemology, and she has taken this interest into the domains of family nursing, nursing ethics, and teaching and learning in higher education. Dr. Doane's major contributions to the discipline have included the retheorizing of 'knowing' and nursing practice within those domains. She enjoys adventures and travels with her children, Pilates and movement awareness classes, singing with a choir, and spending time with friends.

COLLEEN VARCOE was born in Killarney, Manitoba. She holds a Registered Nurse diploma from the Royal Columbian Hospital School of Nursing, a baccalaureate in Nursing, master's degrees in education and nursing, and a PhD in nursing. She currently runs a paragliding school with her partner, runs and works out, gardens, and parties. Dr. Varcoe is currently an Associate Professor at the University of British Columbia School of Nursing. Her scholarship focuses on women's health with an emphasis on violence against women and a particular interest in Aboriginal women's health, and the culture of health care with an emphasis on nursing ethics and ethical practice. Her key contributions to the discipline include the text *Family Nursing as Relational Inquiry* (2005), co-authored with Gweneth Doane, and the edited text *Women's Health in Canada: Critical Perspectives on Theory and Policy* (2007), co-edited with Marina Morrow and Olena Hankivsky.

that has no relevance to the "real" world of practice. This tendency to objectify theory—to separate it out from everyday "real" practice and think of it as a "thing" to be applied and used—has had profound implications for theory development and nursing practice. It has not only constrained the theory-development process but also ultimately served to limit nurses' choices, clinical decision making, and their capacity for ethically responsive practice.[2]

In contrast to this objectifying approach to theory, we concur with pragmatist philosophers who believe that all so-called "theory" is always already practice.[4–6] While this idea is not necessarily a new one to nursing, we believe that its significance has not been adequately examined. Specifically, it is our intent to illustrate the integral role practice experiences play in the ongoing development of theory and the potential a pragmatic orientation has to not only enhance theory development in nursing but also reshape the everyday moments of nursing practice. In this article, we illustrate the utility of pragmatism to nursing by

describing how we have explicitly approached theory development as a practical (and practice) activity of inquiry to attend to diversity in family nursing. Although elsewhere[3] we have explicitly turned our attention to difference and diversity in terms of religion and spirituality, health and healing practices, sexual orientation, ethnicity and race, by way of illustration, we focus in this article on how a pragmatic approach to theory has enabled us to conceptualize "family" and "culture" in ways that support more responsive and socially just nursing practice.

A Pragmatic Understanding of Theory

The term *pragmatism* is derived from the Greek word meaning action, from which the words "practice" and "practical" also come.[7] Roth recounts that pragmatism was first introduced into philosophy by Charles Peirce in 1878, who pointed out that beliefs are really rules for action. Peirce contended that the sole significance of a thought or concept was the conduct it produced. Pragmatism is a process of clarifying the meaning of a thought and rests upon the principle that meaning is determined by unpacking a concept and/or theory with respect to the practical consequences in future experience.[7] So, for example, pragmatism might ask what a particular concept or theory leads us to expect, to focus upon, to attend to, and to do in our nursing practice. As a process, pragmatism attempts to interpret each theory by tracing its practical consequences. Central questions pragmatism asks include the following: What difference would it practically make to anyone if this notion rather than that notion was held to be true? What concrete difference will any idea or theory make in anyone's actual life? What experiences will be different? What is the value of any theory or idea in experiential terms? If no practical difference can be traced, there is no difference and the thought (or theory) is meaningless in that particular situation.[7]

William James further developed the pragmatic perspective, highlighting that all theories are merely approximations—"They are only a man-made (sic) language, a conceptual shorthand." [6(p 147)] James also contended that "truth" is something that *happens* to an idea. Ideas or theories become true, are *made* true by events, "Truth lives for the most part on a credit system. Our thoughts and beliefs 'pass,' so long as nothing challenges them, just as bank notes pass so long as nobody refuses them."[6(p 163)] For example, within nursing there are many theoretical possibilities when it comes to describing and making sense of a particular situation or experience. Any number of rival formulations may be developed and any one of the theories from some point of view might be useful. As James contends, however, theories and ideas become true (are meaningful) just in so far as they help us to get into satisfactory relation with our experiences and *result in more responsive action.*

In contrast to many philosophical or theoretical perspectives, pragmatism does not stand for any special results. It is only a process. But the significance of that process is the fundamental change it offers in our approach to theory development and to nursing practice.

Theory moves beyond an abstraction that is developed in isolation from everyday practice and becomes a practical activity that is central to every nursing moment. The goal of theory development is no longer to develop a truth or doctrine to follow, nor is it considered useful to compare different theories and/or argue which theory is ultimately more true. From a pragmatic perspective, one cannot look on any idea or theory as "more true" and/or as closing the quest for knowledge. Rather, the process involves setting any and all theory to work within everyday practice experiences and engaging in a continual inquiry to determine the value of the different theories to a particular situation in terms of consequences. Subsequently, theory "appears less as a solution, then, than as a program for more work, and more particularly as an indication of the ways in which existing realities may be changed. Theories thus become instruments, not answers to enigmas, in which we can rest. We don't lie back upon them, we move forward, and, on occasion, make nature over again by their aid. Pragmatism unstifles all our theories, limbers them up and sets each one at work."[6(p 145)]

Opening Spaces for Theory Development Through Pragmatic Inquiry

As an approach to knowledge, pragmatism does not look to any particular results but offers an attitude of orientation to take into practice. This attitude involves looking away from static abstractions and categorical ways of thinking and looking toward possibilities. As such pragmatism does not offer new knowledge "content" but rather a pragmatic "practice" process of theory construction that does not limit or confine our theorizing and/or the theoretical possibilities available to us. Berman's description[8] of the nomad who dwells in the midregion of knowing and moves into knowledge in such a way that seeks to destroy static models rather than develop them mirrors a pragmatic process of theory development. "In the nomadic mind . . . the road to truth is always under construction; the going is the goal . . . For nomads "truth is a verb, something you live. No sooner are you at one point than an elaboration or revision suggests itself." [8](p 198)

Engaging in a pragmatic process of theory development involves living a world presence rather than a worldview.[8] Rather than living from a unified, fixed perspective, one is grounded in immediacy, experience, and practice. As James[6] describes, "Pragmatism is willing to take anything, to follow either logic or the senses and to count the humblest and most personal experiences."[6](p 157) Subsequently, rather than being limited to an intellectual activity, theorizing is seen as an embodied, reflexive process of responsive action.[3] As such, theorizing involves tuning into and critically considering bodily sensing, intuitive and emotional responses, existing theories and research, contextual forces, and so forth. These responses and forces are seen as forms of knowing that can in-form and re-form our in-the-moment knowing actions, that is to say, theoretical practice.

Overall, pragmatism inspires an opening up to theoretical possibilities rather than the development of theoretical doctrines and truths. The pragmatic process is a process of inquiry and choice. One inquires into the different possible theories or "truths" to find a theory that works—a theory that will mediate between previous truths and new experiences. As we listen and attend to our experiences, in practice those experiences have "ways of boiling over, and making us correct our present formulas."[9](P 170) Thus, in this way our practice experiences bear the fruits of theory development.

Interestingly, Dickoff and James[10] brought a similar discussion to nursing theory more than 3 decades ago. These authors described 4 levels of theory, including (*a*) factor-isolating theory, (*b*) factor-relating theory, (*c*) situation-related theory (including predictive and promoting/inhibiting theory), and (*d*) situation-producing theory. It is this idea of the fourth level of theory that we are discussing and building upon in this article. Situation-producing theory is practice-minded theory whose purpose is "to allow the production of situations of a desired kind."[10](p 105) Situation-producing theory is developed not only for the sake of producing theory but also for producing a desired reality. These authors contend that situation-producing theory is the highest level

of theory, since it exists and is produced for practice. They have argued (and we concur) that "theory for a profession of practice discipline must provide for more than mere understanding or "describing" or even predicting reality and must provide conceptualization specially intended to guide the shaping of reality to that profession's professional purpose."[10](p 102)

Theory Development: A Process of Inquiry

New truth is always a "go-between, a smoother over of transitions. It marries old opinion to new fact so as ever to show a minimum jolt, a maximum of continuity . . . A new opinion counts as true just in proportion as it gratifies the individual's desire to assimilate the novel in his (sic) experience to his beliefs in stock. It must both lean on old truth and grasp new fact."[9](p 150)

Dickoff and James[10] emphasize the complexity and difficulty of developing situation-producing theory. We offer in this article a description of how pragmatism has helped us in the challenge of this complex and difficult theory development. Specifically, drawing upon pragmatist thought, we suggest a way of proceeding in practice that can support and foster the cultivation of situation-producing theory and ultimately re-create realities, both in the practice of individual nurses and the contexts of healthcare delivery.

Approaching practice with this pragmatic understanding of theory and truth compels us to take an inquiry stance—to pay attention and inquire into our own personal experiences, the experiences of others, existing knowledge such as formal theory and research, and the contextual elements and structures that shape our experiences and practice. Such an inquiry begins with the assertion of the knowledge-making capacity of people—that all people bring self-directing, self-generating, self-knowing, and selftranscending capacities.[11] A pragmatic inquiry supports us to inquire into and question the "knowing" we live in our practice, how that knowing enhances and/or constrains our in-the-moment responsiveness, and, ultimately, to remake that knowing-in-action. This knowing includes development of theory that may illuminate our action, guide and provide our action with meaning, and ultimately reshape "reality." Therefore, central to a pragmatic inquiry are questions of adequacy. Questions a pragmatist might ask as part of the theory development inquiry process include the following: Is our knowledge of things adequate to the way things are? Are our ways of describing things, of relating them to other things so as to fulfill our needs as good as possible?[4] In the context of nursing, we believe that a pragmatic inquiry includes questions such as "Are our ways of describing things, of relating them to other things so as to be responsive to patients as well as possible? Is our knowledge of things adequate to the way things are in nursing practice? Do available theories address and inform the questions and challenges that arise in our nursing work?" These questions of adequacy are essential, as according to James, any truth "has its palentology, and its "prescription," and may grow stiff with years of veteran service and petrified in men's (sic) regard by sheer antiquity."[6(p 15l)] We concur with Dickoff and James'admonition that "a professional is a doer who shapes reality rather than a doer who merely attends to the cogs of reality according to prescribed patterns."[10(p 102)] In a similar vein, Reason and Torbert[11] contend that when we numb ourselves with knowledge (take up static doctrines), we actually become less susceptible to learning, to growth, and to people. Reason and Torbert argue that knowledge development involves learning through risk-taking in living.

As part of our work, we have intentionally engaged in a pragmatic inquiry into nursing practice in experiences of difference and diversity. This intentional inquiry was inspired through numerous experiences where we each (independently) found ourselves deeply disturbed by the inadequacy of our practice, of existing theory, and of healthcare structures and processes to attend to difference and diversity in people/families. Although we each came from different areas of nursing, we felt strongly that many of the truths and theories that dominated understandings of people/families did not do justice to their diverse living experiences and/or did not adequately support nurses to promote the health and

well-being of families in their diverse everyday lives. Sharing an ethic of social justice and believing that nursing decisions and actions should be more than merely health promoting and/or economically viable, we found ourselves asking "so what?" If I do or do not do this, "so what" may the impact be? As nurses, we strive toward the ideals of compassion, respect, equitable relations, and the honoring of all life forms. The intent of our ongoing pragmatic inquiry process is to bring knowledge, compassion, and action together to produce practical knowing—to develop knowledge in service of worthwhile human purposes.[11] We concur with Reason and Torbert[11] who contend that ultimately the purpose of knowledge development is to culminate in compassion. Compassion in this sense is not just emotion but is about action—action that interferes with unnecessary pain, sorrow, and/or injustice. It is compassionate action that is both the purpose and the text of such theory development.

A Pragmatic Inquiry Into Family Diversity

Overall, bringing a pragmatic orientation to our practice has directed us to (*a*) focus on the consequences of ideas and theories; (*b*) draw upon multiple theories, ideas, and perspectives examining their contradictions and complementary contributions in terms of consequences; (*c*) focus on the integrity of theory/practice rather than on the divide between them; and (*d*) remake theory and reality. The process of pragmatic inquiry has supported the development of our thinking regarding family and family nursing, and inspired further thinking about diversity in family nursing. By "diversity" we are referring both to the diversity of experiences and meanings of "family" and to other forms of diversity that relate to those experiences and meanings.

Focusing on the Consequences of Ideas and Theories

Our pragmatic inquiry was initially inspired by our experiences of discomfort in our practice. As we worked with people/families from diverse backgrounds and locations and listened to the inner rumblings of inadequacy we felt in our practice responses, it became increasingly clear that existing theoretical understandings of family that governed family nursing did not do justice to the diverse people/families with whom we worked and did not set us up well to respond in meaningful ways to their health and healing experiences. As we traced our practice experiences and responses back to explore what ideas were informing them, we began to explicitly name the consequences of holding those ideas and practicing from particular theoretical locations.[2,12] For example, as described elsewhere,[3,12] we identified how in seeing family as a literal entity—that is, as a configuration of people—we were missing the essence of family for many of those to whom we provided care and entirely discounting the experiences of many others. Furthermore, by doing so, we were drawn away from making important theoretical connections. For example, given that family is the dominant social organizing structure in society, through our practice experiences it became increasingly clear that all people live and experience family in some way regardless of whether they are part of a literal family at any given moment. Ultimately, our situation-producing theoretical work led us to retheorize family as a socially situated relational experience.[3] At the same time, we began to see ways in which our prior theoretical understanding of family (as a configuration of people) had[13] served to constrain our understanding of people's health and healing experiences and our responsiveness to them. This became evident, for example, when working with women who experience violence. Statements we frequently heard nurses make such as "why doesn't she just leave" reflect an understanding of family as some 'thing' that can be left and decontextualize the complex, relational experience of both family and of violence. Such understanding led nurses to offer very limited choices to women, culminating primarily in advice to leave their partners.[13] Not only does such a limited theoretical perspective shape nursing practice in such a way that significantly hinders nurses' understanding of, and responsiveness to, women/families experiencing violence but it also leaves in place and perpetuates the larger societal discourses and theories that limit the knowing and "reality" of family and of violence.

Seeking to expand our understanding of diversity in relation to family, we have also employed our pragmatic stance as we have turned our attention to culture. We had experienced discomfort in relation to the ideas of culture and cultural diversity in our practice, and, once again, these experiences of discomfort served as points of entry into a deeper inquiry. We traced back the consequences of our ideas to the ideas themselves. That is, the impossibility of learning about the multiple "other cultures" in our multicultural, multiethnic practice settings as well as the variations we saw in people/families who were supposedly from the same culture led us to question the adequacy of how culture and nursing practice in relation to culture have been theorized. For example, drawing on others,[14,15] we began to see the practical impact of the overriding acceptance of culture as shared values and beliefs, as something closely associated with or even equated with ethnicity or nation, and as a "thing" that belongs to groups of people. It became evident that such theoretical understandings direct nurses away from the actual experiences and meanings of families and individuals, and make their thinking vulnerable to stereotypes and assumptions. Conceptualizing culture as a thing that belongs to groups leads to a rather static understanding of culture and fosters a process of "othering"—that is, those who belong to groups in which we as nurses do not claim membership are seen as "other." Although the need to retheorize culture has certainly been addressed in the nursing literature, our pragmatic approach to theory helped us see a way of *interrupting and reshaping cultural theory at the practice level.* With the help of writers such as Swendson and Windsor,[16] we began to see how theorizing culture as shared values and beliefs of groups promoted a sensitivity to customs, habits, food preferences, health beliefs, and so on, but did not draw attention to the way in which social, economic, and political forces shaped these aspects of culture. Because "cultural sensitivity" is fundamentally concerned with learning about "others," often distinguished from self on the basis of race, ethnicity, or nation, and is particularly concerned with learning about the values, beliefs, and practices of certain (usually nondominant) groups, in practice it leaves nurses open to assumptions, stereotypes, and inappropriate generalizations. As we inquired into the adequacy of a cultural sensitivity approach to nursing practice, it became evident that cultural sensitivity served to emphasize difference at the expense of similarities and focus upon the values, beliefs, and behaviours of particular individuals, families, and groups without drawing attention to the larger circumstances of their lives. Furthermore, this way of theorizing culture and nursing practice left Eurocentric thinking[17] unchallenged and promoted nurses to normalize Eurocentric practices and designate anything outside of those normative practices as "other."

Overall, by examining the consequences of our theories and ideas, we were able to evaluate the adequacy of those theories and ideas in everyday nursing practice, and in particular, how they optimized and/or limited responsiveness to diverse families. For example, thinking of a Canadian family as "Vietnamese" drew attention to certain dietary practices, religious practices, and so on, but did not draw attention to the ways in which immigration from Vietnam effected differently various generations of immigrants, the ways in which global politics, war, and economics shape various families' practices and experiences, or how racism might shape the family's health care encounters. Indeed, it became evident that the theory of culturally sensitive nursing practice offers superficial understandings of the experiences of the families and is inadequate when it comes to knowing and responding to experiences of diverse families.

A living example of this was provided by a local hospital publication entitled *The Multicultural Corner.* This periodical publication variously featured particular groups of people. One issue focused upon "Indo Canadians," "listing the "Countries of Origin" as "Pakistan, India, Sri Lanka, Bangladesh, Nepal, Fiji, East Africa, United Kingdom, and Hong Kong"; "Religion and Religious practices" as "Sikhism, Hinduism, and Islam"; and the languages spoken as "English, Hindi, Punjabi, Guharate, and Urdu. Most speak English." By theorizing

culture as something belonging to groups and defining the group of concern in this manner, the authors of this publication grouped together hundreds of thousands of diverse people. The consequences included ideas that might apply to any person, family, or group (eg, "lots of support from family and friends"), ideas that might or might not apply to people within the defined category (eg, "role of women—caregivers, nurturers, generally submissive but respected)," and a tone of objectification (eg, "cleanliness important," "Family spokesperson is usually the most established male"). Rather than offering guidance to greater sensitivity as was apparently intended, the publication yielded generalizations and invited stereotyping.

Drawing Upon Multiple Theories, Ideas, and Perspectives to Examine Their Contradictions and Complementary Contributions

As we came to see the consequences of the theoretical understandings that were shaping our practices, we simultaneously began looking at other theories and perspectives that could expand our view and more adequately reflect the diversity of people/family and their health and healing experiences. For example, we turned to hermeneutic phenomenology to expand our understanding of living experience and to various critical theories to enhance our "knowing" of sociopolitical family experience.[3,18] Seeking a deeper and more complex understanding of culture, we drew on the wide range of theorists who see culture as deeply imbedded within the webs of power, economics, and politics.[19–23] We began to pursue the *practical consequences* of seeing culture in this way, and of seeing culture as dynamic rather than static.

Ultimately, through this pragmatic process of theoretical inquiry, we gradually began to "retheorize our practice." This retheorizing was a highly practical process. For example, as we played with alternative views of "family" and paid attention to the way those views shaped our responsiveness, we found ourselves developing a view of "family" as a relational living experience.[3] That is, looking beyond "family" in its literal sense (as a configuration of people) as we worked with families in practice, we intentionally focused our attention on what it was that was significant to people in *relation* to family. For example, as it became clear that all people live and experience family in some way regardless of whether they are part of a literal family, we found ourselves immediately tuning into the *experience* of family rather than the configuration of people. This opened up our thinking so that we recognized family for *all* people with whom we worked, regardless of whether or not they had a visible, literal family. We began to appreciate, seek out, and understand the experience of family for people even when they were utterly alone in a literal sense. A man who had been estranged from his literal family and lived on the street for years, a woman who had been in prison and moved from town to town since, with no literal family, a youth who after living in numerous foster homes was on his own with no discernable literal family, all had important experiences of family. They characterized some of their experiences of family as experiences of rejection, of loneliness, of "unlove," and these experiences of family were fundamental to understanding how to more responsively promote their health and healing. Furthermore, they each had other important and significant relationships (sometimes fleeting) that would not necessarily have been captured by our previous understandings of family, but were critical to understand in order to be responsive. Thus, our pragmatic inquiry expanded our "knowing" of family theoretically as well as practically. That is, we found that this ongoing inquiry process fostered a deeper knowing of the people/families with whom we worked, cultivated greater responsiveness in our practice, and simultaneously expanded our theoretical understandings.

Congruent with our view of family as a relational, situated experience, we also began to see culture as a relational experience, as something "that happens between people."[15,24] And we saw that understanding "culture" required understanding the social, economic, political, and historical webs of power within which people are embedded. At a very practical level, this led us to "look over the shoulder" of people/families with whom we worked to see the particular webs within

which they had and were currently living. The consequences of this view of culture included widening our understanding of diversity within families and among families, for example, among families within particular ethnic groups. Such a view led to a more complex view than is implied through the use of ethnic or nationalist categories—rather than seeing a family as "Vietnamese," questions were immediately raised regarding the experiences of any given family. We sought to understand immigration and colonizing experiences, experiences of racism, current economic, social, and political life circumstances, and evolving variations between and among individuals, generations, and groups. We sought to understand the values, beliefs, and practices of people/families as dynamic and changing and as embedded within wider social contexts.

Seeing culture as a relational experience shifted our view of nurses in relation to culture. Rather than seeing nurses as outside some of their patients' cultures, we began to see that when nurses enter into relation, they shape and participate in culture, that is, culture is happening as patients and nurses relate. So, when a third-generation Euro-Canadian nurse enters into relation with a family who has recently immigrated from Vietnam, their histories and experiences mingle within the webs of power. They meet within multiple and shifting cultures (eg, the culture of healthcare, colonialist Canadian culture) and have the opportunity to reinforce and reproduce certain aspects of culture rather than others.

In examining multiple theories, ideas, and perspectives in relation to one another, we were led to understand both family and culture in ways that complemented and were congruent with one another. Critically examining the adequacy of our theories within the context of our everyday practice not only enhanced our capacity for responsiveness to people/families but also helped us develop appreciation for the integral relation of theory/practice.

Focusing on the Integrity of Theory/Practice

As our practice experiences fostered our retheorizing (of family as a relational experience) and we began to experience the profound difference this retheorizing made to our understanding of, and responsiveness to, the particular families with whom we worked, we came to more fully comprehend the pragmatist assertion that all so-called "theory" is always already practice.[4–6] Specifically, we came to appreciate how every nursing moment is imbued with theory/practice and is thus an opportunity for theory development—for rethinking the ideas, assumptions, beliefs, and theories that govern our practice by examining the consequences of them. Overall, our "theory" of theory and theory development shifted from a theory of objectification (where theory and practice are separate and there is a "theory-practice gap") to a relational one (where thinking is not separate from action but rather where action is understood to be integral to theory). In such situation-producing theory, action and remaking reality are inherent.

Remaking Theory and Reality

At the center of this "theory/practice" relation is a praxis process—that is, situation-producing theory means that reality is remade in every moment in nursing. It is important to distinguish this pragmatic "praxis" process from the notion of praxis that has tended to dominate nursing—that is, where praxis has been defined as theory informing practice and practice informing theory. While this view of praxis has drawn attention to the reciprocity between theory and practice, we also believe that in some ways it has reinforced the division between them. Therefore, we want to clarify that we are referring to an understanding of praxis inspired by Friere.[25] Similar to Dickoff and James' notion of situation-producing theory,[10] in Friere's definition of praxis as "reflection and action upon the world in order to transform it,"[25(p 33)] action is integral to theory—it is simultaneously with, and the reason for, thinking. Thus, enacting praxis in this sense, means that *every moment in nursing is purposefully about both thinking and action that focus toward the service of worthwhile human purposes.* From this praxis perspective, it is understood that in each moment we are trying out, evaluating, and

revising our ways of thinking/acting/responding in term of ourselves, the people/families with whom we work, and importantly, as we focus "upon the world," the contexts within which we all live. And, at the heart of this praxis process is the purposeful move toward compassionate action that interrupts and addresses unnecessary pain, sorrow, and/or injustice. For example, in moving toward compassionate action to honor diversity in families, we are compelled to expose and address the underlying sociopolitical structures that are advantaging some people/families and disadvantaging others, and the theories and/or ways of knowing that keep inequities intact.[17] As we try out and evaluate the consequences of particular theoretical understandings of family, of culture, of health, and other theories that dominate healthcare practice and organizations, we gain the opportunity to identify how existing structures (for example, healthcare policies) may need revision in order to be equitable and responsive to families, particularly to those families who do not (or cannot) conform to dominant values and/or expectations.

Implications and Conclusions

Overall, a pragmatic perspective of knowledge suggests that everyday nursing practice is a critical site for theory development. The inseparability of practice/theory and the integral role practice experiences play in the ongoing development of theory has implications for how we practice, teach, and develop knowledge. In the particular example of family diversity, pragmatism has helped us explicitly approach theory development as a practical activity of inquiry, to cultivate situation-producing theory, and ultimately to enhance our theoretical practice.

Seeing theory development as a practical activity, and practice as a theoretical activity serves to direct attention to the way in which nurses enter into practice as "knowing" practitioners. It highlights that theory development is not something that is divorced from everyday practice but is integral to it. Seeing theory/practice as inseparable draws attention to every moment of practice as a site of learning (in this example, a site of learning about families and culture). By attending to each nursing moment in this manner, we move beyond looking to see how theory informs practice or how practice informs theory to looking for the consequences of theorizing/practicing in particular ways.

Perhaps one of the most significant implications of a pragmatic approach to theory/practice is that it places "theory development" firmly in the domain of practicing nurses and recognizes the capacity all nurses have to use their inventiveness for knowledge development to address situations and challenges of everyday practice and to create and re-create their knowing in each moment of practice. In addition, such an approach opens space for people/families to inform our knowing and for us as nurses to more consciously and intentionally choose and effect our actions to be more compassionately responsive in each moment of nursing practice.

REFERENCES

1. Liaschenko J, Fisher A. Theorizing the knowledge that nurses use in the conduct of their work. *Sch Inq Nurs Pract.* 1999;13(1): 29–41.
2. Hartrick Doane GA. Am I still ethical? The socially-mediated process of nurses' moral identity. *Nurs Ethics.* 2002;9(6): 623–635.
3. Hartrick-Doane G, Varcoe C. *Family Nursing as Relational Inquiry: Developing Health Promoting Practice.* Philadelphia: Lippincott Williams & Wilkins; 2005.
4. Rorty R. *Philosophy and Social Hope.* London: Penguin; 1999.
5. Thayer-Bacon B. *Relational (E)pistemologies.* New York: Peter Lang; 2003.
6. James W. *Pragmatism. A New Name for Some Old Ways of Thinking.* New York: Longmans, Green & Co; 1907.
7. Roth JK. Introduction. In: Roth JK, ed. *The Moral Philosophy of William James.* New York: Thomas Y. Crowell Co; 1969:1–18.
8. Berman M, *Wandering God. A Study in Nomadic Spirituality.* Albany, NY: State of New York Press; 2000.
9. James W. *Essays in Pragmatism.* New York; Hafner Publishing; 1948.
10. Dickoff J, James PJ. A theory of theories: a position paper. In: Nicholl LH, ed. *Perspectives on Nursing Theory,* Glenview, Il. Scott, Foresman & Co; 1968/1986:99–111.
11. Reason P, Torbert WR. Toward a transformational social science: a further look at the scientific merits of action research. *Concepts Transformations.* 2001;6(1):1–37.
12. Hartrick Doane GA. Through pragmatic eyes: philosophy and the resourcing of family nursing. *Nurs Philos.* 2003;4: 25–32.
13. Varcoe C. Abuse obscured: an ethnographic account of emergency nursing in relation to violence against women. *Can J Nurs Res.* 2001;32(4):95–115.
14. Allen DG. Knowledge, politics, culture, and gender: a discourse perspective. *Can J Nurs Res.* 1999;30(4):227–234.
15. Stephenson P. Expanding notions of culture for cross-cultural ethics in health and medicine. In: Coward H, Ratanakul P, eds. *A Cross-Cultural Dialogue on Health Care Ethics.* Waterloo, Ontario, Canada: Wilfried Laurier University Press; 1999: 68–91.
16. Swendson C, Windsor C. Rethinking cultural sensitivity. *Nurs Inq.* 1996;3:3–12.
17. Ladson-Billings G. Racialized discourses and ethnic epistemologies. In: Denzin NK, Lincoln YS, eds. *Handbook of Qualitative Research.* Thousand Oaks, Calif: Sage; 2000: 398–425.
18. Hartrick G. A critical pedagogy for family nursing. *J Nurs Educ.* 1998;37(2):80–84.
19. Ng R. Multiculturalism as ideology: a textual analysis. In: Campbell M, Manicom A, eds. *Knowledge, Experience, and Ruling Relations: Studies in the Social Organization of Knowledge.* Toronto, Ontario, Canada: University of Toronto Press; 1995.
20. Anderson J, Perry J, Blue C, et al. "Rewriting" cultural safety within the postcolonial and postnational feminist project: toward new epistemologies of healing. *Adv Nurs Sci.* 2003; 26(3):196–214.
21. Bhabha H. *The Location of Culture.* London: Routledge; 1994.
22. Giroux HA. Public pedagogy as cultural politics: Stuart Hall and the "crisis" of culture. *Cultural Stud,* 2000;14(2): 341–360.
23. Gilroy P. *Against Race: Imagining Political Culture Beyond the Color Line.* Cambridge, Mass: Belknap; 2000.
24. Clifford J. *The Predicament of Culture: Twentieth Century Ethnography, Literature and Art.* Cambridge, Mass: Harvard University Press; 1988.
25. Friere P. *Pedagogy of the Oppressed.* New York: Continuum; 1970.

The Authors Comment

Toward Compassionate Action: Pragmatism and the Inseparability of Theory/Practice

This article was inspired by our desire to extend the conceptualization of nursing theory and theory development beyond a "realist" perspective and to illustrate theory as inherently philosophically and practically based. The article grew out of the work we did in developing our textbook *Family Nursing as Relational Inquiry,* published by Lippincott Williams & Wilkins in 2005. In the text, we used pragmatist philosophy and relational epistemology to develop ideas for guiding nursing practice in ways that did not presume a theory/practice gap. This article allowed us to specifically demonstrate the usefulness of a pragmatic approach to nursing theory development. Our intent is to show how pragmatism has helped us to conceptualize "family" and "culture" in ways that we believe foster ethical and socially just nursing practice.

—GWENETH HARTRICK DOANE
—COLLEEN VARCOE

CHAPTER 13

The Practitioner as Theorist

Rosemary Ellis

When Gulliver traveled to Laputa, land in the clouds, he found rapt theorists wandering about construct-
ing useless ideas. And, generally, that is what we think of theorists. This author, though, says that theorists
in nursing are not the ivory-tower thinkers; they are the nurses who work directly with patients. With
every patient, she explains, we select an approach, then use, modify, and expand it—whether or not we
are conscious of doing so. Because theories in a field have a powerful, long-term influence on the direc-
tion that field will take, the author pleads that we struggle to make already-existing, implicit nursing
theories—such as TLC, for example—clear and explicit, so that nursing will develop in the direction of
more skilled bedside care.

Nursing has been called an applied science. It is, in the sense that it is the application of knowledge from the basic sciences. But nursing care, or nursing practice, is something more. It is not the simple transfer of basic science knowledge. The nurse does not practice chemistry, anthropology, or sociology. She must sort out, select, adapt, and infer from her basic science knowledge. She uses some of the knowledge, orientations, processes of study, or models from these sciences as a guide to understanding patients, their pathology, and therapeutic practices.

This selection, adaptation, and sometimes interpolation from the basic sciences must be done by the practitioner. The physiologist or anthropologist cannot predict what specific knowledge or what concepts the nurse will need. The nurse must identify these, because what is

From R. Ellis, The practitioner as theorist, American Journal of Nursing, July 1969, 69(7), 428–435. Copyright © 1969.
Reprinted with permission from Lippincott Williams & Wilkins

About the Author

ROSEMARY ELLIS was born in Berkeley, CA. She received an AB degree in economics and a BSN from the University of California, Berkeley-San Francisco, followed by an MA in nursing education and a PhD in human development from the University of Chicago. At the time of her death in the fall of 1986, she was a Professor of Nursing, a position she held at Case Western Reserve University since 1964. Dr. Ellis authored more than 30 articles, book chapters, and other scholarly works, including four in the *Japanese Journal of Nursing Research*. She emphasized the importance of pursuing questions about the substantive structure and description of nursing. Her metatheoretical writings have had a significant influence on nursing. The 1993 article "Rosemary Ellis' views on the substantive structure of nursing" by Donna Algase and Ann Whall, published in *Image: Journal of Nursing Scholarship, 25*(1), 69–72, addresses this significant contribution to nursing, drawing from both her published and unpublished works.

needed depends on the specific purpose intended. The nurse, for nursing, uses some framework for her selection and adaptation. In this action she is a theorist. That is, some theory—often not made explicit—directs her selection of the knowledge or concepts to apply.

By "theory," I mean a coherent hypothesis, or set of hypotheses, or a concept, forming a general framework for undertaking something. Theory means a conceptual structure built for a purpose. For nursing, that purpose is practice.

But the practitioner cannot just select from a rack of ready-to-wear theories, because the knowledges and theories as we find them in the basic sciences are insufficient for practice. Instead, nursing practice requires that she structure converging, and sometimes conflicting, facts from the many fields which produce knowledge about human beings.

The nurse works within the framework of the inseparability and interdependence of one person's human life, so she attempts to relate aspects not yet clearly related in the separate sciences.

That is, we strive to act holistically, though our knowledge does not come for use from any holistic science of humans.

In this, the practitioner differs from the scientist. The scientist, due to reasons of control, feasibility, and measurement in study (due, as well, to the sheer impossibility of mastering all sciences, or even specialties within one science) isolates aspects for study.

While the scientist may recognize the interrelationships of, for instance, physiologic and psychologic factors in man, he far less commonly studies these as a whole.

The practitioner of nursing, in contrast, may not have a complete science to nurse the whole man, but nurse the whole man is what she is striving to do. And, she sees the problems that result when one aspect or another is left out.

The practitioner of nursing thus finds herself working from a framework somewhat different from that within which knowledge is typically generated in the sciences. In this translation, the practitioner, of necessity, begins to *restructure* theory. She—often, at least—must apply the theory or concept in a way its originator may not have foreseen. She cannot simply take concepts from the sciences and directly apply them and hope to have the key to the biologic and psychosocial factors bound together in a patient, because this very interdependence is often a factor in response to and recovery from illness.

Generalities Don't Suffice

Further, because we attempt to nurse the individual, general theories cannot suffice. General theories of human behavior describe the typical or the norm, not the exception or the individual. Or, sometimes, they describe the extremes and not the middle range.

For example, it is a useful notion that self-preservation, both in a physical and psychologic sense, is a major element in human behavior that accounts for or explains much observed behavior. Yet it is not uncommon to see patients who do not act rationally for self-preservation. They appear to have some stronger motive for action. We also see heroic acts of self-sacrifice which are not easily explained by general theories of self-preservation.

As one moves from general theories about human behavior to those relevant to all of the helping professions, and then to those relevant to patient behavior, there is need for an increasing number of conditional statements. What applies is shaped by the context, roles, and, for patients, the physical status that presents. This is yet another reason why the professional is a theorist: she is the person who must identify the conditional factors; she has to make the conditional statements.

Related to this is the fact that the professional can encounter conflicting theories, with each supported by some evidence. If she is to take some action she must choose a theory, either consciously or not, for her action is not independent of history; it stems from some framework.

For example, the concept or theory that guides the common practice of encouraging patients to talk about their problems often is not made explicit. Verbalization is generally conceived to be a good thing. But does this concept support the practice in all circumstances for all patients, or explain clearly the exceptions? Theoretically, indiscriminate practice would seem to involve some risk. Do the reasons behind this concept identify the risks and the benefits? The practitioner who follows a practice based on theory must appraise and criticize the theory if she follows it in nursing patients. She must weight the risks and benefits in a manner not required of the scholar who theorizes about a phenomenon in the specific or in general, but who does not treat the individual.

The scholar is often concerned with describing and predicting phenomena. He seeks objectivity, so he reduces, to the extent possible, the influence he may have on the variance due to the experimenter. He seeks to eliminate the human, personal element of the investigator.

This is the converse of a practice discipline. As Conant (1967) has highlighted, a practice discipline seeks not only to describe or predict phenomena, but to introduce change. Practice is goal-directed, not to the accumulation of knowledge, but to the prescription and implementation of activity to change natural outcomes to desired outcomes.

Therefore, the clinical testing of a theory is essential if it is used as a guide to practice. It is the professional practitioner who is able to criticize the theory in use, and determine its value for directing actions to achieve defined outcomes. In this she is not only a *user* of theory, but she may be a *modifier* as well. She is also a *chooser* of theory.

Consider a practice of encouraging a patient to verbalize about his operation. Talking about one's operation occurs frequently enough to have become a folk expectation and to have provoked joking. The frequency and persistence of the behavior suggests that there is some potency behind it. One could speculate, too, that there is possibly a folk norm for the time at which such talking is acceptable, excusable, and tolerated by friends and family. There may also be social norms for what content is acceptable. If such norms exist, and the patient exceeds these norms, he runs the risk of being cut off verbally or avoided by others. One hears complaints to suggest this happens.

Can this be avoided through nursing? From one theory it can be argued that if the nurse encourages a patient to talk about his operation, some of the need to continue talking about it can be extinguished, and the risk for the patient of annoying family and friends can be reduced.

But, from another theory, one could argue that if the nurse, an important figure for the patient postoperatively, encourages the patient to talk, conveys the expectation that he will talk—and thus, in effect, rewards, the behavior—she may prolong or reinforce it, causing the patient to risk violating folk norms.

It is not the originators of alternative theories who can solve a possible dilemma for the nurse. It is the nurse as practitioner and user of theory who must resolve the dilemma—in action, in critique of action, and in further theorizing.

A universal practice of encouraging patients to talk about their feelings may be questioned from another orientation. A medical patient recently talked with one of my faculty colleagues about the graduate student who was caring for him. He could not understand what the student wanted of him. This student, in her clinical course work, had time to talk with patients, and had visited with the patient after she had completed the typical morning care activities of bathing and bed making. Her conversations were patient-focused but were not probing. She did not have any specific goal in mind except to interact with the patient and to get to know him.

This patient, however, told the instructor that he was an orphan, who had learned early that people do not do things for nothing. He interpreted the student's talking with him as evidence that she wanted something from him. This man viewed even conversation as something you get or give only in exchange for something or because you want something. For him, the nurse's attempt to learn more about him by talking with him was seen as a sexual advance. He could not imagine any interaction that did not have an exploitative motive. He was, therefore, made acutely uncomfortable by a very casual attempt by a nurse to encourage him to verbalize. Her motives were significantly misperceived, to the detriment of the patient (though one could argue that perhaps we learned more about the patient because of his discomfort).

There may also be instances where attempting to get a patient to talk about his feelings is contraindicated because it may dissipate the feeling. There may be instances where it is important for someone to experience and to recognize feelings *as feelings*. Talking about them may diminish them, objectify them, and so lose them as feelings. Joy is certainly one emotion that can be diminished by talking about it or attempting to explain it. I can recall an obstetrician father who was so profoundly moved by the birth of his own child that he burst into tears. The intensity of his own feeling totally surprised him, as well as his obstetrician colleagues. It seemed important for him to fully experience the intensity of his feeling and not diminish it until he had really felt it and absorbed it as his own feeling.

Lest I mislead, let me hasten to say that, in general, benefits seem to result from the practice of encouraging verbalization, but what are the exceptions? If benefits accrue, how are they explained? Practice could be more selective, and perhaps more effective, if we knew exactly what patient benefits to expect, and what dynamics would achieve them.

For example, benefits might be due to the patient's recognition, through talking, of the specific content of his feelings.

Benefits could also be due to the sense of companionship which can be achieved by talking with another, without regard for particular content. That is, would talking be effective without a listener? If not, what is supplied by a listener, even a nondirective listener, that is essential?

Is benefit derived from the recapitulation of an event which serves in some sense to produce mastery over, or integration of, the event, as in talking about one's operation? Or are benefits due to some reciprocal system where talking serves in place of some other potentially more detrimental form of discharge, such as acting out or somatization? Choose your theory. It is not likely to hold for all circumstances or cases, nor to support an invariate nursing practice of encouraging verbalization. Thus, the professional practitioner must become not simply a user of given theory, but a developer, tester, and expander of theory. This is not for the purpose of scholarship; it is an essential for intelligent practice.

The Need for Theory

It is essential because of the inadequacies in existing theories for the circumstances of nursing.

It is essential because of the need to synthesize, for practice, knowledge from diverse disciplines not yet fully related in theory.

It also is essential because the basic disciplines often are not pursuing the problems of importance to nurse and patient. For example, there is no extensive study, knowledge, or theory about appetite. As nurses we study nutrition, yet many of our observations and concerns with nutritional problems of patients are not solved by knowledge of nutrition. We need to know more about how to enable a patient to partake of the

Whether or not you agree with this view about TLC, it is an example of a concept that exists, that is associated with nursing, that has been felt to be rather specific to nursing, but that we have not yet made explicit, nor yet fully conceptualized. We probably know, at least at a preconscious level, more about it than anybody else, for we can see it in so many diverse actions and situations. It does not seem unreasonable to suggest that theorizing about something as vague and yet as familiar as TLC might be valuable for understanding nursing.

At this stage in theory development I could entertain, even, the use of jargon—in the sense of a special professional language—to express some of the ideas in nursing. For instance, I would endorse the use of this term TLC for the purposes of talking about it until we can more precisely or more elegantly describe what we are talking about.

At this time in theory development it will be profitable to borrow or adapt concepts and theories from whatever source we can, if they will help us to understand and produce nursing. They must, however, be tested for their usefulness in guiding nursing practice in the arena of practice.

Intuitive exploration, speculation, trial and error, introspection, subjective impression—all can be used toward development of theory.

What is needed are attempts to make theory explicit, with tests of theories for nursing *in the practice* of nursing, and with further development or theories emerging *from the practice* of nursing.

REFERENCE

Conant, L. H. (1967). Closing the practice-theory gap. *Nursing Outlook, 15,* 37–39.

The Author Comments

The Practitioner as Theorist

I wrote this article to demystify the then-prevalent ideas that theory should be "grand theory" or that what was needed was some "theory" to justify nursing. As was evident from the literature and conferences at national meetings, there was great confusion concerning uses of theory and why nurses as practitioners needed theory. With their emphasis on theory and research, nurse scientists often rejected or at least ignored the importance of phenomena of nursing practice.

—ROSEMARY ELLIS
1969

CHAPTER 14

Theorizing the Knowledge That Nurses Use in the Conduct of Their Work

Joan Liaschenko
Anastasia Fisher

The authors propose a classification of knowledge that they call case, patient, and person and that reflects the content of the knowledge necessary to the conduct of nursing work. This classification represents an attempt to theorize from their respective empirical research data. Case knowledge is general knowledge of pathophysiology, disease processes, pharmacology, and other therapeutic protocols. Patient knowledge is that knowledge that defines the individual within the health care system, the knowledge expressed in the individual's response to therapeutics, and the knowledge that enables nurses to move the recipient of care through the health care system and along the illness trajectory. Person knowledge is knowledge of the individual as a subject with a personal biography who occupies a certain social space and who acts with his or her own desires and intentions for reasons that make sense to him or her. Two types of social knowledge serve as relational knowledge, or a bridge that links case knowledge to patient knowledge and patient knowledge to person knowledge. Each type of knowledge is accessed differently and the extent to which each is attained and used is determined by the circumstances of the patient's illness and his or her location in the health care system. The authors make a case for why this classification might be useful to the discipline.

In general, our intellectual project is concerned with theorizing the interaction between knowledge and the actions that constitute nursing work. We begin by naming some knowledges relevant to nursing practice; specifically, in this paper, we propose a designation of the content of knowledge used by nurses in direct links the actions of nursing to the knowledge used in the conduct of those actions, thus legitimating them as work. It has the potential to be theoretically more complete and yet parsimonious, because it recognizes and describes the processes constituting nursing work and not merely the outcomes. Most important, it does so in a language that is used by nurses and is understandable to others.

While it is indisputable that nursing requires scientific, biomedical knowledge, the discipline's nearly exclusive focus on this form of knowledge leaves unrecognized other kinds of knowledge necessary to patient care. In an earlier paper, Liaschenko (1998) argued that nurses know much more than a certain portion of scientific knowledge. In addition to the knowledge of anatomy, physiology, pathophysiology, and so forth, nurses know how to get things done; they know how to move patients through a health care system, how to connect patients with resources. This knowledge is not scientific knowledge, but is knowledge absolutely essential to patient care that is organized, continuous, safe, and humane. Of course, nurses are familiar with this type of action; it is commonly referred to as the coordination of care and involves the transmission and coordination of information. Coordination of care is rarely articulated as work and rarely counts in institutional structures as work (Jacques, 1993). The cultural assumption is that the critical work is the scientific work, all other kinds being of secondary importance, of the kind that "just sort of happens." It is further assumed that there is no knowledge involved in arrangements that "just happen."

Jacques (1993), an organizational theorist who studied nurses, noted the critical importance of this work to the functioning of health care institutions, calling attention to the fact that this work is completely external to the reward structures of institutions. Fletcher (1994), another organizational theorist, studied female engineers and found that while they do the interpersonal work essential to the successful completion of projects, this work "gets disappeared" by institutional structures that refuse to recognize these relational practices as work. In her research on the particular household labor of feeding families, DeVault documented that although a major portion of that work consisted of "thought work," it was viewed as so natural that the women themselves failed to see it as work. One consequence of the lack of a commonly accepted, useful articulation of nursing work is that the nurses themselves, like others who do gendered labor, fail to recognize what they do as work (DeVault, 1991). This invisibility is not total, however, as some nurses have shown themselves to be astute observers of what work they are being paid to do and what work they are not being paid to do (Liaschenko, 1997b).

The studies by Jacques (1993) and Fletcher (1994) were studies of practices specifically concerned with the concept of work, including the knowledge necessary for the work. Likewise, our approach is decidedly empirical in that it was generated from research (Fisher, Fonteyn, & Liaschenko, 1994; Liaschenko, 1993). Our designation of knowledge arose from discussions about the empirical studies of nursing practice that we conducted. Fisher and her colleague, Marsha Fonteyn, did ethnographic fieldwork in a psychiatric emergency service, and in cardiovascular and neurosurgical intensive care units, while Liaschenko conducted a narrative study of home care and psychiatric nurses using unstructured interviews. The design, method, and analyses used in these studies are described elsewhere (Fisher & Fonteyn, 1995; Liaschenko, 1993). Although the aims of the respective research were different, with Fisher and Fonteyn studying clinical reasoning and Liaschenko examining moral dimensions of nursing practice, "knowing the patient" was a central feature for the nurses in both studies. We came to see through our discussions, however, that knowing the patient was used by nurses to refer to different types of knowing that they used in the conduct of their work. We labeled these knowledges case, patient, and person (Fisher, Fonteyn, & Liaschenko, 1994; Liaschenko, 1997a). While "knowing the patient" has received increasing attention in the literature, our work shows that "the patient" is understood in ways that reflect the kind of knowledge needed to do the work of nursing in the confines of contemporary health care structures.

Case Knowledge

Case knowledge, which we consider biomedical knowledge, is the generalized knowledge of anatomy, physiology, pathophysiology, disease processes, and therapeutics (see Figure 14–1). It is concerned with the causation of disease and its treatment. It is gained through the principles of science and the scientific method and is generalizable because it is based on statistical probabilities. Elsewhere, Liaschenko (1997a) has claimed that case knowledge is "disembodied" knowledge in that no particular physical body, nor indeed any body, is required to have case knowledge. One could know, for example, all the facts about cardiac disease without seeing that disease as embodied in a particular individual. One could start with the anatomy and physiology of the heart, follow this with the pathophysiology of various disease entities, and proceed through the therapeutics. Biological norms are implicit in the anatomy and physiology, while pathophysiology reveals the disease processes. The

effectiveness of therapeutics is based on the percentage of the population that responds favorably to a given therapeutic. This knowledge is the standard against which the particularities of an individual recipient of care are evaluated. This case, or biomedical, knowledge is the primary knowledge of the contemporary health care system in that it legitimizes the practice of medicine which, in turn, controls this knowledge. It also legitimizes that aspect of nursing work that is concerned with monitoring disease processes and therapeutic responses.

In their research conducted in cardiovascular and neurosurgical intensive care units and a psychiatric emergency service, Fisher and Fonteyn (1995) identified case knowledge as the basic knowledge nurses need to meet the primary goal of stabilizing, maintaining, and moving critically ill patients to another level of care. In these settings, aspects of knowing the case included nurses' knowledge of the disease processes, physiology, clinical protocols, indicators and range of expected patient outcome (i.e., the usual clinical therapeutics and

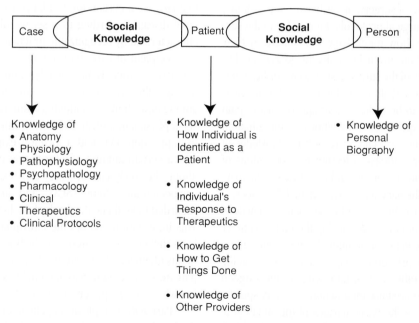

Figure 14–1. *Knowledge that nurses use within the social-temporal-spatial context of their work.*

discourse about his or her particular disease. These are not static entities, but dynamic interactions of social life. The fact that disease and illness will mean different things to different people is particularly important, because it encompasses acquired knowledge and marks the intersection between the work of nursing and an individual's own management of illness. It is the awareness that these factors impact individual lives that constitutes the knowledge that can potentially bridge patient and person knowledge. The link is constructed as the nurse begins to wonder what living with this disease or disability is like for the individual. To ask the question is to visualize that individual as someone more than a patient in a health care system or as something more than an object of biomedical science. This visualization, or imagination, if you will, forms a background, a repertoire of possible explanations that facilitate nurses' formulation of hypotheses regarding the individual's experience and action when this is necessary in the conduct of their work. Once these hypotheses are validated by relevant details of the individual's biography, the nurse can be said to have person knowledge. While we are aware that the choice of "hypotheses" might be cause for objection because of its association with certain philosophies of science, we, nonetheless, use it because it is not entirely inaccurate and it is also understood by working nurses.

Before continuing with person knowledge, it might be useful to compare this type of social knowledge with that previously noted linking case knowledge to patient knowledge. The noteworthy distinction is that the latter is a form of localized and unique knowledge that allows nurses to apply general case principles to an individual in a way that particularizes that individual in order to accomplish nursing work. In contrast, linking patient to person knowledge is generalized and abstract knowledge, but it nonetheless works to further particularize the individual. What makes these two kinds of knowledge the same is that they are both social; that is, they are both knowledge of human beings as social actors in social contexts. Moreover, this knowledge can be accessed only within localized interaction, or, to use Fletcher's (1994) words, "relational practices."

Person Knowledge

In contrast to case and patient knowledge, person knowledge is knowledge of the individual as a self with a personal biography (Brody, 1987; Bury, 1982) who occupies a certain social space and who acts on her or his own desires and intentions for reasons that make sense to him or her (see Figure 14–1). When we know a person, we know something about what it means for the individual to have a specific history, live a particular life, and engage with the world in which he or she is situated. In her paper, *Knowing the Patient?*, Liaschenko (1997a) suggested that knowledge of this engagement included knowledge of how individuals enact their agency within the spatial and temporal dimensions of their lives. Access to this knowledge is by direct interaction with the individual in order over time, either through multiple encounters or over some extended period, and it necessarily involves the subjectivity of the nurse. When the nurse has this knowledge and begins to wonder about the individual's experience along the illness trajectory, the nurse is imagining the position of the individual in order to understand it from his or her perspective, and is not merely applying theoretical knowledge.

As we saw from earlier examples, knowledge of the person is not always possible nor, we would add, desirable. On the other hand, while the nurse may have knowledge of the person, it may not impact in a significant way on the nurse's day-to-day work with that individual. Having said this, we might ask to what end this knowledge of the person, when available, is used in the conduct of nursing work? Liaschenko's research demonstrated that person knowledge was used when there was some conflict or potential conflict between courses of action desired by the individual and those desired by the providers or among the providers themselves. Knowing the person offered a perspective that served to keep the recipient of care central. Interestingly, the imagining of the position of the other seemed a reflexive practice in which nurses were also aware of the position they occupied in the social structure of health care and in their respective institutions. It served as a reminder that neither the nurse nor the recipient of care are separate from or beyond the network of relationships that form the health care system. The nurses in her study saw themselves as institutional representatives of the cultural and personal authority that stands behind scientific medicine and health care institutions (Liaschenko, 1995b, 1997b). In this capacity, they were aware of how easy it was for them to undermine or negate patient agency. Person knowledge is a potent reminder that the life being lived is the life of the recipient of care. Nurses use person knowledge to defend their arguments for an alternative management of disease trajectories and to justify their actions when those actions support an individual's agency, even though this can conflict with established biomedical or institutional courses of action.

Summary

We have theorized a content for the knowledge necessary for the conduct of nursing work that we designate case, patient, and person. This designation originated in discussions of our respective empirical research. Case knowledge is general knowledge of pathophysiology, disease processes, pharmacology, and other therapeutic protocols. Patient knowledge is the knowledge of how an individual becomes identified as a patient, knowledge of the individual's response to treatment, knowledge of how to get things done for the individual within and between institutions, and knowledge of the multiple others who are involved in providing services across time and space. Person knowledge is knowledge of the individual as a self with a personal biography who occupies a certain social space and acts according to his or her own desires and intentions for reasons that make sense to him or her. We suggest that knowledge of social actors and the nurse's work context serve to link case to patient knowledge and patient to person knowledge. Each of these knowledges are accessed in different ways and the extent to which they are attained and used by nurses is determined by the circumstances of the patient's illness and his or her location in the health care system.

Because these knowledges are linked to nursing work, we believe they will make sense to practicing nurses enabling them to think more theoretically about their work and, therefore, to articulate it. Theorizing nursing work has always been a challenge, because much of the work is not scientific; rather, it is concerned with how to get things done within extremely complex systems, work described by Fletcher as relational practices. It is our intention that case, patient, and person knowledge may offer a useful way to begin to theorize about the interaction of knowledge and action that constitutes nursing work, a task that requires the attention of the entire discipline, and not merely of the academics among us. For this reason, we believe the content of this paper has important implications for the what and how of nursing education, a topic for some other time.

Acknowledgments. The authors wish to acknowledge the contributions of Dr. Marsha Fonteyn to early conceptualizations of this work. In addition, we would like to thank Mr. John Paley and especially the editor, Dr. Sara Fry, for their very helpful comments in the preparation of this manuscript. During the preparation of this article Dr. Fisher received support from NIH-NIDA 5T32 DA07257–08.

REFERENCES

Agan, D. R. (1987). Intuitive knowing as a dimension of nursing. *Advances in Nursing Science, 10,* 63–70.

Benner, P. (1984). *From novice to expert: Excellence and power in clinical nursing practice.* Menlo Park: Addison-Wesley Publishing Company.

Benner, P., & Wrubel, J. (1989). *The primacy of caring.* Menlo Park, NJ: Addison-Wesley.

Benner, P., & Tanner, C. (1987). Clinical judgment: How expert nurses use intuition. *American Journal of Nursing, 87,* 23–31.

Brody, H. (1987). *Stories of sickness.* New Haven: Yale University Press.

Bury, M. (1982). Chronic illness as biographic disruption. *Sociology of Health and Illness, 4,* 167–182.

Carper, B. (1978). Fundamental patterns of knowing in nursing. *Advances in Nursing Science, 1,* 13–23.

DeVault, M. (1991). *Feeding the family: The social organization of caring as gendered work.* Chicago: University of Chicago Press.

Fisher, A., & Fonteyn, M. (1995). An exploration of an innovative methodological approach for examining nurses' heuristic use in clinical practice. *Scholarly Inquiry for Nursing Practice, 9,* 263–276.

Fisher, A., Fonteyn, M., & Liaschenko, J. (1994, May). *Knowing: The case, the patient, the person.* Symposium presentation at the International Nursing Research Conference, Vancouver, BC.

Fletcher, J. (1994). *Toward a theory of relational practice in organizations: A feminist reconstruction of "real work."* Unpublished doctoral dissertation, School of Management, Boston University, Boston.

Gadow, S. (1990). Response to "Personal knowing: Evolving research and practice." *Scholarly Inquiry for Nursing Practice, 4,* 167–170.

Jacobs-Kramer, M. K., & Chinn, P. L. (1988). Perspectives on knowing: A model of nursing knowledge. *Scholarly Inquiry for Nursing Practice, 2,* 129–143.

Jacques, R. (1993). Untheorized dimensions of caring work: Caring as a structural practice and caring as a way of seeing. *Nursing Administration Quarterly, 17,* 1–10.

Jenks, J. M. (1993). The pattern of personal knowing in nurse clinical decision making. *Journal of Nursing Education, 32,* 399–405.

Jenny, J., & Logan, J. (1992). Knowing the patient: One aspect of clinical knowledge. *Image: Journal of Nursing Scholarship, 24,* 254–258.

Johnson, J. L. (1994). A dialectical examination of nursing art. *Advances in Nursing Science, 17,* 1–14.

Johnson, J. L., & Ratner, P. A. (1997). The nature of the knowledge used in nursing practice. In S. Thorne & V. Hayes (Eds.), *Nursing praxis: Knowledge and action* (pp. 3–22). Thousand Oaks, CA: Sage Publications.

Liaschenko, J. (1993). *Faithful to the good: Morality and philosophy in nursing practice.* Unpublished doctoral dissertation, University of California, San Francisco.

Liaschenko, J. (1995a). Ethics in the work of acting for others. *Advances in Nursing Science, 18*(2), 1–12.

Liaschenko, J. (1995b). Artificial personhood: Nursing ethics in a medical world. *Nursing Ethics, 2,* 185–196.

Liaschenko, J. (1997a). Knowing the patient? In S. Thorne & V. Hayes (Eds.), *Nursing praxis: Knowledge and action* (pp. 23–38). Thousand Oaks, CA: Sage.

Liaschenko, J. (1997b). Ethics and the geography of the nurse-patient relationship: Spatial vulnerabilities and gendered space. *Scholarly Inquiry for Nursing Practice, 11,* 45–59.

Liaschenko, J. (1998). The shift from the closed to the open body—ramifications for nursing testimony. In S. D. Edwards (Ed.), *Philosophical issues in nursing* (pp. 11–30). Basingstoke, UK: Macmillan.

Meerabeau, L. (1992). Tacit nursing knowledge: An untapped resource or a methodological headache? *Journal of Advanced Nursing, 12,* 108–112.

Meleis, A. (1987). ReVisions in knowledge development: A passion for substance. *Scholarly Inquiry for Nursing Practice, 1,* 5–19.

Moch, S. D. (1990). Personal knowing: Evolving research and practice. *Scholarly Inquiry for Nursing Practice, 4,* 155–165.

Nightingale, F. (1969). *Notes on nursing: What it is and what it is not.* New York: Dover Publications. (Original work published 1860)

Radwin, L. E. (1995). Knowing the patient: A process model for individualized interventions. *Nursing Research, 44,* 364–370.

Rew, L. E. (1988). Nurses' intuition. *Applied Nursing Research, 1,* 27–31.

Rew, L. E. (1989). Intuition: Nursing knowledge and the spiritual dimensions of persons. *Holistic Nursing Practice, 3*(3), 56–68.

Sarvimaki, A. (1995). Aspects of moral knowledge in nursing. *Scholarly Inquiry for Nursing Practice, 9,* 343–353.

Strauss, A., Fagerhaugh, Suczek, & Weiner (1997). *The social organization of medical work.* New Brunswick: Transaction Publishers. (Originally published by the University of Chicago Press, 1985)

Tanner, C. A., Benner, P., Chesla, C., & Gordon, D. R. (1993). The phenomenology of knowing the patient. *Image: Journal of Nursing Scholarship, 25,* 273–280.

Wadel, C. (1979). The hidden work of everyday life. In S. Wallman (Ed.), *The anthropology of work* (pp. 365–384). London: Academic Press.

Wolf, Z. R. (1989). Uncovering the hidden work of nursing. *Nursing and Health Care, 10,* 463–467.

Wolfer, J. (1993). Aspects of "reality" and ways of knowing in nursing: In search of an integrating paradigm. *Image: Journal of Nursing Scholarship, 25,* 141–146.

Young, A. (1993). A description of how ideology shapes knowledge of a mental disorder (posttraumatic stress disorder). In S. Lindenbaum & M. Lock (Eds.), *Knowledge, power, and practice: The anthropology of medicine and everyday life* (pp. 108–128). Berkeley, CA: University of California Press.

The Authors Comment

Theorizing the Knowledge That Nurses Use in the Conduct of Their Work

Our interest has been the actual work of nursing practice. The thrust of our work has been to understand what nurses do for people and what happens to nurses in the complex environments in which they work. Theorizing is our attempt to understand practice, but it is not itself theory. Our goal is to continue theorizing the knowledge, action, and moral stances that constitute nursing work rather than to develop theory. However, should some of our colleagues find our work useful in theory development, we would be pleased—to us, it would mean that we have articulated some aspect of the world of nursing work that makes sense to others.

—Joan Liaschenko
—Anastasia Fisher

CHAPTER 15

Practical Inquiry/Theory in Nursing

Chris Stevenson

Aim. *This paper explores a social constructionist, pragmatist approach to inquiry and theory-building with a view to exploring its relevance for nursing as a practical discipline.*

Background. *Positivist and postpositivist inquiry approaches in practical disciplines have produced 'detached' theories that lack relevance for everyday practice and so sustain the theory–practice gap. Both meta- and mid-range theories tend to see practice as fixed or fixable rather than being enacted in a state of flux.*

Discussion. *Practical inquiry and theory are described structurally and as co-dependent processes. The research process is sensitive to the influence of context and consists of construction rather than capture. Practical theory is judged in terms of whether it helps people to 'go on with' their lives. Practical inquiry/practical theory is superimposed on a previous nursing study in the field of mental health to illustrate how it can account for the processes of clinical research. In particular, the illustration demonstrates the surrender of researcher objectivity in the interests of collaborative understanding that occurs with practical inquiry/theory. Shared meaning arises as rich constructs of the research situation are developed that point to future possibilities for action for all those engaged in the research process.*

Conclusion. *Practical inquiry/theory offers the means to conduct cogent, collaborative, developmental research, although further 'trying out' is required.*

About the Author

CHRIS STEVENSON earned an RMN, a BA(Hons), an MSc(Dist), and a PhD. She is Chair in Mental Health Nursing, Dublin City University. The focus of her scholarship is on describing the nature of meaningful responses to people in psychological/mental health distress, especially suicidality. She has worked closely with Professor Phil Barker in developing and evaluating the Tidal Model of psychiatric nursing, which has a developing profile nationally and internationally. Dr. Stevenson is interested in exploring different routes to knowledge for nursing and other health professions, including how people who are experts by experience contribute. Many articles that she has written challenge orthodox "health wisdom" and the methods by which it is produced. Her hobbies include reading, running, writing, and films.

Introduction

The gap between theory and practice remains alive and well in nursing (Upton 1999). Stevenson (1996) pointed out that the way in which research questions and findings are framed in university contexts may 'miss the point' for practitioners who know only too well what the 'real' issues are for them. On the other hand:

> In practical theory development it is expected that important contributions to theory will come from practitioners in the course of their work and that those who are primarily theorists will engage with practitioners and themselves become involved in applied work. (Cronen 2001, p. 29)

In this frame of reference, the inquiry process is collective and collaborative. Inquiry involves the researcher and research participants in creating meaning in relation to a phenomenon, rather than capturing some pre-existing reality. Dewey (1925/1958) described this as the meaning that arises from synchronized interaction that occurs in an episode of time. The implication is that the inquirer and inquired about are necessarily interlinked, a point I will return to below.

In this paper, I take a radical stance in relation to theory and inquiry, based on the work of Cronen (1984, 2001). Philosophically, Cronen places himself as a systemic, social constructionist, pragmatist: systemic as he prefers to acknowledge the influence of context, social constructionist for seeing the research process as construction rather than capture, and pragmatist in that he judges the value of inquiry in terms of whether it helps people to 'go on with' their lives. In a similar vein, I challenge taken for granted ideas about the superiority of the detached researcher. Detached researchers tend to produce detached evidence, and do not and cannot capture the 'reality' of nursing practices that are enacted in a context of continuous flux. I suggest that judgments about 'good' evidence/theory/research can be made pragmatically rather than with reference to a gold standard, and question the aim of producing meta- or mid-range theory for nursing that is subsequently applied. Theories at the grand end of things tend to be based on positivist ideals (if not actual methodology). They draw together a series of laws or robust relationships or findings. But complex social phenomena, e.g. nursing, are less open to this form of investigation. Mid-range (or substantive) theories tend to be more sympathetic to complexity and are inducted from qualitative data, gathered from a small sample of people who have privileged experience of the phenomenon. Theorists make less grand claims about generalizability, but their theories are still the basis of practice recommendations.

On the other hand, nursing is a practical discipline and so needs practical theory—a term coined by Shotter (1984) and taken up by Cronen (1995, 1984, 2001). Practical theory differs from meta- or mid-range theory. For Cronen (2001), a practical theory consists in instrumentalities (theoretical principles, definitions, descriptions, case examples, models, and methodologies) that grow in richness as the theory is used. Practical theories are a means to improve human systems from the inside, rather than to represent some social or intrapsychic reality. Thus, practical theory is a device that helps conjoint exploration of a situation that is within the actors' view (Cronen & Chetro-Szivos 2001). Practical theory is not the end product of practical inquiry. The two create one another and the process involved consists of 'loops' in which inquiry informs theory and theory informs inquiry. Consequently, I describe them together in the next section, followed by a practical example from my own nursing research experience.

Practical Theory/Inquiry/Theory: Interacting Facets

Traditional definitions have tended to describe meta- or mid-range theory as a 'best guess' about the truth of some aspect of the world, physical or social. The theory presents a formal logic concerning a phenomenon that has lain dormant *within* the phenomenon until unearthed by the detached researcher. The theory then prescribes, either by suggesting hypotheses to test or by dictating action of some kind. Practical theory, paraphrasing Cronen (2001), is concerned with how people create patterns of meaning in their everyday practices that make their 'way of living.' Theory does not precede the action, but is constructed and re-constructed *through* action. In other words, the logic of action is created through people acting together rather than action being the result of a formal system of logic, i.e. a meta- or mid-range theory. This begs the question of why practical theory is useful if it is constantly in flux. Practical theory is useful because it helps to generate *possibilities* for conjoint action, and not because it has a 'truth value'. For example, Stevenson and Beech (1998) consider children playing 'catch.' They have a fixed 'no bounce in between catches' rule (instrumentality) that is subscribed to by the older children. However, when younger ones join in, a new rule emerges (little children can have one bounce in between) that serves to ensure that the game continues.

Practical inquiry does not require theory, although an interactive relationship is helpful:

> The inquirer uses her or his experience, informed by the formal instrumentalities of theory (Cronen 2001).

Equally, 'practical theories are importantly informed by data from practical inquiry' (Cronen 2001, p. 29).

Using Cronen's work, I describe the interacting facets of practical inquiry/practical theory in the following sections.

The Inquiry System

We all share an experimental attitude (Dewey 1929/1938), a desire to know more about our world. But the 'professional' inquirer uses certain 'instrumentalities'—a framework of understanding or practical theories—that are extensions of laypersons' ways of making sense of the world, their *lay* instrumentalities. There are no superior instrumentalities, although in current practice some are privileged and oppress others, e.g. the instrumentalities of science/positivism. Consequently, in practical inquiry the inquirer and inquired about 'pool' their instrumentalities to construct the meaning of a situation. In the inquiry process, everyone is a co-respondent, contributing to the construction of the world that is being 'researched.' The academic researcher brings and takes stories to other domains (Pearce 1999), for example, through academic writing, reports, etc., but is not in any way separate from the research process.

The erosion of the boundary between inquirer and inquired about implies a rejection of objectivity, in the very strict positivist sense. This does not mean, however, that subjectivity is reified instead. The aim is not to know other minds, either the mind of the inquirer or inquired about. Social constructionists deny the concept of mind (Harré 1998). Knowledge, for example clinical diagnosis (considered here as a practical theory), arises through the process of conversational interaction (Birch 1995). Thus, the position of the inquirer—their relationship with others—becomes a central consideration in the process of inquiry.

Recursive Inquiry

Inquiry is not a linear affair. The scientific tradition entails the idea of linear progress towards the 'ideal' society. However, such 'grand schemes' to capture reality exactly have come unstuck (Lyotard 1984). In practical inquiry, the process of inquiry recursively (through folding back on itself) defines the subject, the line of inquiry and the methodology employed (Cronen 2001). Human inquiry is a communication process (Cronen & Chetro-Szivos 2001) constituted of varied conversations (Pearce 1999), and this is why it has the potential to construct rather than reflect reality. The object that we inquire into is changed by the act of our inquiring, that is, by our gazing upon the processes of the system itself (Cronen 2001). This focus differs from that of traditional science, which seeks the hidden laws behind the processes, to *understand*. As the practical inquiry system explores the phenomenon or situation, different aspects may be foregrounded and different methods used to develop *description*.

Instrumentalities Constituting Practical Theory

'Instrumentalities' (as defined by Cronen 2001) are statements about theoretical principles [for example, all nursing takes place within interpersonal relations (Peplau 1952)], definitions (for example, what constitutes 'care'), models (for example, the Tidal Model of Psychiatric nursing, Barker 2000), and methods of data collection, such as focus group interviews (Kitzinger 1995). They can be statements about the subject of the inquiry, about a situation and how its parts articulate together, or about its function. Instrumentalities are not ends in themselves, but are used to make a difference. The practical inquirer seeks to improve relationships between people and their social worlds (Dewey

1929/1938). Consequently, the people engaged in an inquiry must take responsibility for the change that the research achieves.

The Situation-In-View

According to Dewey (1929/1938), we inquire *into* situations. First we identify the situation in view. For Dewey the situations where inquiry is most needed are those that have an element of dysfunction, for example, clinical nursing specialties where waiting times for treatment are too long. However, it is equally possible to look at how a situation may be improved, for example, how a nursing team might improve their treatment approach, which is already currently valued by service users. In either case, we try, in Dewey's terms, to change a dysfunctional or indeterminate situation into a determinate or functional one. Elements of the situation that are unspecified in their relationship with one another (indeterminate) are inquired into, with the aim of converting them into a coherent whole (determinate). We do not necessarily have to look at all the elements of a situation, and what is inquired into may well change through the process of inquiry. Figure 15-1 shows the process by which a situation becomes determinate.

In order to make a situation determinate, we usually begin with some kind of practical theory (a preliminary set of instrumentalities), even if this is implicit. We then need to 'fashion instrumental descriptions and definitions (the emergent practical theory, my addition) for features of the situation and their relationships' (Cronen

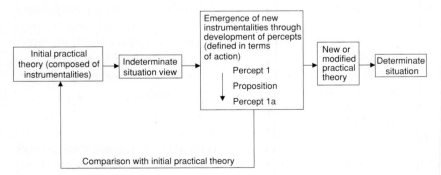

Figure 15-1 *Indeterminate to determinate situation—process.*

2001, p. 21). This achievement occurs through high-lighting certain features of the situation and developing percepts about them.

Percepts (Peirce 1905) differ from concepts, which try to reduce a phenomenon to its essence (James 1909/1996, Cutcliffe & McKenna in press). Concepts are essentialist. Action based in essentialism tends to follow a formula rather than being spontaneous or creative. For example, in using nursing 'care pathways,' diagnosis triggers a set of nursing responses that do not necessarily allow for individual difference, although they may ensure that the minimum standard of care is offered (Jones & Hannigan 2001). On the other hand, percepts involve thick description (James 1909/1996), which includes description of interconnections between aspects of experience (for example, how being a nurse connects with societal ideas about caring). Critically, a percept helps to us to understand a phenomenon by telling us what to *do* in order to be more intellectually or emotionally connected to a phenomenon. In other words, a percept helps to form instrumental descriptions—instrumentalities/practical theory—that enrich, enlarge or amend the initial practical theory that was brought to the inquiry. Thus, practical theory is integral to the inquiry process and does not stand outside of it. For example, a percept of caring might direct us to offer physical and psychological comfort to a patient in distress, to instruct us to imagine being in the other's place, and *through this* we gain an understanding of caring as a phenomenon. An instrumentality that arises might be a model of caring that specifies different domains of caring—physical, psychological, spiritual.

A percept can be treated as a stable object at a point in inquiry, but it has a 'shelf life' as the developing instrumentalities of the practical theory suggest further aspects of the percept. More important than its stability is its function of encouraging reflection, for example, how does it feel to be a 'caring' nurse? When there are expectations about caring, what pressures does the nurse face? Through this process, percepts help to generate propositions or guiding hypotheses, for example, 'The "caring" nurse carries an emotional burden, that is difficult to

because of social expectations, and so needs to
linical supervision to help feel that the care burden
ed.' The development of propositions helps to fur-
evelop percepts. For example, 'caring within nurs-
dependent on a care system, which is broader than
lividual nurse–patient relationship.'

rmination and Beyond

mination' occurs for both the inquirer and
ed about, and is an achievement *of* and *for* the
y system. Stakeholders assess the emergent theory
ab and fit' (Cutcliffe & McKenna 1999) until there
ense of collective 'rationality' or coherence. For
n and Lang (1994, p. 5), speaking as pragmatists,
ality can be thought of as 'grasping something in a
on that has future possibilities,' which allows
concerned to get on with their lives. Thus, deter-
on increases 'grammatical abilities' (Wittgenstein
, (loosely) defined as sets of rules that are co-
d with others and have shared meaning (as in the
le of the children's game, above). Critically,
natical abilities increase the capacity to perform.
; a nursing example, nurses who use a 'tried and
' risk assessment have a set of rules, a grammati-
ility in relation to assessing risk. Over time, they
different level of understanding (coherent deter-
on) of risk through conversations with that
t group. When patients who are presenting in a
e way come to be assessed, nurses find themselves
previously unused assessment strategies.

ment of 'The Good'

rmination (as a coherent set of co-created rules)
e possibilities it points to are judged by their con-
nce rather than with reference to abstract criteria
xample, validity, reliability and generalizability).
itly, if not explicitly, judgement involves compari-
ideed, for James (1904), pragmatism is a way of
g with conflict between ideas. James' pragmatism
; a theory of truth, which derives from the work of
and Schiller:

study that would describe the experience of being in schizophrenia (Aldridge 1998). A full account of the study is found in Aldridge and Stevenson (2001). She chose a phenomenological approach, appropriate to the research question. Although not perceived at the time, the chosen methodology was, in effect, the practical theory we brought to the inquiry. From a practical theory viewpoint, there were three main 'instrumentalities':

- Bracketing off preunderstandings about schizophrenia. As a clinician, Aldridge had been encouraged to think in a negative way about the diagnosis, treatment and prognosis.
- The work of Shingler (2000), an artist who believes that schizophrenia is integral to the human experience, not separate or alien. For this reason, schizophrenia can offer valuable insights into existence.
- The principle of the detached researcher bringing objectivity towards understanding the other's subjectivity.

At this point, the practical theory (phenomenology) was both informing the inquiry and becoming more developed, as illustrated in the comments of one study participant and Aldridge herself:

Participant: Nobody else has ever asked me about schizophrenia. I was able to say my piece . . . I got the chance to say why I believe the things I do . . . it helped me to piece things together in my head. (Aldridge & Stevenson 2001, p. 26)

Aldridge: I became aware of entering each encounter from a not-knowing position, feeling privileged to be invited into the participants' worlds where I found I was connecting on a personal level and developing an insightful understanding of the participants' view-point. (Aldridge 1998, p. 64)

Then one of the participants in the study, Beth (an alias to protect confidentiality), used a particular frame of reference to help her both understand and communicate her experience of schizophrenia, the term being, for her, an unhelpful description. She referenced her-self to Alice in Wonderland (Carroll 1994), and Through the Looking Glass (Carroll 1980) comparing her own perceptions of body distortion with Alice's altered body forms. Aldridge was moved by Beth's account, and in the process of the interview had engaged with her around her poetic framework. The division between the inquirer and inquired about (initial instrumentality) was being eroded—the practical theory was developing as the instrumentality was being refined.

Contemporaneously, Aldridge and I had been studying John Shotter's work on social poetics (Shotter 1998). Holmes (2001) points out that Shotter's social poetics is anchored in the work of Aristotle, Wittgenstein and Bahktin, and is concerned with creating, rather than capturing, understanding. To do this requires a relational practice, meaning that each person responds to the other's words in an engaged way rather than with detached, intellectual or professionalized talk (Shotter 1998). Aldridge and I had been interested in how a different kind of understanding of an unimaginable world (schizophrenia) can arise from tuning in to different channels and forms of communication.

At this point in the research process, we were struggling to maintain a phenomenological approach, seeking the essence of the person's experience. We felt that we were being 'advised by the research process' to embrace a poetic, social constructionist position. Consequently, we decided to change inquiry approach in mid-stream. Retrospectively, we were revising our practical theory to accommodate social poetics with the instrumentalities of social constructionism and Alice in Wonderland. Having adopted a new theoretical approach, we began by revisiting Beth's interview, extending her use of Alice in Wonderland by creating percepts of her individual experience and of psychiatric systems in general. In so doing, we were aware that our constructions were not in any way authoritative, and we urged the readers of our paper to creatively apply Alice's adventures to their own encounters in/with psychiatric systems. However, it is worth quoting an example of how we began to (re)construct our understandings of Beth and her place in psychiatry (Aldridge & Stevenson 2001, p. 23) to illustrate the place of poetics in constructing percepts and instrumentalities:

> At that time . . . I [Beth] wanted a definite diagnosis but now it feels as if I'm being labelled sometimes and people think schizophrenia and violence . . . voices and mad and split personality . . . but schizophrenia is such a wide thing anyway and everybody's different, but it feels like I'm in a little box.
>
> 'I shouldn't know you again if we *did* meet,' Humpty Dumpty replied in a disconnected tone, giving her one of his fingers to shake: You're so exactly like other people." The face is what one goes by, generally,' Alice remarked in a thoughtful tone. 'That's just what I complain of, said Humpty Dumpty. 'Your face is the same as everybody has— the two eyes . . . nose in the middle, mouth under. It's always the same' (Carroll 1980, p. 322)

In relation to practical inquiry/theory, the following instrumentality was developed: The loss of personal identity for Beth is replaced by the identity preferred by 'the system.' Consequently, Beth is restricted in how she can live her life. The system cannot appreciate subtle differences because it uses gross criteria to judge people and so is 'disconnected' from the person. To set the person free from the imposed identity, it is necessary for the system to re-attune to the individual narrative of the experience of schizophrenia.

Previously, Beth's comparisons of her position with that of Alice had not been appreciated. This had led to some strain in the relationships between her and the professional system. When she tried to use Alice to communicate her own experience she was told, 'I'm not talking to you because you're not making any sense.' There was an indeterminate situation. Beth was very positive about her experience of the research process, which was *therapeutic*, because the situation was made determinate—in the sense that Beth and the connected researchers constructed a meaningful rationality concerning schizophrenia and psychiatric systems, and how they can be understood. Beth felt heard and valued and compared this to other occasions. For both Beth and the

rest of the inquiry system (Aldridge and me) there was a sense of different possibilities. The closeness of the encounter between Aldridge and Beth allowed them both to recognize that conventional psychiatry had little to offer her and tended to be empowering for the professional psychiatric system (Stevenson & Aldridge 2001).

The ending of the story is positive in terms of consequences (occurring after the publication of Aldridge & Stevenson 2001). Beth and her Community Psychiatric Nurse (CPN) had struggled in their relationship and she was allocated another nurse. Aldridge spoke with Beth's new CPN about using Alice in Wonderland as a shared frame of reference, and this seemed to allow the CPN to 'go on with the care relationship with Beth.' However, 'engaged' research has an ethical and political domain. Beth's 'regular nurse' expressed concern to Aldridge, remarking that the research might have 'sparked something off.' As part of their education, psychiatric nurses are often advised to avoid talking about the content of 'delusions,' as discussed in a paper about the study:

> Whilst the nurse was caring from within the traditional schizophrenic text, DA was entering Beth's world, conjointly learning from it . . . (Aldridge & Stevenson 2001, p. 26).

Holmes (2001) has criticized the ethics of such engagement, arguing that the promotion of a poetic approach can leave people without the diagnosis that allows them access to health and social care. However, Aldridge and Beth were aware that conventional psychiatry held out little hope for her. The politics of psychiatry are self-serving for the professionals who make decisions about what counts as real or true. The engaged researcher enacted power differently, accepting that multiple realities are possible, although, as argued above, not necessarily equally helpful.

Conclusion

Practical inquiry/theory is a radical approach to addressing the theory/practice gap. It is irreverent to usual boundaries.

developmental research that assists the enactment of the broad church of practice.

REFERENCES

Aldridge D. (1998). *The unique singular self.* Unpublished MSc dissertation, University of Newcastle upon Tyne, Newcastle upon Tyne.

Aldridge D. & Stevenson C. (2001). Social poetics as research and practice: living in and learning from the process of research. *Nursing Inquiry* 8, 19–27.

Barker P. J. (2000). The Tidal Model: the lived experience of person-centred health care. *Nursing Philosophy* 2, 213–223.

Birch J. (1995). Chasing the rainbow's end and why it matters: a coda to Pocock, Frosh and Larner. *Journal of Family Therapy* 2, 219–228.

Carroll L. (1980). *Through the Looking Glass.* Macmillan, London.

Carroll L. (1994). *Alice's Adventures in Wonderland.* Penguin, London.

Cronen V. (1984). Communication theory for the twenty-first century: cleaning up the wreckage of the psychology project. In *Communication: Views from the Helm for the 21st Century* (Trent J., ed.), Allyn and Bacon, Needham Heights, CA, pp. 18–38.

Cronen V. (1995). Practical theory and the tasks ahead for social approaches to communication. In *Social Approaches to Communication* (Leeds-Hurwitz W., ed.), Guilford, New York, pp. 217–242.

Cronen V. (2001). Practical theory, practical art, and the pragmatic-systemic account of inquiry. *Communication Theory* 11, 14–35.

Cronen V. & Chetro-Szivos J. (2001). Pragmatism as a way of inquiring with special reference to a theory of communication and the general form of pragmatic social theory. In *American Pragmatism and Communication Research* (Perry D. ed.), Erlbaum, New York, pp. 27–65.

Cronen V. & Lang P. (1994). Language and action: Wittgenstein and Dewey in the practice of therapy and consultation. *Family Process* 2, 91–112.

Cutcliffe J. R. & McKenna H. P. (1999). Establishing the credibility of qualitative research findings: the plot thickens. *Journal of Advanced Nursing* 30, 374–380.

Cutcliffe J. R. & McKenna H. P. (eds) (in press) *Essential Concepts in Nursing.* Elsevier, Oxford.

Dewey J. [1925 (original)/1958]. *Experience and Nature.* Dover, New York.

Dewey J. [1929 (original)/1938]. *Logic: The Theory of Inquiry.* Henry Holt, New York.

Harré R. (1998). *The Singular Self: An Introduction to the Psychology of Personhood.* Sage, London.

Holdsworth N. (1997). Commentary . . . postmodernity and psychiatric nursing. *Journal of Psychiatric and Mental Health Nursing* 4, 9–14.

Holmes C. (2001). Schizophrenia and the 'disquieting' consequences of social poetics: a response to Aldridge and Stevenson. *Nursing Inquiry* 8, 28–29.

What is Already Known About This Topic

- Underpinning philosophies and frameworks of understanding (postmodernism, social constructionism, pragmatism, systems theory) have been discussed in a range of nursing journals and texts.
- Practical inquiry/theory has been previously developed through integration of philosophies and frameworks into a methodological position.
- Action research shares some methodological assumptions with practical inquiry, such as the cyclical process of research.

What This Paper Adds

- A challenge to orthodox approaches to nursing inquiry and theory generation by re-defining the inquiry 'system,' through challenging linear research models, and through promoting the importance of 'local' rather than grand theory.
- An outline of the structures and processes of practical inquiry/theory, and a demonstration of their application in nursing research.
- A new (to nursing) research approach that can lead to the production of relevant theory for nursing.

However, it needs further application and critical appraisal. It has far-reaching implications, and raises questions that need to be addressed, both within the practice of nursing and in the academy. Who will the researchers of the future be? What will be the spheres of reference for research, both in terms of level and focus? What will happen to traditional research approaches? Will practical theory be counted as evidence? How will it be disseminated (if at all)? Yet, based on the above analysis, practical inquiry/theory may well offer the means to conduct cogent, collective, collaborative,

James W. (1904). *What is Pragmatism? From a Series of Eight Lectures Dedicated to the Memory of John Stuart Mill, A New Name for Some Old Ways of Thinking, in December 1904, from William James, Writings 1902–1920.* The Library of America, New York.

James W. [1909 (original)/1996]. *A Pluralistic Universe.* University of Nebraska Press, Lincoln, NE.

Jones A. & Hannigan B. (2001). Hospital care pathways for patients with schizophrenia. *Journal of Clinical Nursing* 10, 58–69.

Kennedy M. (1979). Generalising from single case studies. *Education Quarterly* 3, 661–678.

Kitzinger J. (1995). Introducing focus groups. *British Medical Journal* 311, 299–302.

Kvale S. (1996). *Interviews: An Introduction to Qualitative Research Interviewing.* Sage, Thousand Oaks, CA,

Lyotard J.-F. (1984). *The Post-Modern Condition: A Report on Knowledge.* Manchester University Press, Manchester.

Pearce W.B. (1999). *Using CMM: The Co-Ordinated Management of Meaning.* A Pearce Associates Seminar, San Mateo, CA, 4 August 1999.

Peirce C.S. (1905). What pragmatism is. *The Monist* 15(2), 161–181.

Peplau H. (1952). *Interpersonal Relations in Nursing.* Putnam, New York.

Shingler A. (2000). *Beyond Reason: An Exploration of Schizophrenia in Images and Words.* Beyond Reason Org, Wirksworth, Derbyshire.

Shotter J. (1984). *Social Accountability and Selfhood.* Blackwell, Oxford.

Shelter J. (1998). Social construction and social poetics. In *Reconstructing the Psychological Subject: Bodies, Practices and Technologies* (Bayer B.M. & Shotter J., eds), Sage, London, pp. 33–51.

Stevenson C. (1996). Taking the pith out of reality. *Journal of Psychiatric and Mental Health Nursing* 3, 103–110.

Stevenson C. & Aldridge D. (2001). Response to Holmes: which reality and who decides? *Nursing Inquiry* 8, 30–31.

Stevenson C. & Beech I. (1998). Playing the power game for qualitative researchers: the possibility of a postmodern approach. *Journal of Advanced Nursing* 27, 790–797.

Stevenson C. & Beech I. (2001). Paradigms lost, paradigms regained: defending nursing against a single reading of postmodernism. *Nursing Philosophy* 2, 143–150.

Upton D.J. (1999). How do we achieve evidence-based practice if we have a theory practice gap in nursing today? *Journal of Advanced Nursing* 29, 549–555.

Wittgenstein L. (1953). *Philosophical Investigations* (Anscombe G. E., Trans.) Macmillan, New York.

The Author Comments

Practical Inquiry/Theory in Nursing

I was aware from my contact with practitioners that there was and is a continuing gap between knowledge produced in the academy and knowledge required in and for practice. For some years, I had been steeping myself in the postmodern/social constructionist literature and came across the idea of practical inquiry/theory in the communication theory/family therapy field. I decided to check out whether this was a useful inquiry approach for nursing through writing the article and making a retrospective analysis of an actual research project. I think practical inquiry/theory has promise for nursing in that local stakeholders produce local knowledge that has immediate application. It allows nurses to be 'natural inquirers' and mitigates against the reluctance nurses have had, to date, to engage in research.

—CHRIS STEVENSON

CHAPTER 16

Intelligent Nursing: Accounting for Knowledge as Action in Practice

Mary E. Purkis
Kristín Björnsdóttir

This paper provides an analysis of nursing as a knowledgeable discipline. We examined ways in which knowledge operates in the practice of home care nursing and explored how knowledge might be fruitfully understood within the ambiguous spaces and competing temporalities characterizing contemporary healthcare services. Two popular metaphors of knowledge in nursing practice were identified and critically examined; "evidence-based practice" and the "nurse as an intuitive worker." Pointing to faults in these conceptualizations, we suggest a different way of conceptualizing the relationship between knowledge and practice, namely practice as being activated by contextualized knowledge. This conceptualization is captured in an understanding of the intelligent creation of context by the nurse for nursing practice to be ethical and effective.

Introduction

In her explorations of time and nursing work, Judy Parker (1997) argues that 'to the extent that there is a weakening of the modernist temporality directed towards the future, there is an opportunity for the nursing voice that articulates the concerns of the moment to be heard. However,' she warns, 'contemporary health care is in the throes of significant change. The nurse is now in the space where everything is happening at once, attuned to the positioning and imperatives of various temporalities. These include not only those of the

gained during education or, much more importantly, the nurse knows how to retrieve it from data banks (Stotts, 1999). This model seems quite logical. We all prefer our nurse to be up to date regarding findings from the newest and best research that relates to the illness that we may suffer from. Through licensure nurses are granted special standing, partly because of their ability to express specialized knowledge under particular conditions (i.e. examinations, reading journal papers, undertaking patient education sessions), which they are expected to keep up to date. This is their contract with the public.

The problem that we find with this particular construction of knowledge is that it relies on a metaphor of dissemination: knowledge is and can be packaged for any situation. The nurse can be taught how to use computer-based technologies to produce the range of available knowledge to apply in any situation. Such knowledge does not seem to rely on any particular space or context for its effectiveness. Knowledge is available and awaits application by the nurse. This model of knowledge and its apparently unproblematic application is clean, powerful, and in that, quite seductive. There is nothing of the messiness of 'the particular' in the discourse of evidence-based practice. Consider again the example of the home care nurse provided above. That example seems overflowing in its depiction of particular circumstances. When the home care nurse asks, 'What do you do with a self-destructive?' she is asking a *very particular* question; she seeks *particular* sorts of answers and she needs these answers in order to continue her practice of appropriate nursing care. While the powerful metaphor of directly applicable knowledge inherent in the discourse of 'evidence-based nursing' circulates in her workplace, its capacities seem irrelevant to the answer she seeks.

As Bruno Latour (1986) reminds us, the relationship between knowledge and action is not simply one of dissemination but rather transformation. The metaphor of 'dissemination' suggests that knowledge remains intact and is simply passed on to the next person in its entirety, unchanged. Latour's argument is that as knowledge moves or spreads through social networks, it is

transformed. It is constantly undergoing change. So, at the juncture between the sort of abstract knowledge represented by the evidence that a nurse might bring to a particular patient care situation, and the actual situation of the patient, the nurse must somehow 'go on' (cf. Giddens, 1984). In our example, the nurse finds it very difficult to 'go on.' She is frustrated with the patient, trying to dismiss her sense of responsibility for him by calling him a 'self-destructive.' She gives us hints of how she has tried to go on in previous meetings with this patient. She has developed plans. She has tried to involve other healthcare providers. In these ways she is transforming the evidence that she brings to the home and in seeking to apply that in this contextualized situation; she also transforms him from an independent person into a 'problem' that she and other healthcare providers must deal with.

Turning back to Parker's comment about ambiguous spaces, in our example the nurse is operating in two knowledge spaces, the decontextualized space of evidence-based practice and the personal space of the patient. She knows about how to screen for depression—the practices she has been taught on this front are relatively consistent and rational. She knows too how to determine if the patient is hypoglycemic or hyperglycemic. Again, the biomedical evidence on diabetes could be very helpful to her. However, she also operates in the very different space of this person's home. She has seen the stash of insulin, she hears his despondency, she recognizes his despair. Seeking to apply the rational evidence in this circumstance, the nurse is 'caught' in the ambiguity of these two apparently distinct knowledge spaces—one created through discourses related to the evidence-based movement, the other created through her interpretations of the man's circumstances of everyday living.

The evidence-based movement has been influential in nursing, but it has also come under considerable critical scrutiny in the nursing literature (Traynor, 1999; Rolfe, 2002, 2005). Clinicians maintain that advocates of evidence-based practice ignore the complex knowledge gained through years of experience. As they point out, to be able to practice competently, the practitioner pays attention to an array of 'evidence,' not just evidence from research. Many of the authors who promote evidence-based nursing practice are aware of the limits of the highly rational and linear understanding of knowledge generation and use inherent in this project and have tried to respond to criticism in different ways, such as by extending the definition of evidence. In addition to being derived from research, evidence is said to come from patient's preferences and from the nurse's work-related experience (Estabrooks, 1998; Kitson *et al.*, 1998). But without the requisite critique of context activating nursing practice, Parker urges us to recognize how very difficult it is for patient's preferences to be known—and once known, to play any sort of role at all in shaping the care provided. It is our contention that evidence-based practice places a primary emphasis on isolating knowledge 'factors' at the expense of the nurses' creative use of that knowledge as a means for 'going on' in her everyday work as a nurse.

Intuition and Emotion Work

In response to the above critique, namely the overemphasis on scientific knowledge as the only legitimate source of knowledge in nursing practice and the rational-technical understanding of practice, a highly influential trend emerged in the last decades of the 20th century celebrating the nurse as the author of knowledge and the primary judge of its legitimacy in clinical situations. This is Patricia Benner's description of the nurse as an **intuitive knower**. Nurses worldwide, having read Patricia Benner's (1984) book *From Novice to Expert* and the follow-up by her in collaboration with colleagues (Benner & Tanner, 1987; Benner *et al.*, 1996), experienced heightened self-confidence and respect for their work. Finally, an academic nurse had articulated the complexities and demands inherent in nursing practice. Those were certainly liberating and empowering times for nurses, but in the long run it has tended to valorize specific heroic actions while at the same time fostering a lack of self-questioning and critique of one's judgements on behalf of the nurse. Many nurses draw on Benner's work—sometimes quite tangentially—to claim expertise base on an intuitive knowledge that is characterized by a troubling lack of public and professional accountability. This trend has led to a subjectivist understanding of nursing knowledge that seems to legitimate and even encourage relativism. There is an overemphasis on the ability of the nurse to know and understand the needs and wishes of her patients, based heavily on her interpretations of the situation.

The faith in the nurse's ability to make correct decisions, based on intuition or insights gained through interaction with the patient, is reflected in the research approach used by Benner and her associates. Examples of expert practice are gained from paradigm cases where the nurses themselves describe what is taken to be highly successful care, without an attempt to validate their inferences in interviews with patients (Purkis, 1994). Their own judgements are taken at face value. This is highly problematic in light of the many studies that have compared nurses and patient's identification of patients' needs and their expectations regarding nursing care, showing considerable discrepancies (Björk, 1995).

Benner is one among many influential nurse theorists who have proposed a form of phenomenological understanding of nursing practice as caring. These theorists share the view that nursing is inherently good and that if nurses are given the opportunity to practise in line with their upbringing all will be well. Magically they will know what is best for the patient. The primary emphasis is on the persona of the nurse and her healing potential as a human being (Boykin & Schoenhofer, 1993).

Nursing, as envisioned in these theorists' writings, aims at something more than providing assistance and comfort. Effective nursing care leads to transcendence, a new understanding of the patient's situation and reconciliation of suffering or pain. This is reflected in Watson's (1985) description of the goals of her theory: 'The goal of the theory ideals are associated with mental-spiritual growth for self and others, finding meaning in one's own existence and experiences, discovering inner power and control, and potentiating instances of transcendence and self healing' (p. 74). The nurse enters into an authentic relationship with the patient, characterized by mutuality, respect, and warmth.

The main difficulties that we see with this understanding of nursing practice is the conflated belief in the nurses' ability to know what is best for the patient, an overemphasis on emotions in nursing practice at the expense of accountable forms of intelligent, informed practice and the way that knowledge relates to practice only ever in a *post hoc* manner. Ultimately, our concern rests on the remarkable neglect of the realities of nursing practice in these accounts. By contrast, we wish to promote an engagement in a debate regarding the ambiguities that become apparent when different forms of knowledge are brought into proximity with one another which, we argue, is responsible for activating the nurse within her practice.

Benner's work demands nurses adopt an identity of the intuitive practitioner. This identity presents opportunities for nurses to selectively point to factors they recall from the care situation when accounting for their practice. All too often, these factors reinforce a model of practice that denies the voice and contribution of the person receiving nursing care and instead, reify the nurse's actions as heroic (Purkis, 1994; Latimer, 2000; Padgett, 2000).

Being Activated by Knowledge

We have engaged in this exploration of knowledge and nursing practice from a position that is skeptical of both of the metaphors discussed above. We are particularly skeptical of their capacity to adequately account for how nursing practice can be said to be knowledgeable. Through engaging in a critical exploration of language use and descriptions of practice we hope to, in what remains of the paper, open up a more productive space within which nursing practice can be understood as being *activated by knowledge*. The argument we set out in this paper rests on an assumption that the metaphors describing nurses as knowledgeable workers come equipped with temporal frames. For instance, where nurses are activated by discourses of 'evidence-based practice,' they will engage in their practice in a linear and future-orientated way, with the aim of reaching predefined outcomes. They are required to structure their care in ways that are future-orientated, driven by goals that they seek to impose into this situation. Meeting on the ground of the patient who endures in an ever-present life, he may seek no future and thus cannot practise in the plan that the nurse has devised.

In the final part of this paper, we would like to explore what might be the implications of Parker's (1997) claim that nurses are 'located in the ambiguous spaces between the competing temporalities' (p. 16). In order to clear a space for expressing different ways of conceptualizing intelligent nursing practice, we want to examine the possibilities and tensions within the practice example in relation to Parker's ideas about time and nursing work. We will suggest ways of conceptualizing the notion of 'context' as a central, but contentious feature of any claim about knowledge and its relations to nursing practice.

Turning back to the nurse in our example above, we can identify broad areas of theoretical knowledge that she as a nurse is expected to possess. She needs to know the most current information regarding diabetes and its treatment; of alcoholism; depression; social isolation and loss; and suicide. In addition, she needs to draw on managerial knowledge to work with the home care aide. Clearly, she 'knew' how to make an assessment of risk for suicide. This would have been one of the ideas she was taught when she was in school, learning to be a nurse. And she clearly had drawn on this knowledge in her attempts to surround this man with sufficient support to help him continue to live. She had the organizational capacity to 'put in home support.' He apparently either acceded to this help or lacked the capacity to resist it.

However, it is the nurse's intelligent use of all this knowledge that makes her an efficient professional who is making the best out of scarce resources. Her work cannot be standardized nor predetermined. It is and will be indeterminate and flexible. As Parker (1997) points out:

> The nurse is in this sense hybrid, able to speak the voices of medicine, nursing, institution and patient. Rather than being confused or disoriented by this multivocality, the nurse can assume a position of 'in between (Parker, 1997, p. 22).

Voicing the Concerns of the Moment

Parker's argument, set out in our introduction, suggests that, in opposition to the sometimes quite simplistic rhetoric in which nurses are encouraged to 'advocate' for their patients, a nursing voice that can articulate the concerns of the patient is contingent on a 'weakening of the modernist temporality directed towards the future.' This future-directed temporality is perhaps most evident in the modern acute-care hospital where patient concerns are so easily set aside by curative technologies. Within that practice setting, nurses must operate in a bicultural manner: able to competently perform the requirements set out by the medical regime but at the same time, aware that this regime may either not be what the person in the bed wants or may represent only one option among many that the person may be aware of. Where there is some awareness of such competing demands, there is also an awareness of possibilities for alternative temporalities, leading in numerous directions towards outcomes unarticulated within a discourse of a medically defined 'future.' Organizing nursing practice around this medically defined future entails occupation of a particular temporality and a setting aside of any other temporality—either a nursing temporality or a patient temporality.

An example can be offered to illustrate the impact of such competing demands. The nurse did the 'right' thing when she entered the patient's home: she took action to rectify the effects of his hypoglycemia. But her interview later in the day indicates that she is aware she could have explored questions of the meaningfulness— or the lack of meaning—of life for this patient. The shift in focus (away from the physical effects of hypoglycemia over to the existential impacts of taking action to rectify the physical effects of hypoglycemia) would take her into a different temporality—and a vastly different range of options for her practice. From this temporality, her actions may no longer be 'right.' Indeed, her confusion about the appropriateness of her actions seems central to her question, 'What do you do with a self-destructive?'

The home can be thought of as 'fracturing' the life world of modern medicine (Habermas, 1984; Liaschenko, 1994). Entering the home, the nurse enters a life world constituted by routines that run on quite different timelines than those guiding the nurse as an employee of a health unit. In our example, the competition around timelines and the power to define them is evident in the nurse's decision to undertake a 'quick' visit elsewhere while the elderly man's blood sugar levels increase. She displays an ability to operate in two different 'time zones,' both very much shaped by her institutional identity as a home care nurse. By contrast, the homemaker who was working away at tidying the kitchen while the patient took his own time to awaken might be read in this example as being 'in time' with the patient. To the extent that low sugar levels impaired his level of consciousness rather than pointing to the possibilities that he has just awakened, being 'in time' with him would not have resulted in a positive outcome—but such evaluation of the value of outcomes can only be made in relation to a modernist temporality directed towards the future. Only if it is assumed the man wants to live can acting on the hypoglycemia be understood as 'good' practice.

Once the nurse returns from her visit, she demonstrates a greater commitment to being with the patient in his time. As her comments reveal later in the interview, she gained an awareness of his 'concerns of the moment' (Parker, 1997, p. 16). She is aware of his despair over losing contact with his friend and how this is experienced by the patient as the last straw in terms of his capacity to perceive meaningfulness in his life. She can only respond to the depth of his despair by asking unanswerable questions about how she is to 'deal' with him now: 'What do you do with a self-destructive?'

Imperatives Embedded in Diverse Temporalities

We have already seen how it is possible for the home care nurse to impose her organizational imperatives to visit numerous patients per day over and against the apparent needs and concerns of individual patients.

But this is not simply a matter of brute power and control. This nurse truly seems to be 'in the space where everything is happening at once' and she is 'attuned to the positionings and imperatives of various temporalities' (Parker, 1997, p. 16). In order to examine how this is so, we need to look at each actor's part in this event.

The Patient

The example provides vivid evidence of the relational character of 'patienthood.' When the nurse enters the house, the homemaker is already present. The homemaker, however, does not read the man as a patient: instead, she makes a reading of him as an elderly man who is groggy from the night's sleep. Coming into his home as a 'service' set up by nurses at the health unit, she focuses on the spaces available for her work: the kitchen and later the living room.

It is with the nurse's entrance to the home that the man becomes constituted as a patient. The nurse makes a reading of the patient's level of consciousness as beyond the limits of what she had come to expect of him at any time of the day. She immediately brings him a glass of juice, *treating* him as someone who may be hypoglycemic. The meaning of being hypoglycemic is not apparent to her at this time. It is only when she returns from the visit that she begins to hear about his despair over losing touch with his friend. Her knowledge of him from previous visits enables her to read this latest blow as one in a series. By the end of the visit, his experiences having been conveyed in slow, dejected tones arising from 'the embodied temporality of endurance' (Parker, 1997, p. 22). He is enduring rather than living his life.

The Nurse

To the extent the nurse recognizes that the patient endures rather than lives, her recognition intersects with expectations she may hold of herself as a home care nurse and with expectations she may know others hold of her in that role. This intersection serves to 'create an uneasy space' (Parker, 1997, p. 22) for the nurse. She may know that the temporality constituting the patient's position in relation to her as a nurse may place demands on her time that will cause problems for her if it results in her not fulfilling her organizational obligations to visit a set number of patients each day. It could be that she recognizes this early on and makes the decision to get one more visit in prior to investigating the patient's situation more fully. But her identity as a home care nurse also provides her with opportunities to leave his immediate space. She is caught between the demands of his endurance and other patients' requirements. In nursing work, there are always numerous others who pull the nurse away *and* enable her to get away. These represent incommensurate demands on the nurse's time. That is, the nurse cannot choose to be in one temporality and then neatly step into the next. She is in *both at the same time—and* the demands of each contradict one another. The 'intuitive' nurse may recognize the patient's existential angst all the while the 'evidence-based' practitioner is taking steps to limit the negative impact of hypoglycemia. These metaphors may offer (competing) descriptive accounts of what we see and hear—and ultimately how we might, *post hoc,* attribute the nurse's actions as representing knowledgeable practice. They do not, however, provide an account of the knowledge upon which the nurse *moves towards* the patient as a nurse: it does not account for her *activation* as a knowledgeable practitioner of nursing.

The Physician

Eventually, there are other 'team' members who enter the event. At the end of the day, the nurse talks about how she thinks of her role as 'bounded' by decisions she can make alone and those she needs to share with others. In this instance, it is her boundary with the physician that comes into play.

By drawing the physician into the relationship, even though he may be, as she claims 'uninterested' in this patient, she diffuses (if even only momentarily) the pressure that builds up for her within this context of competing temporalities. Such diffusion serves to break the disciplinary and ethical obligations that bind her to her patient. The decision to act in particular ways is not hers alone. Other professional care providers share the responsibility for making this decision with her. Of course, in seeking relief from the intensity of making this decision alone, the nurse enters another temporality: that framed by medical practice. We should note here that she does not explicitly consider the fact that she could make the decision together with the patient.

The nurse's conversation with the patient reveals enough of his current situation to suggest to her that he would welcome the release of a death perhaps enabled by an overdose of insulin. However, the medical regime, mediated through the Health Unit which employs the nurse, positions the nurse to ask the interviewer for confirmation that she is right to suspend a patient-centred approach, an approach that is highly valued both in the academy and in practice. Certainly within her workplace, it is a patient-centred approach that would be advocated by managers interested in offloading as much caring work onto patients and families as possible (Purkis, 2001).

The Healthcare System

And here we reveal another layer constituting the spatiotemporal context of home nursing care. On all sorts of fronts, this patient spells 'trouble' for the nurse. Operating in a system fuelled by interests in cost savings, operationalized within the home care sector by a shift in interest towards post-operative surgical patients with predictable outcomes for the nurse to conclude an episode of care, there is simply no telling how long this patient is going to be 'on service.'

> Nurse: We were really, we were so hopeful for Norman (pseudonym). We thought that if we put in this help, kind of gave him that whole . . . I even made a referral to mental health to help him deal with some of the losses that he's had in his life and everything like that. And maybe we could give him a sense of, that, 'Hey! Life is still worth living.' (interview transcript)

The nurse's 'care plan' for this patient involves adding in services such as the homemaker and counselling support—always with a view towards a 'life worth living.' The care plan relies on deeply held views of what help looks like—and notions of evidence that help has been offered. The nurse talks collectively here: 'We were . . . so hopeful for Norman.' The nurse suggests that the nursing team have taken an interest in Norman. Together they devised this plan to help him live. The plan assumes that with referrals to counselling, he might want to live. The help is offered with an intention to have an effect. Such intentionality suggests that the actions are not haphazard. They are strategic and thus knowledgeable.

Having met resistance related to the patient's willingness to take these services up in the temporality they were intended, her labour becomes much more challenging. The strategy did not work. Was the knowledge behind the strategy 'wrong'? Or simply too reliant on the metaphor of evidence-based practice which served to render the patient's wants and desires absent? If patients are not to be entirely dismissed within accounts of knowledgeable nursing practice, then a sufficiently robust account of the context within which practice takes shape *through* knowledge must be generated.

Being Located in Ambiguous Spaces

In the preceding sections, we have opened a typical episode of home nursing care up for critical investigation. Our aim in examining this episode of practice in such detail has been to illustrate the layerings of competing imperatives of time and space within which the nurse engages in her practice.

In Parker's work, we find a way of explicating experiences of acting within ambiguity—which, while not a place of clarity and resolution, is nonetheless a space where competing versions of wants and desires can, under certain circumstances, be heard.

CHAPTER 17

Nursing Theory as a Guide to Practice

William K. Cody

After much deliberation, I find myself more convinced than ever that in the discipline of nursing today, given a forced choice between these two general propositions represented in Dr. Fawcett's questions about theory and practice, it is far more accurate and meaningful to assert that *theory guides practice*. To assert the alternative, that theory arises from practice to an equal or greater extent than theory guides practice, would be a misrepresentation of the contemporary art and science of nursing theory development. In actuality, this assertion has been made widely and, I would venture to say, that is to the detriment of theory development in nursing.

Reflections on Practice: Yes, Guided by Theory

As I reflect on my own experience, I think about the first 10 years of my work in nursing. During those years—the 1970s and the 1980s—nursing was nearly devoid of nursing theory *per se*. In contrast, the next 15 years were inundated with nursing theory. I realize that there always was some identifiable body of knowledge that provided an underpinning to my work. In the early days of my career—and I suspect that this experience is shared with many nurses now around my age, in their 40s and 50s—the knowledge that guided my work could be over-

From W. K. Cody, Nursing Science Quarterly 2003, 16(3): 225–231. Copyright © 2003, SAGE Publications.
Reprinted with permission by SAGE Publications, Inc.

About the Author

WILLIAM K. CODY was born in Hampton, VA, and grew up in North Carolina. He began his career in nursing as a licensed practical nurse and later received ASN and BSN degrees from Regents College; a BS in communication from New York University; an MSN from Hunter College, where he met his mentor, Rosemarie Parse; and a PhD in nursing from the University of South Carolina. He is currently Dean and Professor, Presbyterian School of Nursing at Queens University of Charlotte. He is perhaps best known for his articles on theoretical concerns written for *Nursing Science Quarterly*. As a Robert Wood Johnson Executive Nurse Fellow, 2003–2006, his leadership foci included nurse-managed health centers and community–campus partnerships.

whelmingly categorized as rudimentary knowledge of anatomy and physiology, medicine, pharmacology, physics, chemistry, microbiology, hygiene, psychology, and communication. There was some vague introduction to core ideas (I now know to be) from Virginia Henderson and Dorothea Orem, but their names and the name of any *theory* had been removed from the content. I was simply taught to care for people who were ill in such a way that they could, it was hoped, return to doing as much as possible to care for themselves, as soon as possible.

In the 1980s, I worked in a major urban medical center with a reputation for fine nursing practice. There, my nurse colleagues and I were constantly challenged by the nursing leadership to think critically and to consider the scientific rationale behind every element of patient care. Thus, I found myself obliged to take the rudimentary knowledge that had been the bedrock of my then-biomedical practice and make it broader and deeper, although keeping it almost completely categorizable as anatomy and physiology, medicine, pharmacology, and so on. When I consider these memories from 10 years of intensive bedside nursing, I cannot think of any other domain of life—other than the subsequent 15 years in which my work has been nursing theory intensive—in which my activities (homemaking, my own healthcare, relationships, recreation, participating in the arts, car maintenance, or anything else) have been so *thoroughly* guided by a specified body of knowledge. It was not nursing theory, but it was theory.

Problem-Solving and Common Sense: Guided by, Not Producing, Theories

To be sure, there were many creative ideas that emerged in my shared nursing worklife, ideas that surfaced in direct problem-solving efforts, brainstorming, being asked by my supervisors for input to resolve various situations, and other instances of making-do, jury-rigging, and flying by the seat of one's pants. We came up with different ways of taping intravenous lines to withstand restlessness and confusion, ingenious methods of affixing complicated dressings to large wounds, and clever ways of explaining complex concepts of medicine to lay people so that they might understand what was happening to them. We experimented with different ways of preventing and minimizing pressure sores; we learned when to test serum electrolytes and how to restore fluid, electrolyte, and hemodynamic stability with a minimum of direction from the physician; we organized the work of caring for groups of patients to be more efficient; shared ways of minimizing discomfort while passing various tubes into persons' orifices; and we mentored each other in talking with patients and families about death and dying. I witnessed my associates and myself gradually becoming more and more expert in various aspects of the job.

I admired many of my colleagues for the vast expanse of their knowledge and for their creativity in problemsolving. However, upon much reflection, I would have to say that I do not find it accurate or useful in any way to think of the activities just described as developing, generating, or inventing theory. Indeed, I find that reflecting on my own experiences in light of a robust notion of what constitutes theory development strongly contradicts the notion that *theory arises from practice*. To my knowledge, although I worked with a number of brilliant people and, along with them, solved many hundreds of practical problems with creative solutions, none of those activities rose to the level of generating theory, few were deeply rooted in any philosophy of nursing or anything else except practicality, none were published or widely disseminated, and some were later shown to be misguided by theory development and research.

Applying known principles of science and common sense to activities that are performed repetitively for months or years and coming up with incrementally better ways of doing things, to me, is not theorizing, and it is not useful to think of it as such. It is problem-solving; it is the benefit of practical experience; it is common sense at work. Even if one were to grant that this kind of creative thinking is *theorizing*, if it is neither grounded in a philosophy of nursing nor intended specifically to guide the work that is the specialized mission of nursing, then I see no reason to think of such creative ideas as *nursing* theories. It cannot substitute in any way for the fullness and richness of practice that is guided by nursing theory, and it pales in comparison in meaningfulness and effectiveness in enhancing quality of life.

My view is, to put it simply, that one learns to practice nursing by studying nursing theories, and one learns to practice nursing *very well* by studying nursing theories very intensely over a long period of time. One does not learn to practice in the discipline and profession of nursing by merely practicing what is commonly called nursing but is not specific to nursing, and one does not learn to practice nursing very well by practicing nursing that is bereft of nursing theory, even if it is practiced very intensely over a long period of time.

Contexts of Repression: Likelihood and Limitations

I essentially agree with Dr. Parker when she says that "practice must first be guided by theory, and then the theory can be studied and further developed as a result of expert practice" (Fawcett, 2003, p. 131). The difficulty that resides in connecting higher levels of nursing theory development in general with something called *expert practice* in nursing today is plain to see. By what are today's frontline, bedside nurses guided? I believe that for the most part, now as in the early years of my own career, they are guided by rudimentary principles and empirical generalizations from medicine and pharmacology, with a little social science and an eclectic mélange from a variety of other disciplines as needed for working in their settings and with their populations. Elements of the nursing theories that are taught in schools of nursing are, as often as not, taught sketchily and half-heartedly, and the majority of practice settings do not reinforce, value, or encourage the use of nursing theories. Innate good will, and a modicum of professionalism and ethical reflection upon one's practice can go far toward keeping basic care decent, but these clearly are not substitutes for a coherent vision of one's profession and its unique mission with an articulated practice methodology.

In the United States, nursing practice is carried out in a context of for-profit healthcare that demands skeleton staffing and production-line care, while about a third of the population is uninsured, underinsured, or a paycheck away from being uninsured. It is carried out in a context in which many persons must do without needed medicine because they cannot pay for it. It is carried out in a context in which a sizable proportion of the diagnostic tests performed are ordered as defensive measures against the possibility of malpractice lawsuits. It is carried out in a context in which the majority of the leaders and decision-makers in healthcare and health policy remain straight, White, males from middle- or upper-class backgrounds. And, much of medicine remains prone to the glorification of machismo and dominance in both physician-patient and physician-nurse relationships. The mammoth barrier to nursing theorizing arising in everyday nursing practice is not merely that the dominant ideas that permeate contemporary healthcare are *non-nursing*, although that is certainly the case; the greater barrier is that many of the ideas actually guiding practice (explicitly or implicitly) are alien to nursing's tradition of *caring for whole people where they are and as they are,* and even anathema to such an ideal. Ironically, perhaps, I do see nursing theory-based practice as the primary source of hope for altering these contexts.

The graduate students to whom I teach nursing theory have several common, salient reactions to the proposition that nursing practice should be guided by nursing theory. One reaction is that they (nurses) are far too busy in the chaotic, high-pressure environments of contemporary hospitals to take time to do "all that touchy-feely stuff," as some say. Another is to question why, if this knowledge is important, did the nursing establishment—so famously intent on control of many aspects of nursing education and practice—let them progress through their careers to see themselves and be seen as expert nurses without ever having seriously studied nursing theories? And still another reaction is that it is already hard enough to learn and remember all the medicine and pharmacology, and all the regulations, policies, and procedures required in everyday nursing practice, without trying to remember even more ideas and to practice differently from the habits of thought and action with which they have been indoctrinated over many years. Without a thorough education in nursing theory and the opportunity to engage over time in nursing theory-based practice, these *expert* nurses cannot be expected to develop nursing theory or contribute to nursing theory. This would be analogous to saying that the next great school of thought in psychology is likely to spring up spontaneously from the discipline of engineering.

Contexts of Understanding

I agree with Dr. Parker when she says that "our concepts guide what we 'look for,' and take in . . . and the experience then may be reflected on and described to enhance concepts" (Fawcett, 2003, pp. 131–132), a process she describes as a spiral. It seems that Dr. Parker is picturing something akin to the Heideggerian circle of understanding, which moves circularly or, as Dr. Parker prefers, spirally, from one's current understanding and that which is familiar to that which is new and unfamiliar

and back again, continuously integrating the unfamiliar into one's unfolding experience in accord with one's worldview, values, and beliefs. That which is utterly new to one's experience, completely unfamiliar, incommensurate with one's worldview, or contradictory to one's values and beliefs, is likely to be passed over, rejected, or avoided. I believe this is particularly so when the new idea hovers close to cherished values and beliefs or deeply ingrained patterns of daily life, challenging or contradicting them. We weave the fabric of our day-to-day personal and professional experience using by-and-large the threads and patterns that we know, recognize, and are comfortable with. Yet I deeply wish we (nurse leaders) would better provide young nurses with a deeper familiarity with and appreciation for the richness of the fabrics, yarns, and patterns that constitute *bona fide* nursing philosophy and science, that is, the extant theories and theoretical literature delineating nursing ontologies, epistemologies, and methodologies.

Contexts of Possibilities

When we have a critical mass of bachelor's, master's, and doctorally prepared nurses working in everyday healthcare guided predominantly by theories of nursing—an image that you, Dr. Fawcett, elicited in your exchange with Dr. Parker—perhaps the whole question of whether theory arises from practice will appear different. This would be a nursing workforce that could participate more fully in the work of developing and testing (in the broad sense) nursing theories. I don't believe that this attitude is elitist. I have provided leadership to an ongoing project of teaching the fundamentals of Parse's (1998) theory in a hospice facility staffed with nursing assistants, and I fully believe that the pattern of practice there is grounded in and consistent with nursing theory.

The majority of the contemporary workforce of registered nurses, however, offer a very different challenge to nurse educators, theorists, theoreticians, administrators, and other nurse leaders. They have learned, absorbed, and identified with a body of knowledge and skills that they believe to be nursing—which coincides for the most part with the stark requirements for licensure and the expectations of corporate employers of frontline nurses, and *not* with the body of knowledge that has emanated from 150 years of nursing scholarship rooted explicitly in philosophies of nursing. Naturally, these nurses are prone to respond to their first exposure to nursing theory with the reaction that it has little or nothing to do with *nursing* as they know it. I was one of those nurses for a long time, and in 25 years of working more than full-time in nursing I have met, worked with, or taught thousands of such nurses. The transformation of the educational preparation of nurses and the culture of nursing could yet bring about an environment in which the everyday practice of nursing is grounded in and intersects with *bona fide* nursing scholarship. But what is required to get to that future phase of our development in which "all nurse educators, nurse administrators, nurse researchers, and practicing nurses . . . view nursing from the lens of nursing models and theories" (Fawcett, 2003, p. 133), is nothing short of revolution. This is the revolution that should have occurred in the discipline of nursing, *circa* 1970, with the publication of Rogers' seminal work, *Introduction to the Theoretical Basis of Nursing*, but did not.

The Revolution That Didn't Come and the Potential That Yet Remains

As I refer to something I have called *bona fide* nursing scholarship, I find myself reflecting on exactly what I mean by that. In pondering the meaning, I am reminded of Orem's (1985) early work examining the question of who is a legitimate recipient of nursing services. She eventually came to say:

> Persons with a legitimate need for nursing are characterized (a) by a demand for discernible kinds of and amounts of self-care or dependent-care and (b) by health-derived or health-related limitations for the continuing production of the amount and kind of care required. (p. 31)

Orem's declaration, along with Henderson's (Harmer & Henderson, 1955) famous definition of nurs-

ing, clearly has directly or indirectly influenced the nurse educators who taught me and legions of other students in the 1970s. The beliefs and values reflected in those definitions that were generated in the first decades of self-conscious nursing theory development include the image of the nurse as a kind of surrogate mother. Peplau even stated as much directly in her 1952 book, which was, I believe, the first instance of a nurse deliberately naming her ideas a theory of nursing. Delineated there as one of the roles of the nurse was indeed "mother surrogate" (Peplau, 1952, p. 54). Surely the works of Henderson, Orem, Peplau, and those who carry on their work are *bona fide* nursing scholarship. But I cannot help wondering what may be the lingering effects of the 1950s conceptualization, in that first decade of deliberate and self-conscious nursing theory development, of *the nurse as someone whose central vocational duty is to perform a wide range of personal care for the other in an essentially maternal manner.* To be sure, it is miraculous that a field of human endeavor occupied 95% and led by women was able to assert at all that it was *a science with a unique body of knowledge* in the repressive and sexist era of the 1950s.

The works the early nurse theorists produced were commensurate with the actualities of the everyday work of nurses in their time. Similarly, Orlando (1962) produced a framework that offered as its central contribution a guide to actually thinking through nursing care situations rather than responding automatically. Such conceptualizations, it seems to me, likely merely adduced and formalized dimensions of nursing care embedded in the everyday worklives of nurses and offered a formal structure for implementing the best of then-current nursing practices.

It seems to me that the *next* major wave in nursing theory development, historically, which brought about the radical ideas of Martha Rogers (1970), Paterson and Zderad (1976), Parse (1981), and Watson (1985), got far *ahead* of the vast majority of nurses, leading to a rift between ordinary practice and the leading edge of nursing theory that has continued for 30 years. We will probably never fully understand how or why this happened. My impression is that many nurse leaders in the 1970s,

1980s, and 1990s, without advanced education in nursing theories, deliberately resisted and undermined efforts to advance nursing theory-based practice and research. The federally funded Nurse Scientist programs of the 1960s apparently did much to advance the status of academic nurses in universities, while ironically doing little or nothing to advance nursing science, since the doctorates it supported were all in other fields.

I believe that probably the key dynamic in the non-adoption of nursing theories by nurses has been the over-whelming societal need for professional/vocational caregivers trained for biomedical/technical care in huge numbers, juxtaposed with the immense intellectual challenge, on the other hand, of mastering the creatively synthesized new knowledge generated by a newly emergent discipline. To rise to both of these challenges while also struggling to rise above enforced second-class-citizenship as nurses and as women represents a monumental challenge. And yet a large and growing body of literature continues to emanate from the works of such visionary nurse scholars as Rogers, Paterson and Zderad, Parse, Watson, and their followers. This seems to me a testament to the value of the ideas that have arisen within nursing theory development over the past 50 years. The notions that were born of and are central to nursing—humans as unitary beings, human-environment mutual process, health as much more than wellness alone, life as rhythmic patterning, the centrality of meaning and of interpersonal caring in human experience, the nonlinearity and paradoxicality of human experience, the profundity of the nurse-person relationship, and that relationship as the locus of nursing practice—are all too important to be lost to humanity by a lack of attention to the further development of bona fide nursing science.

The Hijacking of Nursing Science

A glance at the emerging mainstream meaning of *nursing science* is instructive. One might almost think the emergent meaning is being propelled by a reaction against nursing theory. I have before me as I write a list of all the grants funded by the National Institute for Nursing Research (NINR) in fiscal year 2001, retrieved from the World Wide Web (NINR, n.d.). It is easy to see from the titles of the studies that the foci deemed legitimate by the NINR are overwhelmingly those that relate to the kinds of interests that biomedically-trained nurses have held for the past several decades. Some topics of recurring interest to the NINR include arterial disease, hormone therapy, symptoms of angina, thromboembolism, hypertension, hyperlipidemia, nutrition, pulmonary aspiration, mechanical ventilation, genetic testing, smoking cessation, and medication adherence. Upon investigation, one can also ascertain that a small but significant portion of the studies that the NINR funds (perhaps about 10%) are not only conceptually unrelated to nursing but also conducted by non-nurses without any apparent connection to nursing. I also have noted that the American Academy of Nursing now has two disparate and non-overlapping councils, one focused on nursing theory and one focused on something called *nursing science*, which appears to be code for *funded research*. I believe that these two situations, and the thousands of smaller echoes of these situations among groups of nurses all around the world, are the complex multilayered consequences of the rift between theory and practice that occurred many years ago.

As a nurse theoretician, I see this historic rift and its sequelae as first, the emergence of the best that nursing as a discipline has to offer humankind, truly the most original and most important leap forward in the discipline of nursing since Nightingale, and then, the near or complete rejection of that great gift by much of the discipline, after strangely little investigation or effort. The parallel developments over the past 15 years of the nurse practitioner movement, rooted largely in a biomedical perspective, and the non-nursing emphases of the much-coveted NINR funded research would seem to have brought us to the verge of the eclipse of the nursing theory movement.

Can nursing survive as a discipline without a specified body of knowledge of its own? Can a discipline that is fragmented and discontinuous, a discipline with many major stakeholders *within* it who have no real commitment to higher education in nursing and no commitment to the philosophies, theories, or methods specific to nursing survive? I think not. More and more these days one hears academics in healthcare disciplines assert that interdisciplinary research on so-called middle-range theories is where the action is now and that this approach constitutes the wave of the future. Such research is what is most commonly funded by the NINR today. This kind of research is generally focused at a relatively concrete level of scientific understanding, cause-effect in its ontology, and problem-solving in its real purpose.

But the great contributions of any and all disciplines do not reside in the thousands of particular transient projects focused on middle-range or concrete phenomena that its scholars conduct from year to year. Rather, the greatest contribution of a discipline resides in the articulation of its central reason for being, its central mission, and the major conceptualizations of its phenomena of concern. Consider the centrality of the concept of evolution in biology, the concept of the unconscious mind in psychology, or the concept of society itself in sociology. The great contributions of these disciplines to civilizations over centuries do not reside in the experiments in problem-solving on a concrete level that pepper the journals like so many refrigerator drawings, but in the great and lasting ideas central to the discipline. That is what is missing in the so-called nursing science that is not rooted in philosophies and theories of nursing. This is why I am moved to say that the dominant thrust of so-called nursing science today, toward interdisciplinary cause-effect research on concrete phenomena, is in fact detrimental to the future of the discipline. In the unique context of nursing as it exists today, this is tantamount to selling our soul to buy the respect of members of other disciplines—who may never come to know the unique scholarship that resides in the specific literature of nursing philosophy and theory.

Recently, I had experiences with two unrelated, well-respected academics from psychology and audiology. Each, separately, in the midst of conversations, blithely and unabashedly stated something to the effect that "I have read some of that *nursing theory* and I have found it to be nonsense." Actually, one said he found it to be "neither broad nor deep" and the other said it was garbage. Both of these men, by the way, have actually worked closely over time with nurses, but those nurses had no ties to nursing theories. Yet these experiences do not sadden me so much as the fact that a very great many of my colleagues in nursing academia are not only *unwilling* to defend nursing science against such attacks, but are also *unable* to do so, due to their own lack of knowledge.

As a scholar with broad interests, I have read and studied hundreds of books and journal articles from several disciplines outside of nursing. Certainly it would never occur to me (nor, I am sure, to most of our readers) to label and declare a large, heterogeneous, and multidimensional body of knowledge from another discipline to be essentially worthless. I think that the willingness of persons both inside and outside the discipline of nursing to subject the body of knowledge specific to nursing to this kind of ridicule is likely related to the *lack of respect for women and nurses* that is so prominent in our history. It has sometimes surprised me that feminists in nursing have not more assertively defended the body of knowledge that is specific to nursing. (There are, after all, as yet no widely recognized men nurse theorists.) The early 20th century leaders of nursing strongly identified with and interacted with the leading feminists of their day in creating and building the very discipline of nursing. Lillian Wald (1934), a self-described feminist at the turn of the century, later wrote, "The nurse question had become the woman question" (p. 76).

With perhaps one third of nurse academics unable to defend against this kind of disparagement, and possibly another third joining in, it is sometimes hard to be optimistic about the future of nursing theory. I must remind myself that the nursing theory movement is *stronger than ever*, although perhaps *relatively* weaker in relation to other national and international developments, such as the NINR priorities or the nurse practitioner movement. There is more literature on nursing theory-guided practice today than ever before, more nurse scholars are educated in nursing theories today than ever before, and there is a growing number of projects and practice settings (funded by other sources) guided explicitly by nursing theories.

Continuing the Unfinished Revolution

What I find truly most encouraging—and I always come back to this in my musings—is the fact that nursing theory-guided practice can be shown to enhance health and quality of life when it is implemented seriously with strong, well-qualified guidance. Demonstration projects rooted in philosophies and theories of nursing are probably the most valuable means of generating acceptance and buy-in and, in my experience, these *work* brilliantly. Examples include Dr. Parker's (2001) many projects in South Florida, Dr. Gail Mitchell's (see for example, Cody, Bunkers, & Mitchell, 2001) implementation of patient-centered care principles drawn from Parse's theory at Sunnybrook and Women's College Health Science Centre in Toronto, Dr. Sandra Bunkers' many projects in South Dakota (see for example, Cody, Bunkers, & Mitchell, 2001), and our implementation of the Charlotte Rainbow PRISM Model based largely on Parse's theory at the Nursing Center operated by the School of Nursing of the University of North Carolina at Charlotte (Cody, 2003).

What the mid-range problem-solving scholars don't buy into is that *to bring about transformation of healthcare, one needs the whole gestalt of philosophy, theory, and method, aligned with administration and education.* It is much easier to work with unwieldy and stagnant (but powerful) institutions when you merely lay claim to having a circumscribed study or a project that will solve a particular concrete problem for them. What is vastly more challenging but *essential* for the transformation of healthcare is the adoption of a whole different revolutionary way of approaching healthcare. This is what true nursing theory-based practice, after Rogers or Parse or other revolutionary nurse theorists, can do. And it is, however poorly funded or disparaged it may be, still extremely threatening to the powers that be. It may be that *people*—consumers, in today's business-of-healthcare parlance—may be our strongest allies as they become more and more aware of the transformational power of innovative nursing models.

From a global, multigenerational perspective—a very long view—if nursing as we know it does not survive long into the future as an autonomous discipline called nursing, its *loss* does not have to be a catastrophe for humankind. Great ideas, when challenged and repressed, can often seem tenuous, even teetering on the brink of nonexistence, but they are hard to kill. The ideas that are embedded in the great nursing theories of our time may reemerge in some future synthesis that doesn't get called nursing, but they could still be implemented and be of great benefit to humankind. My thinking about this eventuality is simply that it may well happen, given current conditions, and that would be a great pity because these ideas are here, now, ready and available to be put into practice—and when they are, human betterment happens.

Leaders in nursing, especially academics and community-oriented nurses, have long viewed nursing as very much an autonomous profession. Indeed, it has been shown many times in a variety of settings that increased autonomy of nurses is associated with improved quality of care and outcomes (Alfano, 1969; Havens, 2001; Wald, 1934). The truly original, radically visionary nursing frameworks that were put forward by nurse scholars in the 1970s and 1980s offered (and still offer) nurses the best opportunity we have ever had to move into a demonstrably unique and autonomous practice to the greater benefit of humankind. This is a transformational shift, a bold movement toward a new vision of nursing, rooted in concepts and theories that could only have emerged in the unique context of nursing and can only be learned through the extensive study of nursing. Indeed, despite the previously mentioned movement of powerful stakeholders in nursing in the opposite direction, this transformation may still be happening, albeit slowly and quietly, one-by-one, among nurse scholars like those who may be reading this journal. I have not yet known any nurse scholar who, having thoroughly learned how to interpret experience and practice from the perspective of a nursing theory, and having had the opportunity to put the theory into practice in an organization supporting implementation of the theory, to subsequently turn his or her back on nursing theory completely. The value of the turn toward nursing theory is obvious to those who take this path. The power of autonomous nursing practice guided by nursing discipline-specific theories to enhance quality of life in a meaningful way, when experienced directly by practicing nurses, is very persuasive. It is a whole different order of experience from merely implementing various interdisciplinary concrete problem-solving measures based on mid-range research devoid of a philosophical basis in nursing or a coherent vision of nursing and health. Many among us may yet be persuaded to reclaim the uniqueness of nursing.

Full Circle

To come full circle in the discussion, allow me to share my own evolution. I encountered Parse's theory in the 10th year of my nursing career, having by then earned two bachelor's degrees, graduated with honors, climbed a clinical ladder to management, and mentored many new nurses. Yet it still took me 3 to 4 years to learn how to practice well in accord with Parse's theory and method. I am convinced that the vision of nursing theory-based practice that many of us embrace, that of a world in which nursing theory-based practice is universal, is achievable only through a renewed attention to depth in nursing education, greater appreciation of the human condition and our lived experiences, and thorough study of the history and philosophy of nursing, nursing theories, and nursing's unique research and practice methodologies.

Nursing theories guide nursing practice. Nursing theories are more than middle-range problem-solving algorithms. Some nursing theories are revolutionary and transformational. All nursing theories require in-depth study over time to master. Nursing practice will be transformed to the betterment of humankind when all nursing practice is fully autonomous and guided predominantly by nursing theory. A salubrious future for nursing includes a rapid shift toward the vast majority of nurses being educated at the bachelor's level and above, with far greater engagement among nurse scholars in theory development, research, and practice, in a context in which the intellectual domain of nursing is universally recognized as nursing theory. When that time comes, we should perhaps revisit the question of whether theory arises from practice.

REFERENCES

Alfano, G. (1969). The Loeb Center for Nursing and Rehabilitation. *Nursing Clinics of North America, 4,* 487–493.

Cody, W. K. (2003). Human becoming community change concepts in an academic nursing practice setting. In R. R. Parse, *Community: A human becoming perspective* (pp. 49–71). Sudbury, MA: Jones and Bartlett.

Cody, W. K., Bunkers, S. S., & Mitchell, G. J. (2001). The human becoming theory in practice, research, administration, regulation, and education. In M. E. Parker (Ed.), *Nursing theories and nursing practice* (pp. 239–262). Philadelphia: F. A. Davis.

Fawcett, J. (2003). Theory and practice: A conversation with Marilyn E. Parker. *Nursing Science Quarterly, 16,* 131–136.

Harmer, B., & Henderson, V. A. (1955). *Textbook of the principles and practice of nursing.* New York: Macmillan.

Havens, D. S. (2001). Comparing infrastructure and outcomes: ANCC magnet and nonmagnet CNEs report. *Nursing Economics, 19,* 258–266.

National Institute for Nursing Research, (n. d.). *NINR funded grants.* Retrieved March 7, 2003, from http://www.nih.gov/ninr/research/grants_index.html

Orem, D. E. (1985). *Nursing: Concepts of practice* (3rd ed.). New York: McGraw-Hill.

Orlando, I. J. (1962). *The dynamic nurse-patient relationship: Function, process, and principles.* New York: G. P. Putnam's Sons.

Parker, M. E. (Ed.). (2001). *Nursing theories and nursing practice.* Philadelphia: F. A. Davis.

Parse, R. R. (1981). *Man-living-health: A theory of nursing.* New York: Wiley.

Parse, R. R. (1998). *The human becoming school of thought: A perspective for nurses and other health professionals.* Thousand Oaks, CA: Sage.

Paterson, J. G., & Zderad, L. T. (1976). *Humanistic nursing.* New York: Wiley.

Peplau, H. E. (1952). *Interpersonal relations in nursing.* New York: G. P. Putnam's Sons.

Rogers, M. E. (1970). *An introduction to the theoretical basis of nursing.* Philadelphia: F. A. Davis.

Wald, L. D. (1934). *Windows on Henry Street.* Boston: Little Brown.

Watson, J. (1985). *Nursing: Human science and human care.* Norwalk, CT: Appleton-Century-Crofts.

The Author Comments

Nursing Theory as a Guide to Practice

I wrote this article as a part of a dialogue with Marilyn Parker and Jacqueline Fawcett. I was, in-the-main, simply responding to the questions posed by Dr. Fawcett, "Do you think that theory arises from practice? Or, do you think that theory guides practice?" Certainly, I was aware that many before me had provided very scholarly answers to these questions. I aspired to stake out new territory in this piece, by taking a strong stand that *theory guides practice* and providing what I hoped was a cogent and original analysis of some of the contexts in which this occurs. My favorite parts of the article are the most controversial, "The Revolution that Didn't Come" and "The Hijacking of Nursing Science." I believe the comments therein really needed to be said—and still need to be said today.

—WILLIAM K. CODY

CHAPTER 18

The Role of Theory in Improving Patient Safety and Quality Health Care

Barbara A. Mark
Linda C. Hughes
Cheryl Bland Jones

By examining selected research that investigates the relationship between nurse staffing and adverse events, we demonstrate the problems that result from the absence of a strong theory to guide this research. There is considerable work to be done in explicating the theory underlying empirical studies of the relationship between nurse staffing and outcomes. Key constructs must be placed within a theoretical context, proposed causal mechanisms underlying the empirical or hypothesized relationships must be identified, and critical mediating and moderating variables must be recognized.

Theory can be used to mean anything from a simple guess or mere speculation to articulation of a set of interrelated and logical statements that provide explanatory and predictive power. The diverse meanings that can be attributed to the word theory led Merton[1] to suggest that theory has the potential to obscure rather than create understanding. Despite Merton's cautionary note, development of theory that leads to an understanding of nursing's contribution to high quality and safe patient care is of paramount importance. Such theory is essential if we are to develop knowledge that can be generalized from one setting to another, recommend ways of organizing to improve the delivery of quality patient care and, perhaps most importantly, avoid simplistic solutions to the complex problem of insuring safe and high quality patient care in organizational settings.[2]

Successful theory development in the area of health care quality and safety will be reflected in our ability not

Reprinted from Nursing Outlook, *52, B. A. Mark, L. C. Hughes, & C. B. Jones. The role of theory in improving patient safety and quality health care. 11–16. Copyright © 2004 Elsevier Inc. with permission from Elsevier Ltd.*

About the Authors

BARBARA MARK, PhD, RN, FAAN, holds the Sarah Frances Russell Distinguished Professorship in Nursing Systems at the University of North Carolina (UNC) at Chapel Hill. In addition, she is the Co-Director of the Southeastern Regional Health Workforce Center. She is also a senior fellow at the Sheps Center for Health Services Research and the Principal Investigator for the pre- and postdoctoral research training program in Quality Healthcare and Patient Outcomes at UNC-Chapel Hill. Dr. Mark is also a member of the Expert Panel on Quality Health Care of the American Academy of Nursing. Her current research, funded since 1995 by the National Institute of Nursing Research (NINR), focuses on work environments, hospital performance, patient safety, and quality. Another of her projects, funded by the Agency for Healthcare Research and Quality (AHRQ) since 1999, examines the relationships between nurse staffing, hospital financial performance, and quality of care. Her publications have appeared in *Nursing Research, Health Services Research, Health Economics, and Medical Care.*

LINDA CAROL HUGHES, PhD, RN, is a Research Associate Professor at the School of Nursing, UNC-Chapel Hill. Dr. Hughes was born in Purcell, OK, and earned a baccalaureate degree from Oklahoma Baptist University in 1972, a master's degree from Texas Woman's University in 1978, and a PhD from the University of Texas at Austin in 1993. Her dissertation research, funded by an NINR individual predoctoral fellowship, was a multisite survey study to examine the organizational climate for caring among baccalaureate schools of nursing. She recently completed a postdoctoral fellowship in nursing health services research under the mentorship of Dr. Barbara Mark. During this fellowship, Dr. Hughes began her current program of research, which focuses on the relationship between nurses' discretionary work behaviors and patient outcomes in intensive care units. Dr. Hughes has published numerous articles on caring in nursing education, methodological approaches to the analysis of group-level data, and the use of free text nursing intervention data to measure an episode of nursing care.

CHERYL BLAND JONES, PhD, RN, is an associate professor and Health Care Systems coordinator in the School of Nursing, and an Investigator at the Southeast Regional Health Workforce Center at UNC-Chapel Hill. Dr. Jones has devoted her career to understanding nursing workforce issues to improve the nursing work environment, nurse executive practices, and the cost and quality of care. A key contribution of her work has been the development, testing, and refinement of a model to quantify the costs of nursing turnover. Dr. Jones also served as a Senior Health Services Researcher at the Agency for Healthcare Research and Policy (AHRQ) in the U.S. government, where she examined the nursing workforce at organizational and public policy levels, and worked to build health services research capacity in nursing, heighten awareness of nursing health services research, and strengthen the agency's relationship with the nursing research community. Dr. Jones earned a bachelor's degree in nursing from the University of Florida and Master of Science (focus in nursing administration) and Doctor of Philosophy (nursing science, with a minor in economics) degrees from the University of South Carolina. She was inducted as a Fellow in the American Academy of Nursing in 2005.

only to explain why empirical relationships occur but also to predict conditions under which these relationships are most and least likely to hold true. Because formulating "good theory" is so difficult, Sutton and Staw[3] identified examples of what theory is *not*. Theory is not represented by an extensive list of references in which logical relationships are explained elsewhere. Models and variables must be accompanied by logical statements that explain not only how variables are related but also *why* they are related. Similarly, theory is not represented by a description of observed relationships, beta weights, or factor loadings. Data can describe what relationship exists, but cannot explain why the relationship exists. Theory is not a laundry list of variables or a diagram used to depict a structural equation model. Nor is theory rendered in evidence-based clinical practice guidelines or in so-called "best practices." Theory results from a process of systematic and logical reasoning—either deductive or inductive—through which the occurrence or nonoccurrence of some phenomenon can be understood and predicted. Such theory will be useful in building an understanding of the practice of nursing as it is enacted in socially constructed organizational settings.[4] If organizations exist because they can achieve goals that can not be accomplished by individuals alone, then the mere process of organizing introduces a "systemness"[5] to the work of nursing that must be an integral component of any theory that seeks to explain and predict high quality and safe patient care.

In nursing, there are promising beginnings in the effort to better understand the relationship between nurse staffing and patient outcomes. An example is the growing body of empirical research relating nurse staffing to adverse patient events.[6–13] Yet even as dissemination of these findings begins to influence the organization and management of nursing care delivery, the underlying question of *how* nurse staffing affects adverse events remains unexplained. It is only through a clear understanding of the *why* and the *how* that innovative policies and management practices to improve quality and patient safety can be systematically developed, methodically implemented, and rigorously evaluated. In the absence of such understanding, the introduction of policies to guide nurse staffing are likely to be both haphazard and unsuccessful.

In this article we discuss conceptual and methodological issues that are central to the goal of building strong theory that can explain nursing's contribution to patient safety and quality care in acute care settings. This discussion is organized around four questions that reflect the intellectual processes through which causal mechanisms can account for the relationships observed among variables and, in so doing, build theory that has both explanatory and predictive power. These questions include:

- What are the major constructs of interest and how should they be measured within the context of the theory? This places the constructs within a nomological network,[14] a prerequisite to establishing construct validity.
- Why do the constructs relate to each other in the way that is proposed, ie, what are the causal mechanisms underlying the hypothesized relationships?

Theory must also include explanatory frameworks that permit identification of variables that mediate observed relationships as well as contextual factors that moderate the magnitude of those relationships:

- What are the critical mediators in the proposed relationships?
- What are the contextual factors that moderate the proposed relationships?

This article examines these four questions in the context of research investigating the relationship between nurse staffing and adverse patient events. Our purpose is to demonstrate the problems that arise when theory is absent: First, research findings contradict each other, conceptual and statistical power is reduced, and potential effects are masked; and, second, the development of a coherent body of knowledge is hindered and the design of interventions to improve quality and patient safety is made difficult.

What Are the Major Constructs of Interest and How Should They Be Measured Within the Context of the Theory?

In studies investigating the relationship of nurse staffing and patient outcomes, the major constructs seem obvious: Nurse staffing and patient outcomes. While identification of the constructs is, in fact, obvious, their conceptualization and measurement is not. For example, from a theoretical perspective, what does the term "nurse staffing" mean?

Since theory ought to drive measurement, consider the current use of multiple definitions of nurse staffing: (1) actual number of hours of care delivered by RNs (also called "nursing hours"); (2) RN hours as a *percent* of all nursing care hours; and (3) percent of total staff who are RNs. The last two operational definitions are frequently referred to as "skill mix," despite the fact that one measures skill mix in terms of hours and the other measures skill mix in terms of people.[7–9] The fact that "skill mix" is operationally defined differently in different studies makes comparison of findings difficult. Other studies[6,11,13] have measured nurse staffing as the number or percent of RN full-time equivalents (FTEs). These represent different conceptual approaches to measuring different phenomena—they are not multiple indicators of the same construct. Although they have not previously been discussed as such, one can consider a staffing measure that focuses on *hours* of care as a construct reflecting nursing care patients actually receive (assuming that productive hours—not paid hours—is measured). In contrast, staffing as measured by FTEs can be thought of as a unit-level phenomenon reflecting the unit's capacity to deliver nursing care. However, neither of these measures provides information about the actual staffing levels *needed* to deliver safe care; instead, they report only about staffing levels *used* in delivering nursing care.

The importance of distinguishing among these constructs is illustrated in the following two examples. First, imagine the nursing unit with nearly an all RN staff. One would expect that patients on that unit would receive the vast majority of their care from an RN. However, poor management, inadequate support services, and/or poor medication delivery and supply systems might significantly reduce the amount of nursing care actually received by patients, even though staffing—defined as the proportion of staff or staff FTEs who are RNs—is high and presumed to be excellent. Second, use of such different measures may lead to conflicting results that are difficult to reconcile. For example, one recent study[9] found that higher skill mix (ie, a greater proportion of care provided by RNs) was associated with a lower incidence of pneumonia. The study also found, however, that more total licensed hours (ie, the total hours of care delivered by registered and licensed practical nurses) were associated with a *higher* incidence of pneumonia. The discrepancy may be attributed to the inclusion of licensed practical nurses in one measure and

not in the other. The current lack of theoretical development within this particular realm of research makes it difficult to logically integrate these findings.

A theory that proposes clear boundaries for the construct of nurse staffing would help to alleviate the dilemma that results from multiple, overlapping, and conceptually non-distinct measures. Such a theory would also make clear the distinction between "nurse staffing" and "nursing care"—which are often implicitly assumed to be one and the same. Many individual and organizational factors affect the actual delivery of nursing care such that merely having more RNs may not necessarily yield either more care delivered by RNs or higher quality of care. Specifically, more registered nurses may provide better nursing care, which may improve quality and patient safety, but only under certain conditions. For example, more RNs—if they lack the requisite intellectual capacity, skill, motivation, and a caring attitude—would not likely improve quality of patient care simply by virtue of there being more of them. Also, if organizational conditions are such that the environment is not conducive to professional nursing practice, care may suffer regardless of the number of RNs available to deliver care.

Theory is no less problematic when patient outcomes are considered. A great deal of attention is currently directed at "nurse-sensitive" patient outcomes, which have been described, in general terms, as outcomes that are sensitive to "variations." However, it is not clear how the term "variations" is being used. Is it variations in the *amount* of nursing care that is provided? Is it variations in the *quality* of nursing care that is provided? Is it variations in how nursing work is *organized* to provide nursing care? Or is it variations in both quality and amount of care? Additionally, it is unclear at what organizational level—the hospital or the nursing unit—we should measure the relationship between nurse staffing and adverse events. Since we know that nurse staffing varies by unit, how might organizational level variables affect the relationship between nurse staffing and adverse events on a nursing unit? Would we expect certain outcomes to be more (or less) sensitive to changes in numbers of RNs in the hospital, or on the unit, than to changes in the number of hours of care provided by RNs?

Another issue to be considered is that understanding the relationship between nurse staffing and different outcomes, indeed different *classes* of outcomes, may require different theories. Most of the research on nurse staffing, in fact, has examined nurse staffing relative to only one type of patient outcome—adverse patient events. However, different theories might be needed to explain the relationship between nurse staffing and positive patient outcomes, which reflect more than the absence of adverse events. Similarly, different theories might be called upon to explicate the relationship between nurse staffing and the prevention of potential adverse events. New theoretical formulations are beginning to address these issues, but undoubtedly will require additional research. An example is Tucker and Edmondson's distinction between errors (defined as "the execution of a task that is either unnecessary or incorrectly carried out and that could have been avoided with appropriate distribution of pre-existing information," and problems (defined as "disruption in a worker's ability to execute a prescribed task because either: something the worker needs is unavailable in the time, location, condition, or quantity desired and, hence, the task cannot be executed as planned; or something is present that should not be, interfering with the designated task").[15] Thus, gaining a better understanding of the relationship between nurse staffing and patient outcomes, errors and problems, and latent conditions in the practice environment is paramount in demonstrating nursing's contribution to quality and safe patient care.

If we hypothesize that such differential effects might exist, then we move to the next of the four questions posed earlier: how and why do the constructs relate to each other in the way that is proposed?

How and Why Are the Constructs Related to Each Other?

This question addresses the proposed causal relationships among the constructs of interest and explanations for the proposed relationships. In other words, this question focuses on the *theoretical* basis of expecting that changes in nurse staffing will, in fact, result in changes in adverse events. Popular arguments make the case "more RNs, better outcomes"—but this argument only addresses the issue of *what* rather than *why* this relationship holds. That is, why "more RNs, better outcomes"? Why are causal linkages between nurse staffing and patient outcomes as hypothesized? Consider, for example, the following set of theoretical statements:

- RNs' communication with physicians is hypothesized to be more timely, complete and accurate than non-RN staff communication with physicians;
- This "enhanced" communication between physicians and nurses is hypothesized to result in early recognition and intervention in potentially hazardous patient situations;
- Therefore, nursing units characterized by a greater proportion of RN staff will have fewer adverse events than a nursing unit with a lower level of RN staffing.

Given this theoretically derived set of causal statements, the measurement of "nurse staffing" becomes obvious: "nurse staffing" is measured by *the proportion* of RNs to total nursing staff, not the *number of hours of care* delivered by RNs. An explanation for the use of this nurse staffing measure is that the proportion of RN staff is relevant to communication with physicians and unit-level capacity to deliver nursing care. Conversely, the number of hours of care is not an appropriate measure of nurse staffing because this measure would capture data on the nursing care delivered to patients rather than unit level nursing capacity and operations. These theoretical statements do not, however, clearly address—either conceptually or operationally—the identification of appropriate and theoretically relevant adverse events. Thus, theory should guide the development of hypothesized relationships and the selection of measures for both independent and dependent variables, nurse staffing and adverse events, respectively.

In the early stages of theory development, researchers tend to focus on demonstrating the existence of a relationship—broadly conceptualized—between independent and dependent variables, in this case, the hypothesized relationship between nurse staffing and adverse patient events. This is a common progression of knowledge development in any science, but is particularly prevalent in studies of nurse staffing and adverse events.

The wide availability of administrative and other large databases may actually fuel this research strategy: Because data are widely available and accessible, researchers ask the questions that can be answered of the data. It is in the later stages of theory development where researchers begin to address problems in conceptualization, methodologies and conflicting and/or equivocal results.

In the social and organizational sciences, "clean" relationships between independent and dependent variables are unlikely—real social and organizational life is just too complicated to be modeled so simple. Drawing on this assumption would be a useful approach in the study of relationships such as nurse staffing and patient outcomes where complex social and organizational factors likely impact observed relationships. Thus, the next stage of theory development turns to the identification of "mediators" and "moderators"—other variables that in specific ways affect the relationship between the independent and dependent variables. First, we turn to the identification of variables that play a potential mediating role in the relationship between nurse staffing and adverse events; then we discuss possible moderators of this relationship.

What Factors Mediate the Relationships We Observe?

Mediators are variables that explain the mechanism of action that produces the observed relationships between independent and dependent variables.[16] The advantage of testing models in which mediators are specified is that it forces the researcher to consider the *theoretical* basis upon which relationships can be predicted. Mediators thus help explain the relationship between nurse staffing and, for example, variables related to quality or patient safety.

An area of inquiry that has significant potential to inform research in the area of nurse staffing, quality care, and patient safety is being investigated in the field of organizational industrial psychology, where researchers are attempting to unravel the work processes that contribute to employee emphasis on safety issues and a reduction in industrial accidents. In particular, the theory of leader-member exchange (LMX) has been used to explain the motivational process through which employees engage in

voluntary behaviors that have "add-on" value in terms of being beneficial to the organization.[17] The basic premise of LMX theory is that managerial actions that demonstrate positive regard for an employee create a desire on the part of the employee to reciprocate through behaviors that are seen as highly valued by the manager.[18]

The leader-member exchange (LMX) theory is especially relevant to the area of safety and risk mitigation because safety-related behaviors tend to be seen by employees as voluntary and, therefore, as behaviors where "corners can be cut" in order to complete work assignments. According to Weick[19] this tendency results from the fact that, ideally, nothing happens in response to accident prevention behaviors. As a result, it is easy to assume that these behaviors are of lesser importance and can be omitted when time is limited. LMX theory, however, hypothesizes that high quality exchange relationships will result in the performance of safety and risk mitigation behaviors when employees view these behaviors as highly valued by the manager. Hofmann and Morgeson[20] tested and confirmed this hypothesis by demonstrating that, in the context of high quality leader-member exchange relationships, open communication about safety issues was associated with a reduction in work-related injuries.

Based on these findings, one could, for example, hypothesize that the relationship between staffing levels and adverse events is mediated by the quality of the exchange relationship between nurse managers and their staff. In other words, better staffing allows the nurse manager to invest more time and energy in the development of meaningful social exchange relationships with members of the nursing staff. As a consequence, staff nurses who experience a high quality exchange relationship with their manager would be more likely to respond proactively to managerial communication about the importance of safety-related behaviors that contribute to the prevention of adverse patient events.

Figure 18-1 illustrates the proposed role of quality of LMX as a mediator. Four conditions must be present for mediation to be demonstrated.[16] There must first be a statistically significant relationship between the independent variable (nurse staffing) and the dependent variable (adverse events). Second, there must also be a statistically significant relationship between the

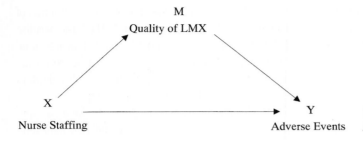

Figure 18-1 *LMX as a mediator of the relationship between nurse staffing and adverse events.*

independent variable (nurse staffing) and the mediator (quality of LMX). Third, after controlling for the effects of the independent variable (nurse staffing), there must be a statistically significant relationship between the mediator (LMX) and the dependent variable (adverse events). Finally, complete mediation is demonstrated when, after controlling for the quality of LMX, the relationship between nurse staffing and adverse events is zero. The more likely scenario in this example is one of partial mediation, where, after controlling for LMX quality, the relationship between nurse staffing and adverse events is significantly reduced. In other words, part of the relationship between nurse staffing and adverse events is explained by LMX. This example provides an illustration of how identification of potential mediators can increase theoretical richness, and may enhance both the predictive and explanatory power of the underlying theory.

What Contextual Factors Moderate the Relationships We Observe?

While mediators illuminate the causal mechanisms that explain why relationships are observed, moderator variables are contextual factors that define the conditions under which such relationships can be predicted.[16] In contrast to mediating variables that explain why independent and dependent variables are related, moderator variables contribute to theory development by specifying factors that affect either the direction or magnitude of the relationship between two variables. Most studies examining the relationships between nurse staffing and patient outcomes acknowledge, at least implicitly, that moderating effects may exist by statistically controlling for some or all of the following variables: Hospital size, urban/rural location, and teaching status. Statistical control affords results that can be interpreted as "all other things being equal." Acknowledgment that statistical control is necessary indicates that results might be different in the absence of such controls.

Variables measured at the nursing unit level may function as moderators in the relationship between nurse staffing and adverse events. Figure 18-2 illustrates such a relationship that was examined in a recently completed study which hypothesized that, because hospitals experience differential financial pressures in markets with varying levels of managed care penetration, managed care penetration might moderate the relationship between nurse staffing and adverse events.[13] Using data from a longitudinal panel of 360 hospitals from 1990–1995, Mark, Harless and McCue[13] found a statistically significant relationship between increasing nurse staffing and decreasing mortality ratio (the ratio of actual to expected deaths) for hospitals located in markets where HMO penetration was greater than 7.5%; no such relationship existed in markets with a lower level of HMO penetration. This demonstration of a moderating effect provides additional information about the conditions under which the staffing-adverse events relationship exists.

Two other studies report better patient outcomes on specialized nursing units where patient admissions are restricted to specific diagnoses.[21,22] The authors speculate that their findings might be explained by the expertise that nurses develop over time when they care for patients with the same or a similar diagnosis. So, it is possible that the relationship between nurse staffing and adverse events may be altered when care is provided on specialized nursing units. Studies to explore the potential moderating effect of a contextual variable like this will require demonstration

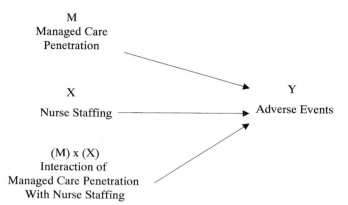

Figure 18-2 *Managed care penetration as a moderator of the relationship between nurse staffing and adverse events.*

of a significant statistical interaction effect in which the relationship between nurse staffing and adverse events is conditioned upon whether patients received nursing care on a dedicated or general nursing unit.

The preceding sections demonstrate why the identification of possible mediators and moderators of the relationship between nurse staffing and adverse events is so important. First, it seems reasonable that hospitals and nursing units that differ from each other in important ways will also differ in how they deploy RNs, and that these differences may ultimately have effects on quality and patient safety. Second, understanding these differences from a theoretical perspective is critical to designing interventions to improve quality and patient safety. It is critical to know what interventions work, why, for whom, and under what conditions. Without this kind of theoretical specificity, interventions to improve quality and patient safety risk being so diffuse that detection of an intervention effect would be unlikely and where an intervention effect is evident, the challenge would be to explain which aspects of the intervention were responsible for its effects.

Summary

In this article, we focused on the research examining the relationship between nurse staffing and adverse events because this area of research has received a great deal of attention, and it allowed us to address four key questions that are critical in developing theory and in advancing knowledge in the area. We have demon-

strated the importance of clearly defining the constructs of interest, explicating hypothesized causal relationships among the variables, and identifying and testing the existence of mediators and moderators of the relationship between nurse staffing and adverse events.

While better documenting and understanding the relationship between nurse staffing and adverse events is critical to patient safety, narrowly focusing on this relationship ignores the intrinsic "systemness"[5] or context in which nursing care is delivered. For example, West[23] suggests that contextual characteristics such as the changing division of labor of health care team members, as well as social barriers to communication may influence knowledge sharing across disciplines, thus affecting the level of risk in the organization. Enlarging the focus of inquiry to take into account this "systemness" increases the likelihood that research findings on the relationship between nurse staffing and adverse events will be successfully integrated into practice.

Weick[24] has argued that people in organizations become so entrenched in pursuit of a particular idea that they either selectively ignore or rationalize evidence that is inconsistent with their perception of the idea—a process he calls "cultural entrapment." In our efforts to understand high quality and safe patient care, nursing as a professional group runs the risk of cultural entrapment through continued emphasis on a narrow set of constructs that adhere to preconceived assumptions about nursing and the way nurses provide care. Our efforts to build theory that is useful for both research and practice will depend on the extent to which we are able to think creatively in terms of identifying constructs that capture the complex interface between the clinical and organizational domains within which nurses practice.

REFERENCES

1. Merton R. On Theoretical Sociology. New York, NY: Free Press; 1967.
2. West E. Management matters: The link between hospital organization and quality of patient care. Quality in Health Care 2001;10:40–8.
3. Sutton R, Staw B. What theory is not. Admin Sci Quarterly 1995;40:371–84.
4. West E. Organizational sources of safety and danger: Sociological contributions to the study of adverse events. Qual Health Care 2000;9:120–26.
5. Berwick DM. Seeking systemness. Healthc Forum J 1992; 25:22–8.
6. Kovner C, Gergen P. Nurse staffing levels and adverse events following surgery in US hospitals. Image: J Nurs Schol 1998;30: 315–21.
7. American Nurses Association. Implementing nursing's report card: A study of RN staffing, length of stay, and patient outcomes. Washington, DC: American Nurses Publishing; 1997.
8. Lichtig L, Knauf R, Milholland D. Some impacts of nursing on acute care hospital outcomes. J Nurs Admin 1999;29:25–33.
9. American Nurses' Association 2000. Nurse Staffing and Patient Outcomes in the Inpatient Hospital Setting. Washington DC: American Nurses Publishing. 2000.
10. Needleman J, Buerhaus P, Mattke S, Stewart M, Zelevinski K. Nurse-staffing levels and the quality of care in hospitals. New Engl J Med 2002;346:1715–22.
11. Kovner C, Jones C, Zhan C, Gergen P. Nurse staffing and post-surgical adverse events. An analysis of administrative data from a sample of US hospitals, 1990–1996. Health Services Research 2002;37:611–30.
12. Cho S. Nurse staffing and adverse patient outcomes: A systems approach. Nursing Outlook 2001;49:78–85.
13. Mark B, Harless D, McCue M. The influence of managed care penetration on the relationship between nurse staffing and quality of care. Health Econ Submitted manuscript. 2003.
14. Cronbach L, Meehl P. Construct validity in psychological tests. Psych Bull 1955;52:281–302.
15. Tucker AL, Edmondson AC. Why hospitals don't learn from failures: Organizational and psychological dynamics that inhibit system change. California Management Review 2003;45: 55–72.
16. Baron R, Kenny D. The moderator-mediator variable distinction in social psychological research: Conceptual, strategic and statistical considerations. Journal of Personality and Social Psychology 1986;51:1173–82.
17. Sparrowe R, Liden R. Process and structure in leadermember exchange. Academy of Management Review 1997; 22:522–52.
18. Setton R, Bennet N, Liden R. Social exchange in organizations: Perceived organizational support, leadermember exchange, and employee reciprocity. J Applied Psych 1996;81: 219–27.
19. Weick K. Organizational culture as a source of high reliability. California Management Review 1987;29:112–27.
20. Hofmann D, Morgeson F. Safety-related behavior as a social exchange: The role of perceived organizational support and leader-member exchange. J Applied Psych 1999;84:286–96.
21. Aiken LH, Sloane DM, Lake ET. Satisfaction with inpatient acquired immunodeficiency syndrome care: A national comparison of dedicated and scatteredbed units. Medical Care 1997;35: 948–62.
22. Czaplinski C, Diers D. The effect of staff nursing on length of stay and mortality. Med Care 1998;36:1626–38.
23. West E. Organizational sources of safety and danger: Sociological contributions to the study of adverse events. Qual Health Care 2000;9:120–26.
24. Weick KE, Sutcliffe KM. Hospitals as cultures of entrapment: A re-analysis of the Bristol Royal Infirmary. California Management Review 2003;45:73–84.

The Authors Comment

The Role of Theory in Improving Patient Safety and Quality Health Care

This article was written as part of the conference "Measuring and Improving Health Care Quality—Towards Meaningful Solutions to Pressing Problems: Nursing's Contribution to the State of the Science," an invitational conference sponsored by the American Academy of Nursing, and held at the University of Pennsylvania in 2002. Our goal was to present a case for stronger theory in better being able to conceptualize problems encountered when doing research on quality of care. We identified components of strong theory and how they can improve the research in this area.

—Barbara Mark
—Linda Carol Hughes
—Cheryl Bland Jones

Transforming Practice Knowledge Into Nursing Knowledge— A Revisionist Analysis of Peplau

Pamela G. Reed

Nursing practice typically has been viewed as applying knowledge. However, currently, there is increasing awareness that nursing practice is also a process of knowledge development. Still, research and practice are not always connected. Analysis of Peplau's works illuminates a scholarship of nursing practice that is relevant today. This paper focuses on a specific strategy and philosophic perspective, as derived from Peplau, for integrating nursing practice more fully into today's knowledge development. Emphasis is on the need for nursing practice-based theory, as well as nursing theory-based practice.

Peplau (1952) fostered a scholarly interest in nursing practice and the nurse-patient relationship that continues to grow today. Although nursing practice generally is not considered a research endeavor, it is in part a scientific and scholarly endeavor (Peplau, 1988). Over the past 40 years, Peplau has described nursing practice as a caring and systematic process that produces knowledge for the benefit of patients and the nursing discipline.

Unfortunately, a "depth of disconnectedness" between current research activities, theory, and practice threatens nursing scholarship (Maeve, 1994; Schmitt, 1994, p. 319).

Analysis of Peplau's ideas can further illuminate the scholarship of nursing practice and the role of nursing practice in contemporary approaches to knowledge development. Of particular interest are Peplau's ideas about nursing practice in reference to the current philosophic

From P. Reed, Transforming practice knowledge into nursing knowledge—A revisionist analysis of Peplau. Journal of Nursing Scholarship, *1996, 28(1), 29–33. Copyright 1996 by Blackwell. Reprinted with permission by Blackwell Publishing.*

About the Author

PAMELA G. REED is Professor at the University of Arizona College of Nursing in Tucson, Arizona, where she also served as Associate Dean for Academic Affairs for 7 years. She is a three-time graduate of Wayne State University in Detroit, receiving a BSN in 1974, an MSN in 1976 (with a double major in child–adolescent psychiatric mental health nursing and teaching), and her PhD (with a major in nursing focused on lifespan development and aging) in 1982. Dr. Reed pioneered research into spirituality and well-being with her doctoral research with terminally ill patients. She also developed a theory of self-transcendence and two widely used research instruments, the *Spiritual Perspective Scale* and the *Self-Transcendence Scale*. Her publications and funded research reflect a dual scholarly focus: Spirituality and other facilitators of well-being and decisions in end-of-life transitions; and nursing metatheory and knowledge development. Dr. Reed also enjoys time with her family, reading, classical music, swimming, and hiking in the mountains and canyons of Arizona.

context for developing nursing knowledge. From a revisionist perspective of Peplau's ideas, practitioners are more than "working scientists," as Peplau (1988) described; practitioners not only "use the knowledge that 'producing scientists' publish" (p. 12), but they, along with patients, create many of the contexts that initiate the formation of nursing knowledge.

Postmodernism and Nursing Knowledge

Revisiting Peplau's ideas about knowledge development is instructive in postmodern 1996. In postmodernism, there is an emphasis on pragmatics and the unadorned events of everyday life as sources of knowledge (Doherty, Graham, & Malek, 1992; Waugh, 1992): Truths, ideals, and overarching conceptual schemes, called "metanarratives," that explain reality as stable, holistic, and universal are criticized and cast aside. These metanarratives, once revered in various disciplines, are being traded for other truths that espouse the instability of meaning, the value-ladeness of perception, and the power of language.

Postmodernism is evident in nursing. Some nurses question the value of nursing theory (King, 1994; Koziol-McLain & Maeve, 1993), particularly "high theory," as found, for example, in the familiar nursing conceptual models or grand theories critiqued in Fawcett (1995a; 1995b) and Fitzpatrick and Whall (1989). These theories

are viewed as too remote or too stagnant for application. Instead some are turning to the culture of nursing practice for knowledge development (Kim, 1994; Maeve, 1994).

Peplau's theory may be one of those nursing theories that seems to lack relevance to today's nursing practice. However, existing nursing theories and conceptual models provide insight into the links between practice, research, and theory. Specifically, a closer look at Peplau's theory demonstrates an approach to knowledge development through the scholarship of practice; nursing knowledge is developed *in* practice as well as *for* practice. In this postmodern era, knowledge development is no longer only a concern of theoretical nursing; it is a concern in practice. Knowledge development increasingly is recognized not merely as a product to apply in practice, but as an activity in the everyday life of the practicing nurse.

Once viewed more narrowly as a psychodynamic theory, Peplau's (1952) "interpersonal process" has broader implications and can bridge nursing's modernist past with current postmodern influences on knowledge development. In modern times, the focus was on identifying universal and unique theoretical concepts that distinguished nursing from other disciplines and provided a scientific base for nursing practice. Peplau's theoretical ideas—such as the interpersonal process between patient and nurse, the developmental capacity of patients, and the centrality of anxiety in health and illness—contributed to a unifying base of knowledge. Peplau's theory also has kept pace with postmodern influences that have reinforced nurses' awareness of the knowledge-laden context of practice, at the level of the patient. Thus, Peplau has provided nursing with a model of scholarship in which knowledge development is nourished by both the practical and the theoretical. It is a scholarship that embraces the unique characteristics of individual patient situations: it employs theoretical insights and generalized meanings that have proven useful to nursing over time.

A Strategy for Linking Knowledge Development and Practice

Peplau's interpersonal process is a strategy for knowledge development that incorporates a modernist emphasis on theory as a source of truth with a postmodern emphasis on the significance of everyday contexts. Although Peplau (1952) made use of the contemporary wisdom of her day, it is equally evident from her 1952 work onward that she applied knowledge in a way that is congruent with recent philosophic trends. Peplau synthesized ideas from the "high theories" of, for example, Harry Stack Sullivan, Abraham Maslow, and Erich Fromm. Yet her approach to inquiry for nursing let the patient and the "voice of nursing" (Johnson, 1993) be heard above the theory. In doing this, Peplau introduced an approach to knowledge development that was anchored in nursing practice, and in the science and art of the nurse-patient interaction. Development and testing of explanations through the interpersonal process between patient and nurse was done for therapeutic purposes. But, by revisiting Peplau's theory, it can be seen that this interpersonal process is also a strategy for generating nursing knowledge, which can then be examined further and refined through research. Steps 1, 2, and 3 describe the strategy of transforming practice knowledge into nursing knowledge.

Step 1:
Observation of Fundamental Units

Knowledge development, according to Peplau, began with observations made in the context of practice. For Peplau,

this context was primarily the nurse-patient relationship. Observation preceded conceptual interpretations. Peplau (1952) outlined various methods of observation that yielded knowledge, including spectator observation, role-playing, and random observation. However, Peplau (1952, 1992a) emphasized participant-observation, in which a nurse uses self as both the instrument and object of observation while participating in the interpersonal process with a patient. According to Peplau (1952), a nurse enters a situation with theoretical understanding, personal bias, and previously acquired nursing knowledge. Patients enter with their knowledge and with the powers and capabilities of a developing human being. Patients possess the principle data for inquiry in the form of underdeveloped or unused competencies, subconscious meanings, and personal knowledge. Nurses possess knowledge of methods to help patients make use of their competencies and to regain well-being.

Peplau (1992c) explained that, while on a philosophic level human beings are not reducible, elements about human beings can be studied and measured to develop nursing knowledge at the theoretic level (p. 88). Relevant units of observation are those that are meaningful and useful to patients, measurable, and definable, and that can be replicated and compared with other data (Peplau, 1952, p. 270). Fundamental units of inquiry within Peplau's theory (1952, 1988) are "processes" and "patterns" and the problems that can emerge from them.

Processes refer to behaviors that develop over time in observable phases (Peplau, 1987, 1992a). Examples include what Peplau called language-thought processes—referring, for example, to development of less ego-centric verbal expressions and thinking. Other examples are personality development, learning processes, and perceiving. Peplau (1992a) also included nursing therapeutic processes, such as the four-phased interpersonal relationship, as that which "co-operates with and assists" other processes to move the patient toward health (p. 125).

Patterns are comprised of separate thoughts, feelings, or actions that share the same theme or aim (Peplau, 1987, 1992a). Peplau (1994), also citing Sullivan (1953), defines pattern as "the envelope of insignificant particular

relationship was the avenue for this to occur. Critical science is concerned not only with the intellectual production of ideas but with practical efforts to transform interpersonal situations (Habermas, 1973; Popkewitz, 1984). Critical science is not unlike a professional discipline, particularly nursing. Emphasis is not on the instrumental use of knowledge for control and manipulation, but on its emancipatory use to liberate a person through enhanced self-knowledge. Congruent with this, Peplau (1952) defined nursing as a "maturing force and educative instrument" (p. 8) for the best interest of patients. Patients may have acquired knowledge of processes and patterns of thinking and acting that constrain their developmental progress and diminish well-being. Insights gained through the critical application of language in nurse-patient relationships often render these views inapplicable and, in this sense, change the world for the patient. The nurse's world changes as well, through self-assessment and personal growth in the relationship (Peplau, 1992a). Mutual learning and self-understanding are considered common outcomes for both patient and nurse (Beeber, Anderson, & Sills, 1990; Forchuk, 1994; Peplau, 1952).

Peplau (1952) proposed a nurse-patient relationship to "facilitate forward movement . . . in ways that displace feelings of helplessness and powerlessness with feelings of creativeness, spontaneity, and productivity" (Peplau, 1952, p. 32). It is a relationship "in which neither nurse nor patient feels helpless" (p. 33). Thus, both process and product of knowledge development are liberating. Patients are encouraged to formulate their own explanations and to "express and amplify their powers" (Peplau, 1952; 1969). Nurses do not presume to have authority over patients (Peplau, 1962; 1992a). Peplau (1952) was cognizant of the imbalances in power in nurse-patient relationships. She embedded strategies to check the nurse's potential misuse of power as well as enhance the patient's sense of power over the course of the investigative process of the relationship (p. 135).

Knowledge generated through the interpersonal relationship, then, reflects a critical theory approach to inquiry. Knowledge is tested for its emancipatory effectiveness throughout Peplau's (1952) four phases of the interpersonal relationship, which outline criteria of emancipatory knowledge for patients. For example, the orientation phase focuses on knowledge that fosters a feeling of acceptance and hope in oneself; the identification phase focuses on enhancing a sense of identity with others and a recognition of inherent capabilities in self and others; the exploitation phase encourages a patient to enact one's powers and make full use of available resources; and the resolution phase fosters a willingness to participate in the ongoing developmental change process. The emancipatory nature of nursing knowledge is evident when participants in the interpersonal process achieve an understanding that is "therapeutic and effects a cognitive, affective, and practical transformation" (Bernstein, 1976, p. 199; 1983).

Tender-Hearted and Tough-Minded

Peplau (1952, 1988) revealed another of her philosophic views in her discussion of "tough-mindedness" and "tender-heartedness." She used these terms to explain a two-parted approach to knowledge development that is incongruent with positivism. Being tender-hearted is being open, accepting, attending to personal knowledge, and sensitive. Being tough-minded is to emphasize critical thinking and reflection, rationality, and verification.

As part of the tough-minded approach, Peplau (1988) cited the importance of objectivity and emotional detachment, but not in the positivist sense that inquiry and values must be independent. Rather, Peplau's use of these terms is more consistent with a hermeneutic understanding of the distance that exists between two people interacting (Allen & Jensen, 1990; Reeder, 1988). Peplau (1952) acknowledged that "in the struggle toward developing a common understanding" (p. 290), not all experiences can be shared or understood. The "text" of the interpersonal relationship must be interpreted with the awareness of inherent differences between two people's social, historical, and personal contexts.

Peplau's (1988) tough-minded stance also incorporates existing theories about regularities and shared experiences. Peplau did not eschew the grand narratives of modern science; theories, for example, from Sullivan on personality development and Maslow on needs gratification were valued for informing nurses about potentially relevant "commonalities in human patterns" (Peplau, 1952). Peplau's (1988) tender-hearted approach was used to translate this existing theoretical information into a more individualized and contextually-based understanding of the "unique and highly personal variations in patterns and problems" of a patient (p. 14).

In this postmodern time, there is an intensified appreciation for the truths found in the everyday contexts of nursing. William James' (1908) original distinction between tender-mindedness and tough-mindedness is becoming blurred (Denzin & Lincoln, 1994). Today, nursing scholarship means embracing the philosophic view that each dimension informs the other in knowledge development. Knowledge gained through tender-heartedness is not subordinated by or reduced to knowledge gained through the more traditional tough-minded approach. Peplau helps nurses see that both are legitimate elements in transforming practice knowledge into nursing knowledge.

Practice in Scholarship

Contemporary nursing epistemology reflects a perspective of knowledge development that Peplau (1952) began over 40 years ago with *Interpersonal Relations in Nursing*. It is increasingly being recognized that practice knowledge as well as other patterns of knowing (e.g., Carper, 1978; Cowling, 1993; Munhall, 1993) are integral to nursing scholarship.

The logical positivist view held by mid-twentieth century nursing scientists may have obscured some of Peplau's contributions to knowledge development. And postmodernist skepticism of nursing models and theories may further relegate the potential insights from these sources to "nursing's intellectual underground" (Rawnsley, 1994). This would be a waste. Nurses in the

21st century should more fully "exploit" nursing meta-narratives of past and present.

Peplau's philosophy of nursing and strategy for developing nursing knowledge provide an original basis for new methods that connect theory, research, and practice. These methods employ the interpersonal relationship as a mode and context for building knowledge; examples are found in Newman's (1990) research as praxis, Boyd's (1993) research practice methods, Kim's (1994) nursing practice theories, and Titchen and Binnie's (1994) action research. The patient's search for truth, as Peplau (1990) envisioned it, is a metaphor for nursing's development of knowledge; both require an interpersonal context, systematic processes, and a combination of science and sensitivity.

Nursing practice is more than a context for applying a tested and refined theory: Practice is a context for initiating and testing theory (Peplau, 1988). In her theory of interpersonal relations, Peplau (1952) operationalized a concept of practitioner that was later described by Ellis (1969) as "not simply a user of given theory, but a developer, tester, and expander of theory" (p. 1438). As such, a practitioner is a participant in a cycle of inquiry that develops nursing knowledge and has a responsibility to make practice knowledge "explicit" (Ellis, 1969). Peplau (1992b) states that she reawakened nursing to the importance of science-based practice after Nightingale.

From this revisionist analysis, it can be seen that Peplau (1952) modeled a philosophy and designed a strategy for practice-based science. As long as what is practiced is nursing, practice will play an essential role in the scholarly transformation of knowledge into nursing knowledge. There is need not only for scholarship in practice, but also for practice in nursing scholarship.

REFERENCES

Allen, M. N., & Jensen, L. (1990). Hermeneutical inquiry: Meaning and scope. Western Journal of Nursing Research, 12, 241–253.

Beeber, L., Anderson, C. A., & Sills, G. M. (1990). Peplau's theory in practice. Nursing Science Quarterly, 3, 6–8.

Bernstein, R. J. (1976). The restructuring of social and political theory. New York: Harcourt Brace Jovanovich, 1976.

Bernstein, R. J. (1983). Beyond objectivism and relativism: Science, hermeneutics, and praxis. Philadelphia: University of Pennsylvania Press.

Boyd, C. O. (1993). Toward a nursing practice research method. Advances in Nursing Science, 16(2), 9–25.

Carper, B. (1978). Fundamental patterns of knowing in nursing. Advances in Nursing Science, 1(1), 13–23.

Cook, T. (1985). Postpositivist critical multiplism. In R. Shotland & M. Mark (Eds.)., Social science and social policy (21–62). Beverly Hills, CA: Sage.

Cowling, W. R. (1993). Unitary knowing in nursing practice. Nursing Science Quarterly, 6, 201–207.

Denzin, N. K., & Lincoln, Y. S. (1994). The fifth moment. In N. K. Denzin, & Y. S. Lincoln (Eds.), Handbook of qualitative research (575–586). Thousand Oaks, CA: Sage.

Doherty, J., Graham, E., & Malek, M. (1992). Postmodernism and the socialsciences. New York: Macmillan.

Ellis, R. (1969). The practitioner as theorist. American Journal of Nursing, 69, 1434–1438.

Fawcett, J. (1995a). Analysis and evaluation of conceptual models of nursing (3rd ed.). Philadelphia: F. A. Davis.

Fawcett, J. (1995b). Analysis and evaluation of nursing theories. Philadelphia: F. A. Davis.

Fitzpatrick, J. J., & Whall, A. L. (1989). Conceptual models of nursing: Analysis and evaluation. Norwalk, CT: Appleton & Lange.

Forchuk, C. (1994). Peplau's theory-based practice and research. Nursing Science Quarterly, 7, 110–112.

Habermas, J. (1973). Theory and practice (J. Viertel, Trans.) Boston: Beacon Press.

Hempel, C. G. (1966). Philosophy of natural science. Englewood Cliffs, NJ: Prentice-Hall.

James, W. (1908). Pragmatism and the meaning of truth. Cambridge, MA: Harvard University Press.

Johnson, R. (1993). Nurse practitioner-patient discourse: Uncovering the voice of nursing in primary care practice. Scholarly Inquiry for Nursing Practice, 7, 143–158.

Kim, H. S. (1994). Practice theories in nursing and a science of nursing practice. Scholarly Inquiry for Nursing Practice, 8, 145–158.

King, M. (1994). Nursing theories outdated (letter to the editor). Journal of Psychosocial Nursing, 32, 6.

Koziol-McLain, J., & Maeve, M. K. (1993). Nursing theory in perspective. Nursing Outlook, 41, 9–82.

Maeve, M. K. (1994). The carrier bag theory of nursing practice. Advances in Nursing Science, 16 (4), 9–22.

Meleis, A. I. (1991). Theoretical nursing: Development and progress (2nd ed.). New York: J. B. Lippincott.

Munhall, P. L. (1993). "Unknowing": Toward another pattern of knowing in nursing. Nursing Outlook, 41, 125–128.

Newman, M. A. (1990). Newman's theory of health as praxis. Nursing Science Quarterly, 3, 37–41.

Peplau, H. E. (1952). Interpersonal relations in nursing. New York: Putnam.

Peplau, H. E. (1958). Interpretation of clinical observations. (Original paper presented at The University of Nebraska College of Medicine, Omaha, NE: In A. W. O'Toole & S. R.

Welt (Eds.) (1989). Interpersonal theory in nursing practice: Selected works of Hildegard E. Peplau, 149–163.

Peplau, H. E. (1962). Interpersonal techniques: Crux of psychiatric nursing. American Journal of Nursing, 62, 50–54.

Peplau, H. E. (1969). Professional closeness. Nursing Forum, 8, 342–359.

Peplau, H. E. (1973). Letter to Geraldine Ellis. Cited in S. R. Welt & A. W. O'Toole (Eds.) (1989). Hildegard E. Peplau: Observations in brief. Archives of Psychiatric Nursing, 3, 254–264.

Peplau, H. E. (1975). Investigative Counseling. (Original paper presented at the University of Leuven, Belgium). In A. W. O'Toole & S. R. Welt (Eds.) (1989). Interpersonal theory in nursing practice: Selected works of Hildegard E. Peplau, 205–229. New York, NY: Springer.

Peplau, H. E. (1987). Interpersonal constructs for nursing practice. Nursing Education Today, 7(95), 201–208.

Peplau, H. E. (1988). The art and science of nursing: Similarities, differences, and relations. Nursing Science Quarterly, 1, 8–15.

Peplau, H. E. (1990). Interpersonal relations model: Principles and general applications. In W. Reynolds & D. Cormack (Eds.), Psychiatric and mental health nursing: Theory and practice (87–132). London: Chapman & Hall.

Peplau, H. E. (1992a). Interpersonal relations: A theoretical framework for application in nursing practice. Nursing Science Quarterly, 5, 13–18.

Peplau, H. E. (1992b). Notes on Nightingale. In J. Watson (Ed.), Florence Nightingale's Notes on Nursing: What it is and what it is not (Commemorative Edition) (48–57). Philadelphia: J. B. Lippincott.

Peplau, H. E. (1992c). Perspectives on nursing knowledge (interview by T. Takahashi). Nursing Science Quarterly, 5, 86–91.

Peplau, H. E. (1994). Quality of life: An interpersonal perspective. Nursing Science Quarterly, 7, 10–16.

Phillips, D. C. (1990). Postpositivistic science: Myths and realities. In E. G. Guba (Ed.). The paradigm dialog (31–45). Newbury Park, NJ: Sage.

Popkewitz, T. (1984). Paradigm and ideology in educational research: The social functions of the intellectual. London: Falmer.

Popper, K. R. (1968). The logic of scientific discovery (2nd ed.). New York: Harper & Row.

Rawnsley, M. M. (1994). Response to "The nurse-patient relationship reconsidered: An expanded research agenda." Scholarly Inquiry for Nursing Practice, 8, 185–190.

Reed, P. G. (in press). Peplau's nursing practice theory of interpersonal relations. In J. J. Fitzpatrick & A. L. Whall (Eds). Conceptual models of nursing: Analysis and application (3rd ed.). Norwalk, CT: Appelton & Lange.

Reeder, F. (1988). Hermeneutics. In B. Sarter (Ed.). Paths to knowledge: Innovative research methods for nursing (193–238). New York: National League for Nursing.

Schmitt, M. (1994). The connectedness of nursing research: Revisiting an old issue (editorial). Research in Nursing & Health, 17, 319–320.

Sellers, S. C. (1991). A philosophical analysis of conceptual models of nursing. Unpublished doctoral dissertation, Iowa State University, Ames, IA.

Sullivan, H. S. (1953). The interpersonal theory of psychiatry. New York: Norton.

Suppe, F., & Jacox, A. K. (1985). Philosophy of science and the development of nursing theory. In H. H. Werley & J. J. Fitzpatrick (Eds.). Annual review of nursing research: Vol. 3 (241–267). New York: Springer.

Titchen, A., & Binnie, A. (1994). Action research: A strategy for theory generation and testing. International Journal of Nursing Studies, 31(1), 1–12.

Waugh, P. (1992). Postmodernism. New York: Edward Arnold.

Whall, A. L. (1989). The influence of logical positivism on nursing practice. Image: Journal of Nursing Scholarship, 21, 243–245.

The Author Comments

Transforming Practice Knowledge Into Nursing Knowledge—A Revisionist Analysis of Peplau

As a psychiatric mental health nurse clinician at the master's level, I was familiar with Peplau's ideas on interacting with patients in a psychiatric setting. Then, as a doctorally prepared nurse interested in the philosophic dimensions of the discipline, I revisited Peplau for her insights into the process of knowledge development. I believed that her statements reflected much more than simply the positivist views of her day and the belief in separation of knowledge development and application. A closer reading of Peplau offered a wealth of ideas on the scholarship of practice and its integral role in nursing knowledge development. I envision a future in nursing where all clinicians are educated to not only apply knowledge but also use their practice to build knowledge.

—PAMELA G. REED

Nursing Philosophies and Paradigms

This unit consists of articles that present a variety of philosophic perspectives conceived within nursing. These philosophies go by different labels, such as 'conceptual system,' worldview, metanarrative, and paradigm as well as 'philosophy of science.' Within a structure of nursing knowledge, paradigms are considered equivalent to conceptual models or frameworks, and are less broad in scope than are philosophies of science. However, what all share in common and why these articles are clustered together, is that they present one or more overarching perspectives of nursing; some perspectives are more local, some more global depending upon the nurse's context of practice or research. And these philosophies and paradigms also represent some level of consensus in thinking about phenomena of interest within the discipline. They are tools or lenses for transcending the immediate context to reflect back upon practice, research, or knowledge and evaluate that context.

Rogers' chapter presents a pandimensional worldview in which is described a conceptual system of sciences, principles, and theories. Reed's neomodernism is a philosophy for nursing science that synthesizes what is useful from modern and postmodern philosophies of science. Other authors present various frameworks or ways of organizing sets of worldviews. Some of these frameworks inform us about the *syntax* of nursing, how science is practiced. Others inform us about the *substance* of nursing, what are the phenomena of concern to scientists and practitioners.

Questions for Discussion

- Is there a place for metanarratives within our postmodern era?
- Is unity, multiplicity, or complementarity in philosophies preferred in nursing?
- Are worldviews constructed or emergent out of some basic nature of reality?
- Are all of the prevailing paradigms in nursing useful for knowledge development?
- Is neomodernism a viable philosophy for research and practice today?
- What new philosophies may be needed for knowledge development in nursing?

CHAPTER 20

Nursing Science and the Space Age

Martha E. Rogers

This article presents the basic elements of Rogers' science of unitary human beings. It defines science, explicates nursing as a science and an art, addresses the meaning of the principles of homeodynamics, and discusses the building blocks of these principles. Several theories arising from the science of unitary human beings are elaborated, and noninvasive therapeutic modalities are discussed as part of nursing practice.

Humankind is on the threshold of a new cosmology transcending an earthbound past. In less than a decade the 21st century will arrive, accompanied by many manifestations of accelerating change. Futurists prophecy multiple scenarios, often in conflict with one another. Genetic engineering engenders a mechanistic explanation of life and spawns ethical issues that far exceed Huxley's (1932) *Brave New World*. Economics, education, health, world affairs, lifestyles, as well as robots, computers, environment, and space travel are just a few of the areas undergoing scrutiny. Interplanetary and intergalactic communication with intelligent life beyond the present purview portends new meanings for citizenship in a space-encompassing world society. These new worldviews also take into account the extraterrestrial.

From M. E. Rogers, Nursing Science Quarterly *1992; 5(1), 27–34.*

About the Author

MARTHA E. ROGERS was born on May 12, 1914, in Dallas, TX. She received her nursing diploma in 1936; a BS in Public Health from George Peabody College in Nashville, TN; an MA in Public Health Nursing Supervision (1945) from Teacher's College, Columbia University, NY; and an MPH (1952) and an ScD (1954) from Johns Hopkins University in Baltimore, MD. Rogers' early nursing practice was in public health nursing in Michigan, and later she established the Visiting Nursing Service in Phoenix, AZ. Dr. Rogers was Professor and Head of the Division of Nursing at New York University for more than 20 years. She was adamant that nursing be recognized as a science with a unique body of knowledge. Dr. Rogers' revolutionary ideas, as expressed in her *Science of Unitary Human Beings* and other writings, have inspired nurses throughout the world. In 1979, Dr. Rogers became Professor Emerita of Nursing at New York University. She was an active member of the nursing community until her death on March 13, 1994. Her vision for nursing continues to play a major role in the evolution of the discipline.

The science of unitary human beings encompasses this human advent into outer space. Today's astronauts are envoys to the human space-directed future. Astronauts, the precursors of spacekind, portend an outward emigration by Homo sapiens and, what is more, their transcendence by Homo spatialis. This transcendence will be an evolutionary, not an adaptive process.

Planet earth is integral with the larger world of human reality. Thus, the space future will not consist of how to use planetary knowledge and skills in space, but an elaboration of a new worldview in which new knowledge and modalities raise new questions, provide new answers, and signify different evolutionary norms. According to Robinson and White (1986), Homo spatialis will transcend Homo sapiens in approximately two generations of space living (about 50 years). Particulate phenomena such as physiological norms are already inadequate for judging the parameters of humankind in space. Even more, the so-called pathology on earth today may signify health for the space-bound.

Homo spatialis looms on the horizon as moon villages, space towns, and Martian communities foretell a new world. Moon-mining and gravity-free manufacturing in space are anticipated within this century. Galactic grocery stores, educational centers, health services, and recreational opportunities are each inevitable inclusions in a space-bound world society.

Increasing space travel capabilities are already manifest in many countries; a new oneness attends planet earth's integration into the space world, a new synthesis in which spinoffs from space exploration mark planet earth's future.

Should all of this seem impossible, one need only recall that in February 1957, Lee DeForest, father of modern electronics, stated: "To place a man in a multistage rocket and propel him into the controlling gravitational field of the moon . . . will never occur regardless of all future scientific endeavors." He compared these proposals to the wildest dreams of Jules Verne (Friedman, 1989). DeForest made this statement just 12 years before the Apollo moon landing.

A New Worldview for Nursing

Nursing's transition from prescience to science has also accelerated, but it must become explicit if nurses are to provide knowledgeable innovative services in a space-bound world society. The explication of an organized body of abstract knowledge specific to nursing is indispensable. The need for such a body of knowledge can be identified in an escalation of science and technology coordinate with public demands for health services of a nature, and in an amount, scarcely envisioned by either the consumers or providers.

A new worldview compatible with the most progressive knowledge available (Lauden, 1977) has become a necessary prelude to studying human health and to determining modalities for its promotion both on this planet and in outer space. The science of nursing is rooted in this new worldview, a pandimensional view of people and their world.

Traditionally nursing's goals have encompassed both the sick and the well, and the consideration of environmental factors has also been integral to nursing's efforts. Education and practice in nursing have been directed toward promotion of health without interruption. The recognition of people as distinct from their parts has characterized nursing from the time of Florence Nightingale to the present.

The introduction of systems theories several decades ago set in motion new ways of perceiving people and their world. Since then, science and technology have escalated. The exploration of space has revised old views, and thus new knowledge has merged with new ways of thinking. Nothing less than a second industrial revolution has been initiated, far more dramatic in its implications and potentials than the first. The pressing need to study people in ways that would enhance their humanness has coordinated with the accelerating technological advances and forced a search for new models. A major hindrance to the evolution of viable models, however, was noted by Capra (1982) when he wrote about the difficulty encountered while trying to apply the concepts of an outdated worldview to a reality that could no longer be understood in terms of these concepts.

The science of nursing was arrived at by the creative synthesis of facts and ideas and is an emergent, a new product. These principles and theories were derived from the abstract system and were tested in the ordinary world. The findings of this research have accumulated and changed commensurate with the new knowledge. A science is open-ended. The elaboration of a science emerges out of scholarly research. Thus, the findings of research are fed back into the system, whereby the system undergoes continuous alteration, revision, and change. A science then, exists only in its entirety, it bespeaks wholeness and unity, and it provides a way of perceiving people and their environment.

The science of unitary human beings has not derived from one or more of the basic sciences. Neither has it come out of a vacuum. It flows instead in novel ways from a multiplicity of knowledge, from many sources, to create a kaleidoscope of potentialities. In turn, fundamental concepts are identified and significant terms are defined congruent with the evolving system. A humane and optimistic view of life's potentials grows as a new reality appears. Then, people's capacity to participate knowingly in the process of change is postulated.

Since nursing is a learned profession, it is both a science and an art. The uniqueness of nursing, like that of other sciences, lies in the phenomenon central to its focus. For nurses, that focus consists of a long established concern with people and the world they live in. It is the natural forerunner of an organized, abstract system encompassing people and their environments. The irreducible, indivisible nature of individuals is different from the sum of their parts. Furthermore, the integrality of people and their environments coordinates with a pandimensional universe of open systems, points to a new paradigm, and initiates the identity of nursing as a science. The purpose of nurses is to promote health and well-being for all persons wherever they are. The art of nursing, then, is the creative use of the science of nursing for human betterment.

A theoretically sound foundation that gives identity to nursing as a science and an art requires an organized abstract system from which to derive unifying principles and hypothetical generalizations. Through basic and applied research, theories are tested, new understandings emerge, and new questions arise. As a result, description and explanation take on new meanings, and a substantive body of knowledge specific to nursing takes form.

A science may be defined as an organized body of abstract knowledge arrived at by scientific research and logical analysis. This knowledge provides a means of describing and explaining the phenomena of concern. A science can also have more than one paradigm or abstract system, but the phenomena of concern remain constant. A worldview is a paradigm from which one can derive principles and theories that may guide practice. More specifically, however, nursing is postulated to be a basic science. Surely, this science does not come out of a vacuum. Neither does it derive from other basic or applied sciences, nor is it a summation of knowledge drawn from other fields. Nursing, instead, consists of its own unique irreducible mix.

Since science is open-ended and change is continuous, new knowledge brings new insights. Thus, the development of a science of unitary human beings is a never-ending process. This abstract system first presented some years ago has continued to gain substance. Concomitantly, early errors have undergone correction, definitions have been revised for greater clarity and accuracy, and updating of content is ongoing. Basic theoretical research, then, continues to be essential for the ongoing development of this field of study.

Both basic and applied research are necessary to nursing's future; basic research provides new knowledge while applied research tests the new knowledge already available. Multiple methodologies that may be used in the pursuit of the new knowledge include quantitative and qualitative methods and encompass philosophic, descriptive, and other approaches. The application of the science of unitary human beings to nursing, from a holistic worldview, also demands new tools and new methods. Moreover, it is only through research that the theoretically sound foundation can continue to evolve.

Historically the term "nursing" has been used as a verb signifying "to do," rather than as a noun meaning "to know." When nursing is identified as a science the term "nursing" becomes a noun signifying a "body of abstract knowledge." Consequently, theories deriving from a science of unitary human beings are specific to nursing, just as theories deriving from biology are specific to biological phenomena, theories deriving from sociology are specific to sociological phenomena, and theories of physics are specific to the physical world.

The study of nursing is not the study of the biological world any more than the study of biology is the study of the physical world. Further, the study of nursing is not the study of nurses and what they do any more than biology is the study of biologists and what they do.

Nursing instead, is the study of unitary, irreducible, indivisible human and environmental fields: people and their world. The complexity of investigatory methodology is not a substitute for substantive content in any field. Downs notes " . . . our research efforts are replete with sophisticated methods applied to unsophisticated content" (Downs, 1988, p. 20). The education of nurses gains its identity by the transmission of nursing's body of theoretical knowledge. The practice of nurses, therefore, is the creative use of this knowledge in human service. Research methods are empty without substance to study. Thus, research in nursing specifies a body of knowledge specific to nursing, and research in other fields is not a substitute.

The uniqueness of nursing, like that of any other science, lies in the phenomenon central to its purpose; people and their worlds in a pandimensional universe are nursing's phenomena of concern. The irreducible nature of individuals as energy fields, different from the sum of their parts and integral with their respective environmental fields, differentiates nursing from other sciences and identifies nursing's focus.

Unitary human beings are specified to be irreducible wholes. A whole cannot be understood when it is reduced to its particulars. The use of the term unitary human beings is not to be confused with the current popular usage of the term holistic, generally signifying a summation of parts, whether few or many. The unitary nature of environment is equally irreducible. The concept of field provides a means of perceiving people and their respective environments as irreducible wholes.

The Science of Unitary Human Beings

The significant postulates fundamental to the science of unitary human beings include energy fields, openness, pattern, and pandimensionality. The development of a science portends the emergence of abstract concepts and a corresponding language of specificity. Scientific language evolves out of the general language. Additionally, terms specific to the system are defined for clarity, precision, and communication so that rigorous

Table 20-1
Key Definitions Specific to the Science of Nursing

Energy Field:	The fundamental unit of the living and the non-living. Field is a unifying concept. Energy signifies the dynamic nature of the field. A field is in continuous motion and is infinite
Pattern:	The distinguishing characteristic of an energy field perceived as a single wave.
Pandimensional:[*]	A non-linear domain without spatial or temporal attributes.
Unitary Human Being: (Human field)	An irreducible, indivisible, pandimensional energy field identified by pattern and manifesting characteristics that are specific to the whole and which cannot be predicted from knowledge of the parts.
Environment: (Environmental field)	An irreducible, pandimensional energy field identified by pattern and integral with the human field.

[*]Formerly titled four-dimensional and multidimensional.

Reprinted with permission from the National League for Nursing, New York, New York. *Visions of Rogers' science-based nursing*, 1990, p. 9. Update 1991.

research can be pursued and replicated. Terminology, except that defined specifically to the system, is interpreted in its general language meaning (see Table 20-1).

Theory concerning a universe of open systems has been gaining support for three quarters of a century. Since the introduction of the theory of relativity, of quantum theory, and of probability, the prevailing absolutism, already shaken by evolutionary theory, has received a critical blow. By the 1920s Selye had proposed adaptation, and by the 1930s von Bertalanffy introduced the idea of negative entropy (Rogers, 1970). Soon after Cannon advanced the idea of homeostasis. Space exploration began in the 1950s, and by the 1960s some physiologists suggested replacing the term homeostasis with the term homeokinesis. As this new knowledge escalated, the traditional meanings of homeostasis, steady-state, adaptation, and equilibrium were no longer tenable. The closed-system, entropic model of the universe began to be questioned and evidence has continued to accumulate in support of a universe of open systems (see Table 20-2).

In a universe of open systems, causality is not an option. Energy fields are open, not a little bit or sometimes, but continuously. A universe of open systems explains the infinite nature of energy fields, how the human and environmental fields are integral with one

Table 20-2
Some Differences Between Older and Newer Worldviews

Older Views	Newer Views
Cell theory	Field theory
Entropic universe	Negentropic universe
Three-dimensional	Pandimensional
Homeostasis	Homeodynamics
Person/environment: dichotomous	Person/environment: integral
Causation: single and multiple	Mutual process
Adaptation	Mutual process
Closed systems	Open systems
Dynamic equilibrium	Innovative growing diversity
Waking: basic state	Waking: an evolutionary emergent
Being	Becoming

Initial development 1968; update 1991.

another, and that causality is invalid. Change, then, is continuously innovative and creative. Moreover, association does not mean causality.

New worldviews abound. Synthesis and holism are predominant among these views. Lovelock (1988) proposed a scientific synthesis in harmony with the Greek conception of the earth as a living whole, as Gaia. Fuller (1981) has argued that earth is a spaceship, and Kenton (1990) emphasizes the fallacy of depending on well-meaning actions and good intentions while people continue to operate with a paradigm that views reality as fragmented. Holistic new worldviews are being proposed by such persons as Bohm (1980), Capra (1982), Sheldrake (Weber, Bohm, & Sheldrake, 1986), and Weber (1986). In addition, Rogers' work focuses on developing a pandimensional worldview by proposing a science of unitary, irreducible human beings that is coordinate with a worldview that includes outer space.

Within this pandimensional view, energy fields are postulated to constitute the fundamental unit of both the living and the nonliving. Field, then, is a unifying concept and energy signifies the dynamic nature of the field. Energy fields are infinite and pandimensional; they are in continuous motion. Two energy fields are identified: the human field and the environmental field. Specifically, human beings and the environment *are* energy fields; they do not *have* energy fields. Moreover, human and environmental fields are not biological fields, physical fields, social fields, or psychological fields. Nor are human and environmental fields a summation of biological, physical, social, and psychological fields. This is not a denial of the importance of knowledge from other fields. Rather, it is to make clear that human and environmental fields have their own identity and are not to be confused with parts. Human and environmental fields are irreducible and indivisible. What may be quite valid in describing biological phenomena does not describe unitary human beings, any more than describing a molecule tells you about laughter.

A science of unitary human beings is equally as applicable to groups as it is to individuals. The group energy field to be considered is identified. It may be a family, a social group, or a community, a crowd or some other combination. Regardless of the group identified, the group field is irreducible and indivisible. The group field is integral with its own environmental field. The environmental field is unique to any given group field. The principles of homeodynamics postulate the nature of group field change just as they postulate the nature of individual field change. They are equally relevant for Homo sapiens, Homo spatialis, and beyond. Furthermore, these principles have validity only within the context of the science of unitary human beings, their meaning has specificity within their definitions, and together they postulate the nature and direction of change.

Pattern is a key postulate in this system (see Table 20-3). It is defined as the distinguishing characteristic of an energy field perceived as a single wave. Pattern is an abstraction, its nature changes continuously, and it gives identity to the field. Moreover, each human field pattern is unique and is integral with its own unique environmental field pattern. In fact, the term "pattern" is used only to refer to an energy field. The characteristics of unitary human beings are specific to unitary human beings. Pattern is not directly observable. However, manifestations of field patterning are observable events in the real world. They are postulated to emerge out of the human-environment field mutual process (see Box 20-1).

Table 20-3
Principles of Homeodynamics

Principle of Resonancy:	Continuous change from lower to higher frequency wave patterns in human and environmental fields.
Principle of Helicy:	Continuous, innovative, unpredictable, increasing diversity of human and environmental field patterns.
Principle of Integrality:	Continuous mutual human field and environmental field process.

Reprinted with permission from the National League for Nursing, New York, New York. *Visions of Rogers' science-based nursing*, 1990, p. 8.

Manifestations of Field Patterning in Unitary Human Beings

The evolution of unitary human beings is a dynamic, irreducible, nonlinear process characterized by increasing diversity of energy field patterning. Manifestations of patterning emerge out of the human/environment field mutual process and are continuously innovative. Pattern is an abstraction that reveals itself through its manifestations.

The nature of unitary field patterning is unpredictable and creative. Change is relative and increasingly diverse. Some manifestations of relative diversity in field patterning are noted below.

lesser diversity	greater diversity	seems continuous
longer rhythms	shorter rhythms	seems continuous
slower motion	faster motion	timelessness
time experienced as slower	time experienced as faster	visionary
pragmatic	imaginative	beyond waking
longer sleeping	longer waking	

■ Reprinted with permission from The National League for Nursing, New York, New York. *Visions of Rogers' science-based nursing*, 1990, p. 9.

Change is continuous, relative, and innovative. The increasing diversity of field patterning characterizes this process of change. Individual differences serve only to point up the significance of this relative diversity. For example, changing rhythmicities possess individual uniqueness. The transition from longer sleeping, to longer waking, to beyond waking is highly variable between individuals. Moreover, further diversity is manifested in so-called "day people" and "night people" as well as in other examples of rhythmical diversity.

Field pattern has been a central idea in this system from its inception over 25 years ago. It is interesting to note that Ferguson (1980) wrote in her book *The Aquarian Conspiracy* that "synthesis and pattern seeing are survival skills of the 21st Century." Ferguson's comment is certainly apropos to the science of unitary human beings. Pattern reveals itself through its manifestations. These manifestations are continuously innovative while the evolution of life and non-life is a dynamic, irreducible, non-linear process characterized by increasing complexification of energy field patterning. The nature of change is unpredictable and increasingly diverse. The rhythms and motion that "seem continuous" refer to a wave frequency so rapid that the observer perceives it as a single, unbroken event. Not only is field pattern diversity relative for any given individual, but there is also a marked increase in diversity between individuals. The implications of this for increased individualization of nursing services are explicit.

Pandimensionality

A universe of open systems underwrites the growing diversity of people and their environments. Pandimensionality characterizes these human and environmental fields and all reality is postulated to be pandimensional. Within this postulate the relative nature of change becomes explicit. The use of the term "pandimensional" to replace the terms "four dimensional" and "multidimensional" does not represent any change in definition. One does not move into or become pandimensional. Rather, this is a way of perceiving reality. Efforts to select words best suited to portray one's thoughts are at best difficult because words are often inadequate to fully communicate the meaning of a particular postulate. One useful analogy of pandimensionality, however, can be found in Abbott's (1952) *Flatland*. Here, the term pandimensional provides for an infinite domain without limit. It

hospital-based sick services. Moreover, the term community-based takes on enhanced meaning as it is defined to include multiple extraterrestrial centers. Supportive services such as hospitals provide an orientation toward pathology, not toward health. Although both community agencies and hospitals provide meaningful services, it is the broad community-based health promotion services that provide the umbrella. As a defined orientation toward health takes place, fewer and fewer people will need the same type of sick services that currently exist. Nevertheless, nothing in this science suggests that humans will be freed from all "disease" and live happily ever after. Disease and pathology are value terms applied when the human field manifests characteristics that may be deemed undesirable. One of today's major health problems is nosophobia, a morbid dread of disease.

Autonomous nursing practice directed by nurses holding valid baccalaureate and higher degrees with an upper division major in nursing science is central to the future. Noninvasive therapeutic modalities are emphasized in this new reality (Barrett, 1990). The practice of therapeutic touch, developed by Krieger (1981), is already in use in many places around this planet. The use of humor, sound, color, and motion also continue to undergo investigation. Additionally, the concept of unconditional love is receiving attention. Attitudes of hope, humor, and upbeat moods have often been documented as better therapy than drugs. Imagery and meditative modalities have much to offer as well. Continued emphasis on human rights, client decision-making, and noncompliance with the traditional rules of thumb are also necessary dimensions of the new science and art of nursing. In addition to this, the noninvasive therapeutic modalities, increasingly emphasized by a range of health care workers, mark the future of nursing practice on this planet and in outer space.

The outcomes of the research in the science of nursing have been reported in the literature and are now finding their way into the practice arena wherever people are (Barrett, 1990; Malinski, 1986; Sarter, 1988). Such research enables one to understand better the nature of human evolution and its multiple, unpredictable potentialities. Description, explanation, and vision strengthen a nurse's ability to practice according to the level and scope of preparation and knowledge in the science of nursing. What is more, holistic trends open up new ways of thinking and spell new worldviews. Other new modalities will emerge out of this evolution toward spacekind that will spark more effective modalities for earthkind.

Caring is one practice modality getting much attention from nurses today. However, as such, caring does not identify nurses any more than it identifies workers from another field. Everyone needs to care; the nature of caring in a given field depends entirely on the body of scientific knowledge specific to the field. Caring is simply a way of using knowledge. Nurses care on the basis of ways they use the science of unitary, irreducible human beings.

Since today's world is rapidly becoming an entrepreneurial society, and nurses continue to move into its mainstream, a substantive knowledge base in a science of nursing has become indispensable. In addition, there is as well a critical need for mutual respect and valuing of differences between all health personnel: between nurses, between health fields, and between the fields of science.

Human beings are on the threshold of a fantastic and unimagined future. In light of this, the potential for human service is greater than it has ever been before. Many nurses have been moving apace to assure that there will be a substantive body of theoretical knowledge specific to nursing to underwrite the practice of nursing. The science of unitary human beings portends a new world in space, the next frontier.

REFERENCES

Abbott, E. A. (1952). *Flatland.* New York: Dover.
Barrett, E. A. M. (Ed.) (1990). *Visions of Rogers' science-based nursing.* New York: National League for Nursing.
Bohm, D. (1980). *Wholeness and the implicate order.* Boston: Routledge & Kegan Paul.
Capra, F. (1982). *The turning point.* New York: Simon and Schuster.
Crum, R. (1989). Why Johnny kills. *New York University Magazine, 4*(2), 34.
Downs, F. (1988). Nursing research: State-of-the-art. *Journal of the New York State Nurses Association, 19* (3), 20.
Ferguson, M. (1980). *The aquarian conspiracy.* Los Angeles: Tarcher.
Friedman, S. T. (1989). Who believes in UFO's? *International UFO Reporter, 14* (1), 6–10.

Fuller, R. B. (1981). *Critical path*. New York: St. Martin's Press.

Huxley, A. (1932). *Brave new world*. New York: Modern Library.

Kenton, L. (1990). Member forum. *Noetic Sciences Bulletin, 5* (1), 6.

Krieger, D. (1981). *Foundations for holistic health nursing practices: The renaissance nurse*. Philadelphia: Lippincott.

Lauden, L. (1977). *Progress and its problems: Toward a theory of scientific growth*. Berkeley: University of California Press.

Lovelock, J. (1988). *The age of Goia*. New York: Norton.

Malinski, V. M. (Ed.) (1986). *Exploration on Martha Rogers' science of unitary human beings*. Norwalk, CT: Appleton-Century-Crofts.

Mallove, E. T. (1989, May-June). The solar system in chaos. *The Planetary Report,* pp. 12–13.

Percival, I. (1989). Chaos: A science for the real world. *New Scientist, 123,* 42–47.

Peterson, I. (1989, July). Digging into sand. *Science News, 136,* 40.

Robinson, G. S. & White, H. M. (1986). *Envoys of mankind*. Washington, D.C.: Smithsonian Institute Press.

Rogers, M. E. (1970). *An introduction to the theoretical basis of nursing*. Philadelphia: Davis.

Sarter, B. (1988). *The stream of becoming: A study of Martha Rogers' theory*. New York: National League for Nursing.

Stewart, I. (1989). *Does God play dice?: The mathematics of chaos*. Cambridge, MA: Brasil Blackwell, Inc.

Weber, R. (Ed.). (1986). *Dialogue with scientists and sages: The search for unity*. New York: Routledge & Kegan Paul.

Weber, R., Bohm, D., & Sheldrake, R. (1986). Matter as a meaning field. In R. Weber (Ed.), *Dialogue with scientists and sages: The search for unity* (pp. 105–123). New York: Routledge & Kegan Paul.

Comments on Author's Behalf

Nursing Science and the Space Age

Martha intended this article to be an up-to-date summary of her work, and that is what it represents. It is comprehensive and includes her most recent thinking. In writing this article, Martha updated her work from the time of her early 1970s book. She was clear that her revisions through the years did not reflect changes in her basic ideas; rather, she said that she just learned better ways of expressing and elaborating on this basic science. Martha often said that there were many pages in the 1970 purple book that she would like to tear out; she hoped that her most recent thoughts would be the ones people used instead of referring back to the 1970 book and some of its outdated terminology. Although Martha did not write another book, she did want this 1992 article to be used to pull together the most important and current ideas in the *Science of Unitary Human Beings*. Although it is not the last thing Martha published, it is her last major treatise on Rogerian Science.

—Elizabeth Ann Manhart Barrett

A Philosophic Analysis of Evidence-Based Nursing: Recurrent Themes, Metanarratives, and Exemplar Cases

Ann L. Whall

Marlene Sinclair

Kader Parahoo

Although Evidence-Based Nursing (EBN) is generally acknowledged as having great potential for nursing practice, philosophic issues regarding EBN are not as yet well-discussed. Unless and until such discussions take place within the discipline, EBN will not be clearly accepted. Philosophic analysis, as one type of philosophic inquiry, is used to address selected issues underlying EBN. This method includes examination of recurrent themes, metanarratives, and presentation of exemplar cases to ground such issues.

The "mantra of the moment" for healthcare professions is how Jennings and Loan describe Evidence-Based Practice (EBP).[1] Within nursing, the recent re-titling of EBP as Evidence-Based Nursing (EBN) has resulted in concern regarding its constituent attributes. Jennings and Loan suggested the need for thoughtful open-minded discussions of EBN. Fawcett et al[2] extended this point, suggesting philosophic examination of important issues. To begin such discussion, a more general definition of EBN was purposefully chosen:

EBN is defined as the conscientious, explicit and judicious use of theory-derived, research-based information in making decisions about care delivery to individuals or groups of patients and in consideration of individual needs and preferences.[3]

Philosophic Analysis as Method

Two decades ago, Ellis[4] emphasized the importance of philosophic inquiry for nursing, suggesting that it be used

Reprinted from Nursing Outlook, *54, A. L. Whall, M. Sinclair, & K. Parahoo. The philosophic analysis of evidence-based nursing: Recurrent themes, metanarratives, and exemplar cases. 30–35. Copyright © 2006 with permission from Elsevier Ltd.*

About the Authors

ANN L. WHALL is a native Michiganian and three-time graduate of Wayne State University in Detroit. She is an Advanced Nurse Practitioner in Michigan and was a Fulbright Distinguished Scholar in the United Kingdom, examining expert nurses' use of implicit memory in dementia care. The focus of her scholarship is gero-mental health, especially improving and/or maintaining the function of persons with dementia. Throughout her career, Dr. Whall has been "driven by the desire to explicate the depth and exquisite nature of nursing knowledge which has historically been unrecognized exterior to nursing." As a diploma graduate, she was denied admittance to graduate programs exterior to nursing on the basis of a belief that nursing was "manual art, not a science." Among her most significant accomplishments is as recipient of the John A. Hartford Doris Schwartz Award in 2003 for "visionary and exemplary contributions advancing the field of gerontologic nursing research" and the ANA Book of the Year awards for her theory development textbooks. Dr. Whall has published widely, held several visiting professorships, and completed multiple research studies and related publications, often with an identifiable emphasis upon the metatheoretical nature of nursing knowledge. Dr. Whall enjoys classical music, golfing, interacting with her three children, and developing international connections within nursing.

MARLENE SINCLAIR, a native of Northern Ireland, has recently become Northern Ireland's first professor of midwifery research at the Institute of Nursing Research, University of Ulster. A personal chair was awarded to her for a specific contribution to research and development, and her profile demonstrates dedication and commitment to building the evidence base for midwifery research. Her research experience spans qualitative and quantitative methods, and she has been involved in research using phenomenology, ethnography, action research, and Randomized Clinical Trials (RCTs). She has worked in partnership with medical colleagues and educationalists locally, nationally, and internationally. Recently she has been elected to sit on the Research and Innovation Committee of Senate at the University of Ulster and the local Northern Ireland R&D Research Advisory Forum. Marlene is the editor of the Royal College of Midwives (RCM) *Evidence Based Midwifery* journal and is a member of the RCM Council.

KADER PARAHOO is Professor and Director of Research at the University of Ulster. He wrote a book titled *Nursing Research: Principles, Process and Issues,* which is in its second edition.

to clarify important issues in the development of nursing knowledge. Philosophic Issues were defined by Ellis as those foundational to the nature and structure of nursing knowledge for/in practice; EBN is clearly one such topic. In an ideal world, philosophic analysis would precede practice usage of EBN. In reality, such disciplinary discussions usually take place after application has occurred.

Edgerton[5] identified 3 major forms of philosophic inquiry: argumentation by analysis, by interpretation, and by logical structure. The steps in philosophic analysis were clarified to some extent by Walker and Avant's[6] discussion of theory analysis, equating analysis to a "breaking into parts" of a theory for the purpose of identifying strengths and weaknesses. The type of topics described as benefiting from philosophic analysis are questions "unanswerable" by the usual scientific means.[7] Although questions regarding EBN do not, at first, appear "unanswerable" in the usual sense, the nature of EBN does depend upon disciplinary values and beliefs which are arguably less answerable by usual scientific means.

The philosophic analyses of Carper,[8] Smith,[9] and Banfield[10] served as a general guide for this analysis. In these earlier analyses, steps included extraction of major themes from selected literature, formation of questions regarding themes, and summarization of major points. These approaches were modified to include: (a) identification of selected themes, (b) examination of EBN discussions from 3 philosophy of science positions, and (c) using nursing metanarratives (defined by Reed as over-arching disciplinary beliefs) to suggest overall "disciplinary fit."[11–13] Exemplar cases were also used to further ground the discussion.

Recurrent Themes

Literature was searched for articles published in nursing and related journals in the last 5 years using Medline and Cinahl and the terms EBN/EBP; 69 initial sources were identified. A panel of 4 nurses with knowledge of EBN selected 5 major themes with philosophic import from these sources. The criteria "philosophic import" was defined by Ellis as issues affecting the fundamental nature of knowledge within a discipline.[4]

The first theme is a pragmatic one, ie, the need for an "adequate infrastructure" for common usage of EBN. The Basford and Slevin[14] discussion describes the need for such infrastructure and suggests that, without it, EBN will not be useable to the clinical practitioner. Such discussions identify the need for ready availability of experts for interpretation and supervision of EBN in practice situations; both safety and ethical issues are evident.

The Ketefian[15] discussion also addresses the infrastructure issue, identifying the gap between production of knowledge and its application. Adequate support to decrease this gap was seen as a generally overlooked issue. Such infrastructure would need to establish not only the clear means for evaluation of "new versus old knowledge," but also the specific identification of the persons and processes empowered to make such decisions. That there are important and substantial resource issues associated with development of such infrastructure is as yet not clearly recognized.

Discussions by Carr and Schott,[16] Ciliska et al,[17] McKibbon and Marks,[18] Mitchell,[19] and Thompson et al[20] suggested a second theme, that of the interplay between "various types of knowledge" in the practice of nursing. In a historic sense, western nursing has always included

more than just empirical/theoretical (or knowing-that) knowledge, but also requisite ethical, aesthetic, personal and experiential (or knowing-how) knowledge.[3,8,21] EBN discussions in general are seen as not adequately addressing the multifarious nature of nursing practice.[22–23] The incorporation of these "multiple ways of knowing" within the definition, let alone practice application of EBN, has yet to be resolved. In nursing, such multifaceted knowledge continues to be greatly esteemed, and support for this position presents somewhat of a conundrum for EBN, at least as it is presently conceptualized.[19] From a historic perspective, a conception of EBN based upon "part knowledge" presents several problems, including aesthetic and ethical issues.

A third theme concerns intuition and the role it plays within EBN. Although "intuition" is related to experiential knowledge, it is seen as less conscious in nature.[24] Cross-disciplinary discussions regarding the use of intuition and EBP have relevance for EBN. Greenhalgh[25] defined intuition in relation to EBP "as a decision making method that is used unconsciously by experienced practitioners but is inaccessible to the novice . . . that (such knowledge) does not follow simple cause and effect logic." Greenhalgh, concluded that the experienced practitioner should generate and follow clinical hunches as well as (not instead of). . . EBP. Although Greenhalgh presents a medical view of EBP, this discussion is helpful in describing how intuition might be included within EBN.

Robinson[26] essentially agreed with Greenhalgh, stating that subconscious computation of all sorts of things . . . based upon past situations . . . leads to rapid conclusions without going through a conscious deduction. Stating that conclusions of more expert clinicians often appear less logical, Robinson's views support the position of Dreyfus: that the expert, in a sense, appears to "discard the rule book."[21] Robinson warned that the best clinical practitioners may become "hemmed in" by protocols and standards and suggests this will result in clinicians developing fewer intuitive skills, leading to more "drone-like" practice.

A concomitant but contrary position regarding intuitive knowledge and its relationship to EBN is less well-identified, (ie, the possible idiosyncratic nature of unconscious intuitive knowing). In clinical application of some practice standards, for example, practitioners might declare themselves possessing intuitive knowledge that must change some aspect of care. The question of evaluation prior to application, and the nature of such evaluation, becomes a vital scientific, ethical, and aesthetic issue. Contrariwise, the outright and automatic rejection of intuitive insights could stifle advancement of clinical practice. That these issues need thoughtful pro/con examination regarding EBN is clear.

A fourth theme concerns practitioners' level of expertise. Although levels of expertise are more discussed within nursing than intuitive knowing, the relationship between level of knowledge and EBN is also uncertain.[24] Dreyfus identified that expert level practitioners may be unable to use their knowledge when restricted by mandated procedures; adherence to method may thus prevent experts from using their expertise to bring about more positive outcomes.[21,27–28] The work of others, eg, Flanagan[29] and Schon,[30] suggests another aspect of this theme: that in critical situations when experts are forced to "stick to the rule book," disastrous results may occur. Examples of airplane pilots' unorthodox approaches saving airliners from crashing are sometimes given for giving experts free-reign in critical situations. The question, then, is how EBN relates to critical/rapidly developing situations in which practitioners believe there is an urgent need to change EBN-based practices.

A fifth theme was termed "less developed questions" to categorize several important but relatively undeveloped points of philosophic import for EBN. One such issue is a concern that nursing practice guided by EBN might over-emphasize technology.[19] That EBN supports a superior view of technology is not clear, however, the technology issue awakens concerns from nursing's past. Past practices within health care may have demonstrated an emphasis upon technology to control behavior. A technological emphasis without requisite ethical examination is thus somewhat of a covert concern.

Another less-developed point concerns practitioners' personal integrity in an EBN era.[23,31] Again, it is unclear that EBN would obfuscate personal integrity in nursing practice, yet the right of practitioners to decline participation in what they consider to be "unsafe" or unethical situations is compelling. The right of patients and families to decline participation in EBN-guided care because of personal or cultural preferences for alternative or no treatment is, likewise, relatively unexplored. A related concern is the impact of EBN upon health care resources. McKenna et al,[32] and Regan,[33] for example, discussed several myths surrounding EBN, most notably, that EBN guarantees improved outcomes of care. Whether EBN leads to improved outcomes and/or is cost effective remains clouded. Such questions affect the general acceptance and usage of EBN, for they raise covert application issues.

Gortner's[34] searches for a common philosophic stance within nursing led her to conclude that the view most commonly held within Western nursing was one of moderate realism. To some extent, this position characterizes these EBN themes, for they reflect a belief that scientific knowledge is relative, variable, and always—to some degree—uncertain; or, as is summarized in a phrase often quoted to new practitioners, "don't ever be too sure."

Placement of Themes Within Philosophy of Science Positions

The dominant philosophy of science position held within any discipline or health care setting affects the daily lives, decisions, and practice of clinicians.[11–12] A central question of philosophy of science is "what counts as evidence" and, the related issue, "who decides what counts."[23] Three philosophy of science positions currently identifiable within practice settings are those of positivism, postmodernism, and neomodernism.

That positivism dominated scientific thought from about the mid-19th to mid-20th century is well accepted.[35] One of logical positivism's major tenets was the verification principle, an aspect of which meant that phenomena were scientifically meaningful only if they were empirically verifiable via sense data.[36–37] There are several characteristics of logical positivism with relevance for EBN, including a tendency to reduce phenomena to their most simplistic level produced in/through scientific efforts.[35] That EBP has been based upon randomized clinical trials (which seek to exclude contextual or seemingly irrelevant concerns) supports this concern. Within Western nursing, however, there has been a historic concern not only for contextual issues, but also for the beliefs of both patients and nurses.

Although positivism was generally considered an important advance over earlier explanatory attempts, it led to acceptance of the verification principle within natural sciences and, later, within nursing. In a strict sense of verificationist objectivity, science would not deal with the subject's views of care, spirituality, or cultural issues. EBN, as currently discussed, appears to value a more holistic view (eg, including patient preferences) and, as such, denies a strict verificationist perspective. A belief in a single viewpoint (even that of EBN) mandated for all health care systems, however, conflicts with Nightingale's historic recognition that health care is dependent upon multiple contextual/environmental factors such as the expertise of available health personnel.

It is worthwhile in discussions of EBN, however, to keep in mind the criticisms leveled at a strict verificationist view, including an emphasis upon producing a single "truth." As Popper observed, "no run of favorable observational data, however long and unbroken, is logically sufficient to establish the truth of an unrestricted generalization."[38] Thus, Popper's point cautions that any one approach supported by EBN might be better viewed as "currently, the best approach."

Postmodern thinking was a reaction to the more restrictive aspects of positivism. Bauman[39] described postmodernism as a "school of thought" and Cheek[40] refers to it as a movement characterized by plurality of thought regarding method, design, art, literature, etc. Postmodernism thus sought a wider view of admissible evidence and a greater appreciation of the individual practitioner's experience as arbiter of "what counts for evidence," and who makes such decisions. One aspect of postmodern thought was the rejection of a universal totality emphasis with its focus upon a singular scientific truth (one goal of positivism).[41]

Postmodern thinking, therefore, was/is much more congruent with nursing's historical perspective.[11] Less of a "top-down" reasoning, the postmodern view took into account the "stand point" of the those affecting and affected by a particular approach to science.[36,13] Evidence-Based Nursing, as currently discussed, does not appear to exclude an individualized "stand point" view so characteristic of postmodernism. Consistent usage of such a viewpoint within EBN would be consistent with nursings' historical focus.

Neomodernism has been described by Reed[13] as a viewpoint which accommodates relevant aspects of both positivism and postmodernism for nursing. Although the beliefs and intra-congruency issues of neomodernism are not currently well described or discussed, at least the tendency to open interdisciplinary discussions supported by such a view is important to EBN. Interdisciplinary practice would seem to demand such an approach, since EBN takes place most often within inter-disciplinary clinical practice settings.[42] In such cases, conflicts between Evidence-Based Medicine (EBM) and EBN will become most evident. The means for resolution of such conflicts, however, has yet to be adequately identified or discussed.

Metanarrative Examination

Rationale for inclusion of metanarrative examination as a component of philosophic analyses relates to the historic perspective of the discipline. Reed[13] defined metanarratives as over-arching and recurring beliefs that have as their source a variety of disciplinary elements. A defining aspect of metanarratives is their traditional acceptance over time as disciplinary and historical ideals. Metanarratives are thus relevant to discussions of EBN, for they serve in a sense as "truth criteria" to guide the application of newer approaches to practice.

The examples Reed[13] gave of major nursing metanarratives were: nursing as patient-centered, health- and pattern-focused, and as valuing the inclusion of patient/family preferences. Nursing metanarratives arguably relate to a commonly identified focus of Western nursing, (ie, a focus upon persons, environment, health, and nursing itself). These concepts deny a focus upon illness alone, a de-emphasizing of the environment in which care (or EBN) is to take place, the ignoring of patient/family opinions and preferences, as well as the notion that the practitioner and patient do not simultaneously affect and/or are affected by the caregiving situation.[43] This broad focus has led to such cherished practices as therapeutic use of self, the examination of empathic pick-up, the valuing of openness in care-recipient relations, and the tailoring of care to culture and developmental stage. The way in which EBN is/will be affected by this view is as yet unclear.

Nightingale's writings, likewise, support a metanarrative for the "valuing of experiential knowledge."[43] A recurrent theme in her writings, Nightingale distrusted theoretic knowledge alone as well as the practice of testing clinical expertise via written examinations.[43] Holding that clinical expertise is best developed via supervised practice, Nightingale valued "know how" or experiential knowledge over "knowing that" or theoretic knowledge. The acceptance within nursing of Polanyi's[44] description of experience as an effective means by which one develops unrecognized or "tacit knowledge," continues to support this view. How such tacit knowledge is to be considered with reference to EBN is yet to be well addressed.

Johnson and Ratner[45] support the combining of empirical, theoretical, and more subjective experiential knowledge. In their discussion, the synthesis of various ways of knowing changes and/or transforms and extends the basis for clinical practice.[21,27–28,46,47] Whether a combination of such knowledge within EBN is feasible is also unclear.

Grounding Philosophic Analysis in Case Examples

Because philosophic analyses by nature are abstract or, arguably, somewhat removed from more concrete situations, 2 prototypical cases are used to clarify philosophic issues regarding EBN. Two case studies presented are congruent with the clinical experiences of 2 of the authors; these examples do not represent, however, any one practitioner, patient and/or clinical situation, and are constructed specifically to represent selected philosophic themes described in this article. Although not specifically focused upon EBN, this first case example presents a potential clinical conflict between EBM and EBN, as well as a conflict between EBM and the traditional nursing value of patient informed practice.

Exemplar Case 1

A nurse midwife (within the United Kingdom midwives are not necessarily nurses) and a physician were working together as colleagues during the delivery of a full-term infant. Both mother and infant were doing well until late in the second stage of labor. Progress had stopped and the infant's heart rate indicated that an instrument-assisted delivery was warranted. Within the given health care setting, the evidence-based practice guideline for instrument-assisted deliveries called for the use of vacuum extraction; in this institution, only physicians were authorized to perform this procedure. The physician attending the patient was not yet expert in this technology, but was expert in the older technology of forceps usage. The time was about 2 AM. There was no other practitioner available who was expert in the newer vacuum extraction process. The attending physician discussed this ethical dilemma with the nurse midwife, ie, complying with the guideline-required technology and increasing the chance of some injury to the infant due to the inexpert skill level of the physician, or using the older technology (the use of forceps) in which the physician was expert. The decision was made (without input of patient preference) to use the older technology and safely deliver the infant as quickly as possible.

Within this example, several philosophic themes are represented. These include: the need for an adequate and supportive system infrastructure, the ready availability of technical experts within the system, ethical issues concerning the physician's lack of updated preparation congruent with the guidelines, the health care system allowing someone without guideline-specified skill to practice, and the mother and/or father preferences not being included in decision-making. Both the nurse midwife and the physician could/would be held responsible for not complying fully with the EBP policy. Not refuting that vacuum extraction has been found safer according to the latest research comparing the 2 procedures, both practitioners' experiential knowledge told them that the infant was at risk and that they needed to act quickly for the safety of the infant. The decision which was made was a pragmatic one, but with a good outcome.

Exemplar Case 2

A woman in her mid-thirties, was admitted at about 10 PM to a maternity hospital for the impending birth of her third child. As was the custom in this community, about 6 weeks prior to the delivery, a birth plan was developed by the mother and a community nurse during a home visit.

The mother had successfully delivered her second child in a squatting position, which the attending midwife at the second birth had recommended and encouraged. The mother preferred this position for the present birth because she found it put less stress upon her back, and with the impending birth she was having lower back pain. The back pain was not mentioned to the community nurse and the birth plan did not include the mother's preference for the squatting position.

On arrival at the hospital, however, the mother explained to the attending midwife that she had back pain and preferred delivery in the squatting position. The midwife did not indicate agreement or her opinion as to this request, nor did the midwife divulge that she was not an expert in assisting delivery with the mother in the squatting position during birthing. As labor progressed, it was evident that the attending midwife did not favor the squatting position, for she deflected such requests, stating that the position would result in more back pain and, further, that she could not see the baby's progress in the birth canal with the mother in that position.

The child was successfully delivered with the mother in a recumbent position. After the delivery, the mother's back pain intensified. She was subsequently given a course of physiotherapy and her back pain resolved.

There are at least 3 philosophical themes present in this situation: the first is that it appears likely the nurse midwife did not know the best evidence for/against the recumbent vs squatting position, including its relationship to back pain. Secondly, even knowing that evidence, the midwife was not experienced with and, therefore, not competent in attending a birth in that position. Finally, there was no discussion of how to resolve the problem when the patient's informed preference conflicted with the preferences and skill of the practitioner.

While the first issue may have been a failure on the part of the infrastructure to make certain that their practitioners know and are competent in practices concerning such positioning, ethically both the practitioner and the system are responsible for assuring such knowledge. A second issue concerns the expertise level of the practitioner and compliance with obtaining such expertise.

Similar to the issue in Exemplar Case 1, the practitioner is faced with 2 opposing choices: (1) to comply with the mother's wishes and risk complications due to lack of practitioner knowledge, or (2) to use the approach with which the practitioner is most familiar and ignore the patient's personal preferences. It is true that someone more familiar with the squatting position might have been accessed, but in critical situations such assistance is not always readily available.

The third issue "negotiating care practices" will arise more frequently as informed patients challenge provider's actions. It is easier for the provider to engage in resolving such conflicts when the provider is the one advocating for the evidence-supported practice, since the weight of the evidence is on the provider's side. In situations such as this, the provider is also required to possess high-level collaborative skill. A caution of Entwhistle[47] has relevance for what is, in essence, a public policy issue that substantial investment of resources may be necessary for EBN to be generally implemented.

Summary

By mid-20th century, Western nursing clearly recognized that clinical practice must be based upon both theoretical knowledge and research findings. The definition of EBN selected for this discussion includes these 2 historically important emphases. There is also little doubt, however, that within the discipline of nursing there is a mandate for the recognition and inclusion of other historically important values and beliefs within the approach known as EBN[19,22–24,31] What is as yet unclear, however, is how these historically important elements may inform and/or influence the important body of knowledge known as EBN.

The authors thank Dr. Julia Seng (Certified Nurse Midwife, The University of Michigan, Ann Arbor), and Dr. Frank Hicks (Associate Professor, Rush University, College of Nursing, Chicago) whose suggestions were incorporated into this article.

REFERENCES

1. Jennings BM, Loan LA. Misconceptions among nurses about evidence-based practice. J Nurs Scholarship 2001;33: 121–7.
2. Fawcett J, Watson J, Neuman B, Walker PH, Fitzpatrick JJ. On nursing theories and evidence. J Nurs Scholarship 2001;33:115–9.
3. Ingersoll G. Evidence-based nursing: what it is and isn't. Nurs Outlook 2000;48:151–2.
4. Ellis R. Philosophic inquiry. Ann Rev Nurs Res 1983;1:211–28.
5. Edgerton SG. Philosophical analysis. In: Sarter B, Ed. Paths to knowledge: innovative research methods for nursing. New York, NY: Nat League Nurs; 1988. p. 169–82.
6. Walker LO, Avant, KC. Strategies for theory construction in nursing. Norwalk, CT: Appleton and Lange; 1995.
7. Kikuchi JF. Nursing questions that science cannot answer. In: Kikuchi JF, Simmons H, editors. Philosophic inquiry in nursing. Newberry Park, CA: Sage; 1992. p. 26–37.
8. Carper B. Fundamental patterns of knowing in nursing. Adv Nurs Sci 1978;1:13–23.
9. Smith JA. The idea of health. New York, NY: Teachers College Press; 1983.
10. Banfield BE. A philosophic inquiry of Orem's self-care deficit nursing theory (dissertation). Detroit, MI: Wayne State University; 1997.
11. Whall A, Hicks F. The unrecognized paradigm shift within nursing: implications, problems, and possibilities. Nurs Outlook 2002; 50:72–6.
12. Whall A, Hicks F. Metanarratives surrounding successful aging. In: Poon LW, Gueldner SH, Sprouse BM, editors. Successful aging and adaptation with chronic diseases. New York, NY: Springer Publishing Company Inc; 2003. p. 220–7.
13. Reed PG. A treatise on nursing knowledge development for the 21st century: beyond postmodernism. Adv Nurs Sci 1995;17: 70–84.
14. Basford L, Slevin O. Theory and practice of nursing: an integrated approach to caring practice. Cheltenham, Glos, UK: Nelson Thomas; 2001. p. 322–6.
15. Ketefian S. Issues in the application of research to practice. Revista Latino-Americana de Enfermagm 2001;9:7–12.
16. Carr CA, Schott A. Differences in evidence-based care in midwifery practice and education. J Nurs Scholarship 2002; 34: 153–8.
17. Ciliska DK, Pinelli J, DiCenso A, Cullum N. Resources to enhance evidence-based nursing practice. AACN Clin Issues 2001: 12:520–8.
18. McKibbon KA, Marks S. Posing clinical questions: framing the question for scientific inquiry. AACN Clin Issues 2001; 12: 477–81.
19. Mitchell G. Evidence-based practice: critique and alternative view. Nurs Sci Quart 1999;12:30–5.
20. Thompson C, McCaughan D, Cullum N, Sheldon TA, Mulhall A, Thompson DR. Research information in nurses' clinical decision-making: what is useful? J Adv Nur 2001;36:376–88.
21. Benner P. From novice to expert: excellence and power in clinical nursing practice. Menlo Park, CA: Addison-Wesley; 1984.
22. Estabrooks CA. What kind of evidence does qualitative research offer cardiovascular nurses? Can J Cardiovas Nurs 1997;8:31–4.
23. Rafael ARP. Evidence-based practice: the good, the bad, the ugly, part two. RNJ 2000;12:7–9.
24. Closs SJ, Cheater FM. Evidence for nursing practice: a clarification of the issues. J Adv Nur 1999:30:10–7.
25. Greenhalgh T. Intuition and evidence—uneasy bedfellows? Brit J Gen Pra 2002;52:395–9.
26. Robinson J. Intuition. Brit J Midwifery 2002;10:670–1.
27. Benner P, Tanner CA, Chesla CA . Expertise in nursing practice: caring, clinical judgment and ethics. New York, NY: Springer Publishing Company Inc; 1996.
28. Benner P, Hooper-Kryiakidis P, Stannard D. Clinical wisdom and interventions in critical care: a thinking-in-action approach. Philadelphia, PA: WB Saunders Company; 1999.
29. Flanagan JC. The critical incident technique. Psycho Bull 1954;51:327–58.
30. Schon D. The reflective practitioner: how professionals think in action. New York, NY: Basic Books; 1987.
31. Rafael ARF. Evidence-based practice: the good, the bad, the ugly, part one. RNJ 2000;12:5–9.
32. McKenna H, Cutcliffe J, McKenna P. Evidence-based practice: demolishing some myths. Nurs Stand 2000;14:39–42.
33. Regan J. Will current clinical effectiveness initiatives encourage and facilitate practitioners to use evidence-based practice for the benefit of their clients? J Clin Nur 1998;7: 244–50.
34. Gortner SR. Nursing's syntax revisited: toward a science philosophy. Internatl J Nurs Stud 1993;30:447–88.
35. Curd M, Cover J. Philosophy of science: central issues. New York, NY: WW Norton Company; 1998.
36. Whall A. The influence of logical positivism on nursing practice. Image: J Nurs Scholarship 1989;21:243–5.
37. Phillips D. Philosophy, science, and social inquiry: contemporary methodological controversies in social science and related applied fields of research. New York, NY: Pergamon Press; 1987.
38. Flew A. A dictionary of philosophy. New York, NY: St Martin's Press; 1979.

39. Bauman Z. Intimations of past modernity. London, UK: Routledge; 1992.
40. Cheek J. Postmodern and post-structuralist approaches to nursing research. Thousand Oaks, CA: Sage Publications; 2000.
41. Abbey R. Charles Taylor: philosophy now. Princeton, NJ: The Princeton and Oxford Press; 2000.
42. Sehon SR, Stanley DE. A philosophical analysis of evidence based medicine. BMC Health Serv Reas 2003;3: 1472–92.
43. Reed P, Zurakowski T. Nightingale: foundations of nursing. In: Fitzpatrick JJ, Whall A, editors. Conceptual models of nursing: analysis and application. Stamford, CT: Appleton and Lange; 1996. p. 27–54.
44. Polanyi M. Knowing and being. Chicago, IL: The University of Chicago Press; 1969. p. 138–157.
45. Johnson J, Ratner P. The nature of the knowledge used in nursing practice. In: Thorne S, Hayes V, editors. Nursing praxis: knowledge and action. Thousand Oaks, CA: Sage; 1997. p. 3–22.
46. Schon D. Educating the reflective practitioner: toward a new design for teaching and learning in the professions. San Francisco, CA: Jossey-Bass; 1991.
47. Entwhistle VA, Sheldon TA, Sowden A, Watt IS. Evidence-informed patient choice: practical issues of involving patients in decisions about health care technologies. Intern J Techn Assessment Hlth Care 1998;14:212–25.

The Authors Comment

A Philosophic Analysis of Evidence-Based Nursing: Recurrent Themes, Metanarratives, and Exemplar Cases

This philosophic analysis was conducted as part of my Fulbright Distinguished Visiting Professorships (2001–2002 and 2003–2005) at the University of Ulster, Northern Ireland, U.K. Dr. Marlene Sinclair was concerned with explicating several practice issues concerning the use of Evidence-Based Practice (EBP) in midwifery practice, and Dr. Kader Parahoo (Research Coordinator) had previously developed materials regarding EBP. I suggested philosophic analysis as a theory clarification strategy to assist in identifying issues related to the use of derived EBP principles within the discipline of nursing. Dr. Sinclair adds that this is a foundational philosophical article that unites thinkers and researchers in nursing, midwifery, and academia across the world in an attempt to put down a serious marker for deeper philosophic inquiry using metanarratives.

—Ann L. Whall
—Marlene Sinclair
—Kader Parahoo

Commentary on Neomodernism and Evidence-Based Nursing: Implications for the Production of Nursing Knowledge

Pamela G. Reed

The Whall, Sinclair and Parahoo[1] philosophic analysis is a vital process in the evolution of the evidence-based nursing (EBN) movement. As a social movement, EBN can generate new ideas about the nature of nursing practice. One step in their analysis was the examination of EBN discussions from 3 philosophy of science positions: modernism, postmodernism, and neomodernism. The first 2 are familiar, but the third, neomodernism,[2] is a relatively recent perspective that has been revisited periodically in the literature since 1995.[3–5] An elaboration of this perspective and its congruence with the EBN themes is offered here, to extend the authors' philosophic analysis of EBN and bring additional insights into the role of practice in nursing knowledge development.

Philosophy of science is in transition, moving beyond modernism and even postmodernism. This transition presents an exciting opportunity to reconsider philosophies of nursing science. Existing epistemologies of science range from Popper's privileged view of scientific knowledge to Rorty's pragmatic and pluralistic views that avoid privileging science above other means of generating knowledge. Pat definitions of scientific knowledge, truth, and progress are no longer taken for granted by nurses and other knowledge builders. It is an important time to participate in the dialogue about nursing philosophy.

Neomodernism

As a basic discipline and a profession, nursing possesses unique resources for generating new approaches to knowledge production. It's likely that clinicians and

Reprinted from Nursing Outlook, *54, P. G. Reed, Commentary on neomodernism and evidence-based nursing: Implications for the products of nursing knowledge, 36–38. Copyright © 2006 with permission from Elsevier Ltd.*

About the Author

PAMELA G. REED is Professor at the University of Arizona College of Nursing in Tucson, Arizona, where she also served as Associate Dean for Academic Affairs for 7 years. She is a three-time graduate of Wayne State University in Detroit, receiving a BSN in 1974, an MSN in 1976 (with a double major in child–adolescent psychiatric mental health nursing and teaching), and her PhD (with a major in nursing, focused on life-span development and aging) in 1982. Dr. Reed pioneered research into spirituality and well-being with her doctoral research with terminally ill patients. She also developed a theory of self-transcendence and two widely used research instruments, the *Spiritual Perspective Scale* and the *Self-Transcendence Scale*. Her publications and funded research reflect a dual scholarly focus: spirituality and other facilitators of well-being and decisions in end-of-life transitions; and nursing metatheory and knowledge development. Dr. Reed also enjoys time with her family, reading, classical music, swimming, and hiking in the mountains and canyons of Arizona.

researchers desire a philosophy of their science that is more comprehensive and congruent with their disciplinary perspective as well as with the inter-disciplinary world they inhabit. Neomodernism[2] is a philosophy of science inspired by notable shifts in philosophy of science and, more importantly, by the unspoken incongruence between values espoused by nursing about the centrality of practice and praxis, and extant science practices and educational standards that have marginalized the majority of professional nurses from knowledge development.

Neomodernism advances ideas derived from the intersection of modernism and postmodernism values of science, several of which originated in the 17th century Enlightenment. These include: a spirit of experimentation; disenchantment with dogmatic views about truth; desire for emancipation from ignorance and authority; creative and critical thinking; tolerance of ambiguity; an open-ended view of nature; and skepticism. Postmodernism departs from modernism in its dispute of: foundationalism, a belief in an unchanging truth; essentialism, the belief in a universal essence in human nature; and realism, belief in a universal reality that exists independent of historical or social context.

Neomodernism builds upon these shared and unshared values. It is also a response to a late 20th century shift in philosophy of science. This shift is evident among philosophers of science as well as scholars from the humanities, economics, literary theory, and professional disciplines such as psychology and medicine;[6–9] these scholars have proposed new philosophic approaches that integrate or sit between modernism and postmodernism, and transcend the science wars.

Philosophic Congruence with EBN Themes

Several themes found in Whall et al's[1] philosophic analysis of EBN are congruent with major tenets in the philosophy of neomodernism. One critical tenet of neomodernism is reflected in 2 EBN themes concerning: (a) the gap between the production and application of knowledge, and (b) the practitioner's level of expertise. An integral relationship between knowledge production and practice, beyond the usual lip service, is a pivotal view within neomodernism. Knowledge development cannot effectively occur without this partnership of roles. In neomodern thought, the nursing practitioner is not merely a knowledge consumer or user, but is a knowledge producer.

This idea derives, in part, from the visionary thinking of nursing scholars found for example in Rosemary Ellis'[10] "practitioner as theorist" idea and Peplau's[11] explication of clinical practice as a scientific method for transforming scientific knowledge into nursing knowledge. Practicing nurses who participate as knowledge builders can generate the theory-based knowledge, which sociologist Andrew Abbott[12] stated was so essential for a profession to achieve "full jurisdiction" over its practice. The current minority of knowledge producers, mostly doctorally-prepared research nurses, alone cannot provide adequate theory-based knowledge needed by all professional nurses to achieve full jurisdiction over practice.

Nursing will face a crisis in knowledge production unless the educational system is reformed to educate nurses for neomodern practice of EBN. In addition, personal integrity and reflective judgment capacity, 2 additional EBN themes identified by Whall et al,[1] are also at risk because of traditional science practices that maintain the gap between the production and application of knowledge.

Another EBN theme identified was the "interplay between various types of knowledge in the practice of nursing." Top-down, linear approaches to knowledge development, whereby the knowledge researchers produce is "handed down" to clinicians for application, is untenable within a neomodern nursing epistemology that calls for the participation of clinicians in knowledge development. To the extent that neither empirical nor ethical theories can directly inform action, there is need for new kinds of theories that evolve out of practice. Modernist philosophy of science separates values and aesthetic experiences from scientific theorizing, and separates the theorist from the context of discovery. Postmodern philosophy eschews metanarratives, such as nursing conceptual models, and undercuts their contribution of historical wisdom to theories about the nature and focus of nursing. Within neomodernism, traditional philosophies of science can give way to new forms of scientific theorizing that provide both an understanding of local meanings and law-like explanations of broadly shared patterns of health in human systems.

According to neomodernist philosophy, scientific theory is not only a form of thinking exemplified by Newton, who transformed natural philosophy into modern science; scientific theory is a process by which practitioner and patient participate in the co-production of knowledge. Neomodern clinicians need to be educated in how to employ various patterns of knowing—from aesthetic and empirical to technologic and sociopolitical—to generate science theories of nursing in practice. To borrow from Kaplan's[13] philosophy of science, "science is enhanced, not contaminated," if nurses "place their theorizing in the context of concrete experience. Such a placing makes theory deeper," by making the entire web of nursing available to mine for knowledge production. EBN reflects this neomodern view when both the practice of nursing and the practice of science are considered essential to and synergistic in building disciplinary knowledge.

Tenets of Neomodernism

The tenets of neomodernism reflect a philosophy of science that is actively engaged within the practice arena. These tenets posit the following epistemologic and ontologic ideas:

- A new empiricism that encourages the use of new tools, methods, technologies to justify knowledge production. It allows for new sources of justification of knowledge that extend or replace direct observation with instruments, as in "instrumental justification,"[14] and other technologies of nursing research and practice.

- A new epistemology in which clinicians are educated to use various patterns of knowing to produce knowledge in practice. With few exceptions,[15] Carper's[16] 4 patterns of knowing and the multiple writings her work has generated have not been fully exploited for innovations in knowledge development. The accomplishments nursing has made in the study of physiological and biobehavioral phenomena through primarily empirical patterns of knowing is laudable as one of many approaches to theory development that nursing epistemology can inspire.

- A critical realism that acknowledges an underlying pattern, a capacity for self-organization, agency, humanism, spirituality, and potential for empowerment. Unlike modernism, neomodernism doesn't distance itself from its romantic roots and, in so doing, allows for a larger, more diverse repertoire of human experiences for building theory about caring for human beings during health events.[17,18]

- Values for difference and for an ongoing critique of oppression. For example, neomodernism shares views of feminist epistemology and critical theory in promoting the pursuit of knowledge as far as science methods will take one, in ways that maximize potential for egalitarianism and freedom from oppression.[19]

- Assumption of universal/shared principles as well as individual uniqueness and local truths. Philosophers of science, for example, are entertaining theory-building strategies that allow for "partial truths" where, before, universal truth was the goal. And they desire theories that are open and have potential to go beyond themselves.[20] All of this theorizing is balanced by an external "corrective" (such as a particular framework or worldview) to inform judgments about what is emancipating, good, healthful, and other value-laden concepts in nursing theorizing.

- Neomodernism champions an ongoing critique that keeps metanarratives, theories and philosophies open, dynamic, and contextually relevant. There is a re-enchantment of nursing science, where the meta-physical matters, but it is balanced by a critical awareness of history, context, and free will that informs knowledge production.[21]

Neomodernism brings together unlikely partners in the practice of science. In his integration of modernism and postmodernism, for example, Davis[22] identified "lines of affiliation" between Enlightenment philosopher Kant and postmodern philosopher Lyotard. Through his analysis of their seemingly disparate epistemologies about the role of performance in knowledge development, he advanced the principle that knowledge is produced as much as it is received by a scientist. Similarly, bringing together transformed roles of clinician, researcher, and theorist can lead to significant advances in knowledge production that enhance basic nursing knowledge and EBN, as well as nurses' personal integrity, judgment capacity, and jurisdiction over practice.

Philosophical analysis of EBN and other practice movements in nursing is a catalyst for clarifying philosophical foundations of science. Emergent philosophies of science, in turn, generate important implications for educating clinicians prepared from baccalaureate through practice-doctorate levels, who can function confidently and effectively as knowledge producers in a neomodern era of nursing practice.

REFERENCES

1. Whall AL, Sinclair M, Parahoo K. A philosophic analysis of evidence based nursing: recurrent themes, metanarratives, and exemplar cases. Nurs Outlook 2005;54:30–35.
2. Reed PG. A treatise on nursing knowledge development for the 21st century: beyond postmodernism. Adv Nurs Sci 1995;17:70–84.
3. DiBartolo MC. Philosophy of science in doctoral nursing education revisited. J Prof Nurs 1998;14:350–60.
4. Whall AL, Hicks FD. The unrecognized paradigm shift in nursing: implications, problems, and possibilities. Nurs Outlook 2002;50:72–6.
5. Spenceley SM. Out of fertile muck: the evolving narrative of nursing. Nurs Philos 2004;5:201–7.
6. Holzman L. Performing psychology: A postmodern culture of the mind. New York, NY: Routledge; 1999.
7. Hands DW. Reflection without rules: economic methodology and contemporary science theory. New York, NY: Cambridge University Press; 2001.
8. Tonelli MR, Callahan TC. Why alternative medicine cannot be evidence-based. Academic Med 2001;76:1213–20.
9. Eagleton T. After theory. New York, NY: Allen Lane; 2003.
10. Ellis R. The practitioner as theorist. Am J Nurs 1969;69:1434–8.
11. Reed PG. Transforming knowledge into nursing knowledge: a revisionist analysis of Peplau. IMAGE: J Nurs Scholarship 1996;28:29–33.
12. Abbott A. The system of professions. Chicago, IL: University of Chicago Press; 1988.
13. Kaplan LD. Family pictures: a philosopher explores the familiar. Chicago, IL: Open Court; 1998.
14. Humphreys P. Extending ourselves. In: Carrier M, Massey GJ, Ruetsche L, editors. Science at century's end: Philosophical questions on the progress and limits of science. Pittsburgh, PA: University of Pittsburgh Press; 2000. p. 13–32.
15. Fawcett J, Watson J, Neuman B, Walker PH, Fitzpatrick JJ. On nursing theories and evidence. J Nurs Scholarship 2001;33:115–9.
16. Carper BA. Fundamental patterns of knowing in nursing. Adv Nurs Sci 1978;1:13–23.
17. Schneider KJ. Toward a science of the heart: romanticism and the revival of psychology. Am Psychologist 1998;53:277–89.
18. Trainer BT. The challenge of postmodernism to the human service professions. J Applied Philosophy 2000;17:75–92.
19. Kourany JA. A philosophy of science for the twenty-first century. Philosophy Sci 2003;70:1–14.

20. Da Costa NCA, French S. Science and partial truth: a unitary approach to models and scientific reasoning. New York, NY: Oxford University Press; 2003.

21. Cooke M. Between 'objectivism' and 'contextualism': the normative foundations of social philosophy. In: Freundlieb D, Hudson W, Rundell J, editors. Critical theory after Habermas. Boston, MA: Brill; 2004. p. 61–76.

22. Davis C. After poststructuralism: reading, stories and theory. New York, NY: Routledge; 2004.

The Author Comments

I appreciated the opportunity Ann Whall gave me through this article to elaborate on the tenets of 'neo-modernism,' a philosophy of science that she used in her analysis of evidence-based nursing. Neomodernism may not have been my best choice in terminology, but it was my initial attempt—in the 1990's when I developed this idea and first wrote about it—to articulate a philosophic view of nursing science that logically integrated the strengths of modern and postmodern thought. Since then I have noticed that other philosophers have expressed similar ideas, including those espousing a "post-postmodernism." I think this view provides a philisophic basis as well as broad guidelines for educating all nurses into being active participants in theory development and knowledge production.

—Pamela G. Reed

CHAPTER 23

From a Plethora of Paradigms to Parsimony in Worldviews

Jacqueline Fawcett

Nursing knowledge development is guided by philosophic claims about the nature of human beings and the human-environment relationship. Those philosophic claims are variously referred to as paradigms or worldviews. Four sets of worldviews have been cited as fundamental to the development of nursing knowledge. One set is the mechanism-organicism dichotomy. The characteristics of those two philosophic approaches to the study of the human-environment relationship were described by Reese and Overton (1970), among others, and are outlined in Table 23-1. Hall (1981) proposed another set of worldviews that reflect philosophic claims about the nature of change in human beings and the human-environment relationship. The characteristics of those views, which are labeled change and persistence, are shown in Table 23-2.

Parse (1987) discussed the features of yet another set of philosophic claims, which she called the totality and simultaneity paradigms. The characteristics of those two paradigms are listed in Table 23-3. Recently, Newman (1992) identified what she claims are the three prevailing paradigms for nursing knowledge development. The characteristics of her three paradigms, the particulate-deterministic, the interactive-integrative, and the unitary-transformative, are summarized in Table 23-4. Newman (1992) explained that "the first of the paired words [in the names of the three paradigms] describes the view of the entity being studied and the second describes the notion of how change occurs" (p. 10).

From J. Fawcett, Nursing Science Quarterly *1993; 6(3), 56–59.*

About the Author

JACQUELINE FAWCETT received her bachelor of science degree from Boston University in 1964, her master's in Parent–Child Nursing from New York University in 1970, and her PhD in Nursing, also from New York University, in 1976. Dr. Fawcett currently is Professor, College of Nursing and Health Sciences, University of Massachusetts, Boston. She is Professor Emerita at the University of Pennsylvania. Starting with her dissertation, Dr. Fawcett conducted a program of research dealing with wives' and husbands' pregnancy-related experiences that was derived from Martha Rogers' conceptual system. Subsequently, she undertook a program of research dealing with responses to caesarean birth derived from the Roy Adaptation Model of Nursing. A third program of research, also derived from the Roy Adaptation Model, focuses on function during normal life transitions and serious illness. Dr. Fawcett is perhaps best known for her metatheoretical work, including many journal articles and several books. Since 1996, Dr. Fawcett has lived in the mid-coast region of Maine with her husband John and a now-tame feral cat, Lydia Dasher. She and her husband own Fawcett's Art, Antiques, and Toy Museum. She swims laps and walks on a treadmill at a fitness center for exercise and relaxation and sails on a windjammer off the Maine coast during the summer.

Table 23-1
Characteristics of the Organismic and Mechanistic Worldviews

Organicism	Mechanism
Metaphor is the living organism.	Metaphor is the machine.
Human beings are active.	Human beings are reactive.
Behavior is probabilistic.	Behavior is a predictable linear chain.
Holism and expansionism are assumed—focus on wholes.	Elementarism and reductionism are assumed—focus on parts.
Development is qualitative and quantitative.	Development is quantitative.

Table 23-2
Characteristics of the Change and Persistence Worldviews

Change	Persistence
Metaphor is growth.	Metaphor is stability.
Change is inherent and natural.	Stability is natural and normal.
Change is continuous.	Change occurs only for survival.
Intra-individual variance.	Intra-individual invariance.
Progress is valued.	Solidarity is valued.
Realization of potential is emphasized.	Conservation and retrenchment are emphasized.

Table 23-3
Characteristics of the Simultaneity and Totality Paradigms

Simultaneity	Totality
Human beings are synergistic; more than and different from the sum of their parts.	Human beings are bio-psycho-social-spiritual organisms.
Human beings are in mutual rhythmical interchange with the environment.	Human beings interact in a linear way with the environment.
Health is a process of becoming; it is living a set of value priorities.	Health is physical, mental, social and spiritual well-being. Human beings strive toward an optimal level of health through manipulation of the environment.

Table 23-4
Characteristics of the Particulate-Deterministic, Interactive-Integrative, and Unitary-Transformative Paradigms

Particulate-Deterministic	Interactive-Integrative	Unitary-Transformative
Phenomena are isolatable, reducible entities with definable, measurable properties.	Reality is multidimensional and contextual.	Human beings are unitary and evolving as self-organizing fields.
Entities have orderly and predictable connections.	Entities are context-dependent and relative.	Human fields are identified by pattern and by interaction with the larger whole.
Change occurs as a consequence of antecedent conditions that can be predicted and controlled.	Change is a function of multiple antecedent factors and probabilistic relationships.	Change is unidirectional and unpredictable.
Relationships are linear and causal.	Relationships move from linear to reciprocal.	Systems move through stages of organization and disorganization to more complex organization.
Only objective, observable phenomena are studied.	Both objective and subjective phenomena are studied, with emphasis on objectivity, control, and predictability.	Emphasis is on personal knowledge and pattern recognition.

Toward Parsimony in Worldviews

An analysis of the characteristics of the four sets of worldviews revealed some similarities and yielded a single parsimonious set of three worldviews: reaction, reciprocal interaction, and simultaneous action. More specifically, the analysis revealed that the particulate-deterministic paradigm is similar to mechanism, persistence, and totality. The combination of characteristics from those perspectives yielded the reaction worldview (Box 23-1).

Furthermore, the analysis indicated that the interactive-integrative paradigm is similar to organicism and

BOX 23-1

The Reaction Worldview

- Humans are bio-psycho-social-spiritual beings.
- Human beings react to external environmental stimuli in a linear, causal manner.
- Change occurs only for survival, as a consequence of predictable and controllable antecedent conditions.
- Only objective phenomena that can be isolated, defined, observed, and measured are studied.

BOX **23-2**

The Reciprocal Interaction Worldview

- Human beings are holistic.
- Parts are viewed only in the context of the whole.
- Human beings are active.
- Interactions between human beings and their environments are reciprocal.
- Reality is multidimensional, context-dependent, and relative.
- Change is a function of multiple antecedent factors.
- Change is probabilistic and may be continuous or may be only for survival.
- Both objective and subjective phenomena are studied through quantitative and qualitative methods of inquiry.
- Emphasis is placed on empirical observations, methodological controls, and inferential data analytic techniques.

BOX **23-3**

The Simultaneous Action Worldview

- Unitary human beings are identified by pattern.
- Human beings are in mutual rhythmical interchange with their environments.
- Human beings change continuously, evolving as self-organized fields.
- Change is unidirectional and unpredictable as human beings move through stages of organization and disorganization to more complex organization.
- Phenomena of interest are personal becoming and pattern recognition.

reflects elements of the totality view. In addition, that paradigm can incorporate elements of both change and persistence. Taken together, those perspectives yielded the reciprocal interaction worldview (Box 23-2).

Finally, the analysis suggested that the unitary-transformative paradigm is similar to organicism but even more similar to simultaneity. Furthermore, the elements of change are most evident in that paradigm. Combining the characteristics of those perspectives resulted in the simultaneous action worldview (Box 23-3).

Conclusion

The triad of worldviews presented in this column represents an attempt to draw together the characteristics of four different existing sets of paradigms or worldviews, representing nine perspectives, in a logical manner. Nursing's early scientific development began with the reaction worldview and evolved through the reciprocal interaction worldview to the simultaneous action worldview. Most contemporary scientific nursing knowledge resides in the reciprocal interaction and simultaneous action paradigms. The schema presented here is a relatively parsimonious structure that reflects the different philosophic claims under-girding nursing's scientific knowledge development. This attempt at drawing existing sets of paradigms together is open to debate, and readers are invited to a dialogue on the issue.

REFERENCES

Hall, B. A. (1981). The change paradigm in nursing: Growth versus persistence. *Advances in Nursing Science, 3*(4), 1–6.

Newman, M. A. (1992). Prevailing paradigms in nursing. *Nursing Outlook, 40,* 10–13, 32.

Parse, R. R. (1987). *Nursing science: Major paradigms, theories, and critiques.* Philadelphia: Saunders.

Reese, H. W., & Overton, W. F. (1970). Models of development and theories of development. In L. R. Goulet & P. B. Baltes (Eds.), *Life span developmental psychology. Research and theory* (pp. 115–145). New York: Academic Press.

The Author Comments

From a Plethora of Paradigms to Parsimony in Worldviews

This article was written in response to what I regarded as a growing diversity of perspectives about worldviews under girding nursing conceptual models and theories. The author's preceding schemata of worldviews failed to acknowledge the existing schemata and, instead, presented their views as if they arose in isolation from what came before. Inasmuch as I believe that knowledge is cumulative and that new ideas come from an understanding of existing ideas, I attempted to integrate the various existing worldviews into a parsimonious schema of three worldviews. I have found my schema particularly useful to my understanding of the philosophic underpinnings of nursing conceptual models and theories. I have incorporated this schema into my frameworks for analysis and evaluation of conceptual models of nursing and analysis and evaluation of nursing theories (see my book, *Contemporary Nursing Knowledge: Analysis and Evaluation of Nursing Models and Theories*, Philadelphia: F. A. Davis; 2005). I believe that a better understanding of worldviews is a crucial component of theory development in the 21st century.

—JACQUELINE FAWCETT

CHAPTER 24

Prevailing Paradigms in Nursing

Margaret A. Newman

The variability and ambiguity of things called paradigms, both within and outside nursing, have left me at times feeling very confused. In nursing we often refer to the medical paradigm as opposed to the nursing paradigm, or curing versus caring, or health as the absence of disease versus health as an evolving pattern of the whole.[1] Parse[2] has categorized nursing theories in what she has labeled the totality paradigm versus the simultaneity paradigm. Others speak to a quantitative paradigm versus a qualitative paradigm. These perspectives reflect to some degree various philosophies of science. What is the basis for the naming of a paradigm: the discipline it represents, the subject matter it addresses, the thought processes it reflects, dimensions of time-space, the nature of the data collected, or what? One of the international doctoral students at Minnesota asked me why nursing is so caught up

in consideration of paradigms. In answer to her question, my thoughts were that it has something to do with the history of the development of nursing science (e.g., our alignment and subsequent disalignment with medicine). When you take a look at the various ways in which we refer to the paradigms, not to mention for the moment the term *metaparadigm,* it is no wonder that graduate students have difficulty sorting it out.

Nursing is not alone in having to deal with the paradigm issue. Guba's recent book, *The Paradigm Dialog,*[3] is based on a 1989 conference devoted to this debate in education and related fields. Guba introduced the discussion with an ontologic, epistemologic, and methodologic analysis of four paradigms he identified as relevant: positivism, postpositivism, critical theory, and constructivism. A resume of the basic belief systems associated with these

Adapted from a paper presented at the 1991 National Forum on Doctoral Education,
Amelia Island, Fla., June 1991. M. A. Newman, Nursing Outlook, *40(1), 10–13, 32. Copyright © 1992 Elsevier Science. Reprinted with permission.*

About the Author

MARGARET A. NEWMAN was born in Memphis, TN, on October 10, 1933. She received her first degree (BSHE, 1954) in home economics at Baylor University. She entered nursing at the University of Tennessee, Memphis, in 1959 and received a BSN in 1962. Her graduate study included an emphasis on medical-surgical nursing at the University of California, San Francisco (MS, 1964) and a further emphasis on rehabilitation nursing and nursing science at New York University (PhD, 1971). Except for a short tenure as director of nursing for the clinical research center at the University of Tennessee, the emphasis of her work has been in education (at New York University, Penn State University, and the University of Minnesota). The focus of her scholarship has been on theory development in nursing. The books *Health as Expanding Consciousness* (1986, 1994) and *A Developing Discipline* (1995) represent her major contribution to nursing theory. She is an avid fan of live theater and music, with subscriptions to two local theater groups' offerings and the St. Paul Chamber Orchestra.

paradigms (Table 24-1) provides a background for sorting out the paradigm issues in nursing.

Extant Views in Nursing Research

A wide range of beliefs about what constitutes reality and how to go about finding it is reflected in the research taking place in nursing. Sime, Corcoran-Perry, and I have developed our own version of the scientific paradigms we see at work in nursing research.[4] We pursued this task for the purpose of delineating how the seemingly disparate work of various members of our faculty can indeed relate to a common focus. We tried not to introduce three new labels, but we did not

Table 24-1
Basic Belief Systems of Positivism, Postpositivism, Critical Theory, and Constructivism

	Ontology	Epistemology	Methodology

Positivism	Realist:
	   Reality exists "out there"
	   Driven by natural laws
		Objectivist:
		   Inquirer adopts distant and non-
		     interactive posture
			Experimental
			Empiric
			Controlled
			Testing of hypotheses

Postpositivism	Critical realist:
	   Same as positivism except cannot
	     be known because of lack of
	     ability to know
		Modified objectivist:
		   Objectivity an ideal that can be
		     only approximated
		   Guarded by critical community
			Modified experimental
			Emphasis on critical "multiplism"
			   (elaborated triangulation)

Critical theory	Critical realist:
	   Reality influenced by societal
	     structures
		Subjectivist:
		   Values mediate inquiry
		   Goal is to free participants from
		     effect of ideology
			Dialogic, transformative
			   Intended to eliminate false
			     consciousness and facilitate
			     transformation

Constructivism	Relativist:
	   Reality is mental construction,
	     socially and experimentally based
	   Many interpretations possible
	   Multiple realities
		Subjectivist:
		   Inquirer and respondent are fused
		     into single entity
		   Findings are creation of process
		     between the two
			Hermeneutic, dialectic
			   Aims to identify the variety of
			     constructions that exist and
			     bring them to as much
			     consensus as possible

Excerpted from Guba EG. The alternative paradigm dialog. In: Guba EG, ed. The paradigm dialog. Newbury Park, Calif: Sage, 1990:17–27.

see our categorizations fitting neatly into those already described. Eventually, rather than referring to them as I, II, and III, we succumbed to assigning descriptive labels to depict the key dimensions in each: I—particulate-deterministic, II—interactive-integrative, and III—unitary-transformative. The idea here is that the first of the paired words describes the view of the entity being studied and the second describes the notion of how change occurs.

From the particulate-deterministic paradigm, which holds closely to the positivist view, phenomena are

> viewed as isolatable, reducible entities having definable properties that can be measured. These entities have orderly and predictable connectedness to each other. Change is assumed to be a consequence of antecedent conditions—conditions that, if sufficiently identified and understood, could be used to predict and control change in the phenomena. Relationships within and among entities are viewed as linear and causal.[4]

From a particulate-deterministic view, only the most objective, observable manifestations of health, such as physiologic parameters, would be considered suitable subject matter for research. A phenomenon such as caring, considered by some as the essence of nursing, either would have to be removed from its context and given an operational definition or would be considered by some as outside the realm of science.

The interactive-integrative paradigm (similar to postpositivism) maintains allegiance to the need for control and predictability in research but views reality as multidimensional and contextual. It acknowledges the importance of experience and includes both subjective and objective phenomena but holds to the objectivity, control, and predictability of the positivist view. It moves away from linearity and acknowledges that in some instances understanding without predictability is enough. Change is viewed as "a function of multiple antecedent factors and probabilistic relationships."[4] Knowledge is context dependent and relative. From this perspective, nursing phenomena are viewed as both objective and subjective in reciprocal interaction.

The unitary-transformative paradigm presents a significant shift in the view of reality. The human being is viewed as unitary and evolving as a self-organizing field, embedded in a larger self-organizing field.

> It is identified by pattern and by interaction with the larger whole . . . . Change is unidirectional and unpredictable as systems move through stages of organization and disorganization to more complex organization. Knowledge is personal, involves pattern recognition, and is a function of both viewer and the phenomenon viewed . . . . Inner reality depicts the reality of the whole.[4]

Nursing would be studied as a unitary process of mutuality and creative unfolding.

Historically we seem to have moved from addressing primarily the health of the body as affected by environmental factors to interplay of body-mind-environment factors in health, and, more recently, to health as an experience of the unitary human field phenomenon embedded in a larger unitary field. These three perspectives, biophysical science, biopsychosocial science, and human science relate to different paradigms. The biophysical sciences are single-paradigm sciences with broad consensus among their members; biopsychosocial sciences involve multiple competing paradigms encompassing both objective and subjective phenomena and relating to different views on the nature of human beings and society.[5] Human science embraces a view of the human being as a unitary phenomenon and represents a major paradigm shift from the previous two (Table 24-2).

Table 24-2
Shift in Emphasis of Nursing Science

Health Focus	Science Category	Paradigm
Body ← environment	Biophysical	Single
Body-mind-environment	Biopsychosocial	Multiple
Unitary field	Human	Emergent

Focus of the Discipline

There is another consideration in nursing science. Nursing science is a professional discipline and as such has a commitment to alleviate the problems of society. The nature of the reality we are dealing with must incorporate knowledge of the process of making things better for society—a knowledge of praxis: "thoughtful reflection and action that occurs in synchrony, in the direction of transforming the world."[6]

What is our commitment then? Some would say "the promotion of health." At least two objections to that focus are that (1) it is phrased in the language of intervention and objectivity and therefore excludes the unitary-transformative paradigm; and (2) it is not an exclusive domain of nursing. Others would say "caring." Similar objections might apply: (1) from a positivist view, caring may not be amenable to scientific study; and (2) it is of a universal nature that is not limited to one discipline.

Sime, Corcoran-Perry, and I found that as we progressed in our exploration of prevailing paradigms, our intent became to identify the unifying focus of nursing as a professional discipline. After much discussion among ourselves and other colleagues and review of the literature, particularly over the past decade, we came to the conclusion that the focus of nursing as a professional discipline can be characterized as "caring in the human health experience."[4] This focus synthesizes the phenomena of nursing at the metaparadigm level and makes explicit the nature of the social mandate of nursing. *Caring* designates the nature of the nursing practice participation. *Human health* experience brings together the focus on *human* health and modifies it to mean the human health *experience*. The experiential dimension characterizes the phenomenon as something beyond the traditional objective-subjective perspective. The whole phrase taken together signifies the social mandate to which nursing has responded throughout our history and circumscribes the boundaries of the discipline.

Each major concept of this focus, taken alone, manifests itself in different ways. Morse and her associates[7] have done a comprehensive review of the variety of ways in which caring has been defined and studied. Their work illustrates the different paradigmatic positions prevalent in nursing today. The same is true for research related to the concept of health. Most of this research emanates from the dominant objective-subjective paradigms.[8] At the same time, research that connects caring and the health experience in a mutual, transformative process is emerging as a powerful force within the explication of our discipline.

Are We a Multiple-Paradigm Discipline?

This question leads to the question of whether the aforementioned focus can be addressed within the objectivist, interventionist tradition. Benner's answer would seem to be "no." Benner[9] points out that within a social scientific context, caring is "decontextualized" and "operationalized" and becomes just one more therapeutic technique. I take that to mean that this way of viewing caring does not capture the essence of caring.

When we[4] began work on "The Focus of the Discipline" paper, we thought of ourselves as each being representative of one of the three paradigms, but the more we discussed the underlying assumptions of each and came to accept the disciplinary focus of caring in the human health experience, the more each of us became convinced of the necessity of the unitary, transformative paradigm for development of the knowledge of our discipline. We ourselves were transformed in the process. We concluded that knowledge emanating from the first two paradigms is relevant but not sufficient for the full elaboration of nursing science.

Others tend to agree. Pender[10] describes the shift in nursing to human science, which views persons as unified wholes and focuses on the *experience* of health. She calls for a unitary perspective but still uses the language of objectivity in calling for valid and reliable measures. Parse[2] says that a discipline encompasses more than one paradigm to guide inquiry, yet clearly takes her stand in what she calls a simultaneity paradigm, one that embraces mutuality and transformation as the nature of human processes.

We seem to be hedging. Are we afraid to give up the certainty in knowing that the positivist view offers? In discussing the movement to new paradigms, Skrtic[5] points out that the "divorce of science from its contemporary raw empiricist base, and its realliance with judgment, discernment, understanding, and interpretation as necessary elements of the scientific process" means giving up the false certainty of logical positivism and facing the anxiety of less certain forms of knowing.

My original intent was to try to fairly, accurately present each of the prevailing paradigms and to say "Let's agree to disagree and go on about our business." Identifying the paradigms is the easy part. The hard part is acknowledging the pervasive nature of a paradigm, the fact that the values inherent in a paradigm are deeply embedded in the adherents and become normative, indicating what is important and what should be done about it. Paradigms have been compared with cultures in that they represent shared knowledge of what is and what ought to be and *adherents cannot imagine any other way to behave.*[11] This begins to explain some of the uneasiness we experience when an adherent of a paradigm other than our own speaks to the importance of that way of thinking and behaving.

Some argue for accommodation among paradigms; others assert that they have nothing in common. Skrtic[5] takes the position that "the point is not to accommodate or reconcile the multiple paradigms . . . ; it is to recognize them as unique, historically situated forms of insight; to understand them and their implications; to learn to speak to them and through them . . . ." Moccia[12] has described the deeper meaning of what is involved in attempts to accommodate different paradigms: the contradiction of trying to control and not to control, the expectation of being able to predict and at the same time acknowledging the process as innovative.

For almost a decade now, thanks to Munhall,[13] we have been aware of the discrepancies between our values as a profession and our practices as scientists. Now it is important to recognize the inconsistencies within our science, inconsistencies we are passing on to students. Lincoln[14] has experienced the same conflicting values:

I have often told questioners that research training programs should be two-tracked, with training in conventional and emergent-paradigm inquiry models, followed by training in quantitative and qualitative methods both, completed with computer applications for both quantitative and qualitative data.

But with what I have intuitively come to understand about the pervasiveness of the paradigm we use to conduct inquiry, I now think that training in multiple paradigms (at least in more than a historical sense) is training for schizophrenia. If we want to change new researchers' paradigms, we must do more than legitimate those paradigms in the inquiry outlets, such as journals. We have to train people in them, intensively. We probably ought not to be dividing their attention with other than historical accounts of conventional science. We probably ought to recognize the profound commitments people make to worldviews and create centers where such training can go on . . . .[14]

A movement has begun within nursing education to create centers with a particular focus—perhaps to emphasize one paradigm as dominant. The question is: Are we willing to allow, even encourage, that to occur? Or do we want to give all of the paradigms equal time and emphasis in all the programs? Or perhaps a third alternative might be to promote pockets of parallel emphases from different paradigmatic perspectives within a single program.

Some think that positivism is dead—others see it as alive and well and still dominating the scientific community. In graduate curricula, for instance, is it not true that most "basic" research courses emphasize the tenets of controlled, objective science? Does that not say that this is the way it is and anything else is alternative or deviant? And how many of our courses on theory development begin with the isolation of concepts, development of propositional sets, and derivation of causal relationships? If a faculty seeks to convey a different perspective, they would need to examine their basic ontologic and epistemologic beliefs and develop courses that are consistent with those beliefs.

A Paradigm Shift

Evidence of a paradigm shift exists in nursing. Johnson's bibliometric analysis of nursing literature since 1966 depicts a shift from a scientific medical model to a model based on holism.[15] Sarter's analysis of four contemporary nursing theories reveals commonly shared themes, emphasizing holism, process, and self-transcendence.[16] She suggests that it represents an emerging paradigm. The shift perhaps has not been as revolutionary as Kuhn would have predicted. A recent headline in the *Brain/Mind Bulletin* is apropos: has various advantages and disadvantages, depending on individual program needs.

"Can you remember where you were when the paradigm shifted?"[17] Assuming that the shift has occurred, it is incumbent on us to reevaluate the values and structures that shape our discipline.

The Challenge

The challenge before us is twofold: the need to identify and agree on the central question in nursing, the focus of discipline, and the need to clarify the scientific values and methods that will address that question.

REFERENCES

1. Newman MA. Health as expanding consciousness. St. Louis, Mo.: CV Mosby, 1996.
2. Parse RR. Nursing science: major paradigms, theories, and critiques. Philadelphia, Pa.: Saunders, 1987.
3. Guba EG, ed. The paradigm dialog. Newbury Park, Calif.: Sage, 1990.
4. Newman MA, Sime AM, Corcoran-Perry SA. The focus of the discipline of nursing. ANS 1991;14(1):1–6.
5. Skrtic TM. Social accommodation: toward a dialogical discourse in educational inquiry. In: Guba EG, ed. The paradigm dialog. Newbury Park, Calif.: Sage, 1990:125–35.
6. Wheeler CE, Chinn PL. Peace & power: a handbook of feminist process. 2nd ed. New York: National League for Nursing, 1989:1.
7. Morse JM, Solberg SM, Neander WL, Bottorff JL, Johnson JL. Concepts of caring and caring as a concept. ANS 1990; 13(1):1–14.
8. Newman MA. Health conceptualizations. Ann Rev Nurs Res 1991;9:221–43.
9. Benner P. Nursing as a caring profession. Paper presented at meeting of the American Academy of Nursing, October 16–18, Kansas City, Mo., 1988.
10. Pender NJ. Expressing health through lifestyle patterns. Nurs Sci Q 1990;3(3):115–22.
11. Firestone WA. Accommodation: toward a paradigm-praxis dialectic. In: Guba EG, ed. The paradigm dialog. Newbury Park, Calif.: Sage, 1990:105–24.
12. Moccia P. A critique of compromise: beyond the methods debate. ANS 1988;10(4):1–9.
13. Munhall P. Nursing philosophy and nursing research: in apposition or opposition? Nurs Res 1982;31(3):176–7;181.
14. Lincoln YS. The making of a constructivist: a remembrance of transformations past. In: Guba EG, ed. The paradigm dialog. Newbury Park, Calif.: Sage, 1990:67–87.
15. Johnson MB. The holistic paradigm in nursing: the diffusion of an innovation. Res Nurs Health 1990;13:129–39.
16. Starter B. Philosophic sources of nursing theory. Nurs Sci Q 1988;1(2):52–9.
17. Can you remember where you were when the paradigm shifted? Brain/Mind Bulletin 1991;16(7).

The Author Comments

Prevailing Paradigms in Nursing

This article is a follow-up to the treatise on the "focus of the discipline" and provides a general paradigmatic background for viewing the nursing paradigms. More importantly, it presents the methodologic and curricular dilemmas posed for students and educators when the unitary-transformative paradigm is acknowledged as essential to the development of nursing knowledge. I no longer see "human" as adequate for describing the science of nursing, because the unitary focus is on a continuous human-environmental field and the praxis nature of the knowledge encompasses the action component of the nurse-patient process.

—MARGARET A. NEWMAN

CHAPTER 25

A Multiparadigm Approach to Nursing

Joan Engebretson

Nursing theory development has made good progress in differentiating the domain of nursing from medicine; many of these theories are categorized as holistic theories. Nursing classification systems are also being developed to organize extant nursing practice. The dissonance between the two has been one of the most difficult contemporary issues for the leadership of nursing. A framework is proposed that would account for these disparate approaches. This proposed framework for the domain of healing is in keeping with the metaparadigm of health and uses a multiple paradigm approach. Nursing interventions are discussed in relation to the framework. It invites a dialogue in keeping with the scholarship of holism. Practice and scholarship implications are discussed.

Nursing theory has, since the 1960s, sought to define the profession of nursing and to differentiate its scope of practice from that of biomedicine.[1] This search has led to some discrepancies between theory development that differentiates nursing action from biomedical nursing practice, the latter of which uses many nursing actions derived from biomedicine. Differentiating autonomous nursing practice was a necessary step, because historically many nursing functions were derived from biomedicine, since nurses have practiced in biomedically dominated settings.

One primary differentiating feature was holism, which was contrasted with biomedical reductionism.

J. Engebretson, A multiparadigm approach to nursing. Advances in Nursing Science *1997, 20(1), 21–33.*
Copyright © 1997. Reproduced with permission of Lippincott Williams & Wilkins.

About the Author

JOAN C. ENGEBRETSON was born in Wisconsin, on November 12, 1943, and grew up in Minnesota. She received a BSN from St. Olaf College, an MS from Texas Woman's University, and a DrPH from the University of Texas Health Science Center at Houston School of Public Heath. She worked as a public health nurse both in Oakland, CA, and Boston, MA, and has been a faculty member at University of St. Thomas, Houston, TX, and University of Texas Health Science Center at Houston, School of Nursing and School of Public Health. Her clinical focus has been maternal-child and women's health. Her academic focus includes health promotion, culture, theory, and qualitative methodologies in research. Her research has included the development of a pacifier for low-birth-weight infants, women's anticipations of hormonal therapy for perimenopause, ethnographic studies of healing, clinical trials of Reiki Touch therapy, patient's beliefs and experiences related to chronic diseases, and the incorporation of complementary therapies and approaches to healing. Her primary focus is related to a better understanding of various perspectives and strategies of healing that nurses can incorporate into patient care to promote health throughout the health-illness continuum. Throughout her life, she has developed interests in travel, cooking, reading, and photography.

The movement to declare nursing holistic is now well accepted; however, a holistic framework must be inclusive of, not only differentiated from, biomedicine. In alignment with holism, the appropriate construct for the nursing profession is healing. Health is a derivative of healing, or making whole, and part of the metaparadigm of nursing.

Another element of professional evolution is the development of diagnostic, intervention, and outcomes classifications systems. These are often grounded in nursing practice and thus reflect both nursing activities as well as predominant sociocultural ideologies. There is often a disjuncture between the differentiating and defining theories and the more pragmatic classifications systems.[2] In an effort to reconcile grand conceptual models and practice, this article presents a conceptual framework for discussion as a step toward the consolidation of a holistic approach to nursing. The intent is to support both unique autonomous actions and to incorporate medically derived actions. Using the construct of healing, a multiparadigm model is presented to incorporate both the medical model and other cultural healing models on which nurses may ground their actions. This integration is at the level of paradigm, which allows the incorporation of and expansion beyond the biomedical model and avoids the pitfalls of the derivative-differentiation polarity.

Nursing has over the past 30 years made great strides in the development of nursing theories and conceptual models. These activities have been necessary to define the professional domain to its members and to society at large. Theory guides the practice and the activities that are unique to the profession, informs research efforts, and provides direction for future development.[3]

Contemporary Controversies

Despite the progress made, the use of nursing theories in practice has been a matter of controversy. One area of controversy is the dichotomy between medicine and nursing, with many theories focusing on unique nursing functions and in some cases redefining actions associated with medical models. This position has often still held the medical model as the orthodox standard against which nursing defined itself by negation or differentiation, thereby maintaining dependence on the medical model.

Closely related to the nursing-medicine dichotomy is the rupture between academia and practice. Academia and much of theory development focused on the autonomous nature of nursing, differentiating it from medicine. Extant nursing practice often eschewed the nursing theories learned in school, and practicing nurses functioned in a more pragmatic manner reflective of the medical model.[4] Many times the praxis of nursing is covertly, if not overtly, aligned with the medical model. This alliance with the medical model is understandable considering the hegemony of the medical bio-scientific model in U.S. culture. Barnum[4] noted that normative theory evolves from practice rather than academic theory development and that inconsistencies develop when practice (theory) is not intellectually analyzed and scrutinized according to logical coherence.

A third, related problem area is the disjuncture between nursing theories and the diagnosis, intervention, and outcome classification systems. The two strongest competitors in the theory business are holistic theories and nursing process,[1,4] which often represent opposing philosophies regarding content, methodology, and interpretation. Holistic theories are global, espouse a transcendental view of humans, and are committed to not viewing subject matter as an accumulation of parts.[4]

Nursing process approaches are much more concrete and practice based and have focused on nursing action and classification systems.[5] The International Council of Nurses,[6] the Omaha Project,[7] the Iowa Project,[8] and separate projects by Grobe[9] and Saba[10] have recently developed nursing classification systems.

Recent debates in nursing have also reflected controversies over the usefulness of a unified theory vs multiple theories. Reed[11] proposed an approach that links science, philosophy, and practice in the development of nursing knowledge. She advocated a metanarrative that involves a dialogue of practice and philosophy. This metanarrative provides an excellent format for the development of nursing theory that is holistic in nature and can integrate multiple paradigms from the patient's perspective and from the nurse. It is in this spirit of inviting a dialogue and providing a format for a dialectic discussion between

paradigms that the author presents the multiparadigm model.

Holism and Nursing

Grand theory, or the concept level of theory development, has evolved into a metaparadigm with four propositional statements related to the concepts person-health, person-environment, health-nursing, and person-environment-health.[12] The global level defines the frameworks within which the more restricted structures develop.

Consistent with the concept heal—health, the related ideologies for nursing theory development would come from healing, rather than be restricted to medicine. Healing and health stem from the root word *hale,* or to make whole.[13] This etymology grounds the concept heal—health in holism. Barnum[4] identified holistic theories as the fastest growing trend in nursing. Holistic concepts in nursing have been evident since the time of Florence Nightingale and evolved in nursing theories through the influence of Teilhard de Chardin, Jan Smuts, and Ludwig von Bertalanffy.[14] Anthropology, another discipline based on holism, provides another source of information on healing that can inform nurses in the development of holistic theory. Traditionally, in many cultures, healers, shamans, and medicine people reflected the broader concept of healing rather than the science-based concept of cure.

Holistic health has recently become very popular among both lay and professional groups. Characteristics of holistic health have been described in many studies.[15–19] Two common mistakes occur in the analysis of holism from a modernist perspective based in a scientific or reductionistic paradigm. Alster's[15] analysis of holistic health is an example of such an attempt; it reaches the syllogistic conclusion that holistic health cannot be studied scientifically because it is not scientific.

The opposite pitfall is to romanticize traditional or primitive healing systems and unfavorably compare science and biomedicine. This antiscience position is often seen in lay literature that attributes all social ills to scientific–rational thinking while extolling a holistic framework as the alternative. A consistent holistic framework incorporates science but does not hold that paradigm as sufficient for explaining the human experience or for bringing about health or healing. The model proposed in this article recognizes the holistic nature of nursing and expands the domain from disease treatment to the broader concept of health by incorporating several paradigms and their adjunctive ideological perspectives on humans, health, and therapeutic actions.

Historical Context of Western Medicine

Healing systems reflect and influence the cultural values of the parent culture. Contemporary biomedicine has been informed by and influential in the development of modernism. Modernity had its philosophical origins in the 17th century with the emphasis on rationality by the protagonists Galileo and Descartes.[20] Kuhn[21] described the shift of vision that enabled people to see and think about phenomena in a different manner and that he labeled a "paradigm shift." Modernity is characterized by the development of science and technology, the valorization of reason and humanity's dominion over nature. The scientific paradigm of modernity has dominated medicine and health care.

The establishment of the scientific model as the foundation for biomedicine paralleled the development of modernity. The scientific paradigm is characterized by philosophical dualism between the material and nonmaterial, and the corresponding designation of matter as the subject of science and the nonmaterial or metaphysical as the domain of religion. Descartes is often credited with conceptualizing the mind–body dualism and the corresponding value of the mind–soul as the superior demarcation of the human.

Throughout the following centuries, especially in England, increasing cultural value was placed on the scientific, material, rational, and technical.[22,23] Metaphysical and nonmaterial issues associated with religion were progressively devalued, especially among intellectuals.[24] Medicine, which historically had been based in a metaphysical model and supported by religion, became the domain of science and was severed from its metaphysical and religious roots. This split allowed medicine to make unprecedented technological advances through the application of scientific reason. But a contemporary surge of public interest in alternative healing modalities suggests that the biomedical scientific approach by itself is insufficient for healing.

Development of the Multiparadigm Model

The multiparadigm model was developed from the author's ethnographic work with healers and nurses. Field work, including participant observation, long interviews, free listing, and pile sorts, was used in a study exploring and comparing the conceptual frameworks of health and healing between nurses and healers.[25] A matrix of healing modalities that incorporated biomedicine and examples of alternative models emerging in the United States in the late 1980s and early 1990s was developed to focus the study on healers using healing touch[26] and used to orient nurse practitioners to alternative healing modalities that their clients might be using.[27]

This matrix was then developed into the Heterodox Explanatory Paradigms Model for health practice that incorporated multiple healing modalities.[28] The philosophical coherence of the model and the related positioning of modalities was presented as a framework for developing integrated health care models. Because nurses and healers have similar conceptual frameworks of healing,[25] this model could be adapted for nursing as a possible framework toward a more holistic model.

Philosophical Design

The multiparadigm model (Fig. 25-1) developed from the author's previous work[25–28] represents a multiparadigm approach to healing. Philosophical dualism between the material and nonmaterial is represented on both axes. Four paradigms of healing are incorporated and philosophically arranged from the most material to the most nonmaterial along the horizontal axis, which represents a philosophical continuum from logical positivism to metaphysics. Consistent with the positivist–metaphysical continuum, the mechanical paradigm is on the extreme left, reflecting the logical positivism of its philosophical scientific foundation. The paradigms are progressively more nonmaterial, ending in the most

Positivist ←──────────────────────────────→ Metaphysical

	Modalities	Mechanical	Purification	Balance	Supranormal
Material ↑	Physical manipulation	Biomedical surgery	Colonics Cupping	Magnetic healing Polarity	Drumming Dancing
	Applied and ingested substances	Pharmacology	Chelation	Humoral medicine	Flower remedies Hallucinogenic plants
	Energy	Laser Radiation	Bioenergetics	Tai chi Chi gong Acupuncture Acupressure	Healing touch Laying on of hands
	Psychological	Mind–body	Self-help (confessional type)	Mindfulness	Imagery
Nonmaterial ↓	Spiritual	Attendance at organized religious functions	Forgiveness Penance	Meditation Chakra Balancing	Primal religious Experience Prayer

Figure 25-1 *Explanatory paradigms.*

metaphysical paradigm, supranormal, at the extreme right. The vertical axis represents the Cartesian body–mind dualism in healing activities. Activities that are most material or physical are at the top. Moving down, activities become progressively less material and more psychological or spiritual.

Horizontal Axis

The four paradigms are mechanical, purification, balance, and supranormal. The mechanical paradigm is best represented by examples from biomedicine, which is primarily a mechanistic, materialistic paradigm exemplified by the focus on discovering explanatory mechanisms to understand a healing activity. The positivist philosophy bases knowing on objective, material data perceived by the senses.[29] It is characterized by determinism, mechanism, and reductionism. Disease is assumed to be reducible to disordered body functions and a disease-specific etiology.[30] Treatment and intervention are disease specific.

The purification paradigm has examples cross-culturally and throughout Western history. This paradigm is characterized by healing actions that cleanse or purify. The name of the prestigious English medical journal *Lancet* is a remnant of the bloodletting and purges that dominated Western medicine before technical advances in surgery and antibiotics in the 20th century. Health and healing activities related to cleanliness or purification either physically or symbolically have been documented in many ritual practices.[31] The hygienic health reform movement of the late 19th century[32,33] incorporated many practices that were understood as cleansing and keeping the body pure.

The balance paradigm is best represented by Eastern or humeral systems. In Eastern systems health–healing is viewed as the proper balance of yin and yang and unimpeded flow of Chi (or Ki or Qi).[34] Humeral medicine, or the balance of vital forces or humors, is evident in Hippocratic, Galenic, and Ayurvedic medicine.[35] Nineteenth-century vitalism also incorporated this approach. Health is attained or maintained by creating a balance in daily living through types of foods, activities, temperature, and so forth. Personality types, environment, and circumstances are considered in determining the corrective balance. One example is the hot and cold classification in Mexican folk medicine.

The balance paradigm is on the right half of the model and therefore cannot be fully understood through a materialist mechanistic paradigm.

The supranormal paradigm incorporates all magicoreligious and psychic phenomena used to promote health or create healing. Spiritual, symbolic, and other nonmaterial understandings of healing are in this column. The supranormal paradigm is philosophically the most metaphysical, going beyond physics, sense experience, or any discipline and involving ultimates.[36] This paradigm incorporates psychic, spiritual, and other types of healing such as prayer, distant healing, and other spontaneous healing that cannot be explained by mechanistic models or one of the other paradigms.

Vertical Axis

The vertical axis describes types of healing activities that progress along the continuum from body to mind–soul, from material to nonmaterial. The first row contains physical manipulations, and examples are given for each paradigm. Physical manipulation may be performed either by the patient or on the patient by a healer.

In row 2 applied and ingested substances are listed according to each paradigm. Such substances include all foods, herbs, and pharmaceuticals that are ingested, inhaled, or topically applied.

Using energy, the third activity, is a concept that is poorly understood in biomedicine but important in other paradigms. Many healing activities are understood and conducted as an active manipulation of energy. The concept of energy, or the transfer from matter to energy to matter, has been proposed by some scientists (eg, Bohm, Capra[37]) as the basis for quantum physics and as a possible link in understanding the material and nonmaterial worlds. This could be a promising area in linking the material, physical body with nonmaterial thought, spirit, and so on. The concept of energy has been proposed by some nurses as the basis for understanding the benefits of touch therapies.[38–40]

Psychological activities deal with functions of cognition and of the mind. Mind to body medicine has been a rapidly growing area of research. With the discovery of neu-

rotransmitters and hormonal–neural pathways, mechanisms have been discovered by which thoughts and feelings can manifest in physiological changes.[41] Theory has been developed and researched regarding the association of personality characteristics with illness, in particular hostility and heart disease.[42] Psychoneuroimmunology is another promising field where theory is developing. Associations have been demonstrated between various personality characteristics and mortality and morbidity.[43,44]

Spiritual activities are at the polar opposite of the continuum from physical manipulation. Spiritual actions are distinct from cognitive activities. Spirituality, being the most distant from the physical or material, is the least understood from a modernist perspective. Some studies have found that attendance at religious activities is related to improved health or healing.[45] Attendance at religious activities represents a mechanistic conceptualization of spiritual activity, whereas a primal spiritual experience as described by Cox[46] would be a more metaphysical approach.

The model has, at present, four paradigms, but others could be added along the continuum. Restriction to a two-dimensional format is often interpreted as containing mutually exclusive cells. A more appropriate geographic conceptualization would be as general areas on a double-axis continuum, with no specific boundary between areas. Modalities in the model are examples only, and many other modalities could fit in each location. The modalities describe healing activities only. An individual practitioner–healer could, and often does, use many modalities.

The positioning of modalities according to philosophical continuums also reflects the degree of passivity or activity of the healer. Starting from the upper left corner, where the modalities are most material, the healer is most active and the recipient most passive. Moving diagonally down and across, the person who is healing is progressively more active and the role of the healer increasingly that of facilitator, consistent with healing philosophy, which posits that real healing is done by the "healee."

One area that is a vital part of the nursing metaparadigm and other healing systems is the environment, especially social relationships. Although not specifically addressed in the model, an additional line at the bottom could be added to address social activities.

Application to Nursing

The multiparadigm model is holistic and avoids the medicine-nursing and practice-academia dichotomies by placing the Western biomedical model in context with other paradigms of healing. It speaks to the domain of healing, which is the stated domain of nursing. This model can provide a framework for nursing diagnoses and interventions that easily integrates biomedical model functions with complementary functions that either are autonomous nursing activities or might constitute appropriate referrals. The model also incorporates paradigms that can be useful in understanding cross-cultural healing practices and systems.

Implications for Practice

Operating from a multiparadigm model allows nurses to adapt whatever paradigm or modality fits the situation.

This flexibility is helpful in working with patients who practice health- and healing-related activities from other paradigms. A multiparadigm approach that incorporates models of health–healing can help providers better understand beliefs and practices of patients that may be poorly comprehended in the biomedical model.

Most health practices originate in the popular sector,[47] which includes family and social networks. This sector has beliefs about health maintenance and hierarchies of resort that direct types of health–healing activities, healer consultants, and adherence to treatments. The orientation of the popular sector often incorporates other paradigms than the scientific–mechanistic approach of biomedicine. By understanding the explanatory paradigm of health practices, the practitioner is better able to communicate and collaborate with the client and family in the management of health–healing.

Many interventions listed in the various nursing classification systems may be positioned in this model. Examples from one of these systems, the Nursing Interventions Classification (NIC),[8] have been identified in Fig. 25-2, along with other modalities that could be

Positivist ◄─────────────────────────────────► Metaphysical

Material	Modalities	Mechanical	Purification	Balance	Supranormal
▲	Physical manipulation	Positioning Exercise therapy Joint mobility	Bathing	Exercise promotion	Intuitive body work[†]
│	Applied and ingested substances	Medication administration	Wound and bladder irrigation Leech therapy	Nutritional counseling	Homeopathic remedies
│	Energy	Laser precautions	Phototherapy	Acupressure Acupuncture[†]	Therapeutic touch
│	Psychological	Cognitive restructuring	Active listening[†]	Counseling*	Simple guided imagery
Nonmaterial ▼	Spiritual	Activity therapy*	Forgiveness and purification rituals	Meditation	Spiritual support*

* NIC listed intervention that could be developed with understanding of the paradigm
† No NIC listing and should be considered as a potential referral or potential development for nursing action

Figure 25-2 *Nursing activities and interventions.*

17. Gordon, JS. The paradigm of holistic medicine. In: Hastings AC, Fadiman J, Gordon JS, eds. *Health for the Whole Person.* Toronto, Ontario: Bantam Books; 1980.

18. Lowenberg JS. *Caring and Responsibility.* Philadelphia, Pa: University of Pennsylvania Press; 1989.

19. Mattson PH. *Holistic Health in Perspective.* Palo Alto, Calif: Mayfield; 1982.

20. Toulmin S. *Cosmopolis: The Hidden Agenda of Modernity.* Chicago, Ill: University of Chicago Press; 1990.

21. Kuhn T. *The Structure of Scientific Revolutions.* Chicago, Ill: The University of Chicago Press; 1972.

22. Tarnas R. *The Passion of the Western World: Understanding the Ideas That Have Shaped our World View.* New York, NY: Ballantine Books; 1991.

23. Lavine TZ. *From Socrates to Sartre: The Philosophic Quest.* New York, NY: Bantam; 1984.

24. Johnson P. *Intellectuals.* New York, NY: Harper Perennial; 1988.

25. Engebretson J. Comparison of nurses and alternative healers. *Image J Nurs Schol.* 1996;28(2):95–100.

26. Engebretson J. *Cultural Models of Healing and Health: An Ethnography of Professional Nurses and Healers.* Houston, Tex: University of Texas-Houston, School of Public Health; 1992. Dissertation.

27. Engebretson J, Wardell D. A contemporary view of alternative healing modalities. *Nurse Practitioner.* 1993;18(9):51–55.

28. Engebretson J. Models of heterodox healing. *Alternat Ther Health Med.* In press.

29. Andrews MM, Boyle JS. *Transcultural Concepts in Nursing Care.* 2nd ed. Philadelphia, Pa: Lippincott; 1995.

30. Freund PES, McGuire MB. *Health, Illness and the Social Body: A Critical Sociology.* Englewood Cliffs, NJ: Prentice-Hall; 1991.

31. Douglas M. *Purity and Danger: An Analysis of the Concepts of Pollution and Taboo.* London, England: Ark Paperbacks; 1989.

32. Brown PS. Nineteenth-century American health reformers and the early nature cure movement in Britain. *Med History.* 1988;32:174–194.

33. Whorton JC. *Crusaders for Fitness: The History of American Health Reformers.* Princeton, NJ: Princeton University Press; 1982.

34. Kaptchuk TJ. *The Web that Has No Weaver: Understanding Chinese Medicine.* New York, NY: Congdon and Weed; 1993.

35. Helman CG. *Culture, Health and Illness: An Introduction for Health Professionals.* 3rd ed. Wolburn, Mass: Butterworth-Heinemann; 1994.

36. Reese WL. *Dictionary of Philosophy and Religion: Eastern and Western Thought.* Atlantic Highland, NJ: Humanities Press; 1991.

37. Horgan J. *The End of Science, Facing the Limits of Knowledge in the Twilight of the Scientific Age.* Reading, Mass. Addison Wesley; 1996.

38. Dossey BM, Keegan L, Guzzetta CE, Kolkmeier LG, *Holistic Nursing: A Handbook for Practice.* Gaithersburg, Md: Aspen Publishers; 1995.

39. Slater VE. Toward an understanding of energetic healing, part 1: energetic structures. *J Holistic Nurs.* 1995;13:209–224.

40. Slater VE. Toward an understanding of energetic healing, part 2: energetic process. *J Holistic Nurs.* 1995;13:225–238.

41. Rossi E. *The Psychobiology of Mind-Body Healing.* New York, NY: W. W. Norton; 1993.

42. Orth-Gomer K, Schneiderman N. *Behavioral Medicine Approaches to Cardiovascular Disease Prevention.* Hillsdale, NJ: Erlbaum; 1996.

43. Dreher H. *The Immune Power Personality.* New York: Dutton; 1995.

44. Schneiderman N, McCabe P, Baum A. *Perspectives in Behavioral Medicine: Stress and Disease Processes.* Hillsdale, NJ: Erlbaum; 1992.

45. Larson DB. Religion and spirituality—the forgotten factor in public health: what does the research share? Presented at the 12th annual meeting of the American Public Health Association, November 18, 1996; New York, NY.

46. Cox H. *Fire from Heaven.* Reading, Mass: Addison-Wesley; 1995.

47. Kleinman A. *Patients and Healers in the Context of Culture.* Berkeley, Calif: University of California Press; 1980.

48. Rogers ME. *An Introduction to the Theoretical Basis of Nursing.* Philadelphia, PA: F. A. Davis; 1970.

49. Watson J. *Nursing: Human Science and Human Care: A Theory of Nursing.* New York, NY: National League for Nursing.

50. Parse RR. *Man-Living-Health: A Theory of Nursing.* New York, NY: Wiley; 1981.

51. Newman MA. *Health as Expanding Consciousness.* 2nd ed. New York, NY: National League for Nursing; 1984.

52. Nagle LM, Mitchell GJ. *Theoretic Diversity: Evolving Paradigmatic Issues in Research and Practice.* Gaithersburg, Md: Aspen Publishers; 1991.

53. McKeon ZK. *On Knowing the Natural Sciences.* Chicago, Ill: University of Chicago Press; 1994.

The Author Comments

A Multiparadigm Approach to Nursing

As a public health nurse, I listened to what people believed about health, disease, and healing, and I became interested in cultural orientations to health. An understanding of these orientations, values, and beliefs that underlie health behaviors is central in working with clients in promoting their health. Conducting fieldwork with lay healers, who incorporated strategies and philosophies from cross-cultural and historical approaches to healing, and exploring related literature from anthropology provided a perspective for the multiparadigm model of healing. This perspective allowed for the development of an integrative healing model that includes the biomedical paradigm as opposed to other approaches that compare all healing methods from the biomedical perspective. Incorporating multiple approaches to healing and understanding the differences at the paradigm level will not only be relevant to providing the best health care to a global society but also provide an inclusive model for nursing that incorporates biomedical approaches rather than distinguishing nursing as oppositional to medicine.

—JOAN C. ENGEBRETSON

CHAPTER 26

Toward a Complementary Perspective on Worldviews

Susan K. Leddy

This column has dual purposes. The first purpose is to argue that fragmentation of knowledge in nursing science can be related to the dominant way of thinking of worldviews as competitive dualities. Then, inspired by a rereading of Bohm (1980), the second purpose is to advance a complementary perspective on worldviews to foster an alternative way of thinking with potential for encouraging creative thinking and knowledge synthesis.

Competitive Dualities and Worldviews

Philosophic beliefs about the nature of the existence of human beings and their environments, the human-environment relationship, what accounts for change and stability, and what constitutes knowledge are basic to the development of nursing knowledge and practice. These beliefs represent diverse worldviews that provide "different ways of being aware of the universe" (Phillips, 1995, p. 149). These beliefs also provide the philosophic base for the conceptual models, or paradigms, that represent various frames of reference that can guide the scientific and practical activities needed to develop knowledge (Fawcett, 1995).

Bohm (1980) also stresses the influence of one's worldview on ways of thinking and the development of knowledge. For example, he says that

About the Author

SUSAN LEDDY was fortunate to have the best nursing education possible, earning a BS from Skidmore College (1960, nursing), an MS from Boston University (1965, teaching M/S nursing), and a PhD from New York University (1973, Nursing Science). She later did postdoctoral work at Harvard University (1985, Educational Administration), and the University of Pennsylvania (1994–1996, Psychosocial Oncology). She was a National League for Nursing consultant; a department, school, and college chair; and a dean. Dr. Leddy taught nursing at all educational levels. Her scholarship was grounded in a unitary worldview and a belief in theory as a foundation for the development of knowledge. Her primary interests were exploration of energy theory and health. Her hobbies included exotic travel, weaving, quilting, knitting, watercolor painting, and enjoying her granddaughter, Katie. At the time of her death on February 23, 2007, she was Professor Emerita at Widener University.

when we look at the world through our theoretical insights, the factual knowledge that we obtain will evidently be shaped and formed by our theories . . . . Given perception and action, our theoretical insights provide the main source of organization of our factual knowledge. Indeed, our overall experience is shaped in this way. (p. 5)

Bohm emphasizes that worldviews and ways of thinking, as well as the nature of knowledge that is generated, are intricately interrelated. In fact, he goes even further to suggest that one's perspective shapes the experience of reality.

An important issue in ontology is whether reality exists or is constructed. The influence of science, so highly valued in our culture, can be attributed to the desire for a rational system of truths from which accurate information about the world can be deduced with certainty and precision. Science values rationality, logical thinking, and numerical measurement. Subjective feelings have little value. It is believed that effects can be attributed to a specific cause. Therefore, given that all "facts" have a specific cause, the cause can be discovered through objective and verifiable observation. Science is based on the belief that it is possible to discover true and accurate knowledge of reality.

In contrast, for Bohm (1980), the nature of reality is essentially a way of looking at the world, or worldview, because for him an underlying and unseen pattern is the

primary order of reality. Bohm (1980) suggests that "a theory is primarily a form of *insight,* i.e. a way of looking at the world, and not a form of *knowledge* of how the world is" (p. 4). In a similar vein, he proposes that the degree of clarity of these insights or theories are domain specific; that is, what is clear within the context of some domains may be less than clear when extended beyond those parameters. Bohm further contends that "our theories are to be regarded primarily as ways of looking at the world as a whole (i.e. worldviews) rather than as 'absolutely true knowledge of how things are'" (p. 5). These conceptions of reality as related to perspective provide an interesting alternative to the dominant scientific paradigm and challenge the assumed superiority of competitive dualistic thinking as a primary mode of thinking.

There are two basic philosophic positions for beliefs about reality. Monistic beliefs, such as in Vedanta philosophy, consider ultimate reality as an individual oneness of being. All phenomena are considered to be illusionary manifestations of one unitary consciousness. If everything is flow and mutual transformation, then everything has multiple aspects. Because there is no time, space, or causation, division is only an illusion. Different aspects of the same thing are considered in terms of relation, not reality. Each requires the other to manifest its total nature. However, according to Ajaya (1983), accepting the monistic assumption of the universe as an illusion does not rule out the possibility of employing a dualistic approach to comprehending "the structure, form and dynamics of this illusion" (p. 38). Ajaya maintains that within the monistic worldview, a dualistic approach can be "useful for describing a limited range of phenomena" (p. 115). However, he states that "the more encompassing perspective recognizes both the uses and the limitations of the more restricted perspective, while the more limited point of view is adamantly intolerant of a viewpoint that is beyond its range of understanding" (p. 116).

Contrasting with the monistic view of reality is a dualistic perspective. In one dualistic perspective such as represented in the predominant Western way of thinking, the opposition of contraries, logic, and critical thinking based on competitive dualities is emphasized. In this reductive approach to thinking, the focus is on distinctions between independent concepts. Through a cognitive interaction comprising contrast and comparison, distinct boundaries between concepts are delineated. According to this logic, contraries are seen as mutually exclusive or diametrically opposed to one another. The thinking is *either/or;* thus, contradictions are not allowed, and both cannot be true. For example, health considered as being "good" and disease considered as being "bad" are frequently viewed as mutually incompatible. Therefore, from an either/or standpoint, a person with a disease diagnosis cannot be healthy.

Competitive dualistic thinking has predominated within nursing as the discipline has embraced science. Inevitably, this ingrained way of thinking has permeated extant discussions of worldviews in nursing science. For example, Newman and colleagues have differentiated a three-part schema of particulate/deterministic-interactive/integrative-unitary/transformative worldviews (Newman, 1992; Newman, Sime, & Corcoran-Perry, 1991). Parse classified worldviews into a two-part schema known as totality and simultaneity paradigms (Parse, 1987; Parse, Coyne, & Smith, 1985). Fawcett (1993) described a different three-part schema of reaction-reciprocal interaction-simultaneous action worldview perspectives. Because these worldviews are independent in the sense that they are not interchangeable, each worldview can be interpreted as competitive relative to the other or others within a given schema. For example, Fawcett (1993) clearly indicates that each worldview in her schema is distinct from the others.

All dualistic forms of thinking "interpret experience as an interaction between two fundamental principles" (Ayaja, 1983, p. 11). However, contrasting with the previous view of contraries as mutually exclusive, independent concepts is the perspective that "pairs of opposites are creations of the mind . . . . Different aspects of the same thing, they are terms of relation, not of reality" (Ajaya, 1983, p. 56). And Sabelli (1989) indicates that "opposites are not extremes in a continuum but separate dimensions in a multidimensional space" (p. 316). As relative phases, they have no fixed values but are different points of view of the same larger reality. Given that neither one could exist without the presence of the other, and given that both come from the same source, truth is always partial (Sabelli, 1989).

Sabelli (1989) describes multiple patterns or modes of dualistic thinking as alternatives to the competitive perspective. For example, in a conflictual mode of thought such as Marxist social philosophy or Darwinist theory, alternatives are not absolute but different, and through dialectic contradiction or struggle, there may be mutual annihilation of both. In a hierarchical mode of thought, the emphasis in the interaction of apparent polarities is on falsification of one position through dominance/submission over the other. Therefore, "truth" overcomes falsity. In contrast, within a harmonic mode of thought, apparent opposites are viewed as complementarities, a *both/and* dialogue in which each contains the other as opposing but interrelated aspects of a whole. The emphasis in a harmonic perspective is on dialogue rather than on conflict.

There are a number of approaches to complementary dualities in the literature. The predominant Eastern way of thinking emphasizes concepts as a synthesis of opposites, or a transformation into one another, in which each thing or phenomenon is both itself and its contrary. For example, health is viewed as a value-free concept that incorporates wellness, illness, well-being, and disease into a larger whole. In the Eastern view, dualities are balanced in mutually supportive, cyclical interplay.

Relational Perspectives of the Whole

From a different point of view known as systems theory, components are perceived in relation to one another. The emphasis in this worldview is on the way components function as a whole. Capra (1996) explains the underlying principle of this way of thinking as a shift from perceiving living systems in terms of distinct parts to perceiving them as integrated wholes whose "essential, or 'systemic,' properties are properties of the whole, which none of the parts have" (p. 36). These systemic properties are said to "arise from the 'organizing relations' of the parts—that is, from a configuration of ordered relationships that is characteristic of that particular class of organisms, or systems" (p. 36). A further characteristic of systems thinking is explained as "the *ability to shift one's attention back and forth* [italics added] between systems levels. Throughout the living world we find systems nesting within other systems" (p. 37).

A most significant perspective that lends support to the thesis of this column lies in the insights of Gestalt psychology, in which objects are perceived in a mutually supportive and reversible relationship between figure and ground. Capra (1996), in discussing this Gestalt perspective using the language of systems, concludes that

> what we call a part is merely a pattern in an inseparable web of relationships. Therefore the shift from the parts to the whole can also be seen as a shift from objects to relationships. In a sense, this is a figure/ground shift. (p. 37)

In other words, Capra disputes a mechanistic approach that considers the relationships of objects as limited to their interactions and therefore of secondary importance in describing reality. Instead, he proposes that relationships are primary: "In the systems view we realize that the objects themselves are networks of relationships, embedded in larger networks . . . . The boundaries of the discernible patterns ('objects') are secondary" (p. 37).

Bohm's (1980) discussion of different ways of thinking, in relation to the subject being thought about, helps to clarify the connection. Allowing for a critical distinction between thinking about concrete issues that have a technical, functional, or practical purpose in comparison to pondering philosophical matters concerned with understanding a self-world reality, Bohm recognizes the validity of different modes of thought. For example, although he concedes that a thinking process that separates or divides is an appropriate as well as useful way of thinking about certain activities that have a limited scope (such as technical or practical issues), he disputes any claims that such ways of thinking can be meaningfully extended to include ideas about persons and their relations with the universe. He proposes that such a worldview eventually leads past perceiving divisions as a convenient way of processing discrete data and becomes an experience of self-world reality. Such a way of consistently perceiving separately existent fragments in oneself and one's world shifts the perspective. Bohm (1980) warns that "being guided by a fragmentary self-world view, man then acts in such a way as to try to break himself and the world up, so that all seems to correspond to his way of thinking" (p. 2).

A competitive mode of thinking can be a strength in the effective explication and clarification of distinctions, such as in worldviews. In teaching doctoral students, I have found that a useful strategy to clarify content and foster critical thinking is a consideration of the specific distinctions between worldviews. Students then can identify which perspective seems closest to their own usually unexamined views of reality. Inevitably, however, students comment that they are steeped, through nursing education and experience, in the dominant ways of thinking, that is, in the totality or the reciprocal-interaction modes. Although the simultaneity and unitary/transformative worldviews appear to have intrinsic appeal, given that students have to choose between the perspectives, they invariably choose to accept what is comfortable because it is familiar.

Thus, one unintended consequence of competitive thinking can be the perpetuation of the status quo worldview in nursing science. Information can become fragmented, compartmentalized into separate bodies of knowledge, "schools of thought" by worldview or conceptual model. Competitive thinking can contribute to divisiveness and possible right/wrong or better/worse thinking. For example, some individuals may regard the totality worldview as an outmoded way of thinking and the simultaneity worldview as a better way of thinking rather than examining them as alternative perspectives. Competitive thinking leads to questions such as, which view of reality is the "right" one? Because reality can only be glimpsed and never really "known," this appears to be an arbitrary and futile exercise. Thinking in opposites can be considered an oversimplification that prevents perceiving the world in its complexity, promotes conflict, and prevents the discovery of creative alternatives (Sabelli, 1989). In contrast, a complementary approach to thinking appears to offer the potential for fostering creative thinking, insight, and the synthesis of a body of nursing knowledge.

Complementary Thinking

Bohm (1980) theorized that the nature of reality is a coherent whole "which is never static or complete, but which is in an unending process of movement and unfoldment" (p. ix). Bohm labeled this whole the *implicate order,* an enfolded "unbroken wholeness of the totality of existence as an undivided flowing movement without borders" (p. 172). However, Bohm also explained that "we can, for convenience, always picture the *explicate order* . . . as the order present to the senses" (p. 186). Thus, the explicate order comprises various patterns of manifestations that are perceived by human beings as recurrent, stable, and separable.

Bohm (1980) said, "The notion that all these fragments are separately existent is evidently an illusion . . . . In essence, the process of division is *a way of thinking about things* [italics added] that is convenient and useful" (pp. 1–2). Again, stressing the significance of the domain perspective, he states that "all our different ways of thinking are to be considered as different ways of looking at the one reality, each with one domain in which it is clear and adequate" (p. 8).

One possible implication of these ideas is to understand extant worldviews as different ways of perceiving reality, rather than as views of differing realities. Each provides partial insight into the whole, because "content and process are not two separately existent things, but, rather, they are two aspects of views of one whole movement" (Bohm, 1980, p. 18). Interpreting that complementary worldview within a nursing science perspective offers a new way of seeing the connections. For example, in a complementary worldview, the totality, particulate/deterministic, and reaction perspectives can be viewed as reflecting content of the perceived explicate order. The simultaneity, unitary/transformative, and simultaneous action perspectives hint of an unending process of movement and unfolding of the implicate order.

As a result, although the observer's perspective may shift between content and process, both are recognized as aspects of reality. For example, both bio-psycho-social-spiritual aspects and unitary pattern manifestations characterize the human being. Cyclical interaction and mutual process can be said to characterize the human-environment interface. Health incorporates functioning, adapting, and becoming, as well as the constructing of meaning. And in the short-term, change may be predictable, while evolution proceeds unpredictably toward increasing complexity.

One way to conceptualize this approach is a ground/figure example from Gestalt psychology. Most people have seen pictures of what appears at first to be undifferentiated dots that can, with concentration, be viewed as a vase or as a profile of a young woman, depending on the focus of the viewer. The whole picture contains both possible figures. By shifting the perspective of the ground, either the vase or the face in profile can be the figure. Such is also the case with content and process. Both are essential for the total "picture," but which becomes the figure depends on the focus of the viewer.

Methods to Promote Complementary Thinking

Dialectical thinking is one method that can be used to develop a complementary perspective on worldviews. In particular, dialectical methods of reasoning can be used "to address apparent contradictions and their synchronization" (Reigel, 1976, p. 689). Rafael (1996) states that "from a Hegelian perspective, dialectic is a logical progression of thought that exposes and examines contradictions and reconciles them through a process of thesis, antithesis, and synthesis" (p. 4). Rawnsley (1993) indicates that Hegel's "underlying assumption of harmony in diversity is postulated as a relationship of essential opposites, a structure or pattern in which what appears antagonistic is merged into a qualitatively different possibility through synthesis into a higher abstraction" (p. 3). The intent of this method of thinking is to synthesize contraries into a more inclusive concept.

Ajaya (1983) uses a different approach to dialectical thinking to describe "progressively more comprehensive frames of reference" (p. 115), in which "the more encompassing perspective recognizes both the uses and the limitations of the more restricted perspective" (p. 116). Given that the perception of dualities as opposites is a creation of the mind, Ajaya proposes that a "more comprehensive understanding that transcends the polarity" (p. 163) be sought. He proposes that a neutral point, not a midpoint, be identified, "encompassing awareness of the extremes, the continuum, and the unifying center from which the polarity emerges" (p. 163). For example, complementary thinking occupies a neutral point that encompasses both separate and unified views.

Paradoxical thinking is another method that can be used to explicate a complementary worldview. Ajaya (1983) portrayed dualistic thought as an intermediate phase between reductive and monistic thought in regard to polarities. In contrast to Hegel and Ajaya, who have different perspectives on dialectics as a method of transforming opposites by synthesizing them into a larger whole, Parse (1992) conceptualizes paradox as "two sides of the same rhythm that coexist all at once . . . . Paradox refers to apparent opposites. These rhythmical patterns are not opposites. Both sides of the rhythm are present simultaneously" (p. 38). As meaning is structured in the process of becoming, the contradiction of opposites is experienced, further

differentiated, and preserved as a rhythmical shifting of views (Mitchell, 1993). Morse, Bottorff, and Hutchinson (1995) also point out that meaning is developed through the examination of a word with its opposite: "For instance, in has no meaning without out, nor up without down. Similarly, comfort has no meaning without discomfort, nor comfortable without uncomfortable" (p. 18).

Parse's approach to paradox can be contrasted with dialectical thinking. In dialectical methods of thinking, differentiating or contradicting characteristics are resolved by being subsumed or synthesized into one more inclusive concept. For example, a 24-hour "day" subsumes daytime, nighttime, twilight, daybreak, and so forth. In contrast, paradoxical thinking preserves the differentiating characteristics in a mutually supportive, cyclical interplay. As paradoxical thinking fosters nuance and a rhythmical shifting of focus between alternatives to clarify continuities and distinctions, sensitivity to paradox should facilitate creative thinking, whereas dialectical thinking promotes synthesis.

Implications for Nursing

I frequently ask students to consider the implications of their proposals, in what has become a trademark, "So what!" Thus, it could be asked, what difference does it make if a complementary rather than a competitive perspective toward worldviews is adopted? What are the advantages for nursing of methods of thinking based on complementary perspectives?

Kim (1996b) has reviewed four different modes with which nursing scientists engage in producing knowledge for nursing practice. A coherence mode refers to a commitment to "a specific philosophical, epistemological, and paradigmatic orientation" (p. 112). A scientist working with a coherence mode is therefore guided by this orientation in knowledge development. Furthermore, Kim maintains that within the coherence mode the focus is on building a paradigm. In contrast, she describes a scientist operating in an integrative mode as seeking to incorporate new knowledge to expand the current foundation for the purpose of increasing the explanatory power of the framework. In addition, Kim describes a scientist working in the pragmatic/eclectic mode as geared toward therapeutic and pragmatic goals that are rational and pragmatic. In this mode, the focus is on solving significant clinical problems. Finally, in the reflective mode identified by Kim, the scientist evaluates viable knowledge in terms of its validity in the practice situation. The focus in this mode "is on knowledge development as a situationally generative process" (p. 112).

It should be made clear that my personal scientific commitment is to the development of knowledge from the perspective of the coherence mode. I believe that an inclusive, overarching, ontological framework is essential as the philosophical basis for synthesis of knowledge from apparently disparate theories and conceptual models into a coherent science. It therefore follows that I would think it desirable, if possible, to accommodate competitive worldviews in such an inclusive, overarching, ontological framework.

Kim (1996a) suggests that pluralism as an approach to nursing knowledge development and the application of theory into practice "points to a possibility, not of coherence and patterning, but of chaos, fragmentation, and arbitrariness" (p. 63). Although competing ontological perspectives are only one probable basis for the current state of the science, Kim states concern that absence of a unifying structure for such pluralism can impede knowledge development and create confusion. She maintains that "nursing must seek or develop a unifying framework that can pull together its effort in knowledge development in order to prevent nursing's demise to an epistemic chaos" (1996c, p. 15).

In addition to providing a comprehensive framework for knowledge synthesis, a complementary perspective on worldviews has the advantage of facilitating the exploration of contextual background and multiple facets of concept, content, and process. The emphasis shifts from competition to inclusion. Instead of bits of incomplete and unconnected information, a much more meaningful gestalt of knowledge can be generated. Therefore, through a complementary perspective, the worldview can provide both a blueprint for developing knowledge and a perspective for synthesizing knowledge into a meaningful whole.

In nursing, critical thinking leading to clinical decision-making is the primary—some might say exclusive—way of thinking taught in educational programs. This is the premise, even though support is lacking for the impact of nursing education on critical thinking. Little evidence links critical thinking to clinical judgment, and support for a strong relationship between critical thinking and success in nursing education is lacking (Kintgen-Andrews, 1991).

Bohm (1980, p. 5) stresses the influence of one's worldview on ways of thinking and the development of knowledge. Given the emphasis on atheoretical rationality and logical thinking throughout their education, is it any wonder that many nurses have fragmented knowledge and therefore practice with rule-based cognitive rigidity? I submit that an overarching ontological framework for theories would make possible education that is more likely to develop a coherent organization of knowledge for nursing practice. Critical thinking is only one facet of integrative thinking (P. Fasnacht, personal communication, August 1999), which is a thinking method that fosters creative tension leading to linkages between concepts, envisioning, and the creation of patterns. Such thinking methods, essential to the development of cognitive flexibility and creativity so necessary for truly professional nursing practice, should be fostered in nursing curricula at all levels.

Summary

In this column, it has been argued that fragmentation of knowledge in nursing science can be related to the dominant way of thinking of worldviews as competitive dualities. To move toward resolving that conflict, the thesis has been set forth to claim that a complementary perspective on worldviews as an ontological framework can promote knowledge synthesis and alternative thinking methods in nursing science. Implications of the potential for a complementary perspective for encouraging integrative and creative thinking for professional nursing practice has been presented.

REFERENCES

Ajaya, S. (1983). *Psychotherapy East and West: A unifying paradigm.* Honesdale, PA: Himalayan Institute.

Bohm, D. (1980). *Wholeness and the implicate order.* London: Routledge & Kegan Paul.

Capra, F. (1996). *The web of life.* New York: Anchor Books.

Fawcett, J. (1993). From a plethora of paradigms to parsimony in worldviews. *Nursing Science Quarterly, 6,* 56–58.

Fawcett, J. (1995). *Analysis and evaluation of conceptual models in nursing* (3rd ed.). Philadelphia: Davis.

Kim, H. S. (1996a). Reflections on building a cumulative knowledge base for nursing: From fragmentation to congruence. In *Proceedings of the Nursing Knowledge Impact Conference* (pp. 63–67). Boston: Boston College.

Kim, H. S. (1996b). Summary of future directions. In *Proceedings of the Nursing Knowledge Impact Conference* (pp. 111–117). Boston: Boston College.

Kim, H. S. (1996c). Viable options for applying theory to practice. In *Proceedings of the Nursing Knowledge Impact Conference* (pp. 15–21). Boston: Boston College.

Kintgen-Andrews, J. (1991). Critical thinking and nursing education: Perplexities and insights. *Journal of Nursing Education, 30,* 152–157.

Mitchell, G. J. (1993). Living paradox in Parse's theory. *Nursing Science Quarterly, 6,* 44–51.

Morse, J. M., Bottorff, J. L., & Hutchinson, S. (1995). The paradox of comfort. *Nursing Research, 44,* 14–19.

Newman, M. A. (1992). Prevailing paradigms in nursing. *Nursing Outlook, 40,* 10–13, 32.

Newman, M. A., Sime, A. M., & Corcoran-Perry, S. A. (1991). The focus of the discipline of nursing. *Advances in Nursing Science, 14,* 1–6.

Parse, R. R. (1987). *Nursing science: Major paradigms, theories, and critiques.* Philadelphia: Saunders.

Parse, R. R. (1992). Human becoming: Parse's theory of nursing. *Nursing Science Quarterly, 5,* 35–42.

Parse, R. R., Coyne, A. B., & Smith, M. J. (1985). *Nursing research: Qualitative methods.* Bowie, MD: Brady.

Phillips, J. R. (1995). Can researchers transcend bad science? *Nursing Science Quarterly, 8,* 148–149.

Rafael, A. R. F. (1996). Power and caring: A dialectic in nursing. *Advances in Nursing Science, 19*(1), 3–17.

Rawnsley, M. M. (1993). Dialectics and the diverse discourse in nursing science. *Nursing Science Quarterly, 6,* 2–4.

Riegel, K. F. (1976). The dialectics of human development. *American Psychologist, 31,* 689–698.

Sabelli, H. C. (1989). *Union of opposites: A comprehensive theory of natural and human processes.* Lawrenceville, VA: Brunswick.

The Author Comments

Toward a Complementary Perspective on Worldviews

This article evolved out of a sense of frustration with the current status quo in nursing science. Students, even at the doctoral level, are unwilling, or unable, to engage in imaginative risk taking, thinking "out of the box." Much current research is atheoretical, with an emphasis on concrete "right or wrong" outcomes. My point in the article is that by reframing thinking perspectives, engaging in dialectical and paradoxical thinking, and renewing emphasis on clear conceptual and theoretical foundations, there is potential to stimulate creative thinking, knowledge synthesis, coherent scholarship, and the development of a real scientific rationale for practice.

—SUSAN LEDDY

- What guidelines can poststructuralist philosophers offer for judging the quality of one's theory?

- Are certain philosophies more useful than others to nursing?

- Should multiple perspectives be entertained in one's research and if so, how?

- Does the existing range of philosophies represent a more or less stable set, or will new philosophies emerge?
  - If so, what perspectives on nursing and science might they indicate to us?

CHAPTER 27

Understanding Paradigms Used for Nursing Research

Kathryn Weaver
Joanne K. Olson

Aims. *The aims of this paper are to add clarity to the discussion about paradigms for nursing research and to consider integrative strategies for the development of nursing knowledge.*

Background. *Paradigms are sets of beliefs and practices, shared by communities of researchers, which regulate inquiry within disciplines. The various paradigms are characterized by ontological, epistemological and methodological differences in their approaches to conceptualizing and conducting research, and in their contribution towards disciplinary knowledge construction. Researchers may consider these differences so vast that one paradigm is incommensurable with another. Alternatively, researchers may ignore these differences and either unknowingly combine paradigms inappropriately or neglect to conduct needed research. To accomplish the task of developing nursing knowledge for use in practice, there is a need for a critical, integrated understanding of the paradigms used for nursing inquiry.*

Methods. *We describe the evolution and influence of positivist, postpositivist, interpretive and critical theory research paradigms. Using integrative review, we compare and contrast the paradigms in terms of their philosophical underpinnings and scientific contribution.*

Findings. *A pragmatic approach to theory development through synthesis of cumulative knowledge relevant to nursing practice is suggested. This requires that inquiry start with assessment of existing knowledge from disparate studies to identify key substantive content and gaps. Knowledge development in under—researched areas could be accomplished through integrative strategies that preserve theoretical integrity and strengthen research approaches associated with various philosophical perspectives. These*

About the Authors

KATHRYN WEAVER, born in North Bay, Ontario, and raised in Shubenacadie, Nova Scotia, received her undergraduate education at Dalhousie University, Halifax, Nova Scotia; her master's degree at the University of New Brunswick, Fredericton, New Brunswick; and her PhD (Nursing) at the University of Alberta, Edmonton. She is Assistant Professor with the Faculty of Nursing, University of New Brunswick, Canada; Postdoctoral Fellow with the Alberta Heritage Foundation for Medical Research, Faculty of Nursing, University of Alberta; and Nurse Psychotherapist with an independent clinical practice counseling women and adolescents suffering from eating disorders. Her teaching interests include qualitative research, psychiatric–mental health nursing, health assessment, community development, and nursing ethics. Her program of research involves qualitative inquiry into individual and family perspectives of eating disorders and ethical sensitivity in professional–client relationships. She is principal investigator and coscript writer of the video documentary *Through True Eyes: Recovery from Eating Disorders* (produced by Atlantic Mediaworks, Fredericton, NB, 2007). She enjoys spending time with her children, gardening, video gaming, and travel.

JOANNE OLSON was born in Willmar, MN. She received her undergraduate education at Augustana College, Sioux Falls, SD; her master's degree at the University of Minnesota (School of Public Health), Minneapolis; and her PhD (Nursing) at Wayne State University, Detroit, MI. She is a Professor and Associate Dean, Undergraduate Programs, in the Faculty of Nursing, University of Alberta, Edmonton, Alberta, Canada. Her teaching interests include nursing theory development, spiritual aspects of nursing practice, spiritual assessment in health promotion, and community health nursing. Her primary research interests include nurse–client interactions, health promotion within faith community settings, nursing practice that addresses the spiritual dimensions of people, and nursing education. She has a clinical faculty practice as a Parish Nurse and has co-authored a book entitled, *"Nursing within a Faith Community: Promoting Health in Times of Transition."* She has offered local, national, and international leadership in the development of faith community nursing and in the Sigma Theta Tau International Honor Society of Nursing.

strategies may include parallel studies within the same substantive domain using different paradigms; theoretical triangulation to combine findings from paradigmatically diverse studies; integrative reviews; and mixed method studies.

Conclusion. *Nurse scholars are urged to consider the benefits and limitations of inquiry within each paradigm, and the theoretical needs of the discipline.*

Introduction

Paradigms are patterns of beliefs and practices that regulate inquiry within a discipline by providing lenses, frames and processes through which investigation is accomplished. The need to clarify the paradigms of nursing research has been identified as one of the top 10 issues facing the discipline (Colorado Nursing Think Tank 2001). Working to achieve further clarity will enable nurse researchers to structure inquiry, making explicit the philosophical assumptions underlying their methodological choices. The purpose of this paper is to examine the paradigms used in nursing research and to make recommendations about conducting disciplinary inquiry. To achieve this purpose, we explore the evolution and influence of the various research paradigms on nursing theoretical and disciplinary development, and we present ontological, epistemological, and methodological similarities and differences among positivist, postpositivist, interpretive and critical theory paradigms. The goals of inquiry, place of theory in the research process, and nature of knowledge sought within each paradigm are described. We recommend a pragmatic approach to conducting disciplinary inquiry and we suggest integrative strategies that clarify the theoretical perspective most needed to build disciplinary knowledge.

Background

Defining Research Paradigms

The task of clarifying the paradigms used for nursing research is complicated by semantic confusion between the terms 'paradigm,' 'disciplinary matrix,' 'research tradition' and 'worldview.' Kuhn (1970) uses the term 'paradigm' (p. 10) to describe a heuristic framework for examining the natural sciences and 'disciplinary matrix' (p. 182) for social sciences. Laudan (1977) defines a 'research tradition' as the 'set of general assumptions about the entities and processes in a domain of study, and . . . the appropriate methods to be used for investigating the problems and constructing the theories in that domain' (p. 81). Kikuchi (2003) equates paradigm with an individual's perceived 'worldview.' It is beyond the scope of this paper to differentiate extensively between these various terms to determine if they all describe the same phenomenon. We will use the term 'paradigm'— despite criticism of its ambiguous and inconsistent use— as it has been most often understood and applied by nurse scholars (e.g. Allen *et al.* 1986).

We understand paradigms to be mechanisms to bridge a discipline's requirements for knowledge and its systems for producing that knowledge. Paradigms are lenses for viewing and interpreting significant substantive issues to the discipline. Issues deemed worthy of pursuit are prioritized; others are suppressed (Cheek 2000). Paradigms are also frames that hold the vocabulary, theories and principles, as well as the presuppositions and values related to an inquiry (Thompson 1985, Moccia 1988, Bunkers *et al.* 1996). We further define

paradigms as sets of philosophical underpinnings from which specific research approaches (e.g. qualitative or quantitative methods) flow.

Paradigms are established by communities of scholars with shared beliefs about the nature of reality and knowledge construction (Jacob 1989, Hinshaw 1996). They are human constructions categorized by differences in beliefs and values (Hamilton 1994). As such, paradigms can be neither proved nor disproved (Moccia 1988, Guba 1990). This may create doubt about how best to initiate inquiry. According to Kuhn (1970), all disciplinary research is conducted within paradigms. The approaches to inquiry open to a researcher within a particular paradigm are defined by the paradigm itself (Laudan 1977).

The paradigms that have been used for nursing research are positivist, postpositivist, interpretive and critical social theory. The positivist paradigm arose from a philosophy known as logical positivism, which is based on rigid rules of logic and measurement, truth, absolute principles and prediction. Postpositivism has emerged in response to the realization that reality can never be completely known and that attempts to measure it are limited to human comprehension. The interpretive paradigm emphasizes understanding of the meaning individuals ascribe to their actions and the reactions of others. The critical social theory paradigm is concerned with the study of social institutions, issues of power and alienation, and envisioning new opportunities (Gillis & Jackson 2002).

It is widely held that adherence to one paradigm predetermines the direction of theory development for a discipline, ultimately delimiting knowledge available for utilization in practice. The different types of knowledge required for nursing practice may be constructed from single or multiple modes of inquiry. Fawcett *et al.* (2001) advocated for multiple modes of inquiry to meet nursing's knowledge needs. Van der Zalm and Bergum (2000) illuminated the empirical, moral, aesthetic, personal and socio-political contributions to knowledge that arise from using a single mode of inquiry. Rather than uncritically prescribing single or multiple modes of inquiry, we support basing research on a clearer, more integrated understanding of the paradigms used for nursing inquiry.

Evolution of Paradigms for Nursing Research

Since the time of Nightingale, nursing has been concerned with acquiring theoretical knowledge for application to practice. Initially, nursing borrowed theories from other disciplines to meet its practice needs (Meleis 1997). Early theoretical ideas unique to nursing were derived mainly from clinical observations, personal knowledge and philosophical thinking (Kirkevold 1997). These early nursing perspectives were useful for articulating the nature of nursing and guiding practice but less useful for guiding nursing research (Hinshaw 1999). The evolution of nursing as a professional discipline necessitated the establishment of a scientific research base (Wuest 1994, Donaldson & Crowley 1997/1978) to increase disciplinary credibility.

The effort to increase credibility has been influenced by factors within and external to nursing. Internally, attention has been directed towards developing a specialized knowledge base that could be taught to students and used to distinguish professional education from technical training. Externally, nursing has struggled to differentiate itself from medicine and to develop the knowledge to respond to changing societal needs (e.g. technological advances, increased scope of nursing practice). To develop a scientific base for nursing and to seek professional status in esteemed medical and academic institutions, nurse researchers at first followed the dominant positivist paradigm (Cull-Wilby & Pepin 1987, Nagle & Mitchell 1991).

Positivism

Positivism, referred to as the received view, uses scientific method to develop general abstract laws describing and predict patterns in the physical world (Suppe & Jacox 1985). Theory is established deductively through formal statistical testing of hypotheses (Lincoln & Guba 1985). Objective generalizable theory is sought via stringent control of contextual variables. The influence of positivism can be seen in the conceptual models of Orem and Roy (Nagle & Mitchell 1991, Barrett 1992) and in such tools as nursing diagnoses and practice standards (Dzurec 1989, Drew & Dahlberg 1995).

Postpositivism

Research in the postpositivist paradigm continues the positivist emphasis on well-defined concepts and variables, controlled conditions, precise instrumentation and empirical testing (Guba & Lincoln 1994). Objective knowledge is sought through replication. The postpositive paradigm is judged appropriate for the study of nursing questions requiring systematically gathered and analysed data from representative samples (Bunkers et al. 1996), technical clinical knowledge about specific interventions (Horsfall 1995), and predictive theories for at-risk individuals and populations (Norbeck 1987).

Interpretive

The Heideggerian view of the nature of being-in-the-world and of humans as self-interpreting has spurred the evolution of the interpretive paradigm (Holmes 1996, Appleton & King 1997). In this paradigm, intersubjectivity (mutual recognition) between researcher and research participants is fostered and valued (Dzurec 1989, Horsfall 1995). Phenomena are studied through the eyes of people in their lived situations. The unitary nature of person-with-environment is congruent with the individualized, holistic practice espoused by the nursing discipline (Drew & Dahlberg 1995). Examples of nursing theories developed within the interpretive paradigm are Parse's (1992) *Human Becoming*, based on the inseparability of humans and their environments, and Leininger's (1988) *Transcultural Nursing*, concerned with culturally competent care for people of similar or different cultures.

Critical Social Theory

Critical social theory, inspired by the writings of Marx, Habermas and Freire, includes feminist, grassroots and emancipatory movements. It is concerned with countering oppression and redistributing power and resources (Maguire 1987, Lutz et al. 1997). A critical theory perspective assumes that truth exists as 'taken for granted' realities shaped by social, political, cultural, gender and economic factors that over time are considered 'real' (Ford-Gilboe et al. 1995). Within the critical theory paradigm, research becomes a means for taking action and a theory for explaining how things could be (Maguire 1987). Process, not product is emphasized (Thorne 1999). A desired focus is praxis, or the combination of reflection and action to effect transformation (Mill *et al.* 2001).

Method

Integrative review of the literature describing the various paradigms was conducted using Ganong's (1987) method of analysis. This method was selected because it provides a structured, practical approach to identifying and understanding relevant themes and differences in a body of literature. The method consists of (a) formulating questions for the review, (b) making decisions about what to review, (c) organizing the characteristics of the literature reviewed and (d) evaluating the reliability of ideas, arguments and findings. The questions we formulated were: What are the similarities and differences in the assumptions underlying the paradigms used for nursing research? What is the significance of paradigms to theory and disciplinary knowledge development? What are the consequences in choosing one paradigm for nursing research over others?

We addressed these questions through study of the theoretical and philosophical literature. Using the keywords research paradigm, research tradition, disciplinary matrix, worldview, nursing knowledge, positivism, postpositivism, interpretive, and critical social theory, material was identified from the computerized databases for nursing, allied health, medical and educational literature (e.g. CINAHL, Medline, Pubmed, EBSCO and ERIC). Primary sources were identified by reviewing the reference lists of the retrieved material. We did not limit the search to a specific timeframe as the history of nursing research and nursing science has been short. The sample consisted of 72 journal articles and chapters published in English.

To organize the characteristics of the literature reviewed and to determine the current state of knowledge, we constructed a table using as columns the categories for comparison that emerged from the reading and as rows the individual paradigms (see Table 27-1). Critical analysis was completed by identifying underlying assumptions, examining the logic of explanations, evaluating the content of each work in light of previous work, and clustering results. We carried out what Kirkevold (1997) defines as a *synopsis review* in that we clarified and portrayed systematized information about each paradigm without attempting to unify the alternative theoretical positions.

Table 27-1
Paradigms Used for Nursing Research

Contributions	Limitations
Positivist	
Generalizability of findings beyond a particular sample (Baker *et al.* 1998)	Context stripping limits application to practice (Schumaker & Gortner 1992)
Produces description and prediction (Allen *et al.* 1986, Labonte & Robertson 1996)	Explanation as well as description and prediction needed to guide nursing intervention (Schumaker & Gortner 1992)
Objectivity enhances credibility. Only directly observable theoretical entities held to exist; researcher role is detachment (Allen *et al.* 1986, Guba & Lincoln 1994, Clark 1998)	Value-free observations impossible as observations based on perception, a function of prior knowledge and experience (Schumaker & Gortner 1992, Playle 1995). Scientists may ensure the status quo (Gould 1981)
Attempts to discover universal truth through verification (Lincoln & Guba 1985, Gortner 1993)	Absolute truth is rarely if ever established (Chinn 1985)
Belief that scientific methods used to investigate the physical world can be used to investigate the social world (Feyerabend 1990)	Humans seen as extensions of nature described via causal mechanical laws (Kleynhaus & Cahill 1991). Ignores possibility that humans actively construct their social world and knowledge (Blummer 1969)

(continued)

Table 27-1
Paradigms Used for Nursing Research (Continued)

Contributions	Limitations
Postpositivist	
Recognizes fallacies of verification. Seeks to falsify hypotheses (Gortner 1993) and establish probable truth (Maguire 1987)	Knowledge claims represent probabilities about human phenomena rather than universal governing laws (Letourneau & Allen 1999)
Attempts holism by including subjective states (Schumaker & Gortner 1992) and multiple perspectives and stakeholders (Letourneau & Allen 1999)	Neglects 'whole' person by studying parts (Pearson 1990, Nagle & Mitchell 1991). Does not make explicit how the views of patients as stakeholders are drawn into the research process
Powerful, i.e. attracts funding (Guba & Lincoln 1994, Cheek 2000)	Theory development controlled by others outside of discipline. Power influences what can and will be known (Dzurec 1989)
Encourages precision, caution and scepticism (Gortner 1993). Credibility through conformity with judgment of peers (Letourneau & Allen 1999)	Conformity with peers within postpositivist paradigm may lead to becoming 'pot-bound'
Logical for study of phenomena such as genetic issues and epidemiology (Norbeck 1987). Defines boundaries of nursing separately from social sciences (Drew 1988, Gortner 1993)	No 'cookbook' techniques for achieving balance of heterogeneous qualitative and quantitative methods (Letourneau & Allen 1999, p. 627)
Interpretive	
Inquiry is means for articulating, appreciating, and making visible the voices, concerns and practices of research participants (Benner 1994)	May ignore ecological, historical, and risk factors (Gortner 1993)
Focus is subjectivity and intersubjectivity (Dzurec 1989, Drew & Dahlberg 1995, Horsfall 1995)	Loss of objectivity limits ability to discriminate patterns that are fundamental to humans (Allen 1985)
Truth viewed as multiple realities that are holistic, local, and specific (Ford-Gilboe *et al* 1995)	Less explanatory power as infinite number of interpretations are possible for a given phenomenon (Berger & Luckmann 1966)
Seeks understanding, shared meaning, and embedded meaning (Allen & Jensen 1996)	Theorizing limited because the human state is not objectified outside of the lived experience and present (Gortner 1993)
Meaning is constructed in the researcher–participant interaction in the natural environment (Guba & Lincoln 1994, Ford-Gilboe *et al.* 1995, Hinshaw 1999)	Discomfort with the uncertainty of the ever-changing nature of knowledge
Critical Social Theory	
Exposes oppression through understanding shared meanings of political, social, historical and cultural practices that impede equal participation (Ludz *et al.* 1997)	Emphasizes rationality while excluding feelings despite the emancipatory potential of feelings (Campbell & Bunting 1991)
Theory and practice closely linked. Research goes beyond description towards action to change inequities (Mill *et al.* 2001)	If researchers know ahead of time that social action is needed, then do not need research to justify this (Gortner 1993)
Ensures representation of diverse and under-represented views (Gortner 1993, Wuest 2000)	The one who critiques is part of the culture being critiqued which suggests complicity (Reed 1995)
Practitioners can develop tacit knowledge from practice via criticism and reflection (Fawcett *et al.* 2001)	Practitioners may not see themselves as researchers or theorists and practice as data (Tolley 1995)
Research process characterized by continual redefinition of problems and by cooperative interaction between researchers and those whose environment is being researched	Focus on problems defined by oppressed groups and collective humanity. May exclude the individual and personal level. Some research team members may have more power than others (Campbell & Bunting 1991)

Findings

Comparing and Contrasting the Paradigms

The philosophical underpinnings of the positivist, post-positivist, interpretive and critical theory paradigms of nursing research were assessed for similarities and differences. The interpretive paradigm differed ontologically from the others because it is based on relativism, a view of truth as composed of multiple local and specific realities that can only be subjectively perceived (Allen *et al.* 1986, Guba 1990). Positivist, postpositivist and critical theory paradigms are based on realism, a view of truth as universal and independent of human perception of it. Postpositivist and critical theory paradigms are based on the assumption that this universal truth may not be accessible to everyone (Allen *et al.* 1986, Guba & Lincoln 1994). Positivist and postpositivist paradigms differed epistemologically from the others in their assumption that observations can be objective and either 'value free' or 'value neutral' (Norbeck 1987, Schumaker & Gortner 1992). Researchers working within interpretive and critical theory paradigms have considered observations as subjective, 'value relative', or 'value mediated' (Lincoln & Guba 1985). In addition, researchers in the interpretive paradigm have sought *intersubjectivity* or shared subjective awareness and understanding within the research relationship. Methodologies associated with each paradigm reflected the ontological underpinnings of relativism or realism and epistemological underpinnings of objectivity, subjectivity or intersubjectivity. For example, the participatory action research approach of critical social theory was developed to reveal hidden power imbalances, learn how people subjectively experience problems, and make this knowledge publicly available.

We further examined the paradigms to distinguish differences in the goals of inquiry, nature of knowledge sought, and the place of theory in the research process. With the overall aim of creating good science, the goals of research within each paradigm varied. The goals of positivist and postpositivist paradigm research were control and prediction (Allen *et al.* 1986, Guba & Lincoln 1994); the goal of interpretive research was

understanding (Ford-Gilboe *et al.* 1995) and that of critical theory was emancipation (Maguire 1987). Theoretical knowledge of truth as an absolute entity was sought in the positivist paradigm, and truth as a probable value was sought in the postpositivist paradigm (Guba & Lincoln 1994, Letourneau & Allen 1999). Practical knowledge to help understand or change the social world was the focus of interpretive and critical theory paradigms. This type of knowledge, co-constructed between researchers and research participants, was subject to continuous revision (Campbell & Bunting 1991, Kim 1999). In the positivist and postpositivist paradigms, theory was established deductively. The positivist focus was on verifying hypotheses and replicating findings (Lincoln & Guba 1985, Morse & Field 1995); the postpositivist focus was on falsifying hypotheses (Guba & Lincoln 1994). In the interpretive paradigm, theory emerged inductively—hypotheses were formulated and tested to generate theory, and established theory was used to explain the data (Lincoln & Guba 1985, Morse & Field 1995). Theory and knowledge in the critical social theory paradigm were closely linked in that theory made shared meanings of social interactions explicit and illuminated embedded barriers to autonomy and responsibility (Allen *et al.* 1986, Mill *et al.* 2001).

Significance of Paradigms to Nursing Theory Development

The evolution of multiple paradigms has sparked extensive debate over the need to determine if one, a combination of several, or any at all is best for nursing research. We assessed the utility of a unitary, pluralist, or anti-paradigmatic approach to guide inquiry through identification of each paradigm's contributions and limitations.

Contributions

Different benefits to nursing theory development were associated with various research studies within the postpositivist, interpretive and critical theory approaches. Nursing research conducted within the postpositivist paradigm contributed to health promotion, illness prevention and professional education. For example, through post-positivist quantitative inquiry, Faye and Yarandi (2004) identified that African American women were at greater risk of depression because of lower income, lesser education and residency in rural committees. Treat-Jacobson and Lindquist (2004) found the intensity of exercise required to receive functional benefit following cardiac bypass surgery to be less than many people realized. A study of the knowledge and attitudes of nurses caring for patients with AIDS (Walusimbi & Okonsky 2004) provided baseline data from which to determine appropriate educational interventions for nurses.

Nursing research conducted in the interpretive paradigm involved different qualitative methods to gain in-depth and detailed description, understanding and explanation of ordinary occurrences as experienced by those in the field. For example, Austin *et al.* (2003) used a hermeneutic phenomenological approach to understand the experiences of nurses attempting to address ethical concerns in patient care within health institutional environments. Through participant observation fieldwork, Ellefsen and Kim (2004) obtained information about how nurses view, interpret and receive the meanings of clinical situations. These findings using the interpretive paradigm research have identified specific strategies nurses use with patients that can inform and improve nursing practice.

Researchers conducting inquiry in the critical social theory paradigm have made it their responsibility to raise awareness of social problems and to ensure that the voices and perspectives of marginalized people are heard. In keeping with this mandate, Georges (2002) called for greater examination of the context of social and political inequities creating and sustaining suffering. Bermann (2003) described the need for researchers who work with children, in which empowerment is a goal, to acknowledge power imbalances in research relationships and to enable children to shape the interviews.

Limitations of the Paradigms

Our review revealed limitations associated with each paradigm (see Table 27-1). Positivist and postpositivist research approaches, in denying social contexts and intersubjectivity within research relationships, may perpetuate technically-oriented practice (Horsfall 1995). Positivism has tended to be inconsistent with holistic practice in its denial of unobservable values, including spiritual aspects and relationships within complex socio-political, ecological environments. Its claims of producing value free observations and discovering universal truth are questionable. The major criticism of postpositivism is its reduction of people to parts and its dehumanization of them to scores and percentages for statistical analyses.

Research within the interpretive paradigm has tended to ignore the influence of biological factors and social structures on individual action. The loss of objectivity (e.g. multiple interpretations of multiple realities, non-objectification of the human state) has limited theorizing. The interpretive approach can be criticized for its underlying assumptions about all being equal. Critical theory, shown to value the collective above the individual, has tended to demean participants asked to respond to shared, pre-existing social orders they had no part in creating. Critical theory researchers have been criticized for their complicity in being part of the culture they critiqued and for suppressing findings incompatible with their beliefs.

Unitary Paradigm

Those who have embraced a unitary or a single paradigm approach for nursing research have asserted that incommensurable ontological and epistemological differences among the paradigms required choosing one over the others for specific research projects. In this way, the set of beliefs about health, relationships of person with environment and goal of nursing knowledge expressed in the paradigm were preserved (Mitchell & Pilkington 1999). Donaldson and Crowley (1997/1978) have explained that a discipline is characterized by 'a unique perspective, a distinct way of viewing all phenomena, which ultimately defines and limits the nature of its inquiry' (p. 242). While they have articulated the need for an overarching framework of values agreed to by members of the discipline, clearly Donaldson and Crowley have not explicitly recommended establishment of a single research perspective. The overarching framework for nursing inquiry could endorse research approaches within diverse paradigms (Northrup 1992, Reed 1995).

Paradigmatic Plurality

Proponents of paradigmatic plurality (combination of several paradigms) have argued that knowledge developed from one perspective could complement knowledge developed from another (Leddy 2000). They recommended harnessing the processes and products from multiple paradigms to meet nursing demands for knowledge for practice (i.e. scientific knowledge, professional judgment in the form of personal knowledge of clients, humanistic connection, and clinical experience to aid ethical decision-making). Rolfe (1998) provided the example of a nurse who found scientific knowledge helpful to determine patient status. However, such knowledge could not direct the nurse about how to respond when a patient asked if he was dying. 'In a discipline that deals with human beings, it is perhaps not feasible that only one theory should explain, describe, predict, and change all the discipline's phenomena' (Meleis 1997, p. 77).

Anti-Paradigmatic Inquiry

An argument for anti-paradigmatic inquiry has been put forward by Kikuchi (2003). She recommended studying only questions that all participants could answer, and approaching questions in 'piece-meal' (p. 13) fashion. We agree that research conducted as a public enterprise towards which all members of a discipline can work may help to enlarge the disciplinary body. However, we are concerned that such research might limit rather than expand the pursuit of some of the types of knowledge needed for nursing practice (e.g. emic perspectives, narratives, issues of power and control). We also question whether this anti-paradigmatic stance is representative of the positivist paradigm, in which research questions are either limited to those that can be posed in terms of independent and dependent variables (Dzurec 1989) or to variables whose existence can be directly verifiable (Schumaker & Gortner 1992, Clark 1998).

Addressing the Paradigms Debate

In order for nursing to resolve the paradigm debate, we believe that nurses must come together and address the thoughtful questions raised by Barrett (1992). These questions are concerned with which paradigmatic philosophy best reflects nursing values, what processes could be used to pursue a unified disciplinary path, who will determine the one right approach, and who will relinquish their own commitment for the sake of unity. Based on our consideration of the literature, we could not justify choosing one paradigm over others when most can inform different aspects vital to nursing practice. Theory arising from postpositivist paradigm inquiry has yielded prescriptive or situation-producing theory, such as interventions for managing specific health or illness threats (Gortner 1993). Theory generated through interpretative paradigm inquiry has enabled nurses to develop insights into unique individual responses within clinical situations that could improve the care of those involved (Van der Zalm & Bergum 2000). Knowledge constructed via critical social theory has benefited people collectively by uncovering and transforming oppressive situations (Mill *et al.* 2001).

We identify a trend in the literature towards using multiple paradigms for nursing research (e.g. Cull-Wilby & Pepin 1987, Monti & Tingen 1999). We do not support anti-paradigmatic nursing inquiry because of its potential to exclude important topics not researchable from all paradigm perspectives. We are concerned that its 'top down' application of general principles to particular cases may limit knowledge construction to existing conceptualizations.

Discussion

Nursing's obsession with the paradigm debate has occupied much space in the literature. Failure to build the nursing knowledge base comprehensively has been assumed to result from the lack of a consensual overarching framework for conducting research. Yet nursing has not pursued 'integration of nursing research from the level of a conceptual framework for a particular study to the level of more general theories and ultimately to that of a unified body of nursing knowledge' (Donaldson & Crowley 1997/1978, p. 237). We must, therefore, ask ourselves and our discipline if the current state of fragmentation of nursing knowledge has been the result of limited nursing inquiry in which individual studies were not related to one another, or if it has been the result of research emanating from an individual paradigm, a collective paradigm, or no paradigm at all.

Pragmatic Approach to Evaluating Disciplinary Inquiry and Theory Development

In research, the purpose and the question guide inquiry and knowledge development (e.g. Burns & Grove 2001, Morse & Richards 2002). The choice of a research paradigm and method are also guided by the current state of knowledge about a particular area of nursing. For example, within a positivist or postpositivist paradigm a randomized controlled study cannot be conducted if the variables to be controlled have not first been defined. There is no need for interpretive paradigm inquiry if we already know what is being hypothesized and what we are apt to find. The participatory action research of the critical social paradigm is inappropriate if the knowledge sought is merely shared views, without opportunity to engage in action to address domination and power inequities.

In addition, two ideas must be kept in mind when considering the choice of research paradigm. The first is that scholars often restrict research questions to those that can studied within the paradigms with which the scholars align themselves. The second is that not all paradigms are afforded equal credibility. Legitimacy is conferred by certain groups (e.g. funding and publication review boards) who regulate what constitutes valid research. Pursuing inquiry in one paradigm may further the interests of a dominant stakeholder, while diverting energies away from developing sensitive methodologies and unique research interests needed for nursing (Horsfall 1995).

To reduce these potential sources of bias, it seems necessary to determine criteria and a process for evaluating disciplinary inquiry. A measure of the effectiveness of an inquiry is its problem-solving ability or usefulness

to those involved (Laudan 1977). It is also recommended that nursing research priorities be situational-specific and practice-based (Dickoff & James 1968, Im & Meleis 1999). Moreover, the basic concern of all nursing research is to improve the health and wellbeing of the people studied (Ford-Gilboe *et al.* 1995, Warms & Schroeder 1999). Thus, theory development in nursing must support service to people and the health of society.

We believe that nursing inquiry may be effectively evaluated through a pragmatic approach. The term pragmatism is derived from the Greek word for action, from which the words 'practice' and 'praxis' originate (Barnhart 1995, James 1907/1998). Pragmatism is determining the value of an idea by its outcome in practice and conduct (James 1907/1998). A pragmatic approach stresses critical analysis of facts, applications and outcomes rather than abstraction and verbal solutions (James 1907). This approach can move nursing beyond the boundaries and restrictions of a single paradigm towards theory construction tailored to fit particular situations (Doane 2003). Surely the tenets of pragmatism (i.e. commitment to what works in practice, appreciation of plurality, and desire for integrated results) are relevant to nursing? Nurse clinicians have identified that theory-practice gaps exist when theory does not address diverse practice demands (e.g. Hanchett 2001). A pragmatic approach calls for theory to be designed and tested in practice. This could counter passive acceptance of inquiry conducted for reasons other than to improve the health and comfort of those whom nursing serves. A pragmatic approach could stimulate inquiry that complements one paradigm with another.

Strategies to Develop Nursing Knowledge

We suggest that inquiry should start with assessment of the existing theoretical base containing findings from diverse, disparate studies. Critical analysis or review and critical appraisal are modes of inquiry that integrate the literature. They can help to determine if research within a single paradigm is sufficient to meet practice demands. To critically analyse or review means to examine the existing literature on a particular topic, determining weaknesses in the research or inconsistencies in findings (Kirkevold 1997). This can identify gaps in available knowledge, areas where existing knowledge is untrustworthy, and areas requiring further information before conclusions can be drawn. The findings from critical analysis or review can assist nurse clinicians to judge if the knowledge base is solid enough for practical application. Critical appraisal involves exploration of pragmatic utility (Morse 2000), and synthesizes key substantive content to direct inquiry towards areas that need development. Overloaded or under-researched areas impinging on and influencing practice can thereby be opened up (Horsfall 1995). Critical appraisal can help to explicate the sociopolitical historical context within which health and illness problems are developed and addressed.

Following critical assessment of the literature, nursing knowledge may need to be developed in under-researched or underdeveloped areas. This reopens the issue of which paradigm to use. As previously discussed, the purpose of the inquiry, in conjunction with the state of knowledge development in the substantive area, should guide paradigm selection. A pluralist approach may have greater utility to nursing because it holds that research from various paradigms can contribute to the development of knowledge needed for nursing practice.

How best to utilize a pluralist approach to inquiry and subsequent theory development without violating the philosophical underpinnings of the individual paradigms is not well described in the literature. One strategy is to design a research program comprised of parallel studies within the same substantive domain, using different paradigms. This preserves the theoretical and philosophical clarity of each tradition (Mitchell & Pilkington 1999). Follow-up integrative techniques, such as conceptual triangulation of research findings (Foster 1997) and integrative review (Kirkevold 1997), could then be implemented to synthesize knowledge from the separate research studies. Conceptual triangulation is a procedure for combining findings from paradigmatically diverse studies in such a way as to safeguard individual study designs. It involves integrating findings from research completed in different paradigms after considering threats to rigour and examining

---

What Is Already Known About This Topic

- Nursing knowledge has been developed from a variety of research approaches within multiple paradigms.
- The need to clarify the paradigms used for nursing research is an important issue facing the discipline.
- Individual research paradigms, while serving to protect the integrity and rigor of knowledge construction within a scientific community, may define and restrict approaches to inquiry.

What This Paper Adds

- Critical analysis of the research approaches within various research paradigms does not justify choosing one paradigm over others.
- The discipline's task of developing knowledge may be enhanced through the use of integrative strategies that maintain the theoretical perspectives of individual research paradigms.
- An anti-paradigmatical approach to research may limit disciplinary knowledge development.

---

the strength of the evidence (Foster 1997). Integrative review enables integration of relevant information from isolated studies into a comprehensive account (Kirkevold 1997). Additionally, mixed methods studies (i.e. using quantitative and qualitative methods from different paradigms in a single study) can help to accumulate knowledge without crossing paradigmatic boundaries if researchers clarify in advance the contribution of each paradigm (Morse 1991). We think these strategies could help to reduce theory–research–practice discrepancies because they respect theoretical perspectives.

Pluralistic integrative approaches can suggest important new lines of research, empowering researchers to address problems which cannot be resolved satisfactorily by adherence to inquiry within a single paradigm. These approaches can be undertaken by communities of scholars who, as Hinshaw (1996) has predicted, will continue the growth of the nursing knowledge base through critique, constructive criticism and challenge of ideas. With attention to theoretical perspectives, we contend that findings within multiple paradigm can be integrated to increase the cumulative knowledge needed for the substance of our discipline and to provide relevant research-based knowledge to clinical nurses.

Conclusion

Integrative review of the major paradigms used for nursing research has allowed us to identify issues that potentially limit theory and disciplinary development. Embracing different paradigms for nursing research, while responding to the need for knowledge to direct nursing practice, had introduced confusion and perhaps intolerance and competition. To understand better the paradigms used for nursing research and to begin to resolve the tension between unitary, pluralistic and anti-paradigmatic perspectives, we have examined the philosophical underpinnings and knowledge development within individual paradigms and assessed the pragmatic utility. No single paradigm emerged as unequivocally superior to another for nursing research. Rather, knowledge resulting from research within each paradigm was sought and valued for its contribution in describing, interpreting, explaining and predicting the complexity of human health experiences and illness responses. Critical assessment of the existing theoretical base will help nurses adequately to understand and address nursing's knowledge needs. We recommend pluralistic approaches that maintain the individual theoretical perspectives of each paradigm because such approaches protect the integrity and rigour of knowledge construction, thus insuring a more worthwhile and valuable contribution to disciplinary development. The practice of situating research within paradigms, as well as the knowledge resulting from research processes, must be considered in the light of their ability to advance the social mission of nursing: to enhance health and wellbeing and alleviate suffering.

Author Contributions

KW contributed to study conception, design and drafting of the manuscript; KW and JO contributed to critical revisions of the manuscript for important intellectual content; JO supervised the study.

REFERENCES

Allen D. (1985) Nursing research and social control: alternative-models of science that emphasize understanding and emancipation. *Image: Journal of Nursing Scholarship* 17(2), 58–64.

Allen M.N. & Jensen L.A. (1996) Knowledge development in nursing. In *Canadian nursing. Issues and perspectives* (Kerr J.R. & MacPhail J., eds), Mosby, St Louis, pp. 85–104.

Allen D., Benner P. & Diekelmann N.L. (1986) Three paradigms for nursing research: Methodological implications. In *Nursing Research Methodology: Issues and Implementation* (Chinn P., ed.), Aspen, Rockville, MD, USA, pp. 23–38.

Appleton J.V. & King L. (1997) Constructivism: a naturalistic methodology for nursing inquiry. *Advances in Nursing Science* 20(2), 13–22.

Austin W., Bergum V. & Goldberg L. (2003) Unable to answer the call of our patients: mental health nurses' experience of moral distress. *Nursing Inquiry* 10(3), 177–183.

Baker C., Norton S., Young P. & Ward S. (1998) An exploration of methodological pluralism in nursing research. *Research in Nursing and Health* 21, 545–555.

Barnhart R.K. (ed.) (1995) *The World Book Dictionary 2 (L–Z).* World Book Inc., Chicago, p. 1635.

Barrett E.A. (1992) Disciplinary perspective: united or diversified? Response: diversity reigns. *Nursing Science Quarterly* 5, 155–157.

Benner P. (1994) The tradition and skill of interpretive phenomenology in studying health, illness, and caring practices. In *Interpretive Phenomenology: Embodiment, Caring, and Ethics in Health and Illness* (Benner P., ed.), Sage, Thousand Oaks, CA, pp. 99–127.

Berger P.L. & Luckmann T. (1966) *The Social Construction of Reality.* Doubleday, New York.

Bermann H. (2003) Getting critical with children – approaches with a disempowered group. *Advances in Nursing Science* 26(2), 102–113.

Blummer H. (1969) *Symbolic Interactionism: Perspectives and Method.* Prentice Hall, Englewood Cliffs, NJ, USA.

Bunkers S.S., Petardi L.A., Pilkington F.B. & Walls P.A. (1996) Challenging the myths surrounding qualitative research in nursing. *Nursing Science Quarterly 9*, 33–37.

Burns N. & Grove S.K. (2001) *The Practice of Nursing Research.* W.B. Saunders, Philadelphia.

Campbell J. & Bunting S. (1991) Voices and paradigms: perspectives on critical and feminist theory in nursing. *Advances in Nursing Science* 13(3), 1–15.

Cheek J. (2000) Setting the parameters. In *Postmodern and Post-structural Approaches to Nursing Research* (Cheek J., ed.), Sage, Thousand Oaks, CA, USA, pp. 1–15.

Chinn P. (1985) Debunking myths in nursing theory and research. *Image—The Journal of Nursing Scholarship* 172, 45–49.

Clark A.M. (1998) The qualitative-quantitative debate: moving from positivism and confrontation to post-positivism and reconciliation. *Journal of Advanced Nursing* 27, 1242–1249.

Colorado Nursing Think Tank (2001) JAN Forum: saving the discipline—top 10 unfinished issues to inform the nursing debate in the new millennium. *Journal of Advanced Nursing* 35, 138.

Cull-Wilby B.L. & Pepin J.I. (1987) Toward a coexistence of paradigms in nursing knowledge development. *Journal of Advanced Nursing* 12, 515–521.

Dickoff J. & James P. (1968) A theory of theories: a position paper. *Nursing Research* 17, 197–203.

Doane G.H. (2003) Through pragmatic eyes: philosophy and the re-sourcing of family nursing. *Nursing Philosophy* 4(1), 25–32.

Donaldson D.M. & Crowley D.M. (1997/1978) The discipline of nursing. In *Perspectives on Nursing Theory* (Nicoll L., ed.), Lippincott. (Original work published 1978 in Nursing Outlook, 26, 113–120), Philadelphia, pp. 235–246.

Drew B.J. (1988) Devaluation of biological knowledge. *Image—The Journal of Nursing Scholarship* 20, 25–27.

Drew N. & Dahlberg K. (1995) Challenging a reductionistic paradigm as a foundation for nursing. *Journal of Holistic Nursing* 13,33 2–3 45.

Dzurec L.C. (1989) The necessity for and evolution of multiple paradigms for nursing research: a poststructuralist perspective. *Advances in Nursing Science* 11(4), 69–77.

Ellefsen B. & Kim H.S. (2004) Nurses' construction of clinical situations: a study conducted in an acute-care setting in Norway. *Canadian Journal of Nursing Research* 36, 114–131.

Fawcett J., Watson J., Neuman B., Walker P. & Fitzpatrick J.J. (2001) On nursing theories and evidence. *Journal of Nursing Scholarship* 33(2), 115–119.

Faye G. & Yarandi H.N. (2004) Depression among Southern rural African American women: a factor analysis of the Beck Depression Inventory-II. *Nursing Research* 53, 251–259.

Feyerabend P. (1990) *Farewell to Reason.* Verso, London, England.

Ford-Gilboe M., Campbell J. & Bermann H. (1995) Stories and numbers: Coexistence without compromise. *Advances in Nursing Science* 18(1), 14–26.

Foster R.L. (1997) Addressing epistemologic and practical issues in multimethod research: A procedure for conceptual triangulation. *Advances in Nursing Science* 20(2), 1–12.

Ganong L.H. (1987) Integrative reviews of nursing research. *Research in Nursing and Health* 10, 1–11.

Georges J.M. (2002) Suffering: toward a contextual praxis. *Advances in Nursing Science* 25(1), 79–86.

Gillis A. & Jackson W. (2002) Introduction to nursing research. In *Research for Nurses: Method and Interpretation* (Gillis A. & Jackson W., eds), F. A. Davis, Philadelphia, pp. 3–36.

Gortner S.R. (1993) Nursing's syntax revisited: a critique of philosophies said to influence nursing theories. *International Journal of Nursing Studies* 30, 477–488.

Gould SJ. (1981) *The Mismeasure of Man.* Penguin, London, England.

Guba E.C. (1990) The alternative paradigm dialogue. In *The Paradigm Dialogue* (Guba E.G., ed.), Sage, Newbury Park, CA, USA, pp. 17–30.

Guba E.C. & Lincoln Y. (1994) Competing paradigms in qualitative research. In *Handbook of Qualitative Research* (Denzin N.K. & Lincoln Y., eds), Sage, Thousand Oaks, CA, USA, pp. 105–117.

Hamilton D. (1994) Traditions, preferences, and postures in applied qualitative research. In *Handbook of Qualitative Research* (Denzin N.K. & Lincoln Y., eds), Sage, Thousand Oaks, CA, USA, pp. 60–69.

Hanchett M. (2001) Where is the theory to support infusion nursing? *Journal of IV Nursing* 24(1), 56–60.

Hinshaw A.S. (1996) Research. Research traditions—a decade of progress. *Journal of Professional Nursing* 12, 68.

Hinshaw A.S. (1999) Evolving nursing research traditions: influencing factors. In *Handbook of Clinical Nursing* (Hinshaw A.S., Feetham S.L. & Shaver J.F., eds), Sage, Thousand Oaks, CA, USA, pp. 19–30.

Holmes C.A. (1996) The politics of phenomenological concepts in nursing. *Journal of Advanced Nursing* 24, 579–587.

Horsfall J.M. (1995) Madness in our methods: nursing research, scientific epistemology. *Nursing Inquiry* 2, 2–9.

Im E. & Meleis A.I. (1999) Situation-specific theories: philosophical roots, properties, and approach. *Advances in Nursing Science* 22(2), 11–24.

Jacob E. (1989) Qualitative research: a defense of tradition. *Review of Educational Research* 59, 229–235.

James W. (1907) *What Pragmatism Means. Lecture 2 in Pragmatism: A New Name for Some Old Ways of Thinking,* Longman, Green & Co., New York, pp. 17–32. Retrieved from http://spartan.ac.brocku.ca/~lward/James/James_1907/James_1907_02.html on 30 September 2003.

James W. (1998) Truth is established on pragmatic grounds. In *Classic Philosophical Questions,* 9th edn (Gould J.A., ed.), Prentice Hall, Upper Saddle River, NJ, USA, pp. 375–383.

Kikuchi J.F. (2003) Nursing knowledge and the problem of worldviews. *Research & Theory for Nursing Practice* 17, 7–17.

Kim H.S. (1999) Critical reflective inquiry for knowledge development in nursing practice. *Journal of Advanced Nursing* 29, 1205–1212.

Kirkevold M. (1997) Integrative nursing research—an important strategy to further the development of nursing science and nursing practice. *Journal of Advanced Nursing* 25, 977–984.

Kleynhaus A.M. & Cahill D. (1991) Paradigms for chiropractic research. *Chiropractic Journal of Australia* 21(3), 102–107.

Kuhn T.S. (1970) *The Structure of Scientific Revolutions.* University of Chicago Press, Chicago.

Labonte R. & Robertson A. (1996) Delivering the goods, showing our stuff: the case for a constructivist paradigm for health -

promotion research and practice. *Health Education Quarterly* 23, 431–447.

Laudan L. (1977) From theories to research traditions. In *Progress and its Problems: Toward a Theory of Scientific Growth* (Laudan L., ed.), University of California Press, Berkeley, pp. 70–120.

Leddy S.K. (2000) Toward a complementary perspective on worldviews. *Nursing Science Quarterly* 13, 225–233.

Leininger M.M. (1988) Leininger's theory of nursing: cultural care diversity and universality. *Nursing Science Quarterly* 1, 152–160.

Letourneau N. & Allen M. (1999) Post-positivistic critical multiplism: a beginning dialogue. *Journal of Advanced Nursing* 30, 623–630.

Lincoln Y. & Cuba E. (1985) Postpositivism and the naturalist paradigm. In *Naturalistic Inquiry,* Sage, London, pp. 14–46.

Ludz K.F., Jones K.D. & Kendall J. (1997) Expanding the praxis debate: contributions to clinical inquiry. *Advances in Nursing Science* 20(2), 23–31.

Lutz K., Jones K. & Kendall J. (1997) Expanding the praxis debate: contributions to clinical inquiry. *Advances in Nursing Science* 20(2), 23–31.

Maguire P. (1987) *Doing Participatory Research.* University of Massachusetts, Amherst, MA, USA.

Meleis A.I. (1997) *Theoretical Nursing: Development & Progress.* Lippincott, Philadelphia.

Mill J.E., Allen M.N. & Morrow R.A. (2001) Critical theory: critical methodology to disciplinary foundations in nursing. *Canadian Journal of Nursing Research* 33, 109–127.

Mitchell G.L. & Pilkington F.B. (1999) Research issues: a dialogue on the comparability of research paradigms—and other theoretical things. *Nursing Science Quarterly* 12, 283–289.

Moccia P. (1988) A critique of compromise: beyond the methods debate. *Advances in Nursing Science* 10(4), 1–9.

Monti E.J. & Tingen M.S. (1999) Multiple paradigms of nursing science. *Advances in Nursing Science* 21(4), 64–80.

Morse J.M. (1991) Approaches to qualitative-quantitative methodological triangulation. *Nursing Research* 40, 120–123.

Morse J.M. (2000) Exploring pragmatic utility: concept analysis by critically appraising the literature. In *Concept Development in Nursing: Foundations, Techniques, and Applications* (Rodgers B.L. & Knafl K.A., ed.), W.B. Saunders Company, Philadelphia, pp. 333–352.

Morse J. & Field P. (1995) *Qualitative Research for Health Professionals.* Sage, Thousand Oaks, CA, USA.

Morse J.M. & Richards L. (2002) *Readme First for a User's Guide to Qualitative Methods.* Sage, Thousand Oaks, CA, USA.

Nagle L. & Mitchell GJ. (1991) Theoretical diversity: evolving paradigmatic issues in research and practice. *Advances in Nursing Science* 14(1), 17–25.

Norbeck J. (1987) In defense of empiricism. *Image—The Journal of Nursing Scholarship* 19, 28–30.

Northrup D.T. (1992) A united perspective within nursing. *Nursing Science Quarterly* 5, 154–155.

Parse R.R. (1992) Human becoming: Parse's theory of nursing. *Nursing Science Quarterly* 5, 35–42.

Pearson A. (1990) *Nursing: From whence to where?* Deakin University Press, Victoria, Australia.

Playle J.F. (1995) Humanism and positivism in nursing: contradictions and conflicts. *Journal of Advanced Nursing* 22, 979–984.

Reed P.G. (1995) A treatise on nursing knowledge development for the 21st century: Beyond postmodernism. *Advances in Nursing Science* 17(3), 70–84.

Rolfe G. (1998) Nursing knowledge. In *Expanding Nursing Knowledge* (Rolfe G., ed.), Butterworth Heinemann, Oxford, pp. 7–39.

Schumaker K.L. & Gortner S.R. (1992) (Mis)conceptions and reconceptions about traditional science. *Advances in Nursing Science* 14(4), 1–11.

Suppe F. & Jacox A.K. (1985) Philosophy of science and the development of nursing theory. In *Annual Review of Nursing Research 3* (Fitzpatrick H.W.J., ed.), Springer, New York, pp. 241–265.

Thompson J.L. (1985) Practical discourse in nursing: going beyond empiricism and historicism. *Advances in Nursing Science* 7(4), 59–71.

Thorne S.E. (1999) Ideological implications of paradigm discourse. *Nursing Inquiry 6,* 123–131.

Tolley K. (1995) Theory from practice for practice: Is this a reality? *Journal of Advanced Nursing* 21, 184–190.

Treat-Jacobson D. & Lindquist R.A. (2004) Functional recovery and exercise behaviour in men and women 5 to 6 years following coronary artery bypass graft (CABG) surgery. *Western Journal of Nursing Research* 26(5), 479–496.

Van der Zalm J.E. & Bergum V. (2000) Hermeneutic-phenomenology: providing lived knowledge for nursing practice. *Journal of Advanced Nursing* 31, 211–218.

Walusimbi M. & Okonsky J.G. (2004) Knowledge and attitudes of nurses caring for patients with HIV/AIDS in Uganda. *Applied Nursing Research* 17(2), 92–99.

Warms C.A. & Schroeder C.A. (1999) Bridging the gulf between science and action: the 'new fuzzies' of neopragmatism. *Advances in Nursing Science* 22(2), 1–10.

Wuest J. (1994) Professionalism and the evolution of nursing as a discipline: a feminist perspective. *Journal of Professional Nursing* 10, 357–367.

Wuest J. (2000) Concept development situated in the critical paradigm. In *Concept Development in Nursing: Foundations, Techniques, and Applications* (Rodgers B.L. & Knafl K.A., eds), W. B. Saunders, Philadelphia, pp. 369–386.

The Authors Comment

Understanding Paradigms Used for Nursing Research

We were told that the paradigm issue was resolved—a "done deal" in 21st-century nursing! Yet, we wanted to see for ourselves the state of understanding of the paradigms used for nursing research. Consequently, this quest began as a position paper prepared by the first author for a doctoral level course in nursing theory development taught by the second author. Intrigued by the tension concerning unitary, pluralistic, and antiparadigmatic perspectives, and fueled by both our own spirited dialogues and the voluminous published discourse, we continued the manuscript as an integrated review of the literature. The project was intended to add clarity to the ongoing paradigm debates and as such it strengthens understanding of the salient issues and contributes our recommendations of strategies for preserving theoretical integrity and philosophical congruence in disciplinary knowledge development.

—Kathryn Weaver
—Joanne K. Olson

Bridging the Gulf Between Science and Action: The "New Fuzzies" of Neopragmatism

Catherine A. Warms
Carole A. Schroeder

Rather than a philosophy, pragmatism is a way of doing philosophy that has major implications for solving disputes involving nursing science, theory, and practice that may otherwise be interminable. Pragmatism weaves together theory and action so that one modifies the other continuously, but both maintain their mutual relevance. Pragmatism emphasizes pluralism and diversity, and depends on an ethical base for determination of what is reasonable. Recently repopularized by the philosopher Richard Rorty and others, pragmatic ideals seem inherent to nursing. We propose that a better understanding of the history and utility of pragmatism will enhance both clinically relevant nursing theory and theoretically relevant nursing practice.

Pragmatism may be the most misunderstood philosophical movement in the history of philosophy. Unlike most philosophy, pragmatism is not based on theoretical notions of truth or falsity, and it refuses to offer a method for discovering truth. Instead, pragmatism is a way of *doing* philosophy. On its most basic level, pragmatism is the theory that the meaning of a proposition or course of action lies in its observable consequences. Moreover, the sum of these consequences constitutes the meaning of the proposition or action. Pragmatism is a method for evaluating philosophical problems by tracing the practical consequences of each question. In the words of William James, "The question is not, "Is that true?" but "*What difference* would it make if that is

About the Authors

CATHERINE ANN WARMS was born in Bremerton, WA, and attended the University of Washington for all her undergraduate and graduate nursing education. She received a BA in social welfare in 1971, a BSN in 1981, an MN in Family Nursing in 1986, and a PhD in nursing science in 2002. She has been a rehabilitation nurse for more than 20 years and has worked in multiple nursing roles, including inpatient nursing, outpatient nurse practitioner, and research study nurse. Currently, she is a postdoctoral scholar in biobehavioral nursing at the University of Washington School of Nursing, focusing on health promotion for people with disabilities and/or chronic conditions, with an emphasis on physical activity, its measurement, and its effect on health in populations with mobility impairments. Her hobbies include gardening, cooking, and reading.

CAROLE A. SCHROEDER was born in the San Francisco Bay Area and grew up in Reno, NV; received her doctorate at the University of Colorado Health Sciences Center; and did postdoctoral study at the University of Washington in health systems before taking a faculty position. She has been a single parent for most of her adult life, an experience that leaves her with a unique understanding of issues of gender, class, power, and privilege. The focus of her scholarship is to promote social justice and decrease inequalities in health and health care access. Her key contributions include her theoretical writings, work with vulnerable populations, and teaching approach using the Peace and Power philosophy and methods developed by Dr. Peggy Chinn.

true?"[1(p112)] For the pragmatist, belief in a truth cannot be separated from intent, performance, and consequences. Considering the immense ethical contradictions inherent in both the theory and practice of nursing, pragmatism may be a way of grounding our work in a new coherence.

The purpose of this article is twofold: (1) to discuss the history of pragmatism as a philosophical movement, and (2) to argue its relevance to the advancement of nursing knowledge and action in a postmodern world. Pragmatism is a way of "doing" philosophy that weaves together theory and action so that they intertwine, each modifying the other, continuously maintaining their mutual relevance.[2] In contrast to the criterion-based conception of reality, which creates a gulf between scientific objectivity and everyday human activity by its continual search for a defined "truth," the pragmatist conception of reality bridges that gap through inquiry that is a continual reweaving of different versions of the truth, one that incorporates new ideas and better explanations in the context of human encounters and activities. Pragmatism may be a means

for nursing to abandon stale theoretical and scientific debates that have inhibited our progress toward philosophical and clinical relevance.

Definition: Confusion and Clarification

The words pragmatism and pragmatic have been co-opted into common usage with meanings that have lost their original richness. Today, pragmatic is commonly used to mean practical or utilitarian. This association of pragmatic with practical assumes knowledge must be limited to promote action. But, as conceived by the early pragmatists, action is creative, complex, knowledgeable, and expansive; it is directed toward new applications of knowledge that bridge the gap between the "actual good and possible better."[9(p43)] The tendency for the term to be used only in its most basic sense of "practical" has separated pragmatism from its history and transformed it into a term of disparagement. A person who is considered pragmatic may also be thought atheoretical, narrow minded, and dogmatic. In actuality, in the philosophical sense of the word, a pragmatic person is very open minded and willing to listen to as many ideas or versions of the "truth" as possible to better solve problems.

History of Pragmatism

Pragmatism began as a uniquely American philosophical movement that appeared near the end of the 19th century, peaked in popularity just before World War II, and then lay dormant for 25 years. In 1977, pragmatism reemerged in a postmodern cloak as neopragmatism, largely because of the efforts of philosophers Richard Rorty at the University of Virginia in Charlottesville, Hilary Putnam at Harvard University in Cambridge, Massachusetts, and Richard Bernstein at the New School for Social Research in New York. As a philosophical movement, pragmatism has been evolutionary in nature, changing with each philosopher who contributes to its tenets. In its earliest stages in the 19th century, pragmatism was popularized by the work of three major philosophers, Charles Sanders Peirce, William James, and John Dewey. We briefly discuss the contributions of each to the development of both pragmatic thought and the pragmatic method below.

Pragmatism was first named by William James (1842–1910) in a lecture given at Berkeley in 1898. In this lecture James presented what he called Peirce's principle of pragmatism, giving Charles Sanders Peirce (1839–1914) credit as originator of the philosophical movement. In 1877, Peirce and several other scientists and philosophers formed the Metaphysical Club in Cambridge, Massachusetts. During discussions with James and others, Peirce began to piece together a method "for making ideas clear."[3(p109)] The earliest versions of pragmatic thought emphasized respect for the views of others and the notion that conversations, not dogma or universal truth, are the basis for developing beliefs.

After James had named this way of "doing" philosophy pragmatism in the Berkeley lecture, Peirce outlined the pragmatic method. This method involved carefully defining conceptual terms and then imagining the practical, ethical, and theoretical consequences of affirming or denying a concept. Unlike previous thought that emphasized definition and preset evaluative criteria, the pragmatic method emphasized that inherent in those *consequences* was the whole of the concept.

Although Peirce has been credited as being the originator of pragmatism, William James popularized the movement. James emphasized that pragmatism was a way of doing philosophy, a method of "settling metaphysical disputes that otherwise might be interminable."[1(p94)] Graduate students in nursing may appreciate James' descriptions of such disputes:

Is the world one or many? Fated or free? Material or spiritual? Disputes over such notions are unending. The pragmatic method in such cases is to try to interpret each notion by tracing its respective practical consequences. *What difference would it practically make to anyone if this notion were true?*[1(p96)]

James claimed pragmatism to be "anti-intellectualist." He believed rationalism to be pretentious, for pragmatism has no dogmas or doctrines, only method. James also coined the term "cash-value," a term that relates to the worthwhileness of a theory, meaning theories are only worth what they can be used for. He stated, "Theories thus become instruments, not answers to enigmas, in which we can rest. Pragmatism unstiffens all our theories, limbers them up and sets each one at work."[4(p27)] He describes this "work ethic" as the standard for value:

Pragmatism is willing to take anything, to follow either logic or the senses and to count *the humblest and most personal experiences*. She will count mystical experiences if they have practical consequences.[1(p111)]

James also tackled the notion of truth, heretically claiming that truths are plastic and made, rather than discovered by using the rigorous methods of science. James' work predated our postmodern relinquishment of the notion of universal truth, handed down by higher authority.

The philosopher John Dewey (1859–1952) was the final member of the founding triumvirate of pragmatism. Dewey was a student of Peirce at Johns Hopkins

University in Baltimore and later taught at the University of Chicago and Columbia University in New York. For Dewey, the essential feature of the pragmatic way of knowing was "to maintain the continuity of knowing with an activity which purposely modifies the environment."[5(p216)] For Dewey, reason was the ability to apply prior experience to a new experience, and a reasonable person kept an open mind.

Although denied entry into academic halls because of gender, Jane Addams (1860–1935) was also extremely influential in pragmatic thought. An early social worker and women's suffrage advocate, Addams opened Hull House, a settlement house that was a community service center for the poor in Chicago. She envisioned Hull House as a place of possibility, one where people, working together, could produce meaningful change. She viewed action as integral to life:

> The settlement stands for application as opposed to research; for emotion as opposed to abstraction, for universal interest as opposed to specialization . . . it is an attempt to express the meaning of life in terms of life itself, in forms of activity.[6(p276)]

Addams' life work exemplified the tenets of pragmatism by her willingness to value humble experiences and disciplinary pluralism, and to examine the ethical and practical consequences of an act.

Richard Rorty, Richard Bernstein, and the Pragmatic Revival

By the 1930s, the popularity of pragmatism appeared to wane. Existentialism, structuralism, Marxism, and psychoanalysis also emerged in the 1930s, and all of these schools of thought competed with pragmatism for public attention. In actuality, pragmatism did not disappear at all, but became so ingrained in the American way of life that its tenets were inherent in all of the major schools of thought and philosophical approaches.

Richard Rorty, a professor of humanities at the University of Virginia, is credited with the recent revival of pragmatism as a way of doing philosophy in the United States. This reemergence of pragmatic thought is popularly referred to as neopragmatism.[7] With the publication of *Philosophy and the Mirror of Nature* in 1979, Rorty successfully adapted pragmatism to the postmodern environment of the late 20th century:

> The aim . . . is to undermine the reader's confidence in the *mind* as something about which one should have a philosophical view, in *knowledge* as something about which there ought to be a theory and that has foundations and in *philosophy* as it has been conceived since Kant.[7(pxxxii)]

Rorty used irony to carry on the anti-intellectualist tradition of William James, and developed his own particular version of pragmatism that is tolerant of alternative views and humanistic, "not in the sense of trying to bring about something already defined, an essential human nature, but in the sense of *creating* something better than what we have known before."[8(p78)]

In 1987, Rorty described 20th century pragmatism as "new fuzziness,"[9] and claimed that pragmatism blurs the distinctions between objective and subjective and fact and value. See Table 28-1 for Rorty's version of pragmatism.[9]

Perhaps the most radical aspect of Rorty's work is a set of moral values, rather than preordained criteria, used by the new fuzzies as the basis for judgment of logic. These values include:

- tolerance
- respect for the opinions of those around us
- willingness to listen
- reliance on persuasion rather than force
- emphasis on communication over agreement or truth.

Rorty promotes broad intellectual tolerance and, above all, leaves room for alternative narratives.

> Rorty qualifies as a legitimate heir to the pragmatic tradition by virtue of his implicit focus on a problematic deeply embedded in the American experience: the fact and consequences of *plurality* in its psychological, social, and political forms.[10(p66)]

Table 28-1
Rorty and the New Pragmatism

Tenet	Explanation
No theory of truth, instead, an ethnocentric view of truth ("work by our own lights," no better lights to work from).	Humans are responsible only to our selves. Each person will hold as "true" those beliefs we find good to believe.[9(p42)] Ethnocentric view is that there is nothing to be said about truth separate from our own descriptions of procedures of justification.
Distinctions between objective/subjective, rational/irrational, true/false unhelpful.	Beliefs can be agreed upon without being true or rational in the methodological sense. The best way to find out what to believe is to listen to as many suggestions and arguments as possible, contrast our beliefs to proposed alternatives and choose that which offers the best solution or answer for that time, place, and situation—not that which is most true.
Redefine inquiry	Inquiry is a matter of "continually reweaving a web of beliefs"[9(p44)]—trying out new beliefs as they are ssuggested and incorporating or discarding them as we see fit. The goal of inquiry is the attainment of an appropriate mixture of unforced agreement with tolerant disagreement in a community which encourages "free and open encounters."[9(p44)]
Pragmatism has an *ethical* base, not an epistemological or metaphysical base.	Pragmatism depends on moral values or virtues for determination of what is reasonable: "tolerance, respect for the opinions of those around us, willingness to listen and reliance on persuasion rather than force."[9(p40)]
Disciplinary diversity is the goal.	All disciplines participate in cooperative human inquiry and all are equally objective if there is unforced agreement. "Fierce competition" between disciplines is vital.[9(p45)]
Redefine progress.	Progress cannot be judged by forward direction but by the fact of richer human activity, the opportunity for humans to do more interesting things and to be more interesting people.

The emphases on plurality and tolerance figure prominently in the works of another neopragmatist, Richard Bernstein. Professor of Philosophy at the New School for Social Research, Bernstein declines to identify a pragmatic essence or a set of propositions shared by all pragmatists, because " . . . there can be no escape from plurality—a plurality of traditions, perspectives, philosophic orientations."[11(p389)] Like Rorty, Bernstein suggests that disciplinary boundaries dissolve so that richer conversations can take place across them. He calls us to

nurture the type of community and solidarity where there is an engaged fallibilistic pluralism—one that

is based upon mutual respect, where we are willing to risk our own prejudgments, are open to listening and learning from other and we respond to others with responsiveness and responsibility.[11(p400)]

Narrative, or dialogue, is the method espoused by Bernstein for encounters between individuals and disciplines. He characterizes a community as "a group of individuals locked in an argument,"[12(p66)] and suggests that a vital pragmatism is "the ongoing process of being locked in argument."[12(p66)] The variety of voices constituting the narratives is the primary basis for vitality. Rather than truth, the reason for inquiry is the *application* and *usefulness* of beliefs held by a discipline.

The history of pragmatism is found in the writings of its founders. Peirce emphasized respect for all viewpoints and conversation as the pathway to developing beliefs. For James, pragmatism was not a philosophy in and of itself, but a way of settling disputes. James believed theories to be instruments, valued only for their utility. James also initiated the important emphasis on pluralism. Dewey added an educator's perspective with his approach to learning as doing, a way of applying experience to life. The neo-pragmatists Rorty and Bernstein revived the notion of narrative, tolerance for all viewpoints, and truth as what we *choose* to believe. They added an emphasis on communication and free and open encounters as methods to achieve interdisciplinary cooperation in human inquiry. Both philosophers remind us that pragmatism relies on an ethical base of moral values, rather than specific criteria to evaluate the worth of knowledge.

> We should relish the thought that the sciences as well as the arts will *always* provide a spectacle of fierce competition between alternative theories, movements, and schools. The end of human activity is not rest, but rather richer and better human activity. We should think of human progress as making it possible for human beings to do more interesting things and be more interesting people, not as heading toward a place which has somehow been prepared for us in the past.[9(p45)]

Pragmatism and Nursing

> the usefulness of theory . . . is ultimately answerable to those whose lives are supposed to be bettered by it.[13(p263)]

The tenets of pragmatism are not new to nursing. Nursing has always attended to the cash value or the worthwhileness of nursing theories to achieve desired results in clinical nursing. Clearly, nurses are interested in doing what works. Donaldson (1995) posits that nurse scholars and scientists who intend to build the discipline of nursing "keep in mind that the centrality

and value of this knowledge will be determined by the nurse pragmatist."[14(p6)] For Donaldson, a nurse pragmatist is willing to use any existing theory or knowledge relevant to the situation, "spanning distinct philosophies, paradigms, and disciplines."[14(p6)] For nursing science to be relevant, it must have utility, usually for the achievement of mutually determined clinical outcomes. For Donaldson, a nurse pragmatist is a nurse in practice, "one who is caring for patients and requires a useful knowledge base from which to make applications to "do" nursing."[14(p10)] Donaldson's discussion of the nurse pragmatist emerges from the early pragmatists' assertions of theories as instruments, learning by doing, and the notion of valuing interdisciplinary knowledge.

Although pragmatism seems embedded in the ideals and reality of nursing practice, it also has great utility for furthering the longstanding debates regarding nursing theory and research. In the following sections, we offer four noteworthy examples from the nursing literature that seem to use pragmatic ideals to solve problems in nursing science.

In a 1992 article, Schumacher and Gortner[15] discuss recent shifts in philosophy that replace the tenets of traditional, positivistic science with so-called scientific realism. Shumacher and Gortner move away from the old view that universal laws apply to all situations regardless of circumstance, to a view of science and research that takes into account the context of the phenomena under discussion. Discussing causality, they assert that the notion of causation in "human science is complex, multifaceted, and possibly multidirectional."[15(p7)] At the same time, they defend the traditional notion of causality, stating it is required to make science clinically relevant and because clinicians need to know "the likely consequences of certain events under given conditions."[15(p7)] This approach is pragmatic, illustrating a pluralistic approach that solves problems using ideas from both traditional positivistic science and scientific realism. Schumacher and Gortner weave their ideas into a conception of nursing science that they believe is relevant and useful for nursing. Our task in nursing becomes one of encouraging free and open encounters while listening to as many conversations as possible to discern the utility of Schumacher and Gortner's ideas for nursing.

Utility is also foremost in the 1995 treatise from Ford-Gilboe et al on the pragmatics of science in nursing.[16] The authors discuss the postpositivist, interpretive, and critical paradigms and the use of qualitative and quantitative methods. They conclude that combining strategies across paradigms enhances the value of a study. Ford-Gilboe et al, like Schumacher and Gortner, seem to believe that "good" nursing science is pragmatic. They expand their argument for a pragmatic nursing science by advocating the critical paradigm as an appropriate perspective for advancing nursing knowledge.[17] Under the umbrella of the critical paradigm, the authors propose methods for the purpose of accomplishing a "critical agenda"[17(p13)] to create knowledge that will be persuasive for the purpose of producing change. They emphasize respect for the opposing opinions and reliance on persuasion rather than force, both moral values inherent in pragmatism.

Missing from pragmatist writings is a comprehensive analysis of the inescapable power dynamics inherent in the process of communication. Henderson opens the conversation in nursing with a presentation of participatory action research as a research method that may reduce power hierarchies between researcher and researched.[18] She describes consciousness raising as a method that precedes other forms of data collection, for it is the format in which research takes place: "By engaging in critical and liberating dialogues, individuals uncover the hidden distortions within themselves that help to maintain an oppressive society."[18(p63)]

Critical and liberating dialogues, similar to Rorty's notion of free and open encounters, are both based in ethical notions of unshackled communication and tolerance for diversity. The ideals of feminism and critical theory could advance pragmatic tolerance by addressing power imbalances that create rifts between the researcher and the researched. The tolerant pragmatist would not object to this agenda as long as she can evaluate its value in the given situation.

Boyd also presents a structure for nursing research that is congruent with pragmatist ideals.[19] Boyd uses multiple approaches to research and emphasizes the utility of each approach for specific types of situations depending on context. Her ideas are pragmatic in their respect for pluralism and notions of theories as instruments. Boyd portrays nursing encounters as opportunities for communication and for constructing theories that will be useful in future encounters. For Boyd, nursing becomes a mutual search for both meaning and action, by "adding a research agenda to one's nursing work merely provides for the communication of what is learned so that other nurses, other patients may profit from it."[19(p20)]

Boyd's approach to nursing science is an example of a willingness to use the "humblest and most personal experiences"[1(p111)] to create a knowledge that is tolerant, inclusive, and contextual in nature.

Nursing at the Crossroads

In a discussion of shifting paradigms in the fields of bioethics and health law, Wolf[20] describes these fields as standing at a crossroads between

> the well trod road of conversations among experts, governed by top-down theory . . . abstract pronouncements, inattentive to differences . . . (and) a new more complex path, wide enough to accommodate multiple proposals and critiques as to method, willful attention to feminist, race-attentive and other contributions . . . teeming with people.[20(p415)]

Nursing stands at that same crossroads. The struggle for nursing science to find itself, to be able to name a tradition or paradigm into which nursing knowledge belongs, has proven interminable and impractical. As nursing science evolves into the millennium, an enhanced willingness to use knowledge from other disciplines and share that knowledge with all disciplines seems to be emerging in nursing.[21] As professional nursing matures, we welcome the fact that our old fascination with long-standing debates regarding appropriate methodologies and methods of inquiry in nursing seems to be waning. Pragmatism is an approach that holds promise for developing innovative and useful nursing knowledge in the future, and we would do well to heed Peirce's words: "The willful adherence to a belief and the arbitrary forcing of it upon others, must both be given up and a new method of settling opinions must be adopted."[3(p10)]

Writing on pragmatism and feminism, Seigfried[13] discusses the interrelationship of theory and practice in words that seem particularly relevant for nursing.

> emancipatory theory arises out of practice as much as it reflects back on it. It is a tool for directing practice, not a privileged insight into reality. As a tool it is instrumental to an outcome desired, rather than a hegemonic imposition of a predelineated order. Therefore, theories should be capable of revision as outcomes surpass or undercut expectations . . . The usefulness of theory, therefore is ultimately answerable to those who lives are supposed to be bettered by it.[13(p263)]

Nurse-philosopher Dr. Sally Gadow (unpublished poem, 1995) says words similar to those of Seigfried in a more poetic form:

Musings on Theory

Theory speaks as if a theorist's words are more
    true, more important,
than the words a particular patient and nurse will
    say with each other
in their experience together.
Ambiguity is the possibility for a different
    meaning: ambiguity is freedom.
Can theory have a different meaning?
Can theory emancipate instead of coerce, open
    instead of closing the door to meanings?
Can there be a critical theory?
I think so—if a theory is just another story,
    one meaning among many,
    without authority,
    always surpassed by the stories each
        nurse and patient compose in their
        situation together.*

---

* Courtesy of Dr. Sally Gadow © 1995.

Pragmatism is proposed as one way of assisting nursing to emerge from the old constraints of modernism, and begin to act on what is known, rather than act upon what has been told. No longer concerned only with the truth or falsity of a proposition or situation, nurses can begin to ask the pragmatists' question, "*What difference* would it make if this were true?" Pragmatism is a way of doing philosophy that weaves together theory and action, each continuously modifying the other and maintaining their mutual relevance.[2] Considering the immense ethical contradictions inherent in the theory and practice of nursing, pragmatism may be a means for nursing to move toward a higher level of philosophical and clinical relevance.

REFERENCES

1. James W. Pragmatism's conception of truth. In: Menand L, ed. *Pragmatism: A Reader.* New York: Vintage Books: 1997:94–131. (Original work by James written in 1907).
2. Mahowald MB. So many ways to think. An overview of approaches to ethical issues in geriatrics. *Clin Geriatr Med.* 1994;10(3):403–418.
3. Peirce C. The fixation of belief. In: Houser N, Kloesel C, eds. *The Essential Peirce: Selected Philosophical Writings, Vol. 1 (1867–1893).* Bloomington: Indiana University Press; 1992:109–123. (Original work by Peirce written in 1877).
4. James W. Pragmatism. In: Burckhardt F, ed. *The Works of William James: Pragmatism.* Cambridge, MA: Harvard University Press; 1975:20–30. (Original work by James published 1904).
5. Dewey J. Theories of knowledge. In: Menand L, ed. *Pragmatism: A Reader.* New York: Vintage Books; 1997: 205–218. (Original work by Dewey written in 1916).
6. Addams J. A function of the social settlement. In Menand L, ed. *Pragmatism: A Reader.* New York: Vintage Books; 1997:273–286. (Original work by Addams written in 1899).
7. Menand L, ed. An introduction to pragmatism. In: *Pragmatism: A Reader.* New York: Vintage Books: 1997: i-xxxiv.
8. Kolenda K. *Rorty's Humanistic Pragmatism.* Tampa: University of South Florida Press; 1990.
9. Rorty R. Science as solidarity. In: Nelson J, Megil A. McCloskey D. eds. *The Rhetoric of the Human Sciences: Language and Argument in Scholarship and Public Affairs.* Madison: University of Wisconsin Press. 1987: 38–52.
10. Hall DL. *Richard Rorty: Prophet and Poet of the New Pragmatism.* Albany, NY: State University of New York Press; 1994.
11. Bernstein RJ. Pragmatism, pluralism and the healing of wounds. In: Menand L. ed. *Pragmatism: A Reader.* New York: Vintage Books; 1997:382–401. (Original work by Bernstein written in 1988).

12. Bernstein, RJ. American pragmatism: The conflict of narratives. In: Saatkamp J. ed. *Rorty and Pragmatism*. Nashville. TN: Vanderbilt University Press; 1995:54–68.

13. Seigfried C. *Pragmatism and Feminism*. Chicago: University of Chicago Press: 1996.

14. Donaldson SK. Nursing science for nursing practice. In: Omery A, Kasper C, Page G, eds. *In Search of Nursing Science*. Thousand Oaks. CA: Sage Publications; 1995:3–12.

15. Schumacher K, Gortner S. (Mis)conceptions and reconceptions about traditional science. *Adv Nurs Sci*. 1992;14(4): 1–11.

16. Ford-Gilboe M, Campbell J, Berman H. Stories and numbers: coexistence without compromise. *Adv Nurs Sci*. 1995; 18(1):14–26.

17. Berman H, Ford-Gilboe M, Campbell J. Combining stories and numbers: A methodologic approach for a critical nursing science. *Adv Nurs Sci*. 1998;21(1):1–15.

18. Henderson D. Consciousness raising in participatory research: Method and methodology for emancipatory nursing inquiry. *Adv Nurs Sci*. 1995;17(3):58–69.

19. Boyd C. Toward a nursing practice research method. *Adv Nurs Sci*. 1993;16(2):9–25.

20. Wolf S. Shifting paradigms in bioethics and health law: The rise of a new pragmatism. *Am J Law Med*. 1994;20(4): 395–414.

21. Moody L. The quest for nursing science. In: Woody LE. ed. *Advancing Nursing Science through Research*. Newbury Park, CA: Sage Publications; 1990:15–46.

The Authors Comment

Bridging the Gulf Between Science and Action: The "New Fuzzies" of Neopragmatism

This article began as a class project for a course on the philosophy of nursing science taught by Carole Schroeder, my first attempt to write a scholarly paper after more than 20 years of practice as a nurse clinician. My need to find a way to bridge my own gulf between my past nursing practice and my hope for a relevant nursing science was clearly addressed by Rorty's writings and the philosophic tenets of neopragmatism that Dr. Schroeder presented in class. Together, we built upon the original class project by merging the ethical basis for pragmatism with the notion of emancipatory theory emerging from and reflecting back on nursing practice. This article presents an approach for development of nursing knowledge in the 21st century that argues for disciplinary postmodernity, diversity, free and open conversations, and tolerance of ambiguity. We hope that by adopting a neopragmatic approach to philosophy, nursing science will evolve beyond truth seeking and instead will find a way to interweave theory and action by developing knowledge that is ultimately "answerable to those whose lives are supposed to be bettered by it."

—CATHERINE ANN WARMS

—CAROLE A. SCHROEDER

Nursing's Syntax Revisited: A Critique of Philosophies Said to Influence Nursing Theories*

Susan R. Gortner

Lodged within the syntax of a discipline are the value systems and research constraints that influence theory development and research strategies. Humanism and postmodern philosophy have challenged natural science philosophical influences on nursing's syntax. This paper examines the construction of nursing's syntax from empiricist, hermeneuticist, feminist, and critical social theory views. In this critique, two requirements are placed on the world views: (1) they must accommodate theoretical (realist) terms important to nursing; and (2) they should provide explanatory power for these terms within nursing's disciplinary substance. Arguments are continued for a "within-the discipline" structure, a substantive and syntactical structure for the discipline of nursing that recognizes the centrality of biobehavioral processes in the practice of nursing [Gortner, IMAGE: J. Nurs. Scholarship 22, 101–105 (1990)].

Introduction

Over a decade ago Donaldson and Crowley (1978) presented a landmark paper before the Western Society for Nursing Research, on the structural and syntactical features of nursing as a discipline, following characterizations developed by Schwab (1964). They identified the "sub-stantive structure" as those conceptualizations, borrowed or invented, which are consonant with the perspective of

---

*Based on an invited paper presented at the First Symposium on Knowledge Development sponsored by the College of Nursing, University of Rhode Island, Newport Beach, U.S.A., 7 September 1990 and revised during a sabbatical as professeure invitée, faculté des sciences infirmières, Universite de Montréal, Canada, Spring 1991.

Reprinted from International Journal of Nursing Studies, *30(6), S. R. Gortner, Nursing's syntax revisited: A critique of philosophies said to influence nursing theories, 477–488. Copyright 1993 with permission from Elsevier Ltd.*

About the Author

After graduating from Stanford University in 1953 with an AB degree in social sciences, SUSAN REICHERT GORTNER enrolled in the generic master's program at Frances Payne Bolton School of Nursing, Case Western Reserve University, graduating with honors in 1957. She completed a PhD in higher education from the University of California, Berkeley, in 1964, which coincided with the births of her children. She relocated with her scientist husband to Maryland and joined the Division of Nursing as a health scientist administrator, first to evaluate the 1964 Nurse Training Act and later to serve as Branch Chief for Research and Research Training. She was the first Associate Dean for Research (Nursing) at the University of California, San Francisco (UCSF). Dr. Gortner's many honors and recognitions include Frances Payne Bolton School of Nursing Distinguished Alumna, UCSF Helen Nahm Research Lecturer, Fulbright Association Lecturer/Research Scholar in Norway (Oslo University), and, most recently, the American Academy of Nursing "Living Legend" award in 2001. Internationally known for her views on nursing science and research, she developed a collaborative program of research on cardiac surgery recovery, examining patient and family treatment choices and outcomes and recovery processes. Dr. Gortner was honored for this work by the National Center for Nursing Research (now NINR) and the American Heart Association. She lived full-time in the High Sierras in California and enjoyed summer and winter sports with her Border Collies. At the time of her death in February 2006, she had joined the Orvis School of Nursing as Endowed Chair to help faculty development in research.

the discipline; in contrast, the "syntax" of the discipline refers to "the research methodologies and criteria used to justify the acceptance of the statements as true within the discipline" (p. 119). Lodged within the syntax are the value systems and research constraints that influence theory generation and research designs; these "function to ensure that enquiry will result in conclusions and statements that are appropriate, valid, and reliable for the purpose of the discipline" (p. 119). Theories are both descriptive and prescriptive in this scheme, as shown in Figure 29-1, and intercept the substance and the syntax in Donaldson and Crowley's representation.

Both the substance and syntax, as the structural elements of the discipline, can reflect the nursing perspective of humanism and concern with the whole person. Yet this perspective can be problematic for the development of the discipline, since holism stands in direct opposition to objectivism and its associated reductionism. Accordingly social philosophy has become increasingly popular as a conceptual base for contemporary nursing. Natural science philosophy, including the philosophy of biology, appears now to have little conceptual value for nursing so that the associated view of humans as living organisms or entities is being supplanted by the view of humans as social beings. Hermeneutics has been proposed as an alternative syntax for the discipline, along with feminism and/or critical social theory and other non-naturalistic world views (Allen, 1985; Moccia, 1988; Benner and Wrubel, 1989; Holden, 1990; Holmes, 1990). What will these modifications of syntax accomplish for nursing as an emerging disciplinary field? How will the questions of substance be formulated and pursued? This is an issue first identified by Donaldson and Crowley in the conclusion of their 1978 paper and subsequently emphasized by Meleis (1987) nearly a decade later. Should particular phenomenological social philosophies continue their ascendancy in nursing, there will be ontological as well as epistemological consequences. The belief systems or ontologies may disallow reality outside of the human, the existence of biobehavioral patterns and regularities, and even theories. The belief systems or ontologies will determine the nature of explanations about phenomena, and whether explanations can become generalizations or not (Collin, 1992).

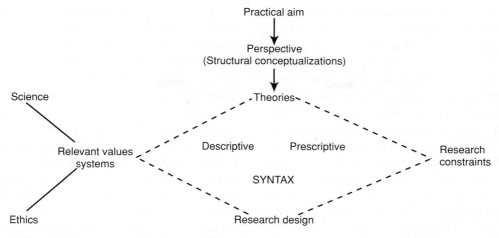

Figure 29-1 *Structure of a professional discipline.*

The purpose of this paper is to re-examine construction of the syntax (the value systems and research constraints), from empiricist, hermeneutic, feminist and critical social theory views. In this examination two requirements will be placed on the world views, in keeping with the author's scientific orientation. The requirements are that world views should accommodate theoretical (realist) terms important to nursing, and they should provide explanatory power for these terms within nursing's disciplinary substance.[1] Scientific realism maintains that theoretical terms and abstractions arising from scientific work exist, refer to the real world, and may or may not be true (Boyd, 1984). Explanatory power is the capacity of a set of propositions not only to account for a given event but to generalize to other events of the same set. Explanations therefore need to be nomothetic (that is law-like or general) as well as idiosyncratic (specific to the case, the particular, the singular). Explanations must cover the phenomena ["save the phenomena" in the van Fraasen (1980) terminology] and also predict what might happen the next time the same set of circumstances occurs (a traditional feature of scientific explanations). In the critique offered in this paper, arguments will continued for a "within-the-discipline" structure, a substantive and syntactical structure for the discipline of nursing that recognizes the centrality of biobehavioral processes in the practice of nursing (Gortner, 1990).

Origins of the Critique

Identification of supposed positivistic influences on nursing's syntax (i.e. theory and research) appears to have arisen from the Suppe and Jacox (1985) critique of nursing theories, in which the requirement of operationalization is said to be positivistic. Jacox subsequently has acknowledged that her earlier writings on theory development (Jacox, 1974) were unduly influenced by positivism. Interestingly, neither Whall (1989) or Meleis (1991) could find direct evidence of positivistic influence on nursing practice (Whall) or theory (Meleis), although Whall (personal communication, 1991) has observed that the "truth criteria" (i.e. are the relationships empirically verifiable)

---

[1] Hesook Kim comments on these requirements, noting that scientific realism and explanatory power "represent major value systems of sciences that have contributed to the empiricist view of scientific knowledge." She suggests that hermeneutics, feminist (relativist) and critical social theory propose a different syntax. Donna Wells agrees, noting that the expectation of scientific realism for nursing's syntax construction gives "immediate primacy to a world view of empiricism." My contention is that these requirements, or some variation thereof, should be imposed on those views proposing a different syntax, to illustrate consequences and to aid in the choice of syntax. I would agree with Wells some conjoint view would be an improvement, as against a primordial view (one asserting primacy).

proposed for evaluation of nursing theories had positivistic overtones. Other critiques of natural science and positivistic science orientations have come from critical social theorists in nursing (Thompson, 1985, 1987; Allen, 1985; Moccia, 1988), from proponents of phenomenological and interpretive views (Benner, 1985; Benner & Wrubel, 1989; Leonard, 1989) and from some nursing philosophers who advocate caring as the leitmotif of nursing (Gadow, 1980; Eriksson, 1990; Newman et al., 1991).

These criticisms contain a central theme that positivism is antithetical to nursing's disciplinary orientation, an orientation or perspective that is framed by humanistic concepts, values and practices. Because of these humanistic intentions, it is argued that the research needs to be humanistic. The position that philosophical viewpoints necessarily should guide and direct research strategy may be termed the "purist" position. The "nonpurist" position has argued for theoretical and methodological pluralism, and toward a consensus regarding nursing philosophy of science (Gortner, 1990; Nagle and Mitchell, 1991). Still another position, "the radical separationist thesis," has been offered by Suppe at a knowledge development symposium (Suppe, 1990). This position argues that a discipline's theory and research are distinct and not necessarily congruent in philosophy (humanistic) and strategy (empiricist or phenomenological). Epistemology provides "no evidential role" for knowledge claims; rather philosophy can play a role in credentialing knowledge claims, a process of legitimatizing the claim into the shared body of information the discipline accepts and uses.[2] This position would allow humanism to be the dominant nursing perspective while allowing scientists to engage other themes and inquiry forms at various levels of analysis (Suppe, 1990).[3]

The stakes are high, for the arguments strike at the very belief systems of nursing scholarship and how we credential, accept as legitimate, the discoveries arising from scholarly work. How will we decide which is the more important question: "How is it that we know?", "What do we know?" or "What does it mean to be a person?" (patient or nurse). The first two questions have been the heart of Ph.D. training in the discipline. The third is raised by those advocating moral, social and political foundations for nursing's epistemology. How we respond will determine whether our conceptualizations can be microanalytic (e.g. cellular, biological) as well as microanalytic (e.g. social or cultural), whether the syntax can be objective and logical as well as interpretive and reflective, and whether we can model the human system/state at various levels (e.g. cell, organ, system) or rest with meanings and motives within the context of culture and society.[4]

Positivism/Empiricism

Suppe and Jacox's (1985) essay on philosophic influences on nursing theory development appears to be the major source for contentions that nursing theory has been influenced by positivism. Whether this contention of influence is accurate, despite assertions in our literature that it is, would depend on evidence that we don't have and preferably would have to be garnered from the theorists themselves. At the conference where this paper was originally presented, both Hesook Suzie Kim and Callista Roy were present; neither acknowledged the supposed influence of positivism on their own writings. Kim believes (personal communication, 1991) that the logical positivist influence on early theoretical works in nursing was selective and circumspective rather than dogmatic. Indeed, the reference by theoreticians to propositions and terms that are capable of empirical demonstration and testability might better reflect a (scientific) realist position rather than a logical positivistic or antirealist position. This skepticism about supposed

---

[2] In her review of this paper, Kim notes that credentialing knowledge claims is a function of syntax, again supporting the importance of syntactical arguments for the discipline.

[3] Ann Whall's response to the "radical separationist thesis" is that such separation would make for a "very disparate and conflicting knowledge base"; perhaps this is what nursing has at present, but "is it a valid and worthy goal?". Probably not, but it does reflect current reality. Could the theories be reframed in the light of the evidence, I ask?

[4] Wells comments that more than meaning and motives would result: patterns of health and illness might be revealed through such examination, aiding explanation as well as understanding.

positivistic influences prompted Whall to examine American nursing practice guides for the period 1950–1970; she failed to find evidence of positivistic influence and commented that it was strange, indeed, to have purported influence in one sector (theory) and not in the other (practice) (Whall, 1989).

In portrayals of philosophical positions, it is important to bear in mind that old distinctions no longer suffice. Much of the critique of positivism has been rendered against the form known as logical positivism, and the Vienna Circle. That form of positivism is no longer extant, and to continue to reference it (e.g. Sarnecky, 1990) is to ignore its demise in the late '60s (Glymour, 1980; Hacking, 1981; Schumacher & Gortner, 1992). Even in Benner and Wrubel's recent portrayal, positivism is equated with empiricism and illustrated through a mechanistic, reductionist principle: "the complex can be best understood in terms of its basic atomic components, components that bear no intrinsic relation to one another" (Benner and Wrubel, 1989, p. 32). This statement about contemporary empiricist views regarding the process of science continues fallacious equivocations of empiricism with reductionism, atomism, and quantification. There is no historical basis for the association of positivism with quantification; statistical theory and practices arose not from philosophy but from agricultural science.

Rather there is a postpositivistic view, a contemporary empiricist view (Schumacher & Gortner, 1992; Gortner & Schultz, 1988; Norbeck, 1986) that continues belief in observables, in careful scientific strategies that bear results that can be corroborated if not confirmed. This modern view has arisen in part through the historicist criticism of Kuhn (1970), Lakatos (1970), Laudan (1977) and others, including the positivists themselves. Contemporary empiricism recognizes the fallacies of the principle of verification, the impossibility of separating fact from theory and thus of making scientific endeavors antirealist (as the logical positivists attempted), acknowledges the theory-ladeness of observation and experience, and does not differentiate the context of discovery from justification in scientific work. Modern empiricists, along with clinical scientists, are concerned with com-

plex phenomenon, some of which can be reduced and partitioned for study and some of which cannot. What guides a research program is a significant problem area, as for example pain or recovery or caregiving strain or postpartal depression, for which explanation and understanding are sought. Extant theory is used generally, hence the hypothetico deductive terminology. Yet generative theory is not ruled out; in fact Roy's experience with brain damaged adults during her Robert Wood Johnson Clinical Nurse Scholar's program is credited with the revisions and adjustments made subsequently in her theoretical position. Her work reflects clearly the thinking of an empiricist scholar (Roy, 1989).

In the following features are reflected the strengths of empiricist scholarship: (1) specification of factors assumed to be key to understanding and explanation of the phenomenon under study and (2) the expectation for theory testing and theory generation. Inherent is the belief that the event under study can be modelled or "objectified" (Schumacher & Gortner, 1992). The relevant syntax for nursing would consist of (a) generalized knowledge based on explanation of kind-phenomena; (b) human phenomena objectively identifiable and observable; and (c) predictions as well as explanation (Kim, personal communication, 1991; Schumacher & Gortner, 1992).

Because of this expectation, contemporary empiricism has the capacity for explanation that is so necessary for clinical practice. The observables (mood state, vital signs, laboratory and radiographic findings) must be linked with the unobservables, those normal and abnormal physiological and psychological processes to suggest causal factors and thus treatment. The efficacy of treatment is judged in terms of outcomes. Clinical practice has become more scientific and technologically dependent because of the need for identifying increasingly complex patient states (presumptive and competing diagnoses), which require prolonged periods of observation and assessment because of their complexity, and for which multiple therapies are needed. Acute care practitioners continually confront these complexities. Their scientific and clinical judgments are analytical, logical and empirical as often as they are intuitive and interpretive.[5,6] The latter forms of reasoning inform and extend the former, but generally lack specificity and logic. They answer the what of the phenomenon, not the why which is the impetus for therapeutic action. They also provide the equivalent of hypothetical counterarguments or counterfactuals, to support or weaken the clinical or scientific explanation.

Empiricism then is criticized for the very features that have made it the mainstay of scientific work. It is particularly relevant for the biological and behavioral sciences, for explicating fundamental human processes of biological and behavioral origin. It has appeal for subspecialties in acute and critical care, in which the human state is objectified and monitored painstakingly. It forces upon the investigator precision, caution and skepticism about outcomes; it seeks associations between theory and fact, acknowledging the importance of *a priori* propositions and hypothesized causal processes.

In the author's view, empiricism has been given short shrift in nursing, because of continued fallacious identification with logical positivism, because of lack of familiarity with primary sources on the perspective, and because of the critiques rendered by hermeneuticists, phenomenologists, and critical social theorists. Our historical reliance on the social sciences for our scientific base contributes to the anti-empiricist or anti-naturalist argument.[7] Also contributing to the critique of positivism is our inclination to adopt a philosopher of the month (Kuhn was our first white knight, followed by Laudan, Habermas, Toulmin and Foucault). We might take seriously Suppe's recent admonition not to take philosophy as dogma (Suppe, 1990).[8]

Hermeneutics

Hermeneutics has a century old tradition in continental philosophy (Palmer, 1969), and together with humanism is gaining appreciable interest in North American circles, especially in departments of philosophy, education, and social science (e.g. Phillips, 1987; Rosenberg, 1988). The reasons for this development are several, not the least of which is belief that the human world is one distinctly different from the natural world. Literary and artistic works are uniquely human creations, societies and cultures are human creations and so, goes the reasoning, are human responses to health and illness. Dilthey was one of the foremost proponents of a distinct human science philosophy in the last century; his "Geisteswissenschaften" was an attempt to set in place an epistemology for the human sciences that would complement that of natural science "Naturwissenshaften" (Dilthey, 1988):

> "The goals of the human sciences—to lay hold of the singular and the individual in historico-social reality; to recognize uniformities operative in shaping the singular; to establish goals and rules for its continued development—can be attained only by the devices of reason: analysis and abstraction" (Dilthey, p. 27).

This perspective on historical consciousness and the value of humanistic and historical knowledge in understanding human existence was an important contribution to understanding and explanation. Dilthey's hermeneutics reflect an accommodation of the "scientific" and the "human"; his anti-naturalism appears less fundamental and dogmatic than that of Heidegger (1962), who took an ontological rather than an epistemological turn with his conception of "Dasein" (Palmer, 1969). It is the power of the ontological senti-

---

[5] Kim comments that this argument "suggests immediate linkages between 'idiosyncratic' features of practice and nomothetic/theoretical knowledge of science."

[6] Whall argues that nursing models need to incorporate physiological patterns as well as organismic relationships; valuing of one over the other will produce variations in outcomes and explanations that are insufficient or incomplete (Fitzpatrick & Whall, 1989, p. 11).

[7] Wells takes issue with this statement, noting that the social sciences have long believed that only empiricist methods will lead to progress in their disciplines. That the critical social theorist arguments were as much against scientism as against positivism is an important observation. I castigate contemporary empiricism and its proponents for the continuing equation of "good science" with "good method." This narrow view of science and scientific quality constrains novel designs and methods and accepts warrantable evidence more readily from programs of biomedical science than those of clinical or social science.

---

[8] Was Suppe "right" or "reasonable," asks Wells. When do we turn to philosophy and under what conditions?

ment of "being as being" (Palmer, 1969) that has brought hermeneutics close to the philosophical orientations of phenomenology, existentialism, and even critical theory. Indeed, the language and semantics requires disciplehood, making intersubjectivity difficult except among disciples (a phenomenon called "communicative entropy" by Suppe, 1990). Further, some proponents of Heidegerrian philosophy have operationalized features as method, contributing to the development of new scholars as well as to programs of scholarship of their own. There are several tenets of contemporary hermeneutics that have influenced nursing theorists and scholars: the appreciation of the human state or essence as supreme; the interactive circle ("hermeneutic circle") between patient and nurse or subject and scientist; shared meaning and embedded meaning, and self-reflection and understanding ("Verstehen") as the basis of knowing.[9] There is a common requirement of social discourse, generating a text or historical record for analysis.

Nursing theories increasingly address biology, behavior, and culture, frequently in interface with one another. They depict associations among factors and may suggest explanatory variables for human health and illness. Some require partitioning, objectification, and specification of relationships, hypothetical and real. The entire area of ecological knowledge known epidemiologically as "host factors" (or "risk factors") cannot be accommodated in a hermeneutic or phenomenology perspective. Human ecology requires identification of an antecedent state in the host/human, interrupting the process of lived experience which is continuous, has no antecedent or consequent, and is the "unit of analysis." Ideologically, hermeneutics captures the ethic of caring identified with nursing; it serves history, sociology, and art well; in this respect, it can frame the artform of nursing in rich and meaningful dimensions. It can frame the nature of human suffering, human health, human recovery in terminology

that can enrich human understanding and thus discourse between sufferer, loved ones and clinicians. Because it will not objectify the human state or model it, it cannot supplant empiricism in explanatory power, only in understanding. Syntax based on this view would value contextual knowledge and understanding from the agent's perspective (Collin, 1992).

Had Dilthey pre-empted Heidegger in the nursing literature, might we have seen more accommodation of the empirical/historical in our writings? Our arguments around philosophies appropriate for the natural or human sciences appear to be classically American (Gortner, 1990). Colleagues elsewhere in northern Europe employ the Diltheyan "Geisteswissenschaften" in their scholarship and are not troubled by an apparent incongruity of philosophy and method as are we. They would appear to illustrate the Suppean "radical separationist thesis."

Feminism and Critical Social Theory

Rational philosophies employing feminist perspectives and critical social theory increasingly challenge traditional epistemology in a number of fields, including the social sciences (Marshall, 1988) and nursing (Allen, 1985; Thompson, 1987; Holter, 1988; Moccia, 1988; Campbell & Bunting, 1991). While these views have quite distinct origins and hold a variety of current positions, they have in common an emphasis on the subjective, on the social construction of reality, on socio-political and economic influences on science, and on the prevalence of racism and sexism in scientific as well as social activities. In recognition of these oppressive mechanisms, both views have an emancipatory purpose with that of critical social theory emphasizing the collective, the aggregate rather than the personal and individual. Here the commonalities cease and distinctions become important.

Critical social theory arose in Germany, specifically in Frankfurt, as a philosophical reaction to early 20th century positivism and natural science and to

---

[9] This requirement and that of the hermeneutic circle, joining investigator and subject, eliminates virtually all of basic biology as a potential scientific base for nursing; does it disenfranchise basic nurse scientists from engaging in theory development and criticism within nursing?

traditional Marxism (Habermas, 1971; Marshall, 1988; Holter, 1988). Assumptions of critical social theory have been stated by Holter (1988), Stevens (1989) and Campbell and Bunting (1991) for the nursing audience. These hold that all research and theory are socio-political constructions, that human societies are inherently oppressive, and that all world interpretations (mythical, religious, scientific, practical and political) are open to criticism (Stevens, 1989). Perhaps the most powerful feature of contemporary critical theory is in the capacity and mandate for the critique; this emphasis on rationality is contrasted with the emphasis on relations, feelings and emotions among some feminist thinkers. While most contemporary scientists would acknowledge the need to consider the political and social consequences of their inquiry, there is not agreement that these features must be part of regular scientific activity (even though it is acknowledged that all theories reflect underlying ideologies and "truth" claims as an anonymous reviewer of this paper has pointed out). Opinions vary on the extent to which scientists should be obligated to consider the socio-political frameworks of their studies. In this respect critical scholars are "up front" in stating clearly for the reader the inherent assumptions governing a given investigation. Critical theorists and critically inclined scientists take seriously the charge for action; for them inquiry is incomplete without the consequential and liberating act. In this key feature critical social theory can become the basis for political and social action; for nursing situations involving group processes and societal organization, the dialectic as rationality and method is appropriate and creative. As rationality, critical theory provides a multidimensional lens for scholarship; as method it requires that oppositional and/or under-represented views on a given problem area are specifically represented. Syntax would acknowledge knowledge as action based.

The number of studies employing critical social theory as perspective is growing in nursing and related fields. As the findings are published and subject to scrutiny (to the process of legitimization and credentialing), the quality of the investigations will be judged.

It is important that the style of presentation and argument be such as to encourage the intended discourse and debate rather than overwhelm and alienate intended audiences. In nursing's literature, critical rationality has taken a more moderate form of expression than was the case several years ago. Yet the requirement for social and liberating action remains and is one of the features this author finds troubling, especially for novice scholars. Why? Because if one knows ahead of time that one is going to undertake social action, then one does not need to carry out the justifying research. One can act as social and autonomous agent without the benefit of science.

Another feature that is troubling is the lack of modeling, and theory respecification, given the stated dissatisfaction with classical social and economic theories. Critical social theory has social, political and economic relations as the units of analysis. This feature has made its empirical application limited to date in our field. So the expectations of realism and explanatory power have yet to be demonstrated. Perhaps a new theory of rationality could be forged, incorporating some of the assumptions of postempiricist philosophy.

The feminist critique of society and science has many of the features of critical social theory, but places its emphasis on the world of women in a male dominated society (patriarchy). It shares with hermeneutics the belief in lived experience and history as the basis of knowing, generating and using language for documentation and analyses. As such it also has a requirement for social discourse and reflexivity among competent persons, presented in the context of the social situation with attendant embedded meanings. Feminist literature in nursing is seen in the writings of MacPherson (1983), Chinn and Wheeler (1985), Duffy (1985), Bunting and Campbell (1990), and Campbell and Bunting (1991). Feminist scholarship appears to be enlarging in nursing theory and research, representing liberal, cultural and radical views, which need to be differentiated for uninformed audiences. Central to the radical view is the belief that oppression (due to the patriarchy) is fundamental and pervasive; here the similarity to critical social theory is clear. Yet one perspective is based in social philosophy, and the other is moving to philosophical statements from sociopolitical arguments. Until recently, critical social theory and feminist theory were not examined for their similarities in social statements, assumptions and methodologies. Several thoughtful comparisons are now available from authors such as Marshall (1988) and Campbell and Bunting (1991). Both perspectives have too heavy a reliance on social relations and actions to serve nursing exclusively. On the other hand, feminism is attractive and meaningful for nursing as a predominantly female profession. Analyses such as that provided by McCormick (1989) and Lips (1989) can provide insights into how nursing science can contribute to improved understanding of human behavior in health and illness without forfeiting science values and strategies. Differences among men and women in moral and scientific reasoning have been demonstrated (Gilligan, 1982) as have gender differences in recovery from illness or treatment (e.g., cardiac surgery) (Rankin, 1990). Would a theory of gender be a major contribution, as Marshall (1988) suggests? Perhaps if it includes the "rapport de force," the social context in which gender is examined (Perreault, 1991). Whether feminist and critical social theory will become part of nursing syntax will depend less on the splendor of the rhetoric and more on the quality of the research and the extent to which the studies have interdisciplinary appeal.

Recapitulation

This critique has set the dual notions of scientific realism and explanatory power as requirements for nursing's developing syntax. Admittedly, these notions reflect empiricist traditions, although they need not be so represented in the position taken by this author. No single world view should have primacy in our syntax; rather the consequences of particular world views for substantive theory development in nursing science need to be considered. The anti-naturalistic positions found within hermeneutics, critical social theory and some feminist views impose limitations on human

science development even more consequential than those of empiricism and empirical inquiry.[10] Common to the hermeneutic position is the foundational place of human agency, an intensionality that has no reality outside the context of the lived experience. Central to the feminist and critical theory arguments is the foundational place of domination (in gender, social class, work place) and emancipation. These features of humanity, gender, class and society are appropriate to contemporary social science and to nursing, in so far as it is a social science. But nursing is not exclusively a social science. It has a biological science component, which it will continue to incorporate in its disciplinary structure until such time as it decides to be an exclusively social activity. Nursing will not be served well by substituting social determinism for biological determinism, any more than feminists will be so served (Marshall, 1988). We are biological as well as social beings; our cell structures and biochemistry exhibit regularities over and over; our social actions barring catastrophes tend to be more regular than otherwise. What is normative for the individual is just that, and should represent "baseline" for contrast against which to judge severity of illness or recovery.

Nursing theories must incorporate the relevant domains, including biology as well as individual and social action and specify the hypothesized links with reality that will encourage theory testing and expansion. Only one of the competing world views, hermeneutics, specifically disallows modeling of the human. In this respect, hermeneutics is an antirealist in its position as was logical positivism earlier in this century. Just as logical positivism expired by virtue of its own constraints, so too may hermeneutics if it disallows realism and explanations beyond the subjective. As Collin has argued recently (1992), an interpetive (hermeneutic) nursing science

---

[10] Antinaturalist is being used here in its original philosophical sense of being distinct from natural science (thus making inappropriate the methodology of natural science for study of the person). Hermeneutics and critical theory are decidedly antinaturalistic given this definition; radical feminism is as well. Hermeneutics also is antirealist, in that the world view does not allow belief in theoretic entities (noumena) external to the lived world.

does not allow theoreticity or the building of theoretical constructs outside of the person and lived experience. A "normative" science structure would, and would use what Collin calls a "third-person" stance to explain "particular quirks in the patient's self-conceptions. Such theories would be causal theories, and we would want them to describe the mechanisms behind distorted self-conception in a way which is both conceptually simple and of general application" (Collin, 1992, p. 23). In essence the case is being made for nomothetic as well as idiographic understandings and explanations. Further, nursing is defined not as idiographic activity but as "individualizing activity" (p. 18), for which theorizing and specifically scientific theorizing is appropriate. "Generalized knowledge will be indispensable in the process of understanding the individual case" (p. 18). For disciplinary fields must build theories about the stuff and substance that intrigues them: for nursing it is the human state during illness and in health, the ecology of human health across the life span. We have acknowledged our need for prescriptive theories, in addition to descriptive ones (Gortner, 1984). Our developing syntax must hold that need intact.

Acknowledgments The author is indebted to Hesook Suzie Kim, Professor of Nursing at the University of Rhode Island, Ann Whall, Professor of Nursing at the University of Michigan, Donna Wells, Assistant Professor of Nursing at the University of Toronto and an anonymous reviewer for their careful readings of earlier versions of this paper. Philosopher of science Frederick Suppe's paper immediately preceded the presentation of the original paper; his observations about 'invisible colleges,' 'credentialling' of knowledge claims, and the 'radical separationist thesis' were important additions to the author's thinking. Colleague and professor of philosophy at the University of California, Riverside, Alex Rosenberg, reviewed the substantive critiques of the world views and reassured the author that her criticisms were valid as presented. Finally, the continued interest of colleagues Karen Schumacher, Inger Margrethe Holter and Afaf Meleis in the author's writings on philosophy of science is gratefully acknowledged. They have been compatriots in the quest for nursing's scientific philosophy and have provided immeasurable assistance.

REFERENCES

Allen, D. (1985). Nursing research and social control: alternative modes of science that emphasize understanding and emancipation. *IMAGE: J. Nurs. Scholarship 17*, 58–64.

Benner, P. (1985). Quality of life: a phenomenological perspective on explanation, prediction and understanding in nursing science. *Adv. Nurs. Sci. 8*, 1–16.

Benner, P. and Wrubel, J. (1989). *The primacy of caring: stress and coping in health and illness.* Addison-Wesley, Menlo Park, CA.

Boyd, R. N. (1984). The current status of scientific realism. In *Scientific Realism* (Leplin, J., Ed.), pp. 41–82. University of California Press, Berkeley, CA.

Bunting, S. and Campbell, J. J. (1990). Feminism and nursing: historical perspectives. *Adv. Nurs. Sci. 12*, 11–24.

Campbell, J. C. and Bunting, S. (1991). Voices and paradigms. Perspectives on critical and feminist theory in nursing. *Adv. Nurs. Sci. 13*, 1–15.

Chinn, P. L. and Wheeler, C. E. (1985). Feminism and nursing. *Nurs. Outlook 33*, 74–77.

Collin, F. (1992). Nursing science as an interpretive discipline: problems and challenges. *Vard I Norden 12*, 14–23.

Dilthey, W. (1988). *Introduction to the Human Sciences. An attempt to lay a foundation for the study of society and history* (Betanzos, R. J., Translator). Wayne State University Press, Detroit, MI.

Donaldson, S. and Crowley, D. (1978). The discipline of nursing. *Nurs. Outlook 26*, 113–120.

Duffy, M. (1985). A critique of research: a feminist perspective. *Health Care for Women Int. 6*, 341–352.

Eriksson, K. (1990). Systematic and contextual caring science. A study of the basic motive of caring and contest. Nursing science in a Nordic perspective. *Scand. J. Caring Sci. 4*, 3–5.

Fitzpatrick, J. A. and Whall, A. (1989). *Conceptual models of nursing: Analysis and application,* 2nd Ed. Robert J. Brady, Co. Bowie, MD.

Fraasen, B. C. van (1980). *The scientific image.* Clarendon Press, Oxford.

Gadow, S. (1980). Existential advocacy. Philosophical foundations of nursing. In *Nursing: Images and Ideals* (Stuart, E. and Gadow, S., Eds). Springer Publishing, New York, NY.

Gilligan, C. (1982). *In a Different Voice.* Harvard University Press, Cambridge, MA.

Glymour, C. (1980). Logical empiricist theories of confirmation. In *Theory and evidence,* pp. 10–62. Princeton University Press, Princeton, NJ.

Gortner, S. R. (1984). Knowledge in a practice discipline: philosophy and pragmatics. In *Nursing Research and Policy Formation: The Case of Prospective Payment.* Papers of the 1983 Scientific Session of the American Academy of Nursing (pp. 5–17). American Academy of Nursing, Kansas City, MO.

Gortner, S. R. (1990). Nursing values and philosophy: toward a science philosophy. *IMAGE: J. Nurs. Scholarship 22*, 101–105.

Gortner, S. R. and Schultz, P. R. (1988). Approaches to nursing science methods. *IMAGE: J. Nurs. Scholarship 20*, 22–24.

Habermas, J. T. (1971). *Knowledge and Human Interests* (Shapiro, J., Translator). Beacon Press, Boston, MA.

Hacking, I. (1981). *Scientific Revolutions*. Oxford University Press, Oxford.

Hagell, E. I. (1989). Nursing knowledge: women's knowledge. A sociological perspective. *J. Adv. Nurs. 14*, 226–233.

Heidegger, M. (1962). *Being and Time* (Macquarrie J. and Robinson, E., Translators). Harper & Row, New York, NY.

Holden, R. J. (1990). Models, muddles, and medicine. *Int. J. Nurs. Stud. 27*, 223–234.

Holmes, C. A. (1990). Alternatives to natural science foundations for nursing. *Int. J. Nurs. Stud. 27*, 187–198.

Holter, I. M. (1988). Critical theory: a foundation for the development of nursing theories. *Schol. Inq. Nurs. Prac. 2*, 223–232.

Jacox, A. (1974). Theory construction in nursing: an overview. *Nurs. Res. 23*, 4–13.

Kuhn, T. (1970). Introduction II, the route to normal science; I, The nature of normal science. In *Structure of Scientific Revolutions* (Kuhn, T., Ed.), pp. 1–34. University of Chicago Press, Chicago, IL.

Lakatos, I. (1970). Falsification and the methodology of scientific research programmes. In *Criticism and the Growth of Knowledge* (Lakatos, I. and Musgrave, A., Eds), pp. 91–196. Cambridge University Press, Cambridge.

Laudan, L. (1977). *Progress and its Problems*. University of California Press, Berkeley, CA.

Leonard, V. W. (1989). A Heideggerian phenomenologic perspective on the concept of person. *Adv. Nurs. Sci. 11*, 40–55.

Lips, H. (1987). Toward a new science of human being and behavior. In *The Effects of Feminist Approaches on Research Methodologies* (Tomm, W., Ed.), pp. 51–69. Wilfrid Laurier Press, Waterloo, Ontario.

MacPherson, K. I. (1983). Feminist methods: A new paradigm for nursing. *Adv. Nurs. Sci. 5*, 17–25.

Marshall, B. L. (1988). Feminist theory and critical theory. *Can. Rev. Sociol. Anthropol. 25*, 208–230.

McCormick, T. (1989). Feminism and the new crisis in methodology. In *The Effects of Feminist Approaches on Research Methodologies* (Tomm, W., Ed.), pp. 13–31. Wilfrid Laurier Press, Waterloo, Ontario.

Meleis, A. I. (1987). Revisions in knowledge development: a passion for substance. *Schol. Inq. Nurs. Prac. I*, 5–19.

Meleis, A. I. (1991). *Theoretical Nursing*, 2nd Edn. Lippincott, Philadelphia.

Moccia, P. (1988). A critique of compromise: beyond the methods debate. *Adv. Nurs. Sci. 10*, 1–9.

Nagle, L. M. and Mitchell, G. J. (1991). Theoretic diversity: evolving paradigmatic issues in research and practice. *Adv. Nurs. Sci. 14*, 17–25.

Newman, M. A., Sime, A. M. and Corcoran-Perry, S. A. (1991). The focus of the discipline of nursing. *Adv. Nurs. Sci. 14*, 1–6.

Norbeck, J. (1986). In defense of empiricism. *IMAGE: J. Nurs. Schol. 19*, 28–30.

Palmer, R. E. (1969). *Hermeneutics. Interpretation Theory in Schleiermacher, Dilthey, Heidegger, and Gadamer*. Northwestern Press, Evanston, IL.

Perreault, M. (1990). Les rapports sociaux de sexe comme fondement d'analyse. Commentaire critique du texte de Gladys Simons "Les femmes-cadres dans l'univers bureaucratique." Sous presse dans le cadre du colloque international: "L'Individu dans l'organization: les dimensions oubliees." Montreal Université.

Phillips, D. (1987). The new dynamics of the sciences. In *Philosophy, Science and Social Inquiry*, pp. 20–36. Pergamon Press, New York, NY.

Rankin, S. H. (1990). Differences in recovery from cardiac surgery: a profile of male and female patients. *Heart and Lung 1*(5), 481–485.

Roy, Sr. C. (1989). Nursing care in theory and practice: early interventions in brain injury. In *Recovery from Brain Injury* (Harris, R., Burns, R. and Rees, R., Eds). Institute for the Study of Learning Difficulties, Adelaide.

Sarnecky, M. T. (1990). Historiography: a legitimate research methodology for nursing. *Adv. Nurs. Sci. 12*, 1–10.

Schumacher, K. L. and Gortner, S. R. (1992). (Mis)conceptions and reconceptions about traditional science. *Adv. Nurs. Sci. 14*, 1–11.

Schwab, J. (1964). Structure of the disciplines: meanings and significance. In *The Structures of Knowledge and the Curriculum* (Ford, G. W. and Pugno, L., Eds). Rand McNally, Chicago, IL.

Stevens, P. E. (1989). A critical social reconceptualization of environment in nursing: implications for methodology. *Adv. Nurs. Sci. 11*, 56–68.

Suppe, F. and Jacox, A. (1985). Philosophy of science and the development of nursing theory. In *Annual Review of Nursing Research* (Werley, H. and Fitzpatrick, J., Eds), Vol. 3, pp. 241–267. Springer Publishing Company, New York, NY.

Suppe, F. (1990). Knowledge development in the context of shifting world views: the philosophy—theory linkage. Paper presented at the first symposium on knowledge development in nursing. Newport Rhode Island, September 1990.

Thompson, J. L. (1985). Practical discourse on nursing: going beyond empiricism and historicism. *Adv. Nurs. Sci. 7*, 59–71.

Thompson, J. L. (1987). Critical scholarship: the critique of domination in nursing. *Adv. Nurs. Sci. 11*, 27–38.

Whall, A. (1989). The influence of logical positivism on nursing practice. *IMAGE: J. Nurs. Scholarship 21*, 243–245.

Whall, A. (1991). Personal communication, 17 April 1991.

The Author Comments

Nursing's Syntax Revisited

This article originally was an invited paper at the first Knowledge Development Symposium at the University of Rhode Island in September 1990. It was further refined during a sabbatical at the University of Montreal in 1991 and is difficult reading. I had been teaching the philosophy of nursing science to first-year PhD nursing students at UCSF and had incorporated postmodern views and arguments along with modern ones. I was concerned that several of the postmodern positions failed to exhibit explanatory power (defined as the capacity of a set of propositions not only to account for a given event but also to generalize to other events in the same set). That theoretic terms and abstractions arising from scientific work may exist and may be true is the position of scientific realism and one that I consider important for the development and credibility of nursing science. Both explanatory power and scientific realism should be accommodated in the theories and worldviews that guide our inquiry. Alternatively, we can develop a "within-the-discipline" philosophic lens that recognizes multiple knowledge domains (biologic, as well as sociologic and humanistic).

—SUSAN REICHERT GORTNER

CHAPTER 30

Unity of Knowledge in the Advancement of Nursing Knowledge

Karen K. Giuliano

Lynda Tyer-Viola

Ruth Palan Lopez

During the past 20 years, we have witnessed an explosion in nursing knowledge providing the discipline with diverse and multifaceted theoretical frameworks and paradigms. One knowledge theme that pervades the dialogue in the scholarly literature is that of multiple ways of knowing. With the acknowledgement that the fundamental nature of nursing knowledge is grounded in the understanding of human nature and its response to its environment, comes an imperative for a consilience of knowledge. The purpose of this article is to present such a unified worldview by articulating a vision of nursing knowledge, a meaning of unity of knowledge, and a challenge to the discipline to embrace inclusive rather than exclusive ways of knowing.

There are many windows through which we can look out into the world, searching for meaning. . . . Most of us . . . clear a tiny peephole and stare through. No wonder we are confused by the tiny fraction of the whole that we see.

—Goodall, 2000, p. 10

The explosion in nursing knowledge over the past 20 years has provided the discipline with diverse and multifaceted theoretical frameworks and paradigms. Within this diversity exists disagreement on both the fundamental nature of nursing knowledge and how that knowledge is known. There is some agreement that

From K. K. Giuliano, L. Tyer-Viola, and R. P. Lopez, Nursing Science Quarterly 2005; 18(3): 243–248. Copyright © 2005 SAGE Publications. Reprinted with permission by SAGE Publications, Inc.

About the Authors

KAREN K. GIULIANO, RN, PhD, FAAN, is currently working as a Clinical Research Scientist at Philips Medical Systems in Andover, Massachusetts. Karen has over 20 years of critical care experience, and her area of research is critical care technology. To her credit, she has numerous publications and national and international conference presentations, which focus primarily on the areas of critical care practice and technology, and creating a more humane critical care environment. Karen's other key contributions to the discipline include publications on statistical methods for nursing research and examining the nature of knowledge of nursing.

LYNDA A. TYER-VIOLA, RNC, PhD, is currently a Clinical Nurse Specialist at Massachusetts General Hospital in Boston, Massachusetts. Lynda has 25 years of high risk obstetrics experience in multiple level III labor and delivery settings. She is also the Co-Director of the Maternal and Infant Health Initiative for Zambia, a World Health Organization–sanctioned program to address maternal and neonatal mortality. Her program of research is stigma and symptom management for HIV-positive pregnant women. She is currently the Yvonne Munn Post Doctoral Fellow in Nursing Research at Massachusetts General Hospital. She is an active member of Sigma Theta Tau and contributes to the discipline of nursing by mentoring Master's and Doctoral students in the clinical setting.

RUTH PALAN LOPEZ was born and raised in Massachusetts. She received her undergraduate nursing education from Boston College, her masters in gerontological nursing from Boston University, and her PhD from Boston College's William F. Connell School of Nursing. She is an Assistant Professor and Coordinator of the Gerontological Nurse Practitioner Program at the Massachusetts General Hospital (MGH) Institute of Health Professions. Her program of research focuses on the comfort needs of dying nursing home residents and their families. In 2005, she was selected as a 2005 John A. Hartford Geriatric Nursing Research Scholar. She has more than 20 years of experience as a gerontological nurse practitioner during which time she has developed and implemented innovative programs to improve the care of older adults in both hospitals and in long-term care facilities.

nursing knowledge should be grounded in the understanding of human nature and its relationship to the environment (Schwartz-Barcott, 1999). In addition, there is some consensus that nursing knowledge should be grounded more practically in the pursuit of describing phenomena, explaining relationships, predicting consequences, or prescribing nursing care (Meleis, 1997). Clearly, these two sets of beliefs are not mutually exclusive, and thus, nursing has come to support the importance of multiple ways of knowing and the value of pluralistic methods of inquiry (Chinn & Kramer, 1999; Forbes et al., 1999). However, simultaneous concern has been expressed that knowledge generated from multiple worldviews or paradigms can ultimately lead to

a fragmentation of nursing knowledge (Taylor, 1997). This notion only strengthens the point expressed by Cody and Mitchell (2002) that "the need for nurses to articulate a coherent philosophical foundation for nursing has never been greater" (p. 4). While the notion of pluralism is certainly widespread in the nursing literature, in most cases this pluralism is seen as relativistic and not as a way of coalescing all nursing knowledge. The purpose of this article is to suggest that the acceptance of pluralism and multiple ways of knowing can be satisfied by embracing Roy's (1997) vision of the unity of knowledge.

The article begins by examining the notion of paradigms and worldviews as currently used in the nursing literature and suggests that the concept of a single paradigm supports a philosophy inconsistent with nursing's goal of building knowledge on the nature of the human response. Next, the strength of plurality in nursing knowledge development, its warrantable evidence, and the concept of a unity of knowledge to support knowledge development and practice is articulated. Finally, the nursing practice implications of this perspective are discussed.

Worldviews and Paradigms

Worldviews and paradigms have been accepted in nursing as essential to researchers' theoretical perspectives, delineation of research questions, and ultimately to the selection of research methods. The search for a nursing paradigm as a means of knowledge development has been extensively reviewed in the nursing literature (Fawcett, 1995; Monti & Tingen, 1999; Newman, Sime, & Corcoran-Perry, 1991; Parse, 1987). Other authors have claimed that nursing knowledge is developed primarily from three slightly different worldviews, post-positivism, interpretive, and critical emancipatory (Jacox, Suppe, Campbell, & Stashinko, 1999). Postpositivism grew out of logical positivism and attempts to identify patterns and regularities and to describe, explain, and predict. The interpretive, humanist, or naturalistic perspective aims to understand meaning. The third worldview, critical emancipatory, strives to address how sociopolitical and cultural factors influence experiences.

The terms *paradigm* and *worldview* are often used interchangeably creating misconceptions regarding their philosophical implications and value. Both terms are used to refer to a cultural group's outlook and beliefs about the world, research traditions, ontology, epistemology, and philosophical perspectives. The terms have also been used in a broad sense to describe a systematic set of beliefs that are held to be true by a scientific discipline (Monti & Tingen, 1999). Worldview can refer to a researcher's general philosophical orientation, belief about the nature of human beings, nursing science, knowledge, and truth (DeGroot, 1988). In addition, worldview can also refer to a point of view from which a field of study is conceptualized, the

assumptions that are inherent in those views, and the basis upon which knowledge claims are accepted (Newman et al., 1991). Parse (2000) made the distinction quite clear that "a paradigm is a worldview; it is the philosophical stance about the phenomenon of concern of a discipline" (p. 275).

The Search for a Paradigm

Kuhn (1970) popularized the concept of paradigm in his description of science in *The Structure of Scientific Revolutions*. Kuhn believed that science was not the steady acquisition of knowledge, but instead, revolutionary based on persuasion, major shifts in thinking, and conversion. According to Kuhn, scientific knowledge is generated by preparadigm inquiry, ultimately leading to the endpoint of a defined paradigm, or a period of normal science. The scientific community defines the standards, beliefs, laws, and theory from which all scientists are to conduct themselves. During a period of normal science, all discoveries are focused on supporting the dominant theory. The process of building support for the dominant theory and essentially discarding evidence that does not conform to the matrix of the dominant theory continues until enough refuting evidence becomes apparent that it can no longer be ignored. Once this occurs, there is agreement that something is fundamentally wrong within the existing paradigm, a crisis ensues, and a revolution occurs. This revolution ultimately results in a major shift in thinking and the acceptance of a new paradigm.

According to Kuhn (1970), the new paradigm is so dissimilar from the earlier paradigm that previously accepted tenets are incommensurable with those defined within the newly accepted paradigm. Incommensurable signifies that the set of scientific concepts, propositions, problems, and solutions have changed so dramatically that they no longer have meaning in the new paradigm. Questions once considered as central to the previous paradigm may no longer be questions at all. Incommensurability is manifested as an inability to translate previous ideas into the new language of the new paradigm.

When first published, Kuhn's (1970) ideas were revolutionary and shook the long held view of progressive scientific development that suggests that each stage of knowledge building in science was based on the accomplishments of its predecessors. Each scientific discipline depends on the findings and interpretations of its predecessors, both inside and outside of the discipline. In the spirit of Aristotle, the underlying assumption is that science is a cumulative, rational process in which justified truth is built upon justified truth (Byrne, 1997). New truths, which are temporally and contextually bound, are defined each time something new is discovered. From this perspective, the purpose of science is to amass knowledge about the world and to grow and progress toward the ultimate truth. Nursing is able to embrace this perspective in each nurse-patient encounter by sharing what is known and the possibility of what can be discovered.

Nursing Paradigms

The nursing literature is replete with a variety of classifications of paradigms and worldviews. From a historical and very broad perspective, nursing knowledge can be considered as falling into two paradigms, the received view and the perceived view (Mindy & Beaton, 1983). The received view represents the positivistic-empiricist approach or natural law approach that is based on a belief in the existence of facts. It is the contention of the received view that there is a body of facts and principles to discover and understand as truth that are independent of historical or social context. This view generates knowledge that is disconnected to any process or being that is interactive. In contrast, the perceived view sees science as primarily historical. Thus, the perceived view is based on the belief that facts and principles are embedded in a particular history or cultural setting. Truth from this perspective is dynamic and found only in interactions among people and their sociohistorical contexts. Therefore, it can be said that truth is bound to a person, place and time, yet has meaning as it is communicated in future interactions.

In addition, three philosophical worldviews can be thought of as having influenced the growth of nursing knowledge: rationalism, empiricism, and historicism (Moody, 1990). Rationalism stresses the importance of a priori reasoning as the primary method of knowledge building. Empiricism embraces the notion that scientific knowledge is derived solely from sensory experience. Lastly, historicism argues that scientific progress takes place in intellectual revolutions and emphasizes the influence of history on science.

Nursing has based growth in knowledge primarily on three distinct views of paradigms: totality-simultaneity (Parse, 1987); paniculate-deterministic, interactive-integrative, and unitary-transformative (Newman et al., 1991); and reaction, reciprocal-interaction, and simultaneous action (Fawcett, 1995) with reference to those that are old and new (Cody, 2000). Within each of these views of paradigms lies support or kernels of truth that enrich practice and generate knowledge. Either due to our lack of defined language or possibly in merit to our ability to see more than there is to see in human interactions, the profession of nursing has generated knowledge from each of these paradigms. However, interpreting nursing knowledge from only one view may limit the value of what is known or the possibilities of what can be discovered.

In the totality paradigm (Cody, 1995, 2003; Parse, 1987, 1991), humans are seen as biopsychosocial and spiritual organisms that interact with the external environment and adapt or attempt to control the external environment. Health is a dynamic process that can be assessed objectively by experts, and the goal of nursing is the maintenance and restoration of norms.

In the simultaneity paradigm (Parse, 1987), humans are seen as more than the sum of different parts, they are open and in mutual process with the universe, and they create their own perception of health through personal knowledge and choice. Health is a process that cannot be objectively assessed and is not limited by norms. Health is achieved through a mutual process between the human and the universe, and the goal of nursing is oriented toward quality of life as defined by the living person (Parse, 1991).

In the particulate-deterministic worldview (Newman et al., 1991), phenomena are viewed as isolatable, reducible entities, with definable properties that can be measured and have orderly and predictable connections. The interactive-integrative perspective is an extension of the worldview and incorporates context and experience. Reality is found within the relationship of the properties. The unitary-transformative worldview considers phenomenon as unitary, self-organizing fields, embedded in larger self-organizing fields.

In reciprocal-interaction (Fawcett, 1995), human beings are active holistic beings as well, and their parts are only to be viewed within the context of the whole. Interactions between human beings are reciprocal, and reality is multidimensional, context-dependent and relative. Participants in this process foster the development of trust in experiencing the continuum of human knowledge and creativity and in giving attention to each other's feelings (Green, 1995). Change is probabilistic, and both objective and subjective phenomena are studied. Knowledge is created through empirical observations, methodological controls, and inferential data analysis (Fawcett, 1995).

The lure to define a nursing paradigm is supported by Kuhn's (1970) assertion that the "acquisition of a paradigm and of the more esoteric type of research it permits is a sign of maturity in the development of any given scientific field" (p. 11). In contrast, Meleis (1991) suggested that nursing knowledge has not developed through a revolutionary process as described by Kuhn, but instead has progressed through an integration that accounts for the accommodation of multiple paradigms and theoretical pluralism within the discipline. Meleis proposed that pluralism is important in nursing because of the discipline's focus on the *whole person* and the impact and interaction of people and their evolving environments. To disavow what has been described as knowledge from within the lived experience perspective would be in one sense disavowing the existence of the lived experience. The ideology that new knowledge is incommensurable with existing knowledge as described by Kuhn is counterintuitive to nursing's acceptance that what is known paves the way for what is to be discovered or what can be known.

Pluralism in Nursing

Historically, nursing has embraced many philosophies from other disciplines. Although diversity in approaches to nursing knowledge development is suggestive of vitality, Kim (2001) has also argued that it has created disarray and a disorganized collection of knowledge bits in nursing. Meleis (1991) suggested that it is desirable for knowledge to develop from different perspectives but that it must be integrated in some way if nursing is to avoid being forever fragmented and divided. According to this view, a unification of methodologies is not what is required, but instead, the acceptance of a broader unifying perspective that allows nurse scholars to integrate and organize different kinds of nursing knowledge under a broader framework.

Kirkevold (1997) believed that full comprehension could be achieved by collection, analysis, and integration of related research findings into a meaningful whole to achieve clarity in practice (Kirkevold, 1997). Hinshaw (2000) supported collectivism as a means of advancing nursing in the 21st century. Hence, according to some contemporary scholars, the discipline of nursing can benefit through the understanding and embracing of multiple perspectives. In addition, there is a strong if not foundational belief throughout most of the contemporary nursing paradigms that the whole of nursing knowledge is greater than the sum of its parts. Variation in theories does not necessarily lead to different bodies of knowledge, but perhaps only to different aspects of a single body (Donaldson & Crowley, 1978). Pluralism of theories promotes productivity and without testing a wide variety of theories, progress toward truth is more difficult to make (Donaldson & Crowley).

What Is Warrantable Evidence for Nursing Knowledge Development?

If one is to accept, as the authors here suggest, that pluralism in nursing is the best path for the development of nursing knowledge, then the notion of what constitutes warrantable evidence must be seriously addressed.

It must be clearly understood that acceptance of pluralism does not signify the endorsement of a relativistic perspective. Each piece of new knowledge needs to be scrutinized critically for its merit and credibility within the context of nursing practice and by each practitioner within each patient encounter (Fawcett, Neuman, Walker, & Fitzpatrick, 2001). Evidence should be generated and validated in multiple forms. Rycroft-Malone and colleagues (2004) stated, "The practice of effective nursing, which is mediated through the contact and relationship between individual practitioner and patient, can only be achieved by using several sources of evidence" (p. 81). The multiple bases of evidence are those from the more acknowledged research and clinical experience, and the less informed, patients, clients and providers, and local context and environment (Rycroft-Malone et al., 2004). To assure knowledge development is robust, concerted effort needs to be made to assure that each of these knowledge bases is included and more importantly, evidence from each is examined for its contribution to care and scientific rigor.

To assess the scientific value of knowledge generated from multiple sources, the authors agree with the three common warrants proposed by Forbes and colleagues (1999). The three warrants are scrutiny of findings and methodological strategies, corroboration, and scope of evidence. The *first* warrant rests on the degree to which the research followed procedures accepted by the community of research and the logical derivation of conclusions from the evidence. The *second* warrant is that the evidence can be corroborated and open to public scrutiny. In the quantitative paradigm this may be accomplished by reproduction of research findings. In the interpretivist paradigm, this may be accomplished by corroboration with research participants. Additionally, corroboration is sought from the research and scientific community. The *third* common warrant is whether the scope of evidence is adequate to address the phenomenon under study. More importantly, does the evidence contribute to a greater body of knowledge (including that which is significant or not) by filling a gap, or debunking dogma. Using knowledge developed from multiple sources and methods lends additional scope to knowledge and further supports this warrant.

Roy's Perspective on Nursing Knowledge

If one accepts the belief that pluralism is necessary for the development of knowledge in nursing, how then can nursing synthesize and integrate knowledge from multiple perspectives and worldviews without ending up with an amalgamation of contradictions? The authors believe that Roy's (1996, 2001) vision of knowledge as both unity and diversity provides the necessary theoretical, philosophical and epistemological support to integrate nursing knowledge. Roy's assumptions support multiple theories and research methods and provide nurse scholars with a vast array of possibilities for organizing nursing knowledge. Roy's integrative and cumulative approach offers the position that knowledge is generated from a multidisciplinary perspective and not as divergent paradigms. Two central ideas, unity in diversity and the existence of universal truths, have important implications for the integration of knowledge developed from multiple perspectives.

Unity in Diversity

In 1996, at the Nursing Knowledge Impact Conference, Roy set the stage for the idea of unity of knowledge by exploring the practice issues raised by the philosophical perspectives of realism, relativism, interpretivism, and humanism. Roy's philosophical assumption of unity demonstrates how one can find unity in diversity and is supported by noted philosophers and scientists. Citing Aristotle, she contended that all knowledge is of the universal (Roy, 1996). All things known are in relation to others both before them and to come. Roy asserted that everything is one substance with different attributes creating abroad and unified force. Roy proposed that nursing can find unity in diversity and that knowledge requires a full unveiling of all the diverse ways of seeing the whole (Roy, 1996).

If Roy's conception of unity in diversity can be accepted as central to nursing practice, then it can provide a perspective for uniting seemingly diverse paradigms in nursing. Cody (2003) explored human diversity by explaining human existence as coexistence and how understanding this relationship across diversities leads to "an infinite range of possibilities" (p. 196). Nursing embraces all things known in relation to others by its unique fundamental principle of caring. Cody said it is "not those who are familiar, who are our own or closely resemble our own—but those who are truly different, unfamiliar, and *other* to ourselves" (p. 196). When this perspective of welcoming that which is not familiar is applied to raising one's awareness to a new level in uncovering knowledge, awareness of boundaries dissolves and things become increasingly more unified. In addition, as knowledge boundaries disappear, each smaller level is a reflection of all other levels. Consequently, one can simultaneously possess both unity and diversity. What is seen depends on where one chooses to focus or for whom one chooses to care (Cody). Rawnsley (2003) expressed a similar sentiment in her support for multiple paradigms for nursing as well as her suggestion that nursing has a desperate need for a unifying vision that allows for divergent points of view.

Universal Truths

The idea of the existence of universal truths is fundamental to Roy's conception of knowledge. Roy (1996, 2001) viewed the pursuit of truth as an evolving notion, understood at one moment and undefined at the next. This supports the need for multiple ways of knowing in order to define and understand the whole of nursing knowledge. Knowledge viewed from this perspective provides the middle ground between the positivist who searches for the one true reality and the interpretivist who searches for multiple realities. Roy (1988) suggested that the rationalist bases truth on empirical facts and the relativist knows truth only in relationship to the thinking person. Since the mind of the observer is influenced by perceptions and theoretical presuppositions, taken to its extreme, one could argue that all observa-

tions are mind-dependent, influenced by multiple realities, and relativistic.

One of the most compelling aspects of Roy's (1996, 2001) perspective is that it makes room for all knowledge because within the belief in the existence of universal truths is the idea that no simple insight is enough, in and of itself, to disclose the whole truth. From Roy's (1996, 2001) perspective, nursing knowledge is both discipline-specific and open to validation and expansion through multidisciplinary scrutiny. Roy's perspective (1996, 2001) contradicts the view of Fawcett (1999) who proposed that all nursing knowledge should be discipline-specific. Knowledge derived from interdisciplinary inquiry allows the discipline to operate in an open rather than closed system model. Furthermore, it enhances a social responsibility for being open to public scrutiny as well as the goal of further and more widespread understanding. This broadened perspective is what makes nursing's multiple ways of knowing accessible to other disciplines. Finally, while there may be a strong belief that the whole of nursing knowledge is greater than the sum of its parts, scholars have no alternative but to select a small portion of potential truth to examine and a small perspective from which to study it. Because of this limitation in scientific inquiry, it is incumbent upon nurse researchers to recognize that, at best, any knowledge generated from a single episode of inquiry represents only a small piece of knowledge and only a part of a larger truth. As a practical consideration, it is necessary to break knowledge into manageable chunks in order to study it, improve our understanding of what is found, and generate more knowledge for future examination. Therefore, one of the most important tasks of nurse scholars is the responsibility to be honest and explicit with regard to the depth and breadth of the current scope of inquiry, as well as interpretation of the findings within the appropriate scope. The challenge for contemporary nurse scholars is to put the knowledge parts together in a way that is integrative, not simply additive, and not irresponsibly dismissive of opposing views without investing in a full understanding of those views.

Conclusions

It is the authors' contention that nursing knowledge is developed from multiple perspectives and lenses. Nursing knowledge development should not support an epistemology in which empirical knowledge is the pinnacle or *gold standard* for knowledge development. Rather, empirical knowledge simply represents one type of warrantable evidence. This position is critical if scholars are to prevent the devaluation of other types of knowledge so integral to nursing. Plurality of methodological approaches and ways of generating nursing knowledge are necessary to reflect the many facets of nursing science and to illuminate the complex phenomena present in nursing practice situations. No one view is sufficient to embrace or drive nursing knowledge in its totality. As Carper (1978) suggested, nursing must be the discipline that uses knowledge and evidence generated from multiple sources as an integral part of evidence-based nursing recommendations. Nursing's position on evidence for practice should demand that knowledge of a phenomenon include data generated from multiple methods and sources. This approach ensures the most comprehensive and unified view possible, and one that best serves the people. When taken from this perspective, data that refutes dogma, so prevalent in nursing, will illuminate gaps in knowledge and areas in need of further knowledge development.

In conclusion, the worldview of knowledge as unity provides an opportunity for nurses to participate in interdisciplinary research and knowledge development and still retain and emphasize the core dimensions of nursing. Based on the complexity of humans and their response to the environment, wide-ranging development and advancement of nursing knowledge is not possible without the integration and use of multiple ways of knowing.

REFERENCES

Byrne, P. H. (1997). *Analysis and science in Aristotle*. Albany: State University of New York Press.

Carper, B. A. (1978). Fundamental patterns of knowing in nursing. *Advances in Nursing Science, 1*(1), 13–23.

Chinn, P. L., & Kramer, M. (1999). *Theory and nursing: A systematic approach* (5th ed.). St. Louis, MO: Mosby.

Cody, W. K. (1995). About all those paradigms: Many in the universe, two in nursing. *Nursing Science Quarterly, 8,* 144–147.

Cody, W. K. (2000). Paradigm shift or paradigm drift? A meditation on commitment and transcendence. *Nursing Science Quarterly, 13,* 93–102.

Cody, W. K. (2003). Diversity and becoming: Implications of human existence and coexistence. *Nursing Science Quarterly, 16,* 195–200.

Cody, W. K., & Mitchell, G. J. (2002). Nursing knowledge and human science revisited: Practical and political considerations. *Nursing Science Quarterly, 15,* 4–13.

DeGroot, H. A. (1988). Scientific inquiry in nursing: A model for a new age. *Advances in Nursing Science, 10*(3), 1–21.

Donaldson, S. K., & Crowley, D. M. (1978). The discipline of nursing. *Nursing Outlook, 26*(2), 113–120.

Fawcett, J. (1995). *Analysis and evaluation of conceptual models of nursing*. Philadelphia: F. A. Davis Company.

Fawcett, J. (1999). *Theory and research*. Philadelphia: F. A. Davis.

Fawcett, J., Neuman, J. B., Walker, P. H., & Fitzpatrick, J. J. (2001). On nursing theories and evidence. *Journal of Nursing Scholarship, 33,* 115–124.

Forbes, D. A., King, K. M., Kushner, K. E., Letourneau, N. L., Myrick, A. F., & Profetto-McGrath, J. (1999). Warrantable evidence in nursing science. *Journal of Advanced Nursing, 29,* 373–379.

Goodall, J. (2000). *Through a window: My thirty years with the chimpanzees of Gombe*. Boston: Houghton Mifflin.

Green, M. (1995). *Essays on education, art and social change*. San Francisco: Jossey-Bass.

Hinshaw, A. (2000). Nursing knowledge for the 21st century: Opportunities and challenges. *Journal of Nursing Scholarship, 32,* 117–123.

Jacox, A., Suppe, F., Campbell, J., & Stashinko, E. (1999). Diversity in philosophical approaches. In A. S. Hinshaw, S. L. Freeman & J. F. Shaver (Eds.), *Handbook of clinical nursing research* (pp. 3–17). Thousand Oaks, CA: Sage.

Kim, H. S. (2001). Directions for theory development in nursing. In N. L. Chaska (Ed.), *The nursing profession: Tomorrow and beyond* (pp. 273–285). Thousand Oaks, CA: Sage.

Kirkevold, M. (1997). Integrative nursing research: An important strategy to further the development of nursing science and nursing practice. *Journal of Advanced Nursing, 25,* 977–984.

Kuhn, T. (1970). *The structure of scientific revolutions* (2nd ed.). Chicago: University of Chicago Press.

Meleis, A. I. (1991). *Theoretical nursing: Development and progress*. Philadelphia: J. B. Lippincott.

Meleis, A. I. (1997). *Theoretical nursing: Development & progress* (3rd ed.). New York: Lippincott.

Mindy, B. T., & Beaton, J. L. (1983). Toward a new view of science: Implications for nursing research. *Advances in Nursing Science, 5*(2), 27–36.

Monti, E. J., & Tingen, M. S. (1999). Multiple paradigms of nursing science. *Advances in Nursing Science, 21*(4), 64–80.

Moody, L. E. (1990). *Advancing nursing science through research* (Vol. 1). Newbury Park, CA: Sage.

Newman, M. A., Sime, A. M., & Corcoran Perry, S. A. (1991). The focus of the discipline. *Advances in Nursing Science, 14*(1), 1–6.

Parse, R. R. (1987). *Nursing science: Major paradigms, theories and critiques*. Philadelphia: Saunders.

Parse, R. R. (2000). Paradigms: A reprise. *Nursing Science Quarterly, 13*, 275–276.

Parse, R. R. (1991). Human becoming: Parse's theory of nursing. *Nursing Science Quarterly, 5*, 35–42.

Rawnsley, M. (2003). Dimensions of scholarship and the advancement of nursing science: Articulating a vision. *Nursing Science Quarterly, 16*, 6–13.

Roy, S. C. (1988). An explication of the philosophical assumptions of the Roy adaptation model. *Nursing Science Quarterly, 1*, 26–34.

Roy, S. C. (1996, October). *Knowledge as universal cosmic imperative*. Paper presented at the Nursing Knowledge Conference, Boston, MA.

Roy, S. C. (1997). Knowledge as universal cosmic imperative. In D. R. Jones (Ed.), *Knowledge impact 1996: Conference proceedings* (pp. 95–117). Chestnut Hill, MA: Boston College Press.

Roy, S. C. (2001, October). *Knowledge as cosmic imperative and impact on the health care system*. Paper presented at the Knowledge Impact Conference 2001, Newton, MA.

Rycroft-Malone, J., Seers, K., Tichen, A., Harvey, G., Kitson, A., & McCormack, B. (2004). What counts as evidence in evidence-based practice? *Journal of Advanced Nursing, 47*, 81–90.

Schwartz-Barcott, D. (1999). Adaptation as a basic conceptual focus in nursing theories. In H. Kim & I. Kollak (Eds.), *Nursing theories: Conceptual and philosophical foundations* (pp. 9–22). New York: Springer.

Taylor, J. (1997). Nursing ideology: Identification and legitimation. *Journal of Advanced Nursing, 25*, 1365–2648.

The Authors Comment

Unity of Knowledge in the Advancement of Nursing Knowledge

The inspiration for our work emanated from coursework for an Epistemology course taught by Sister Callista Roy at Boston College. We were asked to synthesize and critique knowledge for nursing practice. We considered the various ways of developing knowledge for nursing practice, the strengths and weaknesses of various paradigms, and whether knowledge developed from these paradigms with unique assumptions were commensurable. After much debate, we agreed that knowledge to inform nursing practice requires a theoretical framework that integrates and unifies knowledge developed from multiple paradigms. Roy's concept of veritivity, the highest level of knowledge, provides this consilience. This worldview contributes to nursing theory in the 21st century as it provides the discipline with a worldview that unifies diverse and multifaceted theoretical frameworks.

—Karen K. Giuliano
—Lynda A. Tyer-Viola
—Ruth Palan Lopez

find alarming, however, is that the form of the discourse no longer represents a lively dialogue from which diverse conceptual standpoints serve to advance our collective understanding of nursing complexity. Rather, the debate seems to have deteriorated into a binary argument within which theorists are presumed to be either 'for' or 'against' certain coherent theoretical movements. Those who still read within this literature will have noted a disturbing strand of argumentation consisting of what is positioned as the inherent supremacy of one particular form of theorizing over others. Proponents of conceptual models writing in the genre of what they call *simultaneity* theories persistently set their claims against what they collectively refer to as *totality* frameworks. These terms (with their unfortunate connotations of immediacy and relevance as opposed to dominance and control) were coined to distinguish and advance the simultaneity perspective (Cody, 2000) and, to our knowledge, have not been used for purposes other than creating the impression of mutually exclusive binary oppositional intentionality on the part of nursing theorists.

The 'languaging' of this model discourse relies heavily on paradigm terminology, invoking the traditional Kuhnian connotation of revolution by creative new forms of thinking over the dominant, controlling, normative scientific mainstream. As the simultaneity—totality discourse inevitably places the majority of nursing theorizing within the totality paradigm category, with all of the paternalistic, reductionistic, and linear baggage that categorical definition implies, referencing simultaneity as the intention positions an argument as holding intellectually and morally superiority within the disciplinary science. In this context, insistence on positioning nursing theories as paradigmatically incompatible has created a binary impasse within which anything other than uncritical acceptance is interpreted as harsh opposition.

From our perspective, the pattern of these arguments is grounded in a set of false premises about the motivations and purposes underlying the original theoretical developments. Aside from the obvious reality that the majority of these conceptual models emerged during a historical era in which nurse scholars had access to far fewer philosophical and scientific frameworks from which to obtain guidance, it seems illogical to presume that theorists experimenting with ideas such as general systems theory were opposed to holism and subjective experience in favour of reductionism and objectivity. However, in positioning a binary argument in favour of simultaneity, it has become popular to ascribe somewhat sinister motives to those original conceptual framework builders. From our perspective, this form of reasoning seems analogous to attributing sexist intent to those scholars whose writings about humankind preceded our collective access to the gendered language conventions we enjoy today. Attribution of intentionality on the basis of linguistic distinctions that are not commonly accessible seems an entirely weak and illogical form of argument, and one that we ought to expose and challenge in our current intellectual discourse.

As we reflect on these problematic aspects of nursing theoretical discourse, we recognize that the global ideological context since 9/11 has heightened our sensitivity for how our alignment to various ideas can be used strategically to create a conviction of fundamental difference among and between us. In this context, we feel increasingly uncomfortable with the tone and form in which some of nursing's theoretical arguments are articulated, and we are disturbed by what has been constructed as an insoluble paradigmatic divide between nurses of diametrically opposite theoretical orientations. Although this form of argumentation has for the most part been ignored as a 'fringe element' by mainstream academic nursing, we remain concerned that its unchecked proliferation as a legitimate form of 'nursing science' damages the general credibility of our discipline's intellectual project (Johnson, 1999). We recognize from the larger global context that ignoring tensions among ideological positions creates complicity in their escalation. In this analysis, we explicitly challenge not the ideas inherent in the models themselves but the binary form in which they have been positioned and have become entrenched. In so doing, we fully recognize that we expose ourselves to being discounted as inherently unenlightened in some quarters, and embarrassingly uncharitable in others.

Alternatives to the Binary Form

Because nursing is an inherently socially relevant discipline, it seems self-evident that we ought to demand of ourselves an intellectual climate within which critical intellectual inquiry is both nurtured and celebrated. We believe this to mean that we ought to encourage thoughtful reflection about the various manifestations of logic and reason within our disciplinary knowledge discourse. Ideally, then, we would foster an intellectual culture within which we focus on exploration of ideas from the perspective of understanding their inherent coherence, the degree to which they illuminate disciplinary phenomena, their implications for a practice profession, and their congruence with the core values that underpin our disciplinary mandate. In such a climate, ideas positioned as inherently better than other ideas, or expressed with the intention of advancing a particular conceptual framework or ideological stance within our discipline, would seem fundamentally suspect and invite explicit challenges as to who is being alienated or what is being obscured.

What we suggest, then, is a heightened expectation within our nursing scholarly products for sophistication in the manner in which we structure our arguments and the logical forms within which we render our disciplinary discourse. In keeping with an understanding of nursing's inherent complexity, we categorically reject the form of science in which there is only one correct answer, and favour an intellectual culture in which multiple truths can be openly examined for their possible contributions to disciplinary wisdom. When we abandon the search for absolutely right answers and move beyond our traditional relationship to binaries, we make viable the notion that all ideas may contain within them a germ of possibility that can be taken forward by another thinker, another generation, to develop something of value to our discipline.

Various knowledge traditions reveal quite different assumptions about the proper relationship between people and their ideas. For example, Judaic tradition, as encoded in the Talmud, requires that one reflect on the implications of an idea before offering another. Each idea is explicitly understood to represent a distinct angle of vision, a way of thinking about the original text or interpretation. Further, the scholarly documentation of that tradition preserves the sequence of thought so that each new idea does not replace, but builds upon, those that have gone before. There is an inherent value in the variation, and a corresponding assumption that, in the process of documenting the ideas in an iterative relationship with one another, a context will emerge in which ideas move from their original association with certain individuals who articulated them and become part of the sacred heritage of the communities privileged to wrestle with their meaning. In retaining the form of a sustained analytical argument, the text imparts to those who engage with it 'a character of intellectual refinement and personal responsibility' (Neusner, 1995, p. xi). In the tradition of Socrates and Plato, this kind of dialectic welcomes diversity into the conversation in order to create and capitalize upon the inherent value of conflict among ideas (Elbow, 1993).

According to Elbow (1993), the problems associated with our customary affinity for ideas expressed within the binary form cannot be resolved by simply striving for multiplicity, because that too can become a strategic device by which one position strives to achieve dominance. In the Hegelian notion of a dialectic, binary thinking becomes the driver through which the nonresolution of two binaries creates the conditions under which a third and more unifying option can emerge—that 'thesis and antithesis are . . . harnessed to yield synthesis' (Elbow, 1993). However, an older understanding of the dialectic, which predates Hegel and can be found in early sources as diverse as Confucius, Maimonides, and Socrates, rejects a presumption that the opposite ideas must somehow be resolved; rather, in this form of dialectic, the explicit goal is lack of resolution. To achieve this, one must accept the possibility that two claims that seem completely contradictory might both have some usefulness and relevance to our understanding about a phenomenon or, as Elbow speculatively conceives of it, to uphold an 'epistemology of contradiction'. This form of dialectic relies upon opposing ideas in a manner that extends beyond the rhetorical and engages the existential.

For us, the nursing academic community would do well to embrace that sort of engagement in the inherent tensions between ideas. Moving beyond the cultural form of oversimplifying and then discounting the relevance of all prior work (a logic structure that we seem to have mastered all too well in articulating the rationale for our next research project), we favour an intellectual climate in which we can begin with recognizing that 'there is an idea . . . .' and then internalizing each subsequent idea until we have reflected upon it and enlarged upon our thinking in relation to different ideas about the same problem or phenomenon. Setting different ideas in juxtaposition to one another, we would recognize their value in generating insight rather than expecting that each new truth, in the tradition of conventional scientific advancement, would eclipse those that had come before. In so doing, we would create a means by which to fully embrace the mystery and complexity that is nursing.

While we would not go so far as to take the position that there are no inherently 'bad' ideas, we do believe that our disciplinary fear of ambiguity, uncertainty, and suspended judgement may have created an academic culture in which we routinely seek premature closure on truth. Thus, if the intellectual community within nursing can begin to understand itself as inherently operating within the delightful world of competing ideas, then we stand a far better chance of realizing our collective contribution towards some higher purpose on this planet. In this way, nursing inquiry might more fully reflect the 'actualization and celebration' of our human intellectual capacity, and reflect 'our place in the scheme of things' (Reason, 1996, p. 19).

We therefore call upon those engaged in the domain of nursing theorizing to remain conscious of contributing to a legacy that may shape the next generation of thinking within our discipline. Will nurse scholars of the future continue to stake claims on theoretical positions that are divisive and inflammatory? Or will they create a community of thinkers capable of wrestling with ideas and imagining new relationships to truth?

We recognize that binary arguments will likely remain an inevitable presence within some sectors of our scholarly discourse. However, instead of falling prey to them, circumventing them with polite avoidance, or assuming that academic credibility will derive from uncritical adherence to one position or the other, we encourage the nursing scholarly community to demand of its members a renewed rigorous and lively engagement in considering the implications of ideas for our purposes. Instead of coming to loggerheads because of opposing views, we ought to capitalize on them as an opportunity to stimulate our reasoning, to annoy us into further exploration, or to inspire us into conceiving of new angles from which we might wrestle with the social and moral complexity that is the matter of nursing science. Arguments that present themselves in the binary form can be a signal to us that there is something important to consider, and new discoveries to be made. When we accept that, then perhaps we will have taken our rightful place in the world of ideas as a unique and coherent academic discipline.

REFERENCES

Cody W.K. (2000) Paradigm shift or paradigm drift?: a meditation on commitment and transcendence. *Nursing Science Quarterly*, **13**(2), 93–102.

Elbow P. (1993) The uses of binary thinking. *Journal of Advanced Composition*, **31**(1), 51–78.

Johnson M. (1999) Observations on positivism and pseudoscience in qualitative nursing research. *Journal of Advanced Nursing*, **30**(1), 67–73.

Lloyd G.E.R. (1966) *Polarty and Analogy: Two Types of Argumentation in Early Greek Thought*. Cambridge University Press, New York.

Neusner J. (1995) Forward. In: *Everyman's Talmud: The Major Teachings of the Rabbinic Sages* (ed. A. Cohen), pp. ix–xxviii. Schocken Books, New York.

Pilkington F.B. & Mitchell G.J. (2003) Mis-takes across paradigms. *Nursing Science Quarterly*, **16**(2), 102–108.

Reason P. (1996) Reflections on the purposes of human inquiry. *Qualitative Inquiry*, **2**(1), 15–28.

Thorne S., Canam C., Dahinten S., Hall W., Henderson A. & Reimer Kirkham S. (1998) Nursing's metaparadigm concepts: disempacting the debates. *Journal of Advanced Nursing*, **27**, 1257–1268.

Thorne S.E.; Reimer Kirkham S. & Henderson A. (1999) Ideological implications of paradigm discourse. *Nursing Inquiry*, **6**, 123–131.

Voss K.-C. (2002) *Shattered Illusions*. Learning in the Crucible, Centre International de Recherches et Etudes Transdisciplinaires (Paris, Feb/2002). http://perso.clubinternet.fr/nicol/ciret/bulletin/bl6/bl6cl6.htm Accessed August 12/03.

The Authors Comment

The Problematic Allure of the Binary in Nursing Theoretical Discourse

We were inspired to write this article when we perceived that the form of argument in expressing certain theoretical positions within our disciplinary literature seemed, at times, to be deteriorating toward over-simplification and polarization. Our intent was to challenge nurses to more readily detect and challenge this form of faulty argumentation, thereby encouraging a more thoughtful and complex rendering of our disciplinary disputations. We framed this problematic logic form as setting up "binary" arguments in which one's position becomes right simply because the opposite is expressed in an extreme and untenable form, noting that this unfortunate style of argument had also become frighteningly common within the public domain in recent years. However, in so doing, we may have inadvertently allowed for the impression that we saw no place for real binaries within our disciplinary thinking—a challenge that June Kikuchi has since taken up with our work as seen in her 2006 article, "The binary: An obstacle to scholarly nursing discourse?" in *Nursing Philosophy, 7,* 100–103. Through our article, we hope that we have thrown down a gauntlet for rigorous and balanced argumentation on our various positions within nursing's theoretical challenges so that we might distinguish among issues for which our differences are fundamental rather than merely perspectival, and thereby advance our collective thinking into maturity.

—Sally E. Thorne
—Angela D. Henderson
—Gladys I. McPherson
—Barbara K. Pesut

CHAPTER 32

Nursing as Means of Governmentality

Dave Holmes
Denise Gastaldo

Background. *This paper conceptualizes nursing as a health profession in transformation at the beginning of the 21st century. We frame our analysis using Michel Foucault's concept of governmentality. While extensively quoted and used in other disciplines, the work of the late French philosopher has been cited infrequently in the nursing literature. Yet a closer look at his work reveals how Foucault offers a relevant entry point for revisiting nursing theory and nursing practice.*

Aim of paper. *The aim of this paper is to reflect on nursing practice as it is inscribed within the state's modus operandi. We discuss the prevalent notion that nurses are powerless and suggest they do exercise power in many ways and that they are a powerful group.*

Results. *In this paper we show how nursing is a means of governmentality of individuals and of the population because its practices contribute to the management of society through a vast range of power techniques. These techniques range from disciplining individuals to promoting discourses that construct desirable subjectivities. Within this perspective, the emergence of political aspects of nursing theory and nursing practice are made explicit.*

Conclusion. *We explore the limits and potentials of the concept of governmentality to the understanding of nursing as a health profession. This concept can generate a form of critical immobilism, but also promotes a more politically complex understanding of nursing practice.*

About the Authors

DAVE HOLMES currently lives in Montreal, Canada. He received his BScN from the University of Ottawa, Canada, and his MSc and PhD (nursing) from the Faculté des Sciences Infirmières, Université de Montréal, Canada. He currently holds a position as Associate Professor at the University of Ottawa, Faculty of Health Sciences, School of Nursing, where he teaches at the undergraduate and graduate levels. He is also a nurse researcher at the Douglas Hospital Research Centre in Montreal, a teaching psychiatric hospital affiliated with McGill University. He is completing his postdoctoral studies at the University of Toronto, Canada. His main contributions to nursing are poststructuralist analysis of nursing practice in forensic psychiatry and public health.

DENISE GASTALDO is an Associate Professor at the Faculty of Nursing and Centre for International Health, University of Toronto, Canada. She was born in Brazil, where she obtained her BScN and MA degrees. Dr. Gastaldo completed her PhD in the United Kingdom, where she studied health promotion and sociology of health at the University of London. Subsequently, she completed postdoctoral studies at the Faculté des Sciences Infirmières, Université de Montréal, Canada. Her main contributions to nursing are international capacity building for research, critical analysis of nursing and health promotion from a poststructuralist perspective, and exploration of interdisciplinary perspectives on gender and health.

Nursing and Health Care in the 21st Century

Traditionally, nurses have described themselves, and have been depicted by others, as a powerless professional group, which lacks social prestige, is poorly paid, and experiences very limited professional autonomy because of physicians' socially dominant role in providing health care to the population (Lunardi Filho, 2000). In this paper, however, we adopt a different perspective. Employing a Foucauldian notion of power, we draw on the concept of *governmentality* to reconceptualize nursing as an internationally recognized profession of fundamental importance to the provision of health care in the Western world. In many countries, nurses are the largest professional group working in the health field. In qualitative terms, preceding decades witnessed nursing's consolidating higher education degrees and offering more alternatives to graduate studies at master's and doctoral levels (Arruda & Silva, 2000). Increasing numbers of graduate programs are producing more knowledge, and efforts towards providing evidence-based care are being made in many countries (MacGuire

1990, Martin & Forchuk 1994, Francke *et al.* 1995, Gastaldo 2000). Concurrently, nurses have achieved more management positions and political roles, which lead to political influence.

In advanced liberal societies, neoliberal policies have attempted to downsize governmental provision of health care services. For example, in the last decade in Canada length of stay in hospitals has been reduced and family caregivers have been involved in home care activities that were previously provided by health care professionals. Meanwhile, in countries like Brazil that are under the influence of the International Monetary Fund, relying on private health insurance has become a common practice among the middle class. The concentration of resources in the private sector and the globalization of the economy have been reshaping the health field. In some countries, health care has become a commodity that one should be able to afford through insurance [in the United States of America (USA), for example], while in others [such as Australia, Canada, United Kingdom (UK) and Sweden], access to health care is still perceived as a basic right for all citizens. Presently, globalized markets do not translate into global rights for

In short, government means to conduct others and oneself, and governmentality is about how to govern. 'The concept of government implies all those tactics, strategies, techniques, programmes, dreams and aspirations of those authorities that shape beliefs and the conduct of population' (Nettleton 1991, p. 99). Hence, government is an activity that aims to shape, mould or affect the conduct of an individual or a group, that is, to conduct the conducts of people (Gordon 1991). According to Foucault, this *governmentalization* of the state relies on a specific security apparatus that links all together in a very specific complex of procedures and techniques: diplomatic-military techniques, the police, and pastoral power, such as the care of others.

Diplomatic-military techniques, the first dimension of the security apparatus, allows the state to protect itself against external threats and to preserve its territorial integrity through diplomatic representations, a permanent armed force, and established war policies (Gros 1996). In addition, to protect itself against internal threats, the state is endowed with a police force. Finally, pastoral power achieves care of others through various therapeutic regimes while ultimately helping to shape the self so that it fits within an appropriate, 'normalized' way of living (Dean 1999). The normalized way of living refers to a conformity to a set of social rules and ways of concerning oneself and others. The power of normalization imposes homogeneity by setting standards and ideals for human beings (Rose 1998).

Governing is as much about practices of government as it is about practices of the self because the concept of governmentality deals with those practices that try to shape, mould, mobilize and work through the choices, desires, aspirations and needs of individuals and populations (Rose & Miller 1992). Governmentality connects the question of government and politics to the self (Dean 1999). In our discussion, we will explore how nursing is a constitutive element of governmentality by looking at power over life as the governance of populations and individuals (Gastaldo 1997, Gastaldo & Holmes 1999).

Nursing and the Governance of the Population

Nursing as a profession and a discipline is inherently political because it deals with biological existence and generates knowledge about it. Shaping the population for economic and social purposes demands supervision and intervention over biological processes (Foucault 1990). Hence, nursing is a constitutive element of governmentality because it takes part in this management. Currently, nursing's role in managing the population is centred on promoting life and recuperation from illness. Life is governed in a variety of ways, but we will explore two particular methods in this section—knowledge production and social policy.

As one of the largest professional groups in the health field in many countries, nursing plays a major role in the population's health education. Nursing's academic gains and political development have meant that many professionals now serve as professors, researchers, policy makers, consultants and evaluators. These positions give them opportunities to gather information and create policies to be implemented from the local to the international level (Gastaldo et al. 2001).

Acknowledging nursing's influence in managing the population does not mean that nurses work in unison, or that they share a Machiavellian plan to rule society. Nursing, like any other profession, is divided by distinct philosophical and political positions, and it is often motivated by members' self-interests and personal agendas. Any attempt at producing a discourse to promote health is challenged by other discourses, and the governance of society occurs within a constant struggle of conflicting interests. As with any other exercise of power, dominant discourses in nursing face resistance (Gastaldo 1997). As power is the multiplicity of force relations extant within the social body, one specific manifestation of power will encounter another one resisting it. According to Foucault, we are continuously involved in struggles, because struggle for power is pervasive in every society:

> Power is not something that is acquired, seized, or shared, something that one holds to or allows to slip away; power is exercised from innumerable

points, in the interplay of nonegalitarian and mobile relations . . . there is no binary and all encompassing opposition between rulers and ruled at the root of power relations . . . (1990, p. 94)

Social policy constitutes its objects; it helps to give meaning to abstract concepts, such as health and caring. Policies about health generate new understandings of health. As Hewitt (1991) pointed out:

Social policy plays a co-ordinating role in forming 'the social.' It promotes and organizes knowledge, norms and social practices to regulate the quality of life of the population, its health, security and stability. (p. 225)

Health is considered a desirable asset in most societies and health policies tend to involve measures designed to promote health and recuperation from illness. Therefore, nursing is a profession that is well perceived (even though not prestigious), and its interventions are generally well accepted by the public. Since the 1980s, the health promotion movement has linked health to most aspects of public and private life. Moreover, healthy public policy may include issues such as housing, pollution, and violence, among others (Gastaldo 1997).

Two examples illustrate how nurses create policies and knowledge. In Canada, nurses have been instrumental in advancing the health promotion and home care movements during the last decades (McKeever 1996, Stewart 2000). Through research and political action, nurses have helped to de-institutionalize long-term care and to reframe health as a socially determined construct. While claiming to promote a humane and socially grounded care, these movements also reinforced the importance of self-care and self-responsibility for health, and they produced norms for the good citizen, the caring mother, and the acquiescent chronically ill or disabled person. The expectation created by these discourses fosters comparisons between individuals and groups. "The comparisons allow nurses to establish 'normality.'" As a consequence, the "deviant individual becomes a target for surveillance and intervention" (Gastaldo & Holmes 1999, p. 21).

Governmentality also depends on access to knowledge. Those governing society need to understand the politics of everyday life. Epidemics, fertility, and life expectancy are at the core of the rationalities of government (Foucault 1990). Nursing research provides knowledge about the population and helps to decide priorities in funding. "Research findings have provided scientific authority to justify policies that have saved huge amounts of public money by minimizing institutional costs and shifting many of the costs of long-term care to family caregivers" (McKeever 1996, p. 203).

In the case of the home care movement, McKeever (1996) argued that policies also reflect a particular notion of family and home. The home has become the most important site for health care and health promotion in our society, and women the main producers of such services. But this place and worker remain rarely conceptualized in research (McKeever 1996). What prevail in research are samples of 'white' and nuclear families, where the psychological burden of caregivers is stressed over social and economic issues, such as social class, ethnicity, occupational history, and power relations between family caregivers, care recipients, and professionals (McKeever 1996). The home care movement naturalized the home as the optimal site for long-term care (institutional care is now seen as impersonal) and as a private space, where family provision of care is free and therefore saves public funds. As a consequence, long-term care recipients who do not have a family become a burden to society and families that do not provide care according to standards usually proposed by nurses are a problem—somehow they challenge the norm. These situations require management as difficult cases (McKeever 1996).

In the case of health promotion, the discourse of risk reduction for society, once again, takes women's work for granted as free labour. The genderless health promotion discourse assumes that healthy diets will be cooked and served to families without asking by whom. Currently, 'good women' not only provide physical and emotional care, but also promote the health of their families. Furthermore, many of the changes in lifestyle proposed by the health promotion movement will take example, in psychiatric care, nurses are actively involved in this form of power through therapeutic communication in individual therapy.

Data from a grounded theory research study showed that nurses working in a correctional psychiatric setting used both types of power to govern inmates with psychiatric problems (Holmes 2001). On a daily basis nurses, accompanied by correctional officers, participated in rounds where they inspected inmates' cells in order to evaluate their degree of conformity to rules regarding hygiene and allowed content. Nurses working in this setting met inmates/patients once a week for a formal evaluation of their mental health status. It is through this 'therapeutic encounter' that nurses obtained information about the inmates they cared for. But for nurses to know, inmates have to share information about themselves. Confession constitutes the major tool of pastoral power that allows nurses to gather information. The therapeutic encounter is also a privileged moment where inmates/patients can share their feelings, fears and suffering. Pastoral power is also effective because it raises inmates' awareness regarding their condition and thus constitutes the first step to self-regulation.

So, although nurses are using disciplinary techniques such as surveillance, control of activities, punishments, and rewards in order to achieve obedience from inmates, they are also caring for them through pastoral care. In nursing theories, caring traditionally is viewed as being apart from disciplinary regimes in which social control is pervasive (Gastaldo & Holmes 1999). These research findings, on the contrary, confront us with the fact that there is no such paradox between disciplining and caring. To punish and forbid do not exclude treatment, care, reform, rehabilitation and transformation. Indeed, in this correctional psychiatric setting, disciplinary techniques rely on nursing care, while the latter relies simultaneously on the former.

As we can see, nurses use and often combine these two forms of power in their clinical practice. The previous examples illustrate how nurses are directly involved in the governance of individuals through disciplinary and pastoral power.

Governmentality and its Implications for Nursing

As Foucault stated, the concept of governmentality creates a new way of regarding the conduct of humankind; its aim is directed at 'the domains of ethics, government, and politics, of the government of self, others, and the state, of practices of government and practices of the self, of self-formation and political subjectification, that weaves them together *without a reduction of one to the other* (emphasis added)' (Dean 1994, p. 158).

Governing now implies going beyond the state and its official institutions or figures. Based on Foucault's idea, government can be understood as 'an active process which joins political rationalities . . . with governmental technologies' (Curtis 1995, p. 575); a process in which some ideals of social life set the conditions and create fields for intervention in most aspects of everyday living (Simon 1993, Curtis 1995). The articulation of political rationalities with technologies of government is ensured by a specific form of knowledge (scientific *savoir*) and the presence of an expert (nurse) who mediates between the political objectives and the object of intervention (population and individual). The state should now be considered as a 'network of institutions, deeply embedded within a constellation of ancillary institutions associated with society and the economic system' (Hall 1986, p. 17). Power operates within tiny, subtle and complex ramifications established by competent authorities. In an era of governmentality, power is pervasive and it relies on agents who can ensure the optimal functioning of this new art of government (Curtis 1995).

Nurses are health care professionals who are in direct contact with individuals, groups, communities, and populations. They are a powerful group of experts upon whom the state and its institutions rely. Working at the junction of the individual and collective body within power relations that promote and recuperate life, nurses are able, through their interventions, to mould, conduct or affect people as well as to construct, with the help of other health care professionals, people's subjectivities. This is accomplished through a vast range of techniques such as gathering information, producing and disseminating knowledge, and engaging in therapeutic encounters. Similar practices are undertaken by physicians, psychologists and social workers, to name a few. However, nurses are the biggest professional group of the Western world health care systems and the ones who are frequently made invisible, feel unimportant and victims of the organizations and groups that they help to create, sustain, and manage. The traditional framework used by nurses to analyse their practices helps to perpetuate the impression of a powerless profession.

According to Foucault's definition of governmentality, we believe that nurses constitute an important group that helps the state to govern at a distance. Nurses also form a critical group that challenges the status quo and works for a more equitable society. However, we believe that nurses predominantly conceive of health care as a neutral and apolitical practice (Meyer 1998, Freed 1999). Yet nurses' privileged position close to patients and communities allows them to act upon these individuals and groups. Through education, they normalize and discipline; through care, they alleviate the suffering of vulnerable individuals and communities and participate in the construction of patient identities as sick bodies or healthy bodies. They possess a scientific *savoir* that is generally accepted as true knowledge and are able to influence patient behaviours regarding their health, illness, and well-being. Nurses, as good translators of sophisticated medical and nursing terminology, are close to the public's needs and have their confidence.

Indeed, nurses are a group able to exercise power as health care providers, despite the fact that they seldom reflect about their own ways of exercising power or rarely perceive health care as a political activity. Nurses operate within a web of power relations defined by a society (also constituted by nurses) ruled by disciplinary and pastoral power strategies which are the main tools to govern conduct in our contemporary era. Despite the well known rhetoric regarding nurses' powerlessness, we believe that nurses constitute a powerful group of health care professionals located at the crossroad of the state's rationalities and patients' bodies and souls. This understanding situates them as an agency of governmentality.

Final Remarks: Exploring the Limits and Potential of Governmentality

Rethinking nursing through the concept of governmentality could be perceived by many as a threatening experience. We have commented previously that the use of Foucauldian concepts 'can generate a form of critical immobilism' (Gastaldo & Holmes 1999, p. 23) because governmentality links together repressive and constructive ways of exercising power. The deterministic nature of 'power everywhere' and the sense of being governed, even through our freedom, generate strong and emotive responses such as a need to escape, especially because moral attributes traditionally have been attached to different ways of governing. We are used to searching for "the right way' of practising nursing care and of being ethical in our interpersonal relationships or when governing society. For instance, compliance through disciplinary power becomes an imperative for patients suffering from life-threatening diseases, which can be managed by medication. However, the concept of governmentality challenges many assumptions taken for granted in nursing: ethics becomes politics, patient empowerment becomes a call for self-regulation, and in many ways nursing research serves the economic elites to the detriment of social equity.

The concept of governmentality should be seen as a valuable tool for deconstructing nursing as an apolitical practice and a powerless profession. However, it should also help us to envision alternative ways of practising nursing. To insist on a single unified identity as powerless professionals means many times that no criticism can be raised against nurses; it represents the creation of an analytic shield that protects and explains the current arrangements of power. Critical perspectives are seen as unreasonable or victim blaming. To conceive nurses as professionals who exercise power serves a two-fold purpose: it allows for a more complex conceptualization of practice and it can potentially reveal some of the elements that perpetuate nurses' underprivileged position in society.

Being historically situated in a nonpriviledged position to negotiate working conditions or to benefit from social prestige does not mean that nurses do not exercise power or that they are not powerful. The examples presented in this paper illustrate some of the ways in which nurses exercise power in their everyday practices. What remains is the need to articulate power exercises with political rationalities to which groups of nurses subscribe and to analyse the governmental technologies we develop and support. This process should be guided by critiques that emerge from considerations of governmentality because this concept reminds us that competing discourses, even among nurses, are constantly reshaping ideas and practices regarding nursing and health in the social, economic, and political arenas. Personally and as professionals, we have been exploring the potential of combining ideas about governmentality with critical social theories such as emancipatory feminism (Manias & Street 2000). To understand power without being able to identify 'possible transformations' (Meyer 1998) derived from this Foucauldian perspective will not lead nursing into critical political action. However, the concept of governmentality sheds light on the impossibility of a single strategy to achieve more social recognition for nurses and reminds us that we are powerful at the same time that we are situated historically in a nonpriviledged position.

Acknowledgments The authors would like to thank our colleague Dagmar Meyer from the Faculty of Education, Federal University of Rio Grande do Sul, Brazil, for many discussions on the subject of the paper and the scholars from the St Bartholomew School of Nursing and Midwifery, City University, UK, for their comments on this paper, which were shared after a presentation in November 2000. The authors are also grateful to the anonymous reviewers for their comments.

REFERENCES

Arendt H. (1995) Idéologie et terreur: un nouveau type de régime. *Les Origines Du Totalitarisme—Le Système Totalitaire.* Seuil, Paris.

Arruda E. & Silva A. (2000) Perspectiva internacional cerca de indicadores de qualidade em cursos de doutorado em enfermagem. *Revista Basileira de Enfermagem* **53**, 63–73.

Clinton M. & Nelson S. (1999) Recovery and mental illness. In *Advanced Practice in Mental Health Nursing* (Clinton M. & Nelson S. eds), Blackwell Science, Oxford, pp. 260–278.

Curtis B. (1995) Taking the state back out: Rose and Miller on political power. *British Journal of Sociology* **46**, 575–589.

Dean M. (1994) A social structure of many souls: moral regulation, government, and self-formation. *Canadian Journal of Sociology* **19**, 145–168.

Dean M. (1999) *Governmentality.* Sage, Thousand Oaks, CA.

Deflem M. (1998) Surveillance and criminal statistics: historical foundation of governmentality. *Studies in Law, Politics and Society* **17**, 1–28.

Foucault M., ([1975] 1995) *Surveiller et Punir: Naissance de la Prison.* Tel/Gallimard, St-Amand.

Foucault M. (1979) Governmentality. *Ideology and Consciousness* **6**, 5–21.

Foucault M. (1980a) Truth and power. In *Power/Knowledge and Selected Interviews and Other Writings 1972–1977 by Michel Foucault* (Gordon C. ed.), Pantheon Books, New York, pp. 109–133.

Foucault M. (1980b) The eye of power. In *Power/Knowledge and Selected Interviews and Other Writings 1972–1977 by Michel Foucault* (Gordon C. ed.), Pantheon Books, New York, pp. 146–165.

Foucault M. (1990) *History of Sexuality 1: An Introduction.* Penguin Books, London.

Foucault M. (1994a) *Dits et Écrits, tome 4.* Editions Gallimard, Paris.

Foucault M. (1994b) *Dits et Écrits, tome 3.* Editions Gallimard, Paris.

Foucault M. (1997) *Il Faut Défendre la Société.* Seuil/Gallimard, Paris.

Francke A., Garssen B. & Huijer Abu-Saad H. (1995) Determinants of changes in nurses' behaviour after continuing education: a literature review. *Journal of Advanced Nursing* **21**, 371–377.

Freed L. A. (1999) Power, politics and public policy. In *Community Health Nursing: Caring in Action* (Hitchcock J., Schubett P. & Thomas S. eds), Delmar Publishers, Boston, pp. 745–764.

Gastaldo D. (1997) Is health education good for you? Re-thinking health education through the concept of bio-power. In *Foucault, Health and Medicine* (Petersen A. & Bunton R. eds), Routlege, London, pp. 113–133.

Gastaldo D. (2000) Caring beyond nursing: politics from the South—Editorial. *Nursing Inquiry* **7**, 73.

Gastaldo D., De Pedro J. & Bover A. (2001) El reto de investigar en enfermería: una reflexión sobre las universidades españolas y el contexto internacional. *Enfermería Clínica* **11**, 220–229.

Gastaldo D. & Holmes D. (1999) Foucault and nursing: a history of the present. *Nursing Inquiry* **6**, 17–25.

Gordon C. (1991) Governmental rationality: an introduction. In *The Foucault Effect* (Burchell G., Gordon C. & Miller P. eds), The University of Chicago Press, Chicago, pp. 1–51.

Gros F. (1996) *Que Sais-Je? Michel Foucault.* Presses Universitaires de France, Paris.

Hail P. (1986) *Governing the Economy: The Politics of State Intervention in Britain and France.* Cambridge Polity Press, Cambridge.

Hewitt M. (1991) Biopolitics and social policy: Foucault's account of welfare. In *The Body: Social Processes and Cultural Theory* (Featherstone M., Hepworth M. & Turner B. eds), Sage, London, pp. 225–255.

Hindess B. (1996) *Discourses of Power: From Hobbes to Foucault.* Blackwell Publishers, Oxford.

Holmes D. (2001) Articulation du contrôle social et des soins infirmiers dans un contexte de psychiatrie penitentiaire. Thèse de doctorat, Université de Montréal, Montréal.

Lukes S. (1974) *Power: A Radical View.* Macmillan, London.

Lunardi V. (1999) *A Ética Como O Cuidado de Si E O Poder Pastoral Na Enfermagem.* Editoras Universitárias UFSC/UFPel, Florianópolis.

Lunardi Filho W. (2000) *O Mito Da Subalternidade Do Trabalho Da Enfermagem Á Medicina.* Editoras Universitárias UFSC/UFPel, Florianópolis.

MacGuire J. (1990) Putting nursing research findings into practice: research utilization as an aspect of the management of change. *Journal of Advanced Nursing* **15**, 614–620.

Manias E. & Street A. (2000) Possibilities for critical social theory and Foucault's work: a tool box approach. *Nursing Inquiry* **7**, 50–60.

Martin M. & Forchuk C. (1994) Linking research and practice. *International Nursing Review* **41**, 184–187.

Marx K. (1946) *Capital-Volume 1.* George Allan & Unwin, London.

McHoul A. & Grace W. (1993) *A Foucault Primer: Discourse, Power and the Subject.* New York University Press, New York.

McKeever P. (1996) The family: long-term care research and policy formulation. *Nursing Inquiry* **3**, 200–206.

McNay L. (1994) *Foucault: A Critical Introduction.* Continuum Publishing, New York.

Meyer D. (1998) Espaços de sombra e luz: reflex?es em torno da dimens?o educativa da enfermagem. In *Marcas Da Diversidade: Saberes E Fazeres Da Enfermagem Contemporânea* (Meyer D., Waldow V. & Lopes M. eds), Artes Médicas, Porto Alegre, pp. 27–42.

Moss J. (1998) *The Later Foucault.* Sage, Thousand Oaks, CA.

Nettleton S. (1991) Wisdom, diligence and teeth: discursive practices and the creation of mothers. *Sociology of Health & Illness* **13**, 98–111.

Ransom J. S. (1997) *Foucault's Discipline: The Politics of Subjectivities.* Duke University Press, Durham, NC.

Rose N. (1998) *Inventing Ourselves: Psychology, Power and Personhood.* Cambridge University Press, Cambridge.

Rose N. & Miller P. (1992) Political power beyond the state: problematics of government. *British Journal of Sociology* **42**, 173–205.

Simon J. (1993) *Poor Discipline: Parole and the Social Control of the Underclass, 1890–1990.* University of Chicago Press, Chicago.

Stewart M. (2000) *Community Nursing: Promoting Canadians' Health,* 2nd edn. W. B. Saunders, Toronto, ON.

Weber M. (1986) Domination by economic power and by authority. In *Power* (Lukes S. ed.), New York University Press, New York.

Weberman D. (1995) Foucault's reconception of power. *The Philosophical Forum* **26**, 189–217.

The Authors Comment

Nursing as Means of Governmentality

We have entered the 21st century, a time of global markets and fast information flow, and nurses are probably the most important group of health care providers in the world. Despite this assertion, nurses often describe themselves as powerless. Intrigued by this issue, we decided to write two articles (the first one, published in *Nursing Inquiry,* in 1999, was entitled "Foucault & nursing: A history of the present") to illustrate an alternative way to conceptualize power and demonstrate how nurses exercise power, even though they are frequently viewed as a group of professionals in an underprivileged position.

—Dave Holmes
—Denise Gastaldo

Judgements Without Rules: Towards a Postmodern Ironist Concept of Research Validity

Gary Rolfe

The past decade has seen the gradual emergence of what might be called a postmodern perspective on nursing research. However, the development of a coherent postmodern critique of the modernist position has been hampered by some misunderstandings and misrepresentations of postmodern epistemology by a number of writers, leading to a fractured and distorted view of postmodern nursing research. This paper seeks to distinguish between judgemental relativist and epistemic relativist or ironist positions, and regards the latter as offering the most coherent critique of modernist/(post) positivist nursing research. The writings of poststructuralist philosophers, including Barthes, Lyotard, Derrida, Foucault and Rorty are examined, and a number of criteria for a postmodern ironist concept of research validity or trustworthiness are suggested. Whilst these writers reject the idea of Method as a guarantee of valid research, they nevertheless believe that value judgements can and must be made, and turn to notions of ironism, différance, and the differend!. Ultimately, the postmodern ironist reader of the research report must make a judgement without criteria, based on her own practical wisdom or 'prudence.'

The past two decades have seen the gradual emergence of what might be called a postmodern sensibility in the arts, media and (to a lesser extent) science (Lister 1997).

More recently, a number of writers have begun with some success to explore and apply a postmodern perspective to nursing research (for example, Parsons 1995; Fahy 1997;

From G. Rolfe, Judgments without rules: Towards a postmodern ironist concept of research validity, Nursing Inquiry 2006, 13(1), 7–15.
Copyright 2006 by Blackwell. Reprinted with permission by Blackwell Publishing.

About the Author

GARY ROLFE was born in London and studied for a degree in philosophy at the University of Surrey, before training in Portsmouth as a psychiatric nurse. After working for several years in acute psychiatry, he took his Master's degree and doctorate in the Department of Education at Southampton University. Gary lectured at the University of Portsmouth for many years before taking up a Chair in Nursing at Swansea University in Wales, where he currently lives with his wife and three children. Gary has published over 100 books, chapters, and journal articles, and has conducted research in the field of practice development and evidence-based practice. His current writing interests include postmodern philosophy, research methodology, and epistemology.

Traynor 1997; Holmes 1998; Cheek 2000; Holmes and Warelow 2000). However, other attempts have been hampered by an inadequate consideration of the philosophical (and in particular, the epistemological) underpinnings of postmodernism, portraying it simply as a more or less complete relaxation of the rules and methods of modernist science. Watson (1999), for example, seems to suggest that postmodernism is a branch of new age philosophy, making reference in her book *Postmodernism and beyond* to 'the body as a sacred mirror' (159), Chinese Taoism (236), yogic Chakras (75), and 'the Zen of bedmaking' (237). Others, such as O'Callaghan and Jordan (2003), equate postmodernism with 'natural remedies, antiscience sentiments, holism, rejection of authority, individual responsibility and consumerist attitudes to health care' (29). Indeed, for some, postmodernism is regarded not so much as *post* modern, but as *pre* modern or *anti* modern.

This distortion of what is actually a well-developed critique of the modernist position leads to particular problems when it comes to postmodern considerations of validity in nursing research. If we take this naïve antimodernist 'anything goes' view, then validity is simply not an issue. While this rejection of validity as a consideration for nursing research might be acceptable to those researchers who are already sympathetic to the postmodern position, it is unlikely to win any new converts, because it portrays postmodernism as intellectually and philosophically lacking. Furthermore, it portrays it as a theoretical black hole in which decisions

about research can be reached idiosyncratically without any appeal to reason or logic. As Traynor (1997) memorably put it: 'no grounding or privilege, just free-floating trouble making'.

The purpose of this paper is therefore to sketch out some of the reasoning and beliefs that underpin a postmodern view of research and, in particular, its position on validity. The term 'validity' is highly contested in nursing research (see Graneheim and Lundman (2004) for a recent review of the literature), and its relation to concepts such as 'truth' has generated a great deal of debate in the wider research community (Sparkes 2001; Flaherty et al. 2002). However, for the purpose of this paper, I will employ the term 'validity' in its most widely used sense of the 'truth value' of the study. In other words, this paper explores the question of the criteria (or lack of them) that the postmodern reader might employ in deciding whether or not to accept the findings and conclusions of a research report. (For a rather different approach to the postmodern position on validity see Kvale 1996.) It has already been suggested that part of the problem lies in a sweeping and very loose definition of the term 'postmodernism' to describe a broad alliance of philosophers, writers, artists, architects, critical theorists and literary critics who have moved beyond or reacted against the modernist movement. Before we can progress any further, it is therefore necessary to explore and clarify some of the confusing and contradictory terminology surrounding the subject.

A Short Note on Terminology

A great deal of paper and ink have been consumed in futile attempts to define postmodernism, and we might almost say that part of its definition is its resistance to definition (Simons and Billig 1994). Perhaps the best we can do, then, is to say what it is not. Postmodernism is *not* modernism, although there is debate about whether it is the successor to modernism or merely a critique of it (see, for example, Lyotard 1992). Modernism (what postmodernism is *not)* is generally associated with the Enlightenment project which began in the eighteenth century and which 'emphasised a belief in human progress towards some ideal state through rationality and the methods of science' (Rolfe 2001, 39).

Modernism is undoubtedly the dominant paradigm in nursing at the present time, and is closely associated with the research paradigms of positivism and/or post-positivism. Positivists believe that there is a single and potentially knowable reality, which exists completely separately, and independently from ourselves, about which we are able to make more or less objective judgements, and which can be accessed through the application of the scientific method. This 'naïve realist' position gives rise to the correspondence theory of truth, in which a statement is true if and only if it corresponds to an object or event in the 'real world' (Austin 1950). Many writers now accept that positivism in its pure form is untenable, and suggest that most 'hard' scientific researchers are postpositivists. The postpositivists generally adopt a 'critical realist' position which, while also admitting to an objective and independent reality, is more sceptical of our ability to access it first-hand in any kind of accurate fashion. Both of these positions can be seen as variations on the doctrine of 'scientific realism' (Okasha 2002).

In opposition to this modernist/realist/(post) positivist stance is a broad grouping of what might loosely be referred to as postmodernist thinkers. As this paper is concerned with the issue of validity, it will be useful to distinguish between those who advocate an extreme relativist position (usually the postmodern artists, architects and cultural theorists) and those who believe that

we can and must continue to make judgements and distinctions, but who reject the modernist criteria on which they are made (usually the writers, literary critics and some of the philosophers).

Bhaskar (1979) referred to these two positions as judgemental and epistemic relativism, while Denzin and Lincoln (1998) termed them postmodernist and post-structuralist. While both positions are largely antirealist in believing that reality is constructed by (and to some extent dependent on) people, there are nevertheless important differences between them. The poststructuralists, who include Derrida (1974), Deleuze (1994), Foucault (1980) and the later Barthes (1977), as well as self-styled postmodernists such as Lyotard (1984), are epistemic relativists insofar as they adopt a questioning stance towards taken-for-granted assumptions about truth and its origins. In particular, they reject the structuralist claims that there are underlying structures or patterns linking the phenomena of human life (and especially language), which obey predictable and determinable laws.

However, these writers are not out-and-out relativists in the sense of believing that there is no independent and objective reality. But, whilst they accept the notion of an objective world 'out there,' the idea of a single objective truth which describes that world is simply untenable, because truth is dependent on language and language has no logical relation to reality. As Rorty puts it:

> To say that truth is not out there is simply to say that where there are no sentences there is no truth, that sentences are elements of human languages and that human languages are human creations (Rorty 1989, 5).

Denzin and Lincoln's postmodernists go much further in questioning not only the notion of a single truth, but also the idea of a single reality 'out there' in the world, claiming rather that reality is constructed separately by each individual. As we have seen, this judgemental relativist position stands in contrast to the former poststructuralist or epistemic relativist position in which judgements are still possible. In my discussion of research validity, I am naturally more interested in the epistemic relativists, because for the judgemental relativists the notion of any form of collective agreement on validity is virtually meaningless, and judgements, if they are made at all, are subjective and unique.

For the remainder of this paper, holders of this poststructuralist/epistemic relativist position will be referred to as 'postmodern ironists' (after Rorty 1989). Ironists accept that they can never fully justify their judgements to others or to themselves, but nevertheless maintain them in the belief that they are the best that are available at the present time. As Rolfe (2000b) argues, the ironist 'simply *believes* her project to be the best, at the same time knowing that there is no epistemological substance to her belief' (64).

Validity and the Ironist Researcher

For the judgemental relativists, truth is subjective, multiple and fractured, and the concept of validity as an indicator of truth-value therefore has little meaning. For the epistemic relativist or ironist, however, it is not the issue of truth that is at stake, but rather our access to it. The ironist, unlike the judgemental relativist, does not question the existence of an external reality 'out there' (as Rorty would say), nor even the existence of an external 'truth,' but is concerned rather with how we might come to know that reality and be able to verify the truth-value of such knowledge. As Rolfe (2000b) has pointed out:

> Unlike the out-and-out relativist, then, the ironist is not denying the existence of a real(ist) world, nor is she necessarily claiming that we can never 'know' that world, simply that we can never know that we know it (173).

The truth might well be out there, and our research study might well have uncovered it, but the ironist would argue that we can never really know whether we have uncovered the truth or not.

Against Method

For the positivists and postpositivists, validity is guaranteed by a close adherence to method. For example, valid findings from randomised controlled trials (RCTs) depend on the researcher conforming to the rules of sample selection, double blinding, correct administration of data collection tools, and so on. Judgements about the validity of these modernist methodologies therefore focus on the methods section of the research report, rather than on the findings themselves. The findings are assumed to be valid if and only if there are no flaws in the design and implementation of the method. This notion of validity presupposes either that there is one and only one 'gold standard' methodology for any particular type of research question (for example, the RCT is usually considered to be the gold standard for research that addresses issues of treatment effectiveness) or that if there is more than one valid(ated) methodology, each will produce broadly similar findings.

This notion of a single scientific method (*the* Method) which is superior to all others has already been challenged from within the scientific community itself in both the 'hard' sciences (Kuhn 1962; Feyerabend 1970) and the social sciences (Phillips 1973). In putting forward his idea of 'methodological anarchism,' Feyerabend (1970) noted that:

> The idea of a method that contains firm, unchanging, and absolutely binding principles for conducting the business of science gets into considerable difficulty when confronted with the results of historical research. We find, then, that there is not a single rule, however plausible, and however firmly grounded in epistemology, that is not violated at some time or other (21–2).

The idea that validity can be guaranteed by method is also challenged by postmodern ironists. First, they believe that research (that is, knowledge generation) is a creative process and that rigorous adherence to method tends to stifle creativity:

> The invariable fact is that a piece of work which ceaselessly proclaims its determination for method is ultimately sterile: everything has been put into the method, nothing is left for writing; the researcher repeatedly asserts that his text will be methodological but the text never comes. No surer

way to kill a piece of research and send it to join the great waste of abandoned projects than Method (Barthes 1977, 201).

For Barthes, the 'truth' or meaning of the text is in the 'writing' rather than in the method (or, as Barthes prefers, Method). Writing is the creative process in research: 'writing teaches us what we know, and in what way we know what we know [. . .] not until we had written this down did we quite know what we know' (van Manen 1997, 127). As Barthes warned us, if all our effort is put into Method, nothing is left for writing, and the creative process is stifled. And as Feyerabend (1970) added, rigid and rigorous application of the scientific method results in 'the inhibition of intuitions' such that '[the researcher's] imagination is restrained and even his language will cease to be his own' (20).

Second, and more importantly, the postmodern ironists argue that the idea of a single 'gold standard' methodology makes no sense. Not only do different methods produce different findings, but the same method employed on different occasions in different situations will also have a different outcome. Furthermore, there is no objective way of making validity judgements between these different data sets. Thus, the replies given to interview questions will depend on the setting, the occasion, the events immediately preceding the interview, as well as the age, gender, social class and ethnic origin of the interviewer. For example, Clark, Scott et al. (1999) found that mental health service users responded differently when interviewed by other service users to when interviewed by professional researchers, even though the interviews were all conducted in a rigorous fashion. One explanation for the discrepancy might be that the respondents gave more accurate or more truthful answers to other service users, perhaps because they felt able to speak more freely or were less likely to feel judged (Faulkner and Morris 2003).

This, of course, has important implications for the modernist researcher. As a realist, she will believe that the truth exists independently of the interviewer and the research setting, and she will therefore wish to conduct the interview at the time, place and with the interviewer

who will generate data that most closely resemble that truth. The questions she would therefore ask of herself are 'which is the more valid method?'; 'who is the more reliable interviewer?'; and 'which is the more accurate response?'. The ironist researcher, on the other hand, would regard such questions as meaningless, arguing that the responses are merely *different,* and that none is more or less accurate or valid than any other.

The Elusive Self

Modernist researchers aim to neutralise the effects of person and place. Quantitative researchers test for interrater reliability and attempt to decontextualise and depopulate the setting in which the research is taking place (see Billig 1994). Even qualitative modernists such as phenomenologists require the interviewer to 'bracket' off her own attitudes towards the research issues in order to get at the 'true' lived experience of the respondent. Debate continues about the extent to which bracketing is possible, and in any case, it is quite impossible for the researcher to control for the effects of her age, gender and so on.

Despite this, phenomenologists often talk as though they are bringing to light the 'true' lived experiences of their interviewees, and invoke the notion of 'trustworthiness' in support of their claim (Sandelowski 1993). Trustworthiness is usually regarded as an assurance that the researcher has adhered to the rules and method dictated by the paradigm she is following. Thus:

> Research findings should be as trustworthy as possible and every research study must be evaluated *in relation to the procedures used to generate the findings* (Graneheim and Lundman 2004, 109, italics added).

So, for example, the trustworthy phenomenologist is one who has bracketed off her own views about the phenomenon under investigation and conducted the research according to the rules of phenomenological interviewing. For the ironist researcher, however, such a reassurance is not only illusory; it is an indication that the study actually *lacks* validity. The researcher who presents her method as though it was conducted 'by the book' in a trustworthy fashion is not to be trusted. The researcher who claims to have successfully bracketed off her own views so that they do not influence the data is deluding herself and her readers. The researcher who claims to have accessed the 'lived experiences' of her subjects is to be regarded with suspicion.

Ironist researchers argue that there can be no 'true' or 'core' lived experience because there is no true or core self that has the experience and that can accurately reflect and report on it. Rather, they argue that self is relational or dialogical (Bhaktin 1986). In other words, it only makes sense to talk about self in relation to other selves, whether internal or external. I only become aware of my self when I am in dialogue with others or with myself, and this self will respond differently depending on my perception of those other selves. I create and reveal my own self through dialogue as I go along, and what I create and reveal varies from moment to moment and from person to person. The interviewee will therefore create and reveal different selves to different interviewers on different occasions and in different circumstances, although none of these could be said to be the 'true' self.

This is equally the case for internal dialogue or reflection. Depending on the circumstances, different selves (or aspects of the self) within the same person will engage in reflective dialogues with different outcomes. I will come to different conclusions about the same issue depending on whether I am angry, tired, elated, and so on. The modernist might argue that a reflection made whilst I am angry is not a 'good' or 'true' reflection, but the postmodern ironist would claim that there is no 'neutral' or quiescent state of mind that produces better or more accurate reflections than at other times. If we accept this position, then there is no core 'lived experience,' which I can reliably access and accurately express to another person. There is no authoritative version of any research data.

The Death of the Author

If there is no authoritative or 'true' version of research data, if the data are relative to the conditions under which they are collected, then the findings reported in the research report cannot be said to be valid in the sense usually understood by the modernists. However, ironist researchers question the authority of the report in a far more fundamental way. If there is no stable and unchanging self, then the self of the author of the report is also called into question. For example, the report is likely to be written differently depending on which self is writing it and with which other internal selves it is in dialogue with as it writes. Furthermore, the self of the author that later re-reads or reviews her earlier writing is likely to regard it differently from the self that wrote it. Thus, the author of the text has no more authority with regard to its 'true' meaning than any other reader, leading Barthes (1977) to proclaim the 'death of the author,' (142). Barthes took this observation to its obvious conclusion, and argued that we therefore have no way of discovering the 'authorial' or authorised interpretation of the text, that is, the meaning originally intended by the writer. Thus, the authorial voice is no more privileged than the interpretations given to the text by its many and varied readers. (For an ongoing debate on this issue from a nursing perspective, see Rolfe 1997; Closs and Draper 1998; Rolfe 1999; Burnard 1999; Rolfe 2000a.) Meaning is therefore created by the reader rather than the writer of a text and, in this sense, the author as the creative force in literature is dead:

> Once the author is removed, the claim to decipher a text becomes quite futile. To give the text an Author is to impose a limit on that text, to furnish it with a final signified, to close the writing [. . .] the birth of the reader must be at the cost of the death of the Author (Barthes 1977, 147–8).

Although Barthes was concerned primarily with Literature (with a capital L) and the novel, Jacques Derrida broadened out Barthes' thesis to apply to *all* writing. Furthermore, 'the concept of writing exceeds and comprehends that of language' (Derrida 1974), so that the impact of the death of the author extends well beyond the written word and applies to all forms of expression and all attempts at communication. From Derrida's perspective, then, there is no authorial/authoritative central position from which to judge the meaning of a text (in its broadest sense), and there are as many valid readings as there are readers. We live therefore in a 'decentred universe' (Derrida 1974) in which all attempts at validation are personal and subjective.

Knowledge and Power

Jean-Francois Lyoard made a similar point when he defined the postmodern as 'incredulity toward metanarratives' (Lyotard 1984, (xxiv)). Metanarratives are narratives or stories with a legitimising function, that is, stories that define the rules by which other stories can legitimately be told. So for example, science can be seen as a metanarrative that sets the rules according to which research can be designed, funded, carried out and disseminated: science (and scientists) determines what does and does not count as valid research. Science is therefore a game comparable to other games such as chess. The rules of chess are, to a large extent, arbitrary. There is no natural law that says that the bishop must only move diagonally; rather, it is an agreed rule that has no meaning outside the overall rules of the game. Similarly, Lyotard would argue that there is no natural law that says the RCT is the gold standard for evaluating treatment outcomes; rather, it is an arbitrary agreement between scientists that has no meaning outside of the game of science.

If Lyotard is right, then self-proclaimed metanarratives such as science have no natural authority to make validity claims. Science has achieved its position as a metanarrative not because it somehow reflects the laws of the natural world, but because influential scientists have awarded themselves rule-making powers, and have agreed to abide by their own rules. The authority of science derives not from epistemology, but from power and politics. Thus:

> Knowledge and power are simply two sides of the same question: who decides what knowledge is, and who knows what needs to be decided? In the computer age, *the question of knowledge is now more than ever a question of government* (Lyotard 1984, 8–9, italics added).

Foucault (1980) concurred with this view when he observed that 'we are subjected to the production of truth through power and we cannot exercise power except through the production of truth' (93). Science is essentially authoritarian rather than authoritative. When poststructuralists express their incredulity towards science, they are not dismissing it or refuting its claims; they are simply acknowledging that other competing narratives such as reflection or fictional literature have (or should have) equal status as ways of generating and disseminating knowledge. The author is dead, and the validity of the research text should be judged by each individual reader.

Judgements Without Rules: Towards A Postmodern Ironist View of Validity

For the ironist researchers, the validity of research texts is subjective and the truth claims made by the writer have no more authority than those of the many readers. But if this is the case, then according to what criteria are judgements to be made? At first sight, this looks very much like a recipe for an extreme relativist position in which anything goes and all judgements are equally valid. This is the position taken by some postmodernist writers, but the ironists do not argue that all judgements are equally *valid*, but rather that all have an *equal right to be heard*. In other words, we should not automatically discount certain narratives simply because they disagree with, or do not conform to the rules of, the dominant metanarrative of science. There are two questions to be addressed here. First, how are we to judge *between* the truth claims of the various paradigms; between, say, science and reflection? And, second, if validity judgements are made by the readers of the research report rather than by the writer, then what of competing judgements *within* the same paradigm?

Validity Judgements between Paradigms

Lyotard was particularly interested in the first of these questions. In his early work he distinguished between knowledge generated and disseminated through the method of science, and knowledge generated and disseminated through narrative forms such as story telling, pointing out that 'it is . . . impossible to judge the existence or validity of narrative knowledge on the basis of scientific knowledge and vice versa: the relevant criteria are different' (Lyotard 1984, 26). He later extended this critique to all competing paradigms, referring to the impossibility of judgement as a *differend* (Lyotard 1988).

For example, a RCT and an ethnography might generate conflicting data and arrive at different conclusions about the same phenomenon. If we attempt to settle the dispute between them by appealing to criteria such as sample size or test-retest validity, we will clearly favour the RCT. If, on the other hand, we employ criteria of subjectivity and verisimilitude, we will favour the ethnography. There is no neutral position from which to make a judgement, and 'a wrong results from the fact that the rules of the genre of discourse by which one judges are not those of the judged genre or genres of discourse' (Lyotard 1988, xi). The notion of the *differend*, in which one paradigm asserts its power over another, is exemplified by Gournay and Ritter's statement about nursing research that, 'there is of course a place for qualitative methods, but such research needs to use a rigorous approach *and should be linked to quantitative methodologies . . . for it to have any meaning*' (Gournay and Ritter 1997, 442, italics added).

There is no rule-based solution to this impasse that does not disadvantage one of the parties to the dispute. However, that is not to say that a judgement cannot be made, only that it will necessarily be a judgement without rules. Lyotard invokes Aristotle:

> insofar as he recognises . . . that a judge worthy of the name has no true model to guide his judgements, and that the true nature of the judge is to pronounce judgements, and therefore prescriptions, just so, without criteria. This is, after all, what Aristotle calls prudence. It consists in dispersing justice without models (Lyotard and Thebaud 1979, 25–6).

Judgements between the truth claims of different paradigms or discourses can only be made on an individual basis through the application of prudence or practical wisdom.[1] Judgements of research reports are made by individual readers based on their own individual experiences. Different readers will judge differently, but that is only to be expected, as each will have her own ideas about the 'truth' of the matter.

This might appear at first sight to be a judgemental relativist doctrine in which any one judgement is as valid as any other, but paradoxically, the most important implication of this position is that *not* all judges are equally equipped to make claims about the validity or truth of the research. For the modernists, judgements about validity can be made by *anyone* who can read and understand the relevant criteria. We can see this, for example, in many undergraduate research assignments, where the student with little or no experience of conducting research is nevertheless expected to be able to produce a critique of a research paper simply by following a set of criteria related to sample selection, methodological rigor, and so on.

For the ironist researcher, however, a degree of experience or even practical expertise (prudence) is required both in the research process and in the substantive content of the topic being researched. For the ironist, then, research is a *practice* with all that this implies (see, for example, Schon 1983), rather than merely a procedure. Just as nursing practice can only be evaluated and critiqued by experienced nurses, so research practice can only be evaluated and critiqued by experienced researchers. Furthermore, these evaluations are always contingent, and we can never offer any hard justification to support the choices we make, either to ourselves or to others. We therefore choose ironically, recognising that our judgements cannot be logically defended, nor that they are necessarily right for everyone. They are merely the best judgements we can make at the time.

---

[1]Although prudence is nowadays most often associated with caution or discretion, its root lies in the word 'providence', meaning divine guidance. It is in that sense of intuitive or experiential knowledge without recourse to the intellect (what Dreyfus (2001) referred to as expertise or practical wisdom) that it is used here.

Validity Judgements Within Paradigms

This general principle applies equally to validity disputes *within* paradigms. Two ethnographic research projects might arrive at very different findings, each claiming that theirs is the 'truth' of the matter. For Derrida (1982) there is no contradiction here. What is required is not an agreement about what is the 'real' truth, but an agreement to differ, what he refers to as an attitude of *différance*. The word *différance* is a neologism that combines the meanings of the French verbs 'to differ' and 'to defer.' To approach a dispute with an attitude of *différance* is to accept the differences between the two sides but to defer indefinitely any attempt to choose between them. This entails stepping outside of the traditional western Aristotelian logic of 'either-or': to hold an attitude of *différance* entails holding two contradictory meanings in your mind at the same time.

For example, the English word 'cleave' means both to cut in two and to join together. Although the two meanings are contradictory, this does not usually present us with a problem, because when the word is used in a sentence it always takes one meaning or the other, and the correct meaning can usually be determined by the context. As Wittgenstein (1953) tells us, meaning is not fixed, but is derived from the way the word is *used*. When we read the sentence 'the carpenter cleaved the wood,' we understand it to mean *either* that she cut it in two, *or* that she joined two pieces together, depending on the context; we cannot assign both meanings at the same time. Similarly, when faced with two contradictory research reports, the modernist researcher would accept either one or the other (or neither), but not both. However, an attitude of *différance* requires us to do exactly that. As the architect Robert Venturi (1966) put it, the postmodernist prefers 'both-and' to 'either-or.'

This might appear to be a profoundly antiscientific attitude, but in fact scientists are regularly required to adopt this 'both-and' attitude. For example, in certain physics experiments light behaves as a wave, whereas in other experiments it behaves as a stream of particles. A modernist 'either-or' attitude is of little help in understanding these contradictory properties of light. We know that the findings from the different experiments are contradictory, that logically light cannot be *both* a wave *and* a stream of particles, and yet that is how it behaves. The physicist must therefore adopt an attitude similar to Derrida's *différance* by accepting the findings from both studies, by holding two contradictory ideas in her head at the same time and forever deferring judgement between them.

Conclusion

It should be clear by now that, for the postmodern ironists, there can be no checklists of rules or criteria to determine the validity of a research study. That is not to say that they reject the concept of validity outright as having no meaning for researchers. However, unlike the modernists, they do not accept that the rigorous application of Method to the research process will provide any guarantee that the findings will be either valid or reliable. On the contrary, rigour stifles creative research, and to paraphrase Sandelowski (1993), rigor mortis quickly sets in.

One of the problems with challenging the concept of rigour is that it has become a term of praise synonymous with scholarship and good research practice. However, for the ironist, this is merely another example of an arbitrary rule being imposed on the 'game' of research. There is no natural law that equates rigour with validity, and we have seen that the keynote of ironist research is, in fact, the very opposite of rigour. Whereas a rigorous approach suggests a close and rigid adherence to Method, the ironists promote flexibility and reflexivity. Rather than tying themselves to a predetermined method, they will attempt to respond to the ongoing challenges presented by the messy reality of the research project in what Schön (1983) called the 'swampy lowlands' of practice.

Such deviation from the rigours of Method does not, however, compromise the validity or trustworthiness of the study, as the data are *already* fatally compromised. No matter how rigorously the method for producing the research data was conducted, the data themselves will vary according to a myriad of other criteria that can never be controlled for. Postmodernists believe that knowledge is socially and situationally constructed, and that the same situation never occurs twice. However, this is of little consequence, as they also argue that the validity/trustworthiness of the study is in the writing rather than in the method. It is in writing more so than in data collection or data analysis that knowledge is constructed from data. Thus, trustworthiness is concerned *not* with whether the data have been rigorously collected, but with their interpretation and presentation. Paradoxically, any attempt to present the research findings as objective or 'truthful' (that is, as the best or only interpretation of reality) will be seen as untrustworthy. However, if knowledge is created by the researcher through writing the report, then it is *recreated* anew in each reading. Furthermore, each reading results in a rewriting (even if it is only in the head of the reader), and the published text has no greater claim to authority than any of the many rewritings of that text.

Such a statement should not be seen as making any claims about the relative truth of these readings/ rewritings, but rather about their right to be heard. Postmodern ironism is not a judgemental relativist doctrine; it is not arguing that all readings of a text are equally valid, but rather that each has an equal right to a fair hearing. This is a political point rather than an epistemological one, and supports the poststructuralist belief that science has achieved its dominant position through the exercise of power rather than through rational argument. Ultimately, we *have* to make validity judgements about the competing claims of different research paradigms and individual studies. In the absence of any objective criteria, all we have are prudence, our subjective experience and our practical wisdom. Perhaps the best we can do is to judge ironically and without rules, to keep an open mind, and to agree to differ and defer, both with each other and with ourselves.

REFERENCES

Austin J. 1950. Truth. *Proceedings of the Aristotelian society* 24 (supp.): 111–28.

Barthes R. 1977. The death of the author. *Image, music, text.* London: Fontana.

Bhaktin MM. 1986. *Speech genres and other late essays.* Austin: University of Texas.

Bhaskar R. 1979. *The possibility of naturalism.* Brighton: Harvester Press.

Billig M. 1994. Sod Baudrillard! Or ideology critique in Disney World. In *After postmodernism,* eds H Simons and M Billig, 150–171. London: Sage.

Burnard P. 1999. A response to Rolfe's reply to Gloss & Draper. *Nurse Education Today* 19:598.

Cheek J. 2000. *Postmodern and poststructural approaches to nursing research.* Thousand Oaks, CA: Sage.

Clark C, A Scott, KM Boydell and RN Goering 1999. Effects of client interviews on client reported satisfaction with mental health services. *Psychiatric Services* 50:961–3.

Closs S and P Draper. 1998. Commentary: Writing ourselves. *Nurse Education Today* 18:337–41.

Deleuze G. 1994. *Difference and repetition.* London: The Athlone Press.

Denzin NK and YS Lincoln, eds. 1998. *Strategies of qualitative inquiry.* Thousand Oaks, CA: Sage.

Derrida J. 1974. *Of grammatology.* Baltimore: Johns Hopkins University Press.

Derrida J. 1982. *Margins of philosophy.* New York: Harvester Wheatsheaf.

Dreyfus HL. 2001. *On the internet.* London: Routledge.

Fahy K. 1997. Postmodern feminist emancipatory research: Is it an oxymoron? *Nursing Inquiry* 4:27–33.

Faulkner A and B Morris. 2003. Expert paper: User involvement in forensic mental health research and development. *NHS national programme on forensic mental health research and development.* Liverpool: University of Liverpool.

Feyerabend PK. 1970. Against method: Outline of an anarchistic theory of knowledge. *Minnesota Studies in the Philosophy of Science* 4:17–130.

Flaherty M, N Denzin, P Manning and D Snow. 2002. Review symposium: Crisis in representation. *Journal of Contemporary Ethnography* 31:478–516.

Foucault M. 1980. *Power/knowledge.* Brighton: Harvester Press.

Gournay K and S Ritter. 1997. What future for research in mental health nursing? *Journal of Psychiatric and Mental Health Nursing* 4:441–6.

Graneheim U and B Lundman. 2004. Qualitative content analysis in nursing research: Concepts, procedures and measures to achieve trustworthiness. *Nurse Education Today* 24:105–112.

Holmes C. 1998. Postmodernist science in the origins of the theories of Watson and Newman. *Asian Journal of Nursing Studies* 4:1–9.

Holmes C and P Warelow. 2000. Some implications of postmodernism for nursing theory, research and practice. *Canadian Journal of Nursing Research* 32:89–101.

Kuhn TS. 1962. *The structure of scientific revolutions.* Chicago: University of Chicago Press.

Kvale S. 1996. *Interviews: An introduction to qualitative research interviewing.* Thousand Oaks, CA: Sage.

Lister P. 1997. The art of nursing in a 'postmodern' context. *Journal of Advanced Nursing* 25:38–44.

Lyotard J-F. 1984. *The postmodern condition: A report on knowledge.* Manchester: University of Manchester Press.

Lyotard J-F. 1988. *The differend: Phrases in dispute.* Minneapolis: University of Minnesota Press.

Lyotard J-F. 1992. *The postmodern explained to children.* London: Turnaround.

Lyotard J-F and J-L Thebaud. 1979. *Just gaming.* Minneapolis: University of Minnesota Press.

van Manen M. 1997. *Researching lived experience.* Ontario: Althouse Press.

O'Callaghan F and N Jordan. 2003. Postmodern values, attitudes and the use of complementary medicine. *Complementary Therapies in Medicine* 11:28–32.

Okasha S. 2002. *Philosophy of science: A very short introduction.* Oxford: Oxford University Press.

Parsons C. 1995. The impact of postmodernism on research methodology: Implications for nursing. *Nursing Inquiry* 2:22–8.

Phillips DL. 1973. *Abandoning method.* London: Jossey-Bass.

Rolfe G. 1997. Writing ourselves: Creating knowledge in a postmodern world. *Nurse Education Today* 17:442–8.

Rolfe G. 1999. Rewriting myself. *Nurse Education Today* 19:295–8.

Rolfe G. 2000a. On not being clear: A response to Burnard. *Nurse Education Today* 20:449–52.

Rolfe G. 2000b. *Research, truth and authority: Postmodern perspectives on nursing.* Basingstoke: Macmillan.

Rolfe G. 2001. Postmodernism for healthcare workers in 13 easy steps. *Nurse Education Today* 21:38–47.

Rorty R. 1989. *Contingency, irony and solidarity.* Cambridge: Cambridge University Press.

Sandelowski M. 1993. Rigor or rigor mortis: The problem of rigor in qualitative research revisited. *Advances in Nursing Science* 16:1–8.

Schon D. 1983. *The reflective practitioner.* London: Temple Smith.

Simons H and M Billig. 1994. *After postmodernism.* London: Sage.

Sparkes AC. 2001. Myth 94: Qualitative health researchers will agree about validity. *Qualitative Health Research* 11:538–52.

Traynor M. 1997. Postmodern research: No grounding or privilege, just free-floating trouble making. *Nursing Inquiry* 4:99–107.

Venturi R. 1966. *Complexity and contradiction in architecture.* New York: Museum of modern art.

Watson J. 1999. *Postmodern nursing and beyond.* Edinburgh: Churchill Livingstone.

Wittgenstein L. 1953. *Philosophical investigations.* Oxford: Basil Blackwell.

The Author Comments

Judgements Without Rules: Towards a Postmodern Ironist Concept of Research Validity

This article was written as a contribution to a growing postmodern perspective on nursing science, but also out of frustration at what I perceived to be a misunderstanding, misrepresentation, and misapplication of postmodern theory in nursing. In particular, I wished to challenge and refute the idea of postmodernism as a regression to a premodern antiscience, to a new-age mysticism, or as giving license to an 'anything goes' approach to research and theory. The article focuses particularly on the problem of making postmodern judgements about the validity or truth value of research studies, and argues that while there can be no single authorial reading of any research report, the authority of the experienced nurse or researcher should take precedence over the rigorous application of pre-agreed rules or criteria about validity.

—GARY ROLFE

Paradigms Lost, Paradigms Regained: Defending Nursing Against a Single Reading of Postmodernism

Chris Stevenson
Ian Beech

Within nursing, postmodernism has been seen as both a freeing influence and a philosophy of rejection and relativism. Within this paper we consider readings of postmodernism that have been presented and offer a re-reading that retains the idea of 'the good' and is neither relativist nor rejectionist. Local knowledge is to be judged by the relevant community and theoretical knowledge becomes nursing knowledge through reflexivity and improvization in practice. A story is good if it allows people to go on with their lives.

Introduction and Foreword

In considering nursing texts (by which we mean text in its broader sense of a set of signals, whether written, spoken or enacted, that may be read) as part of our academic lives, we have become aware that postmodernism creates philosophical angst and moral panic. Postmodernism has been described as ' . . . a time of paradigms lost' (Reed, 1995, p. 71). There have been attempts from those positioning themselves outwith the postmodern turn to defend nursing from the postmodern hoax (Kermode & Brown, 1996). The three essential themes often ascribed to postmodernism, and the perceived threats, are:

- acceptance of multiple realities with loss of generalizable knowledge as local knowledge of nursing is foregrounded, so that an anarchistic 'anything goes' attitude prevails (Holdsworth, 1997);
- relativism (Porter, 1996): creating an ethically free zone within which guidelines are not possible and

About the Authors

CHRIS STEVENSON earned an RMN, a BA(Hons), an MSc(Dist), and a PhD. She is Chair in Mental Health Nursing, Dublin City University. The focus of her scholarship is on describing the nature of meaningful responses to people in psychological/mental health distress, especially suicidality. She has worked closely with Professor Phil Barker in developing and evaluating the Tidal Model of psychiatric nursing, which has a developing profile nationally and internationally. Dr. Stevenson is interested in exploring different routes to knowledge for nursing and other health professions, including how people who are experts by experience contribute. Many papers that she has written challenge orthodox 'health wisdom' and the methods by which it is produced. Her hobbies include reading, running, writing, and films.

IAN BEECH was born on September 30, 1960, and has earned an RMN, an RGN, and a BA (Hons). Mr. Beech is a PGCE Senior Lecturer in Mental Health Nursing in the University of Glamorgan, Wales, United Kingdom. His primary interests within nursing are working with people in depression using a logotherapeutic approach, spiritual aspects of people's lives and suffering, and the relationship between nurses and people receiving nursing care. Mr. Beech has conducted research into some of these areas using phenomenology and contributed widely within the UK to the debate on research methodology in mental health nursing. He is also facilitating the introduction of the Tidal Model within three separate clinical areas locally. Throughout his life, Mr. Beech developed interests in Buddhism, reading, playing folk music on Tenor Banjo and Octave Mandola, and walking the dogs.

health professionals are able, for example, to ignore the reality of abuse (Minuchin, 1991);

- a philosophy of rejection and destruction. For example, postmodernism signals the 'last post' for psychiatric nursing, leaving uncertainty and fragmentation (Clarke, 1996).

While respecting the issues that learned colleagues have raised, we think that some criticisms of postmodernism within nursing have been based on a single reading which, ironically (for postmodernists at least), purports to capture its *essence* as anarchistic, relativist and amoral, and destructive.

We think that this particular reading has its foundations in the ideology of positivist science. Shotter (1993) notes that when conversations become formalized into a particular discourse, ideological processes are likely to benefit some groups over others. Thus, when there is an orthodox, legitimated approach to knowing about the world, other approaches become subjugated. For example, elsewhere we have narrated

our experiences of ethical and research awarding committees' lack of an understanding of qualitative research proposals because they do not value the kind of knowledge that would be generated (Stevenson & Beech, 1998). When one position becomes dominant, interesting questions arise in relation to epistemological hegemony (Birch, 1995). Do traditional ideas about truth become a normative imperative for all researchers? *Who* are the authentic voices in knowledge production? What benefits do they gain? How do nontraditionalist researchers establish their authority? Lather (1991) points out that traditional ways of knowing and being known necessarily involve a political dimension which includes some self serving bias. Cooper & Stevenson (1998) note that scientific knowledge in our society is seen as legitimate and disciplines adopting scientific methods are seen as respectable. In relation to psychology, they argue that this leads to a 'tidying away' of discrepant forms of knowledge, by overlaying them with science. For example, lay and folk psychological beliefs have been denigrated. We consider the critiques of postmodernism outlined above to be attempts to traditionalize nursing and as such are '. . . a self-descriptive, externalizing of the ideology of the day' (Rorty, 1982, 1–2). We suggest also that postmodernists are not insensitive to the 'real' world and its dilemmas. In the interest of balance, we revisit these 'dilemmas' and offer alternative, postmodern readings. However, we do not want to simply present another authorized version (grand narrative) of the nature of knowledge, from the academy. To do so would be to present a different marginalizing discourse. According to Lyotard (1984), what counts as knowledge is less important than an analysis of how the decision is made about what is classed as real, of who has the authority. For what is classed as not real becomes *second* class. Research falling within the postmodern turn points up the contradiction and presuppositions implicit to the production of any authorized version of the world, including its own (Heslop, 1997). Our aim is to keep the debate about postmodernism in nursing fluid. First, however, we set out what we mean by postmodernism in the context of this paper.

'What Are We Calling Postmodernity? I'm Not Up To Date.'

(Foucault in Schrag, 1992, p. 16)
Postmodernism has been seen as the modern turning upon itself to re-read its texts, reassessing their value in relation to current context.

> Postmodernism does not completely break with modernism . . . postmodernism 'begins' when the present ceases to be informed by the past. (Clarke, 1996, p. 257)

Bauman (1990) argues that postmodernity is not a successor regime to modernity rather modernity undergoing self-examination and resolving to change on the strength of that examination. Problematizing modernity from within modernity is what Habermas (1981) described as the uncompleted project of modernism.

For example, whilst Popper accepted the Humean objection to scientific inductivism, he used it as the foundation for a new logic of modernist science, i.e. falsificationism. For Habermas, the errors of modernity can be corrected by the use of reflective reasoning.

In common with Rolfe (2000), we reject the idea of postmodernism as modernism reflecting upon itself. We think that postmodernism entails a rejection of the values of modernism and this makes it more than the uncovering of contradictions within modernist science. We do not attempt to be definitive about postmodernism, because to do so would be contrary to the spirit of the postmodern turn. We prefer to give our *personal* description of postmodernism, drawing on the work of Stevenson & Reed (1996). Postmodernism is a rejection of the modern, post-Enlightenment concern with the rational and scientific. It is a movement away from grand theories or narratives that try to explain the world towards local and specific knowledge. Although there is much variation in postmodernism, there is sharing of nonfoundationalist ideas. For example, truth is seen as problematic and not necessarily progressively accessible through scientific exploration or logical reasoning. Complexity and ambiguity are celebrated and inconsistencies, paradoxes and contradictions are not of concern, because knowledge is inseparable from the specific context in which it comes into existence. We concur with Wittgenstein (1953) in his work *Philosophical Investigations* that language cannot be separated from a physical reality that it represents. In common with Wittgenstein, we see language as forming the world in which we live. What we know about our world lies in the relationship between the knower and the other. People co-create stories that are treated as negotiated or 'soft' realities which allow them to 'go on with' their lives. For example, this paper is itself a story that allows us to go on with our lives as academic researchers, in a context where there is disagreement about the value of different theoretical (or antitheoretical) inquiry positions. We think that our version of postmodernism can address the reading of postmodernism as antirealist, relativist, rejectionist and destructive, which we examine in the following sections.

One Truth or Multiple Realities?

There are many existing critiques of positivism (e.g. Chalmers, 1999). In a sense, positivism can be seen as a straw person, easy to criticize in its attachment to objectivity, representationalism, etc. when applied in the social sciences. However Rolfe (2000) suggests that some philosophers of science, e.g. Feyerabend and Kuhn, have taken a postpositivist position in criticizing the *methods* of positivist science whilst retaining a commitment to the *ideals* of science. If modernism and postmodernism are incommensurable, as argued above, then there is no way of formulating a description of modernist scientific knowledge within the postmodern *or* of criticizing the postmodern from within the modern. Lyotard (1989) described this impasse as *le différend*. Put simply, there are no rules equally applicable to each position that would allow a comparison between the positions. In such circumstances, decisions about what is 'good' or 'true' are based more on values as Rorty (1982) has argued. Yet, the reading of postmodernism outlined above ignores *le différend*. There are less traditional approaches that try to bridge the discrepant positions of modernism and postmodernism, engaging with the ideas of both. Critical realism, as developed by Bhaskar (1989a), entails the position that there is a real world 'out there.' Although Bhaskar rejects the idea that his view is positivist or empiricist, we would see him as occupying a postpositivist position, since he argues that the reality cannot be theorized about in an entirely objective way because of the limitations of human perception and cognition. Additionally, theoretical objectivity is impossible because of the collaborative process by which people make sense of their world. In this, Bhaskar accepts the social construction of knowledge. But critical realism was developed as an antidote to the perceived relativism inherent in some more 'anarchistic' approaches to 'knowledge' production (Bhaskar, 1989b). It entails an acceptance of an ontological reality, and so a scientific methodology in that there are rational grounds for preferring one belief to another. Truth is that which most closely *approximates* to the ontological reality.

Whilst Bhaskar massages concerns about what can be known, we believe that our world is not simply mediated by discourse, as in critical realism, but created through it. As Rorty (1982) describes it:

> So the real issue is not between people who think one view is as good as another is and people who do not. It is between those who think our culture, or purpose, or intuitions cannot be supported except conversationally, and people who still hope for some other support. (pp. 166–167)

Derrida (1978) challenged the taken for granted view that language is capable of expressing views without changing them. All language is metaphorical, referring to something that is not. By this we mean that language does not represent the world in a straightforward way. As an example we take the metaphorical language of AIDS/HIV:

> The papers are full of new drugs and new theories. The T-cell, it appears, far from being decimated by an HIV awakened from the languor of a 10-year slumber by some internal alarm clock, instead fights tooth and nucleus in a war of attrition against the invading virus, and then, after years of bloody battle, collapses in exhaustion as an army of replicants conquers the corpuscles. (Moore, 1996, pp. 74–75)

The inevitability of metaphor makes multiple meanings possible because, as de Saussure (1983) tells us, there is always a gap between the signifier (the word or act) and the signified (the concept to which the signifier refers). The signifier and the signified together make the sign that points to the object that is the reference. But because of the *inevitable* gap, gauging 'fit' against an external reality, as in positivism and postpositivism, is no longer a way of evaluating beliefs or interpretations. The power of language is demonstrated by an analysis of what happens when communication breaks down. We have given a clinical example elsewhere of a situation where a person encounters a professional and tells the story of being controlled by extra-terrestrial forces (Stevenson & Beech, 1998). The professional has a choice. In following the language game (Wittgenstein,

1953) implicit in professional training, delusional or hallucinatory content is not discussed for fear of reinforcing the presentation of illness. In this circumstance, the person and professional usually enter into stalemate broken by the administration of medication. In entering into a discussion about the meaning of being controlled rather than a disagreement about the nature of reality the possibility for the co-creation of a new story emerges between the person and the professional with new possibilities for progress.

We accept that some readers may be unconvinced by our schizophrenia example given the debates ongoing within the scientific community on schizophrenia, in particular, the search for a marker gene for schizophrenia, the *disease*. Therefore, we offer an alternative example of diabetes mellitus, within which we use the work of Barthes (1977). Barthes rejected the idea of

> . . . the voice of a single person, the *author* 'confiding' in us. The aim of literary criticism was therefore no longer an attempt to arrive at the 'true' meaning of the text as intended by the author. (Rolfe, 2000, p. 38)

The death of the author allows the birth of the reader in the sense that responsibility for making sense of the text lies with the person making a personal interpretation. From our position, there are many different readings of, for example, diabetes mellitus. We do not dispute the body's failure to produce insulin in the way that might be expected. This need not dictate the nurse's approach to the person diagnosed as diabetic. Mitchell (1995) illustrates the approach of a nurse guided by a fairly traditional, scientific knowledge of diabetes to someone who planned to wean herself off insulin. In Mitchell's example, the nurse contacted the physician about the pending non-compliance and arranged a teaching session on the importance of insulin for the woman. After this intervention had been carried out the woman found herself in conflict with the nurse and doctor and, in spite of being educated about the importance of insulin continued to plan to stop taking the drug. A nurse adopting the postmodern approach (advocated by Parse,

1995) entered discussion with the woman. Instead of finding that the woman was ignorant of scientific knowledge about insulin and its importance to her physiology, the nurse found that the woman, while being knowledgeable, did not value that particular story. Neither was the woman suicidal. She had made plans both to cut sugar from her diet and to keep detailed checks on her blood sugar levels. It emerged that the woman's father had died as a result of insulin and she now carried a conviction that insulin might kill her. The ongoing relationship between the nurse and the woman, rather than being based on an 'I'm right, you're wrong' monologue, enabled a set of future possibilities to develop. Superficially, the example is consistent with a realist analysis. The woman had a personal theory, or imperfect interpretation of the world, that guided her intention to stop taking insulin. However, a critical realist analysis invites a pathologizing discourse concerning the woman's case. Specifically, it allows a view that the woman's 'faulty' interpretation needs fixing. Some postmodernists acknowledge that there is a family resemblance (Wittgenstein, 1953) between nursing situations. In discussing diagnostic frameworks, Cronen & Lang (1994) note that there are similarities between people who are labelled as, for example, schizophrenic. However, and critically for these authors, the differences between these people are as great as the sameness and local nursing knowledge is needed. With this perspective there is less attachment to fixing pathology and more room to treat the individual albeit against a background of assumed similarity.

An emphasis on language is problematic for those outwith the postmodern turn. If there is no longer representationalism, then how can one version be better or worse than any other—anything goes with the tyranny of choice. We turn to this issue in our discussion of relativism and pragmatism.

Relativism and Pragmatism

A question arising from the single reading of postmodernism is 'What constitutes "good" postmodern nursing?'

that can easily be generalized from one situation to another. Relativism seems inevitable. Few nurses would claim that the reality of working in an area one day was identical to that of the next/previous day, but they have to make responses and have them judged in a local framework of evaluation and hope that the response will be acceptable and accepted. Reed (1995) argues that good research is useful research in terms of certain patient important dimensions, e.g. informing about healing environments, inner human potential and the developmental/contextual nature of health. A similar set of dimensions might describe *useful* nursing practice.

Reflexivity, based upon critical, ironic reflection, can be the source of ethics. Nurses who reflect on their own contribution to the production of knowledge are placing their values and ideologies centre stage. In such circumstances, nurses can be held socially accountable for the distinctions that they make (Krippendorf, 1991).

Summary of the Postmodern Response to the Three Themes

In returning to the three themes that we identified at the start of this paper, we consider that postmodernism has been presented as: lacking in generalizability and giving primacy to local knowledge; relativist in its permissiveness for anything to be allowed; a philosophy of deconstruction that breaks down truth without replacing it with anything.

In response to the first theme of lacking generalizability we have shown that nursing ideas and nursing research are good if the stories they tell allow nurses and people in care to get on with their lives. If the story is useful it is used, if not it is rejected. While there is no overall generalizability there are family resemblances between stories that have resonance for practitioners.

The second theme alleges that postmodernism is relative and allows anything to go, including abuse. However abuse would be neither good nor useful to nurses and people in living their lives and would not be judged as such by nurses within the postmodern turn.

The third theme considers postmodernism to be destructive in its deconstruction of ideas. We have indicated that deconstruction should not be conflated with destruction and that the reflexive practitioner can improvise around the theme of existing theory while still deconstructing that theory.

So as a means of summarizing the paper's arguments, we want to offer our responses to the question, 'What is "good" postmodern nursing?'. Watson (1995) envisages nursing using the free-floating era of postmodernism as a means of nursing moving away from a reactionary worldview. Lister (1991) values postmodernism as an antidote to the unthinking application of models of nursing. Stevenson & Reed (1996) note that practitioners influenced by postmodern ideas may give the person in psychiatric distress more space to tell her/his story, because the professional is less attached to a single version of the truth of mental illness. If what counts as good nursing is less rule bound than is usually thought, nurses can take responsibility for their own practice based upon reflection in and on action.

REFERENCES

Andersen T. (1987). The reflecting: dialogue and metadialogue in clinical work. *Family Process, 26,* 415–428.

Atkinson B. & Heath A. (1987). Beyond objectivism and relativism: implications for family therapy research. *Journal of Strategic and Systemic Therapies, 6,* 8–17.

Barthes R. (1977). *Image Music Text.* Fontana, London.

Bauman Z. (1990). *Modernity and Ambivalence.* Polity, Cambridge.

Bhaskar R. (1989a). *Reclaiming Reality.* Verso, London.

Bhaskar R. (1989b). *The Possibility of Naturalism: a Philosophical Critique of the Contemporary Human Sciences.* Harvester Wheatsheaf, Hemel Hempstead.

Birch J. (1995). Chasing the rainbow's end and why it matters: a coda to Pocock, Frosh and Larner. *Journal of Family Therapy, 2,* 219–228.

Chalmers A. (1999). *What Is This Thing Called Science?,* 3rd edn. Open University Press, Buckingham.

Clarke L. (1996). The last post? Defending nursing against the postmodernist maze. *Journal of Psychiatric and Mental Health Nursing, 4,* 257–265.

Cooper N. & Stevenson C. (1998). New 'science' and psychology. *Psychologist, 11,* 484–485.

Cronen V. & Lang P. (1994). Language and action: Wittgenstein and Dewey in the practice of therapy and consultation. *Human Systems, 5,* 5–43.

Derrida J. (1978). *L'Écriture and Differance.* (tr. A. Bass). University of Chicago Press, Chicago.

Foucault M. cited by Schrag C. O. (1992). *The Resources of Rationality.* Indiana University Press, Bloomington, MD.

Habermas J. (1981). Modernity—an incomplete project. *New German Critique, 22,* 3–15.

Heslop L. (1997). The (im) possibilities of poststructuralist and critical social inquiry. *Nursing Inquiry, 4,* 48–56.

Holdsworth N. (1997). Postmodernity and psychiatric nursing: a commentary. *Journal of Psychiatric and Mental Health Nursing, 4,* 309–312.

James W. (1907). *What Pragmatism Means.* http://www.marxists.org/reference/subject/philosophy/index.htm (accessed 27/02/01).

Kermode S. & Brown C. (1996). The postmodern hoax and its effects on nursing. *International Journal of Nursing Studies, 33,* 375–384.

Krippendorf K. (1991). What should guide reality construction? In: *Research and Reflexivity* (ed. F. Steier). Sage, London.

Kuhn T. (1970). *The Structure of Scientific Revolutions.* University of Chicago Press, Chicago.

Lather P. (1991). *Getting Smart. Feminist Research and Pedagogy with/in the Postmodern.* Routledge, London.

Lister P. (1991). Approaching models of nursing from a postmodern perspective. *Journal of Advanced Nursing, 16,* 206–212.

Lyotard J.-F. (1984). *The Post-Modern Condition: a Report on Knowledge.* Manchester University Press, Manchester.

Lyotard J.-F. (1989). *The Differend: Phrases in Dispute* (tr. G. Van Den Abbeele). University of Minnesota Press, Minneapolis.

Minuchin S. (1991). The seductions of constructivism. *Family Therapy Networker,* September/October, 47–50.

Mitchell G. (1995). The view of freedom within the human becoming theory. In: *Illuminations: the Human Becoming Theory in Practice and Research* (ed. R. Parse). National League for Nursing, New York.

Moore O. (1996). *PWA: Looking AIDS in the Face.* Picador, London.

Parry A. & Doan R. (1994). *Story Re-Visions: Narrative Therapy in the Postmodern World.* Guilford Press, New York.

Parse R. (ed.) (1995). *Illuminations: the Human Becoming Theory in Practice and Research.* National League for Nursing, New York.

Peplau H. (1988). *Interpersonal Relations in Nursing.* MacMillan, Basingstoke.

Porter S. (1996). Real bodies, real needs: a critique of the application of Foucault's philosophy to nursing. *Social Sciences in Health, 2,* 218–227.

Reed P. (1995). A treatise on nursing knowledge development for the 21st century: beyond postmodernism. *Advances in Nursing Science, 17,* 70–84.

Rolfe G. (2000). *Research, Truth and Authority: Postmodern Perspectives on Nursing.* MacMillan, Basingstoke.

Rorty R. (1982). *Consequences of Pragmatism.* University of Minnesota Press, Minneapolis.

de Saussure F. (1983). *Course in General Linguistics.* Duckworth, London.

Schön D. (1987). *Educating the Reflexive Practitioner.* Jossey-Bass, San Francisco.

Shotter J. (1986). Speaking practically: Whorf, the formative function of communication and knowing of a third kind. In: *Contextualism and Understanding in Behavioural Science: Implications for Research and Theory* (eds L. Rosnow & M. Georgoudi). Praeger, New York.

Shotter J. (1993). *Conversational Realities.* Sage, London.

Stevenson C. & Beech I. (1998). Playing the power game for qualitative researchers: the possibility of a postmodern approach. *Journal of Advanced Nursing, 27,* 790–797.

Stevenson C. & Reed A. (1996). Editorial. *Journal of Psychiatric and Mental Health Nursing, 4,* 215–216.

Watson J. (1995). Postmodernism and knowledge development in nursing. *Nursing Science Quarterly, 8,* 60–64.

Wittgenstein L. (1953). *Philosophical Investigations* (tr. G.E.M. Anscombe). Blackwell, Oxford.

The Authors Comment

Paradigms Lost, Paradigms Regained: Defending Nursing Against a Single Reading of Postmodernism

Entering the 21st century, we were concerned with the growth in rhetoric in the United Kingdom about evidence-based nursing practice. It occurred to us that a narrow definition of evidence was being used, based largely in positivist or postpositivist ideas. In parallel, we noticed that there was a robust critique of postmodern ideas in nursing. However, to our (collective) mind, the critique was based in a reading of postmodernism through a traditional scientific lens. We wanted to argue that postmodernist nursing is not condemned to anarchistic relativism and retains a pragmatic notion of what is "good," that postmodernist nursing defines knowledge as transformable by nurses in everyday practice according to "peculiar" situation, and is what will enable them to sensitively help patients meet their needs.

—Chris Stevenson

—Ian Beech

Epistemologies, Evidence, and Practice

This unit was inspired by seminal and contemporary articles on nursing epistemology coupled with the emphasis on evidence-based practice. The focuses of epistemology, evidence and practice come together to make important statements about our disciplinary knowledge. Transformations in the way we think about nursing knowledge and theory can be tracked historically across seminal thinkers, from Florence Nightingale to Hildegard Peplau to Martha Rogers. In addition, thirty years ago, Barbara Carper initiated an important change in nursing epistemology that is still being realized today. Writings about the roles of professional knowledge, aesthetics, the personal, and critical reflection in knowledge development suggest a movement toward greater epistemological diversity than currently what may be warranted as evidence in practice. And the context of practice is a central consideration for inventing new approaches to theory generation.

Nursing knowledge production in the 21st century will require innovative thinking among theorists and researchers as well as require the leadership of practitioners and involvement of patients. Perhaps the most important message in this unit concerns the importance of *theory-based* knowledge as evidence for practice.

Questions for Discussion

• What role can practice play in knowledge production beyond being the place where nurses identify research problems, or apply and evaluate ideas from theory and research?

- Has nursing epistemology evolved beyond what Nightingale envisioned?
- Has nursing epistemology evolved beyond what Carper envisioned?
- What should be warranted as 'evidence' for practice?
- What are the critical dimensions of nursing knowledge?

CHAPTER 35

Evidence for Practice, Epistemology, and Critical Reflection

Mark Avis

Dawn Freshwater

Evidence-based practice (EBP) has become a critical concept for ethical, accountable professional nursing practice. However, critical analysis of the concept suggests that EBP overemphasizes the value of scientific evidence while underplaying the role of clinical judgment and individual nursing expertise. This paper explores the empiricist position that valid evidence is the basis for all knowledge claims. We argue against the positivist idea that science should be regarded as the only credible means for generating evidence on which to base knowledge claims. We propose that the process of critically reflecting on evidence is a fundamental feature of empirical epistemology. We suggest that critical reflection on evidence derived from science, arts and humanities and, in particular, nursing practice experience can provide a sound basis for knowledge claims. While we do not attempt to define what counts as evidence, it is argued that there is much to be gained by making the processes of critical reflection explicit, and that it can make a valid contribution to expert nursing practice, without recourse to irreducible concepts such as intuition.

Introduction

In recent years, evidence-based practice (EBP) has become identified with accountable, professional nursing practice. Sackett *et al.* (1996, p. 71) characterize EBP as follows: 'the conscientious, explicit and judicious use of current best evidence in making decisions about the care of individual patients . . . integrating individual clinical experience with the best available external evidence from systematic reviews.' In its broadest sense,

From M. Avis and D. Freshwater, Evidence for practice, epistemology, and critical reflection, Nursing Philisophy *2006, 7, 216–224.*
Copyright 2006 by Blackwell. Reprinted with permission by Blackwell Publishing.

About the Authors

MARK AVIS is currently chair in Social Contexts of Health at the School of Nursing at the University of Nottingham in the U.K. After a year in practice in acute mental health care, he took up a place at Kings' College, University of London, to study philosophy, where he was supervised by Peter Winch, best known for his text '*The Idea of a Social Science*.' After graduating in philosophy, he returned to nursing practice, working in a variety of health care of the elderly settings and also taking a part-time Master's degree in the Sociology of Health and Illness. He joined the academic staff at the School of Nursing at the University of Nottingham in 1990. His research career has focused on the use of qualitative research techniques to explore people's experiences of health and social care, and he has also drawn on his philosophical studies to write about the epistemology of qualitative research. His current research work is on processes in self-help and the contribution that self-help makes to health and well-being, with particular reference to the way that people use their experiences in promoting mutual support and learning.

DAWN FRESHWATER holds a bachelor of arts in nursing and education with Honors from Manchester University and the Royal College of Nursing. She received her doctorate in 1998 from the University of Nottingham and also holds a Diploma in Clinical Supervision (counseling and mental health) and a diploma in Jungian psychotherapy. Since the early 1990s, Dawn has maintained an interest in the application and evaluation of transformational research, critical reflexivity, pragmatism, reflective practice, and clinical supervision (in particular, its relation to evidence-based practice and the therapeutic alliance). In 2002, Professor Freshwater was awarded Fellow of the Royal College of Nursing for her outstanding contribution to nursing through research, reflective practice, clinical supervision, and practice development in mental health. This contribution has led to the development and appraisal of a variety of approaches to evaluating the provision and delivery of health care, with particular emphasis on mental health. She is a marathon runner and a keen cyclist.

EBP is a process for grounding knowledge of how to practise on empirical evidence; as such, it draws on a familiar tradition of scientific empiricism. There have been a number of criticisms of the concept of EBP, suggesting that it can overemphasize the value of scientific evidence while underplaying the role of clinical judgment and individual expertise in knowing how to practise (French, 2002). Indeed, making a distinction between external evidence, gained from the methodical application of scientific procedures, and individual clinical experience may be misleading. As Benner, and many others, have pointed out, knowing how to practise is a matter of expertise (Benner, 1984; Benner & Wrubel, 1989; Rolfe, 1998).

Expertise embodies an approach to intuitive and reasoned decision making that employs a variety of evidence (Gregson *et al.*, 2002). In our view, a misleading distinction between hard, external, scientific evidence and the softer, value-laden stuff of personal experience can obscure an underlying logic which requires critical reflection on all the evidence in order to determine how we *ought to* practice.

In this paper, we have two objectives. We want to isolate and preserve what is valuable in the concept of EBP and separate out these beneficial features from versions of scientific empiricism that undervalue personal experience. Second, we want to outline an epistemology for critical reflection that does not leave us attributing the knowledge of expert practitioners to an irreducible or mysterious concept of 'intuition.' Our argument will be that what is worth defending in the idea of empiricism is the emphasis it places on a critical examination of experiential evidence in the light of theory. If we are right, then critical reflective practice, properly conducted, would have an epistemological pedigree to stand alongside randomized controlled trials as evidence for practice. Practitioners who use critical reflection on their experience to understand and improve their practice are being good empiricists. In which case, evidence from systematic reviews, arts and humanities, and individual clinical experience can all make a valid contribution to *knowledge*-based practice.

Empiricism and Evidence

We will start by examining an empiricist view of knowledge that appears to support EBP. Empiricists take the view that evidence, ultimately obtained through the senses, provides a valuable source of information about the world (Blackburn, 1994). However, there are some deep-rooted problems with the idea of evidence as a basis for knowledge. First, we have to consider what counts as good, robust, and supportive evidence for a belief. This is a question of how we provide a justification for our beliefs and claims about the world. Second, we should reflect on whether a belief that is well justified should be regarded as true. In the main, we will be focusing on the first of these questions, the attempt to provide justificatory criteria for belief.

An influential attempt to answer the question of justification is provided by positivism. It is an intuitively attractive view that holds that some beliefs are simply justified by observation or experience, independently of any other beliefs. At the heart of positivist epistemology is a foundationalist principle that we can separate evidence from beliefs; that the evidence of our senses provides a raw, uncontaminated, pre-reflective material out of which we construct our beliefs (Hacking, 1983). The claim that 'It is raining' is justified by observations of rain falling and people and pavements getting wet, what could be simpler.

However, many philosophers have argued, in their different ways, that all evidence must arise in the context of a particular set of beliefs (van Fraasen, 1980; Quine, 1980; Putnam, 1982; Rorty, 1991; Hollis, 1994). Even the simplest observations about rain are dependent upon a complex set of beliefs about the meaning of

terms and the causes of falling water, as well as a belief that the observer is not dreaming, hallucinating, or just mistaken. As the American philosopher Donald Davidson (2001) reminds us, nothing can act as a reason for holding a belief except another belief. Therefore, evidence cannot be separated from the beliefs that influenced its production and interpretation. Sophisticated empiricists, such as Quine (1980) and van Fraasen (1980), argue that beliefs can still be justified, but only because of how they fit with a network of beliefs and evidence. They argue that the mistake made by positivists, in attempting to provide a justification for knowledge, was to treat each belief as an isolated individual, each with its own determinate empirical content. They argue that we must treat our beliefs and experiences as an interconnected whole. The point to note is that, contrary to the central idea of the foundationalist view of justification, no belief is directly linked to an empirical observation that gives it meaning and determines if it is true or false. Each belief is part of a network of beliefs; its meaning and truth depends upon its position in this web of interconnected beliefs. Some of the more abstract beliefs at the centre of the web are integral to interpreting those beliefs most closely linked to experience at the edges of web. For example, a belief based on direct observation and measurement of a patient's health state will depend upon more abstract, interrelated beliefs about health behaviour, physiology, and cultural influences on behavioural expression.

This version of the justification of beliefs has been termed the coherentist view, as it holds that justification depends upon the coherence of each belief with a network of interconnected beliefs. An important aspect of the coherentist view of justification is the recognition that no belief is immune from revision. Beliefs based on observation and experience can be reinterpreted in the light of new beliefs, and that beliefs can be re-evaluated to account for new evidence. In the course of debates about the best course of action in tackling an issue, it is often claimed that there is 'incontrovertible evidence' that one approach is better than another. Coherentists will deny that there is any such thing as evidence that cannot be re-evaluated in the light of a particular context or new ideas. There is no way to step outside our beliefs and establish that a particular piece of evidence corresponds to the facts.

There are a number of important criticisms of the coherentist view of knowledge. Not least is the observation that any justification of knowledge appears to rest on a circular set of claims, a series of beliefs that support other beliefs that in turn support other beliefs without any way of breaking out of the cycle of self-justification. Indeed, several recent philosophers of science (Putnam, 1982; Hacking, 1983; Rorty, 1999; Davidson, 2001) have suggested that the holism thesis and a coherentist view of justification call into question whether there is anything worth preserving in the concept of empiricism as epistemology.

There are a number of responses to this question, and worries about the need to head off these responses before they get started. While some writers such as Rorty (1999) have welcomed the chance to escape from an epistemological straitjacket and spend more time examining the social practices that have led to ideas becoming established and then overthrown. Others writers, such as Haack (1993), have tried to construct alternative criteria for justifying beliefs in order to head off the relativism and loss of authority for empirical science that these radical ideas would encourage. We would observe, as Davidson (2001) and Hacking (1983) have pointed out, that it is difficult to conceive of the possibility that this interconnected network of beliefs and evidence could turn out to be entirely false or allow the possibility of competing conceptual schemes. It does not make sense to seek a means to justify particular basic beliefs in our network of beliefs in order to provide support for the totality when it is the totality of beliefs that provides the background for justification.

We wanted to show that critical reflective practice and empirical science both use evidence as a basis for knowledge. However, the relationship between evidence and belief turned out to be more complex than a foundationalist version of epistemology could allow. Although experience may play a role in causing us to hold certain beliefs and assist us in evaluating the consistency of our beliefs, it proves impossible to hold the view that experience alone can provide a foundation for holding particular beliefs (Hacking, 1983; Haack, 1993).

Science and Epistemology

Over many years, the scientific method has become the most important means of generating evidence about the world and human society, and considerable effort has been devoted to improving the reliability of scientific evidence. However, as the limitations of the foundationalist view of knowledge show, evidence on its own cannot provide necessary and sufficient reasons for holding a belief. Improving the quality of evidence through better measurement techniques, greater objectivity, or improved reliability, cannot overcome the relevance of a whole network of beliefs in determining whether the results of empirical observations might constitute knowledge. In science and EBP, therefore, we have to recognize that a range of beliefs, some of them not evidence-based, will play a role in deciding whether the results of a particular study or series of studies constitute knowledge or even a sound basis for practice.

This is not to deny that attention to obtaining good quality evidence is an important feature of scientific success or EBP. It is simply that the success of science as a means of generating evidence that enlarges our stock of beliefs is not reducible to the employment of protocols that eliminate bias and subjectivity. We agree with Rorty (1991) that the aspects of science that make it so successful as a problem-solving activity are the human qualities of caution, critical reflection, and rational debate. Without a straightforward foundationalist justification, and recognizing that evidence is constructed rather than given by our experiences, what really matters in scientific enquiry is the critical exploration of coherence between beliefs. Therefore, evidence must be treated as open to question, in particular through a careful examination of the beliefs that are integral to interpreting and making sense of that evidence. Therefore, what lies at the heart of the success of empirical science as a means of generating knowledge about the world is the quality of critical reflection upon the evidence that the scientific methods produce.

The character of science is given through the process of working in a spirit of caution, formulating and testing new beliefs and hypotheses to explain the evidence, and sharing and debating these hypotheses with others in a spirit of open enquiry. Empiricists, whether they are scientists or reflective practitioners, search for the best fit between their hypotheses, the evidence, and the background of accepted beliefs. They engage in dialogue, present their evidence, and scrutinize each others' beliefs for consistency, usefulness, and coherence. In this way, the network of beliefs that provides the context for scientific activity is not the individual researcher or practitioner but a community of fellow enquirers.

The Logic of Analysis and Interpretation

Scientists and practitioners are being good empiricists when they subject the evidence gained through experience to a critical thought process in a way that is open to scrutiny and contributes to a community of fellow thinkers. In our view, this process of critical reflection on the evidence is a familiar activity that draws upon a common and, to a large extent, on the recognizable logic of hypothetical reasoning (Follesdal, 1979; Gower, 1997; Freshwater & Avis, 2004). Hypothetical reasoning involves building or inventing hypotheses as plausible ways of explaining evidence from which we can deduce testable consequences. The beliefs which are arrived at by this means should be logically coherent and consistent with all our experiences.

In our view, this mode of thinking is not exclusive to the science method but an intuitive method we use to check the consistency of our beliefs. In our everyday conversations and discussions with others, we produce conjectures, anticipate possible outcomes of courses of action, and rationalize the behaviour of others by attributing to them particular beliefs and desires; we test the success of these beliefs by examining them for consistency and coherence with how events turn out. These predictions help us decide whether a hypothesis is useful or not in explaining our experiences. Follesdal (1979) in a classic paper provides an account of hermeneutic reasoning as based on hypothesis testing applied to all meaningful material including actions, works of art, and texts. He argues that the process of understanding meaningful materials can be seen as an application of the hypothetico-deductive method; we propose hypotheses concerning the subject matter that is being studied and test them for consistency with our other beliefs, assumptions, and interpretation in order to form a comprehensive system of belief that is logically coherent. Pragmatic criteria, such as consistency, convenience, and simplicity, provide reasons to accept those hypotheses that help us to make the most sense of our experience in the context of our other beliefs, including those provided by our scientific and cultural heritage. In most cases, a hypothesis will be accepted where it enhances consistency within our beliefs, by either making new connections or confirming existing ones. However, this should not exclude the possibility that a hypothesis could be accepted that overturns existing conventions.

When hypothetical reasoning is applied to the process of critical reflection on evidence, we suggest that it is based on three identifiable steps. The process contains analytic procedures that use a hypothesis in order to reduce the evidence to its basic elements. In this sense, a hypothesis is like a chemical reagent that causes other substances to appear, use of a hypothesis allows specific features of experience to become apparent. Critical reflection on the evidence also includes interpretation, using inductive logic to build new insights and conceptual explanations from the identification of basic elements of the evidence. Finally, we employ theory-testing procedures, deducing the consequences of new theoretical insights by examining their coherence with further evidence (Freshwater & Avis, 2004). It must be stressed that the above steps are not intended to describe a straightforwardly sequential process; it is iterative, idiosyncratic, and cyclical.

It would be useful to illustrate these steps in hypothetical reasoning applied to critical reflection by drawing on an example. The following example is taken from the reflective journal of Jane, a nursing student on placement in elderly care, brought to clinical supervision during her involvement in a research study (Freshwater, 2000). Reflection was guided by one of the author's

(D.F.) who acted as clinical supervisor. Rather like Howard Becker's (1998) reflections on his seminal work 'The Boys in White,' Jane's example is evidence of socialization into nursing practice. Thus, the advantage of using this as an example is that it captures the connections between epistemology, critical reflection, and social investigation. Jane reads the incident from her journal:

> As I was walking out from hand over I saw Brenda in the dining room. She had put her blouse on back to front and her trousers were undone and therefore falling down. She was wearing no underwear. I went over to her and when she saw me she rushed over and put her arms round me. She looked so pleased to see me, tears came to her eyes. She said that she couldn't get her blouse off and none of the other nurses would help her. She said she had asked for help from the night staff before they went home and been ignored. We were in the ward dining room with other patients looking on and there was a staff nurse sitting at a table. It was 07.45 AM and the night staff had just handed over.
>
> I was very angry that no one had helped Brenda, but I managed to stay calm. I took Brenda to her room and helped her to get dressed. All the time she was thanking me for helping her which evoked two emotions in me. Anger that one of the night staff had not helped Brenda maintain some of her dignity. And humility and some embarrassment, as I realized that my presence had meant so much to her. My knowledge of Brenda's illness caused to me feel distress as I knew that she was going down-hill and that this was not the right way to treat her.
>
> When I returned from Brenda's room I saw the staff nurse who had been sitting at the dining table, she didn't even look up and said 'you don't believe what these patients tell you, they can be really manipulative, she probably has just got out of bed and not even seen a nurse yet this morning. I bet the night staff let her have a sleep in, she's confused. She knows you're a new nurse and she's trying it on.' I didn't say anything in response, just smiled. I was left wondering if this kind, loving elderly lady was pulling the wool over my eyes and I even started to feel angry that I had been so naïve, Brenda must have known that I was a new nurse on the ward and made a beeline for me.

To many practitioners working in elderly care, this might appear to be a fairly unremarkable event, certainly the concept of the 'manipulative patient' was instantly recognized by the supervisor, as was the cynicism of the qualified nurse and the dilemma Jane was experiencing. The supervisor, on hearing the reflection, believes the idea of a manipulative patient to be significant in some way, and begins to analyse why it could be important, applying a piece of theory that had come forth, namely, that when confronted with uncaring acts in the context of caring, it is easier to identify the patient as the problem than to fully experience the act of uncaring. Further, this is compounded where there is a hierarchical and dependant relationship.

Through supervisory processes, using critical reflection, Jane was goaded into offering accounts of her caring beliefs; this sort of questioning drives the outer person to expose their inner contradictions, taking them closer to their essence. With prompting, Jane realized that she would prefer to believe that the patient had been manipulative, than to have to confront the fact that her colleagues had not been able to care in that moment. She said:

> I could not allow this thought as I felt it would be criticizing the trained members of staff which I did not feel able to do. Instead I kept my feelings and my beliefs to myself. This is more to do with my feelings about being inexperienced and needing to get along with people. I suppose one of my beliefs is that I do not know enough about caring to challenge the experts. They know about caring, after all they have done it for years. I think I also want to care for the staff or maybe protect them, they all seem tired. But in caring for the patient and protecting the staff I did not care for myself and my own beliefs and values.

Interestingly, the supervisor describes the process of recognizing the significance of the reflection in the context of a useful piece of theory, in this case, pertaining to the concept of (un)caring. The application of the theory and the identification of the significance of the idea of a manipulative patient/caring nurse occur together. In other words, it is having a theory in mind that makes particular features of experience apparent. Having recognized the importance of the reflection, the supervisor tries to check out the nature of the concepts involved, and how they are applied in practice. She begins to develop and test her hypothesis by getting Jane to reflect further on the incident, which leads to an exploration concerning the concept of caring and its relationship to expertise.

The supervisor has used a piece of theory to isolate an interesting feature of experience and, through a process of testing the application of the theory against experience, she is beginning to identify the concept of (un)caring and its application in the context of manipulative patients and expert nurses. But why is it important? An interpretation of the concept depends upon trying to weave it into other beliefs about medical practice. Interpretation requires consideration of the utility of this idea in explaining the value that Jane was learning about caring:

> I know I could have challenged the staff nurse and talked about the lack of caring that I felt Brenda had received. This would have given me the opportunity to discuss the contradiction between my beliefs about Brenda's care (desirable care) and the actual care. It would also have given me a chance to express my feelings. But I actually started to believe that Brenda had manipulated the situation and my initial intuition about Brenda being treated badly was put aside.

During the iterative process of analysis and interpretation, the supervisor refines and develops the hypothesis by looking for examples of how the idea of caring gives further insight into the values implicit in nursing practice. She begins to identify how values associated with students' experience of caring are connected with a wider network of beliefs and values. Without getting involved in the content about whether Brenda was manipulative or the staff abusive, she challenges Jane to reflect more upon her own caring beliefs:

Perhaps it is hard for to accept that alongside the loving caring part in carers, there may be a part which is neglectful and not so caring, particularly when the nurse is worn out, just like it was hard for you to hold the fact that maybe Brenda is a wonderfully warm and responsive person as well as perhaps needy and manipulative.

Jane agreed, explaining that she also found it difficult to be seen as caring, hence her embarrassment at Brenda's display of affection. This was a cue to move to a deeper level of work and theory testing with Jane. Jane explained that she felt acutely aware of being seen to be special by Brenda in front of the other qualified staff: It could be argued that Jane had experienced being there with the patient, being personally involved, which felt right to her but that a conflicting message was telling her that these were not the actions of a professional nurse. The contradictions appeared to be between what constituted caring behaviour and what was felt to be professional (ethical knowledge). Notwithstanding the need to belong and conform to social norms and practices in the socialization process.

This highlights an important and characteristic feature of contemporary nursing practice, the preference for personal experience over scientific publications as a source of the wisdom used to guide practice. And as Becker (1998) observed, 'even faculty who themselves published scientific papers would say, in response to a student's question about something reported in a medical journal, "I know that's what people have found but I've tried that procedure and it didn't work for me, so I don't care what the journals say".'

This example serves to illustrate the logic of hypothetical reasoning when reflecting critically on evidence. The supervisor uses theory to identify important elements of experience, develops hypotheses that could offer explanations of observations, and goes on to test the hypotheses in new situations and by making connections with existing theory. While this is not meant to be a consummate example, rather it aims to show that the real trick is in subjecting our experience to a critical examination through the use of theory we can bring hitherto unnoticed features of our experience to light. Indeed, it may be that it is through the explicit use of theory that we can 'make the familiar strange' and, in the process, reveal underlying beliefs and values that explain social phenomena.

The example of hypothesis testing provided here is somewhat sanitized by retrospective narration, and we should make it clear that we do not consider the process to be linear, neat, or conclusive. The process can be messy and may involve many false starts and wrong turns. We agree with Popper's (1959) view that thinking up and applying hypotheses is a creative and imaginative process, and also with his belief that ideas must be tested in some way against experience. Where we sharply differ from Popper, and some versions of EBP, is in thinking that the scientific method provides a definitive means for producing the evidence to test a hypothesis against experience, and that this method of hypothesis testing demarcates science from other forms of enquiry.

Critical Reflection and Epistemology

We have used the example above to illustrate the process of critical reflection on the evidence. But the epistemological question remains: can a hypothesis entertained during the process in critical reflection constitute knowledge? The view of knowledge that we have defended suggests that a hypothesis can only be established as knowledge if it can be evaluated against the evidence and established within a network of beliefs. It requires argument to demonstrate that accepting a particular hypothesis is consistent with both the evidence and all our other well-supported beliefs. Follesdal (1979) suggests that simplicity is an important criterion for determining which hypotheses should be believed. He argues that the simplicity of the total set of hypotheses should be considered decisive; the more evidence that can be accounted for by the same set of hypotheses provides a reason to believe those hypotheses. Where we take issue with some con-

ventional views of EBP is over the emphasis placed on techniques of research. Perhaps a lingering faith in a foundationalist view of knowledge can lead to a kind of methodolatry where adherence to procedures designed to enhance reliability and validity of the evidence are accepted in lieu of arguments that examine critically the coherence of evidence and belief, or the simplicity of the set of hypotheses. It is the quality of the arguments that are be put forward to support a claim that matter most, although it is evident that the quality of the evidence will play an important part in establishing that claim.

Once we have discounted foundationalist versions of empiricism, which have erroneously associated the scientific method with the only justification for knowledge, we find that critical reflection on evidence, using hypothetical reasoning, provides a common logic for the ways that qualitative and quantitative researchers, as well as expert practitioners, justify the findings of their enquiries.

Critical Reflection as Expert Practice

We accept that judicious use of the results of good-quality research is a vital aspect of expert practice. The randomized controlled trial remains one of the best means we have to decide whether one form of care is better than another. However, it is worth reminding ourselves that a randomized controlled trial is simply an evaluation technique, and we have argued that knowledge cannot be reduced to the application of a procedure to produce evidence. Knowing how to practise involves an understanding of the results as well as the limitations of relevant research studies; it also requires an awareness of the background theories that influenced particular research studies. Benner and others (Benner, 1984; Rolfe, 1998; Freshwater & Rolfe, 2001) have observed that expert practice involves having to make decisions in a particular context where there may be incomplete or inadequate research evidence, and where there are no obvious rules for the application of that evidence. Of even more significance, they note that research evidence cannot resolve decisions about how the goals and values implicit in health care should be negotiated in each individual healthcare encounter. Providing individualized nursing care requires insight into the beliefs, motivations, and values of individuals in order to decide how to apply what research evidence there is in any particular context. Therefore, expert practice also requires the application of the contextual and idiosyncratic evidence gained through individual healthcare encounters.

Expert practice depends upon the use of critical reflection to interpret a range of evidence in order to decide how to act in each individual healthcare encounter. This kind of complex and intricate evaluation of the evidence should be regarded as quintessentially rational. Perhaps one of the reasons that expert practice has been thought to be based on intuition is precisely because the idea of rationality has been associated with a form of procedural, methodical, and instrumental reasoning regarded as synonymous with a positivist epistemology. The critical reflection and debate with colleagues that is required to make a convincing case for action using the varieties of beliefs and evidence at our disposal cannot be reduced to following a set of procedures. Equally, it should certainly not be placed in a black box labelled 'intuition.' We can use critical reflection, based on hypothetical reasoning, to explicate the tacit knowledge that informs our thinking and decisions when we act on the basis of 'gut instinct' or intuition. While the results of critical reflection on the particulars of experience do not have the same kind of generalizability as the results of research, they do have an intrinsic transferability as we apply the beliefs and hypotheses in new situations in order to evaluate their usefulness. While we do not attempt, within this paper, to define *what* counts as evidence, our argument is that expert practice supports individualized nursing care, and it should be based on a rigorous process of critical reflection on *all* the evidence we have obtained through individual healthcare encounters, including reading novels, watching films, observing art, and reviewing scientific papers.

REFERENCES

Becker H. (1998) *Tricks of the Trade: How to Think about Your Research while You're Doing It.* University of Chicago Press, Chicago, IL.

Benner P. (1984) *From Novice to Expert.* Addison-Wesley, Menlo Park, CA.

Benner P. & Wrubel J. (1989) *The Primacy of Caring: Stress and Coping in Health and Illness.* Addison-Wesley, Menlo Park, CA.

Blackburn S. (1994) *The Oxford Dictionary of Philosophy.* Oxford University Press, Oxford.

Davidson D. (2001) *Subjective, Intersubjective, Objective.* Oxford University Press, Oxford.

Follesdal D. (1979) Hermeneutics and the hypothetico-deductive method. *Dialectica,* 33, 319–336.

van Fraasen B. (1980) *The Scientific Image.* Oxford University Press, Oxford.

French P. (2002) What is the evidence on evidence based nursing? An epistemological concern. *Journal of Advanced Nursing,* 37, 250–257.

Freshwater D. (2000) *Transformational Learning Through Reflective Practice.* Nursing Praxis, Portsmouth.

Freshwater D. & Avis M. (2004) Analysing interpretation and reinterpreting analysis. *Nursing Philosophy,* 5, 4–11.

Freshwater D. & Rolfe G. (2001) Critical reflexivity: a politically and ethically engaged research method for nursing. *NTResearch,* 6, 526–537.

Gower B. (1997) *Scientific Method: An Historical and Philosophical Introduction.* Routledge, London.

Gregson R., Meal A. & Avis M. (2002) Meta-analysis: the glass eye of evidence based practice. *Nursing Inquiry,* 9, 24–30.

Haack S. (1993) *Evidence and Inquiry: Towards Reconstruction in Epistemology.* Blackwell, Oxford.

Hacking I. (1983) *Representing and Intervening: Introductory Topics in the Philosophy of Natural Science.* Cambridge University Press, Cambridge.

Hollis M. (1994) *The Philosophy of Social Science.* Cambridge University Press, Cambridge.

Popper K. (1959) *The Logic of Scientific Discovery.* Hutchinson, London.

Putnam H. (1982) *Reason, Truth and History.* Cambridge University Press, Cambridge.

Quine W. (1980) *From a Logical Point of View* 2nd edn. Harvard University Press, Cambridge, MA.

Rolfe G. (1998) *Expanding Nursing Knowledge.* Butterworth-Heineman, Oxford.

Rorty R. (1991) *Objectivity, Relativism and Truth.* Cambridge University Press, Cambridge.

Rorty R. (1999) *Philosophy and Social Hope.* Penguin Books, Harmondsworth.

Sackett D., Rosenberg W., Gray J., Haynes R. & Richardson W. (1996) Evidence based medicine—what it is and what it isn't. *British Medical Journal,* 312, 71–72.

The Authors Comment

Evidence for Practice, Epistemology, and Critical Reflection

This article developed out of the argument that the active, self-conscious use of hypotheses to create meaning and patterns in evidence and experience was common to both scientific practice and critical reflection. We then pushed this argument about the logic of critical reflection into the arena of epistemology to raise questions about how nurses obtain the knowledge that guides their practice. The growth of the evidence-based practice movement had insinuated that hard evidence should be the bedrock of good nursing practice. We thought that if we could chisel away the hardened secretions of positivism that had built up around evidence-based practice, we would be able to use our observations on the nature of critical reflection to try to reveal an underlying logic in reflecting on evidence that united scientific empirical practice with critical reflection. Like science without positivism, critical reflection also focuses on the quality of analysis rather than the hardness of the evidence. One of our motivations for trying to get this argument out into the open was to bring out the value of reflection on subjective and personal experience and the imaginative application of theory to analyze that experience in generating knowledge. We wanted to raise critical reflection up from its inferior position, and to make clear that the underlying logical processes of reflecting on experience using theory are the same for the scientist as for the critically reflective practitioner. However, one difference that we do want to draw attention to is that scientists tend to reduce the need for complex analysis by designing protocols that limit their exposure to unexpected experiences, whereas practitioners have to find a way of applying critical reflection to the inherent diversity and complexity of their experience, as well as research evidence, in generating the knowledge they need to practice.

—Mark Avis
—Dawn Freshwater

Knowledge Development and Evidence-Based Practice: Insights and Opportunities From a Postcolonial Feminist Perspective for Transformative Nursing Practice

Sheryl Reimer Kirkham
Jennifer L. Baumbusch
Annette S. H. Schultz
Joan M. Anderson

Although not without its critics, evidence-based practice is widely espoused as supporting professional nursing practice. Engaging with the evidence-based practice discourse from a vantage point offered by the critical perspectives of postcolonial feminism, the incomplete epistemologies and limitations of the standardization characteristic of the evidences-based movement are analyzed. Critical analysis of evidence is suggested, such that it recognizes the evidence generated from multiple paradigms of inquiry, along with contextual interpretation and application of this evidence. We examine how broader interpretations of evidence might contribute to nursing knowledge development and translation for transformative professional nursing practice, and ultimately to address persistent health disparities within the complex context of healthcare delivery.

Nursing knowledge development is largely understood as generating the evidence required for professional nursing practice. Evidence-based practice (EBP) is currently the primary approach to knowledge uptake for professional practice, and is believed to support efficiency and ensure that practice decisions result in the provision of effective treatment.[1,2] Best practices based on sound research-based evidence are undisputedly needed given the complexity of today's healthcare environments, with their reliance on rapidly evolving technology, corporate priorities with a focus on efficiencies, and diverse sociopolitical milieus characteristic of the

From S. R. Kirkham, J. L. Baumbusch, A. S. H. Schultz, and J. M. Anderson, Knowledge development and evidence-based practice: Insights and opportunities from a postcolonial feminist perspective for transformative nursing practice. Advances in Nursing Sciences, 2007, 30(1), 26–40. Copyright © 2007. Reproduced with permission of Lippincott Williams & Wilkins.

About the Authors

SHERYL REIMER KIRKHAM, RN, PhD, is Associate Professor in the Nursing Department and Coordinator Scholarship Initiatives in the Master of Arts in Leadership program at Trinity Western University, Langley, British Columbia. She is an investigator with the Culture, Gender, and Health Research Unit at the University of British Columbia (UBC) School of Nursing. Her scholarship is in the area of culture and health pursuing themes related to social justice, intersectional differences, and the social context of health and illness, as related to health care services delivery, health professional practice, and education. Her doctoral dissertation examining the social organization of intergroup relations in health care received the prestigious Governor General's Gold Medal and the Elizabeth Kenny McCann Outstanding Dissertation Award. Current research includes a nationally funded project on the negotiation of religious, spiritual, and cultural plurality in health care, a national survey of nursing programs regarding the utilization of nontraditional clinical placements in Canada, and a collaborative knowledge translation project.

JENNIFER BAUMBUSCH, RN, PhD(c), is a Doctoral Candidate at the School of Nursing, University of British Columbia (UBC). Jennifer's background is in gerontological nursing, and she has held a variety of roles in nursing administration, education, and practice in this area. Since beginning her doctoral studies in 2002, Jennifer has been engaged in an exploration of participatory approaches to knowledge translation. Her doctoral dissertation is a critical ethnography in long-term residential care. Jennifer has been supported during her doctoral studies by the Elizabeth Kenny McCann Doctoral Award, a Killam Doctoral Award, and a Canadian Institutes of Health Research (CIHR) Canada Graduate Scholarship Doctoral Award.

ANNETTE S. H. SCHULTZ, PhD, RN, currently holds a Post-doctoral position at the University of Manitoba, Faculty of Nursing. Her career as a nurse, spanning more than 20 years, has included working clinically in direct patient care positions, conducting policy research focused on the practice of newly graduated RNs for the College of Registered Nurses in British Columbia, and conducting tobacco control research. Her emerging program of research primarily focuses on tobacco control in the context of health care, which draws on her mixed-methods dissertation study that focused on the nurses' role in tobacco control. Future work will include focusing on patients experiences of tobacco control during health-care interaction, specifically while in hospitals with "smoke-free grounds" policies. Additionally, future work will explore individual and contextual factors influencing practitioners' engagement in addressing tobacco use. She is a Mentor with the CIHR Strategic Training Program in Tobacco Research and an alumni member of NEXUS: Researching the Social Context of Health Behaviour at the University of British Columbia.

JOAN M. ANDERSON, RN, PhD, Professor Emerita, School of Nursing, University of British Columbia (UBC), currently serves as the Health Research Coordinator in the Office of the Vice President of Research, UBC, and University Delegate to the Canadian Institutes of Health Research, the Government of Canada's health research funding agency. Educated as a nurse and sociologist, she completed her undergraduate studies at McGill University and her graduate studies at UBC. She was honored with the Elizabeth Kenny McCann Professorship in 2001–2005, and was the first recipient of the UBC Killam Award for Excellence in Mentoring in 2004, given in recognition of outstanding mentorship of the graduate students whose research she supervised. She was a Distinguished Scholar in Residence, Peter Wall Institute for Advanced Studies, UBC, during 2003. Professor Anderson's research career spanning some 25 years has been devoted to understanding the social, economic, political, and cultural context of health, illness, suffering, and healing of people from different ethnocultural backgrounds. With colleagues, she is currently engaged in the translation of research findings into policy and practice, and draws upon a post-colonial feminist and humanist perspective in her research and writing.

broader society.[3] However, there have been wide-ranging critiques of EBP, from concern with the definition and breadth of evidence, to how this approach erodes the autonomy of nursing practice.[4-8]

In this article, we engage with the EBP discourse from another vantage point—that offered by critical perspectives such as postcolonial feminism (PCF)—with the aim of examining how this interpretation of evidence might contribute to knowledge development and translation for transformative nursing practice, and ultimately to address persistent health disparities within the complex context of healthcare delivery. This effort is not to replace the current discourse on evidence, but rather to add another dimension or analytic perspective. Our interest is both epistemological and pragmatic, as we question: "What is evidence?" "How might evidence be conceptualized within different paradigms of inquiry?" "Can different conceptualizations of evidence complement one another?" Driving these questions is a pragmatic concern that traditional notions of evidence, based in Western science, may not sufficiently address the types of deep-rooted factors underlying health disparities, such as poverty and material life circumstances, nor fully account for the complexities of people's everyday lives that ultimately shape health and illness to a significant extent. For example, we have put forward the argument[9,10] that it is not "culture" in some narrow sense that organizes the ways in which people manage an illness, but rather the complex mediating circumstances of their lives. Certain interpretations and use of EBP tend to turn our attention away from these social factors to focus on individualistic models of health with biomedical solutions,[11] in effect bypassing complex problems. Indeed, such complexities may well require that evidence derived from multiple sources, through various modes of inquiry, be considered to support clinical practice.

We begin our engagement with EBP discourses by providing an overview of EBP, and the critiques leveled against it. We then employ the theoretical perspective of PCF as a point of engagement with the EBP movement. Finally, drawing on our programs of research, we apply these insights to a discussion of the reciprocal processes of knowledge development and knowledge translation that serve as a foundation for the transformative knowledge necessary to support professional nursing practice, with the contention that multiple forms of intersecting and complementary evidence are required to address current complexities in health and healthcare.

Précis of Critical Questions About Evidence-Based Practice

The evolution of the EBP movement within healthcare has taken place over the last 3 decades. Reflecting its roots in evidence-based medicine, as envisioned by Sackett,[12*] nursing's equivalent of EBP has been defined as "the integration of best research evidence with clinical expertise and patient values to facilitate clinical decision-making."[13(p4)] Underlying this beginning was the belief that epidemiological and statistical research findings could be useful for influencing the effectiveness of clinical practice.[5,6] The reflection of this origin is present in EBP tools today; for instance, best practice guidelines usually display a set of criteria—strongly favoring evidence from random clinical trials (RCTs) over other studies[14,15]—regarding validity of research findings.

In tandem with the evolution of EBP, we have witnessed a rise in concern about economics and the costs of healthcare. This concern has resulted in the goal of providing efficient care, in that decisions about

---

* Sackett defined *evidence-based medicine* as "the conscientious, explicit, and judicious use of current best evidence in making decisions about the care of individual patients. The practice of evidence-based medicine means integrating individual clinical expertise with the best available external clinical evidence from systematic research. By individual clinical expertise, we mean the proficiency and judgment that individual clinicians acquire through clinical experience and clinical practice. Increased expertise is reflected in many ways, but especially in more effective and efficient diagnosis and in the more thoughtful identification and compassionate use of individual patients' predicaments, rights, and preferences in making clinical decisions about their care. By best available external clinical evidence, we mean clinically relevant research, often from the basic sciences of medicine, but especially from patient-centered clinical research into the accuracy and precision of diagnostic tests (including the clinical examination), the power of prognostic markers, and the efficacy and safety of therapeutic, rehabilitative, and preventive regimens."[12(p71)]

healthcare practice often require a cost-benefit analysis component, yet how we define "benefit" is not always clear. Healthcare management's adoption of EBP processes has been used to support resource allocation decisions.[2,7] Economic restrictions have resulted in shifts toward decentralization of governance and the subsequent requirement for management tools related to clinical practice decisions.[4] Therefore, while ensuring that professional practice is based on the latest scientific evidence, the evolution and adoption of the EBP movement has also supported economic restrictions and decentralization of governance, which rests on the values of *effectiveness, efficiency,* and *standardization* of care. As we argue later in the article, we are not quarreling with these notions, *but rather in their interpretation and use,* particularly when these concepts are used as recipes, without attentiveness to context. Although we would all support the notion of efficient care, the complexity of this concept is often overlooked. For care to be efficient, it has to be effective, and for care to be effective, it means that it has to be appropriate to the context.

Nursing, along with other healthcare professionals, has been faced with integrating this approach to EBP into care delivery. The push toward adopting EBP within nursing has met with critical questions; here, we highlight three interrelated positions within the academic dialogue that are particularly germane to our engagement, later in this article, with EBP.

The first position, articulating an epistemological concern, focuses on the limited view of nursing knowledge characteristic of EBP. It is argued that EBP, with its reliance on RCTs and systematic reviews, provides limited guidance to critically consider evidence from the diversity of research methodologies found within nursing literature and other related disciplines relevant for nursing practice.[6,14] Furthermore, other sources of knowing such as personal experience or expert knowledge are de-emphasized in clinical decision making, yet nurses clearly rely on knowledge beyond that which can be empirically verifiable.[16] Included in these "ways of knowing" are Carper's[17] personal, aesthetic, and ethical knowledge. Representing these types of concerns, nurse scholars have argued that the very nature of nursing as relational practice does not lend itself to "highly rationalized frameworks of perception, let alone intervention."[7(p151)]

The second position raised in nursing literature relates to concerns about the translation of research findings into practice[5] and the relevance of research studies, especially RCTs, which control contextual factors that might be influencing the variable being studied. There is concern that applying context-stripped findings to a context-rich clinical setting makes the application irrelevant. For example, a clinical guideline for pain management may be of limited usefulness when the contexts in which pain occurs are not explored.[16] Underlying such a concern is the ongoing debate regarding the application of evidence to particular or individual circumstances, given the inferential mechanisms of evidential knowledge by which particularities (eg, individual variations) have been averaged out.[16] Research studies, such as random control studies, result in an ability to predict a specific behavior or treatment outcome at a population level. However, what they do not tend to provide is a complete explanation of a behavior or treatment outcome, in particular, an integration of individual variations or contextual factors.

The final position raises concern in relation to nurses' professional practice. Given the complexity of nurses' work environment, nurses need to acquire information or evidence from sources, such as philosophic or aesthetic knowledge, other than research findings to support professional practice.[18] The concern stated here is that EBP tools do not acknowledge or address the reality of nurses' work environment, and so will have, at best, limited utility. Barnes,[4] for example, raises the possibility that this limited utility could well result in the erosion of nurses' autonomy and authority within their current scope of practice. The concern then is that if the practice expectations defined within an evidence-based tool become the norm for practice, these tools will begin to reshape nurses' work. Notably, other scholars[19] tell us that EBP has been embraced within the health professions as a means to improve professional status by making visible their "scientific" knowledge base. These critical issues highlight the complexity of bringing together a narrow view of evidence, such as that traditionally advocated for by EBP, with the realities of nursing practice. While we offer our own critical analysis of EBP later in this article, our response to this concern regarding the erosion of professional practice puts forward a somewhat different interpretation; another way of looking at this is that these tools, in and of themselves, do not address the complexity of patients' lives. We would argue that it not EBP, per se, that risks eroding nurses' autonomy. Rather, autonomy is eroded if nurses use evidence as recipes, without drawing on their professional knowledge and clinical judgment to interpret evidence, and make decisions about *best evidence* in context—this is the core of professional practice.

In summary, although healthcare systems and the profession of nursing have adopted EBP, there are philosophical and practical concerns regarding how EBP is used to guide professional nursing practice. Proponents of EBP refute these concerns as ill-founded misconceptions, and argue that when correctly operationalized, EBP integrates the best research evidence (derived by various research methods) with clinical expertise and patient values to facilitate decision making, implying a thoughtful and critical use of knowledge.[13] Given the complexity of practice and the persistent presence of health disparities, we contend that although the EBP perspective has considerable merit, different ways of looking at evidence are nonetheless needed, not to jettison the work that has been done, but rather to broaden the scope of how evidence is constructed. Furthermore, we would stress that a key issue relates to how nurses interpret and use evidence. The problem arises when evidence is seen as driving clinical decision making, rather than as a tool to be used by the professional nurse as he or she assesses, and makes decisions about best practices within a given context. PCF, we suggest, offers one framework that might help to further our understandings of evidence and EBP. We suggest that rather than replacing evidence generated from a scientific perspective, PCF complements EBP by enriching contextual understandings, and underscoring pro-

fessional responsibility and accountability to use this knowledge to work toward equitable healthcare for all people. As such, it provides another angle on doing science that reframes our ways of constructing what counts as evidence.

A Postcolonial Feminist Reading of Evidence-Based Practice

Postcolonial theory, joining other critical social theories that have at their core the analysis of relations of power, represents a broad based and rapidly expanding domain of scholarship. Said to have originated in the 1960s and 1970s, led by the influential work of anticolonial scholars such as Frantz Fanon[20] and Edward Said's *Orientalism,*[21] postcolonial theory deals with the relations and aftermath of the colonial period and ongoing neocolonialism characterized by oppressive tactics, economic and cultural hegemonies, and totalizing global expansions. Postcolonial feminist theory and black feminist theory, particularly that of scholars such as Patricia Hill Collins,[22] bell hooks,[23] Toni Morrison,[24] and Rose Brewer,[25] direct attention to multiple intersecting oppressions, inclusive of gender, class, and *race* oppression to reveal the multiple dimensions of oppression within societies, and the unequal effects of racism on certain groups of people (eg, women and children). Feminist theory also contributes sustained critique of issues of identity, voice and difference, and the politics of representation; and the articulation of clear methodological direction for both research and practice.

A growing body of nursing scholarship informed by postcolonial feminist theories provides rich analyses of the historical, economic, cultural, and social dynamics at play within healthcare (see, for instance, references 9, 10, 26–34) and demonstrate the salience of these perspectives for nursing scholarship. These works not only attempt to examine the complex intersections between different social relations that have a profound impact on the experiencing of health and illness but also hold up to scrutiny taken-for-granted assumptions about different ethno-cultural communities. Indeed, like Ahmad,[35] these scholars challenge notions of culture as static and determining, and draw attention, instead, to the context in which cultural meanings are constructed, to issues of racialization, systemic racism, and other forms of oppression. Perhaps, most important, no one form of oppression is privileged, but there is the continuous search to understand how intersections operate in everyday life, and in everyday social encounters. This growing postcolonial feminist scholarship builds on earlier integration of critical theories such as feminist and antiracist theories into nursing, as exemplified by Allen et al,[36] Barbee,[37] Campbell and Bunting,[38] and Webb,[39] and shares the agenda of other nurse scholars committed to pursing social justice through critical analyses of how the social construct of race is employed.[40–44]

Postcolonial feminist theory, with its cogent critique of oppressive structures that tend toward standardization, representation of majority view, and erasing of experiences of racialization, classism, sexism, ageism, and homophobia, expands EBP's scientific discourses to be inclusive of various social relations, and in doing so transforms our notions of science. As both academics and practitioners, we have grappled with the application of postcolonial feminist perspectives to practice, and, in particular, to current management discourses and practices. Recognizing the entrenchment or perhaps the inevitability of these discourses and mechanisms, we seek to examine critically current EBP discourses, and offer alternative interpretations that might equip healthcare workers for professional practice and assist in the creation of practice environments that nurture such practice. In doing so, we are working toward opening up spaces for an enriched dialogue regarding evidence as it is generated and applied in practice, with the understanding that EBP itself is not a single entity but rather can be taken up in various ways to support professional practice.

In our effort to reappraise EBP, we join together the deconstructive and constructive imperatives of postcolonial feminist theorizing. PCF approaches are disruptive and resistive in their primary intent, seeking to uncover theoretical, moral, and political inadequacies through lenses of race, class, gender, age, sexual orientation, and other forms of oppression. Simultaneously, the PCF project opens up new sites for the legitimation of currently delegitimated knowledge,[45] and offers new possibilities for professional practice within current practice environments that have become increasingly restrictive. Salient to our discussion here are those features of PCF that hold up for scrutiny of epistemological claims that derive from and maintain the hegemonic center (in this case, the Western center). Equally valuable in the tenets of postcolonial feminist theorizing is the attention to power relations along a shifting and intersecting variety of axes, including race, religion, gender, and class. Our critique focuses on 3 themes made visible through the PCF lens: the problem of incomplete epistemologies; the shortcomings of uncritical standardization; and the everyday realities of race, class, gender, age, and sexual orientation as they operate within contexts of EBP. Together these themes point to the need for a shift toward a more inclusive, reciprocal approach to knowledge development and uptake.

Incomplete Epistemologies as the Basis for Evidence-Based Practice

A PCF reading reveals how the knowledge upon which EBP is based can, unwittingly, be racialized, gendered, ageist, classist, and homophobic. Notably, a PCF lens does not mean one sets out to criticize science itself, rather we raise questions about *how* science is practiced by those who conduct and fund research to perpetuate racialized, classed, and gendered approaches to study design. Furthermore, we are not arguing against empirical knowledge as foundational to professional practice, but do caution against segregating science from the humanities and social sciences in our knowledge generation and application.

Randomized clinical trials (RCTs) serve as the criterion standard of evidence for EBP.[14,15] However, for various reasons such as the complication of seeking interpretive services and the ethical implications of conducting research with people who might be vulnerable for a variety of reasons, researchers have traditionally conducted RCTs with the most accessible dominant majority populations. Yet, the findings of these studies have routinely been generalized as though they represent a universal experience.[11] Similarly, many of the research instruments, interview questions, and tools used today have been developed by and for the majority population and therefore may not capture the experiences of those marginalized within mainstream society.[11,46] Furthermore, the types of research questions that gain funding have traditionally been reflective of the interests of the dominant majority (eg, cardiovascular disease in white men) rather than the needs of groups that have been marginalized. According to a study by the Global Forum for Health Research, health research continues to reflect the priorities of the rich, with 90% of research funding investigating the diseases of 10% of the world's population.[47] Moreover, current values in the scientific community see the favoring of efficient research approaches that require homogeneous study populations, consequently excluding those who find themselves on the margins.[11,46]

The inclusion in our research of social groups that have been marginalized is an important step in developing knowledge to support nursing practice. However, inclusion alone is not sufficient—the nature of our questions, the research methods we use, and the theoretical lenses informing research carry considerable importance in the types of knowledge that result. Meleis and Im[46] observe that while nursing scholarship has moved to study diverse ethnocultural populations, a culturalist and relativist approach has resulted in knowledge that remains essentialist and incomplete through the application of dichotomous thinking that constructs difference as irrevocable and acontextual. They explain,

> By dividing into dichotomies, we may be maintaining categories that have historically defined each culture and each gender. Dichotomies such as male/female, immigrant/nonimmigrant, and African American/Euro-American have helped us to value interstice patterns and responses, but the dichotomies may be preventing us from recognizing the socio-political forces that inhibit us from changing the status quo.[46(p96)]

To counter these historically embedded incomplete epistemologies, a shift in research agendas is needed,

such that researchers not only study cultural knowledge but also situate such knowledge against the historically bound and contextually situated processes and effects of marginalization.

A growing body of evidence from across the globe demonstrates that social inequities in health are widespread, both within and between countries. Whitehead et al[48] note that overall gains in a nation's health frequently mask significant and worsening health outcomes for some population groups (often along lines of gender, geographic region, ethnicity, or socioeconomic characteristics). Many of the causes of inequities in health are social in origin, reflecting income and education disparities, differential exposure to health hazards, and systematic variations in life opportunities for healthy lifestyle or reasonable access to essential goods and services. As Whitehead et al[48(p313)] explain, "Individual lifestyles are embedded in social and community networks, and in living and working conditions, which in turn are related to the wider cultural and socioeconomic model." How is this convincing body of evidence regarding the crucial influence of social determinants of health taken up in the realm of health policy and healthcare services, including at the point of care? Is this type of evidence amenable to the heavily relied upon tools of EBP? Kemm is cautious in the application of the EBP model to public health policy:

> Taking communities rather than individuals as the unit of intervention and the importance of context means that frequently randomized controlled trials are not appropriate for study of *public health* interventions. Further, the notion of a "best solution" ignores the complexity of the decision making process. *Evidence* "enlightens" policy makers shaping how policy problems are framed rather than providing the answer to any particular problem.[49(p319)]

From a PCF perspective, then, the mediating circumstances of what are often referred to as the "social determinants of health" need to be integrated into our nursing knowledge. This inclusion is particularly urgent in the area of culture and health. Given the rise in diversity and the implications this diversity carries for healthcare delivery, considerable nursing scholarship energy has been invested in describing various cultural beliefs and practices, with the hope of improving healthcare services, and, in turn, health outcomes, for ethnocultural communities. Yet, this focus on the individual as a member of a circumscribed cultural group often overlooks the evidence offered by population-based studies pointing to the root causes of health disparities. Put another way, our knowledge development and concomitant knowledge uptake need to extend beyond "culture" per se as a static determinant of health, to account for the complex intersectionalities with the social, historical, economic, and political forces, in determining health and health outcomes. The individual experience must be linked to the social context.

How this accounting of social determinants of health is accomplished is fraught with its own set of challenges. Deriving from a Western empiricist paradigm reliant on operationalization and measurement of discrete variables, health and social sciences have for some time used race as a variable of study, citing the possibility of identifying, tracking, and eliminating health disparities as reason to do so. Yet, race as a biological category has been contested, and, by and large, discounted as a biologically based and meaningful category. In its place, race has been recast as fluid and socially constructed, varying across time and place as a function of historical circumstance.[50] This latter line of argument resonates with the postcolonial feminist conception of race that acknowledges the salience of the term, not in a reified or essentialized fashion, but as a signifier of social relations. While the collection of health statistics by ethnicity continues, and increases in some contexts,[51] the concurrent trend to identifying more specific indicators for health disparities studies stands to offer improved explanatory capacity regarding the mechanisms behind health disparities. Estroff and Henderson explain,

> When factors such as individual lifestyle and behaviours, cultural beliefs, physiologic measures, geographical location, insurance coverage, education, and income are included in studies, the remaining health differences may be attributed to the effects of racial bias or discrimination.[50(p19)]

Underlying such racial bias/discrimination is the context of broader historic and contemporary social and economic inequality. A PCF reading of EBP thus, necessarily, warns against this type of operationalization of variables such as race (and its metonym, ethnicity).[42] Where race is adopted uncritically as an indicator or a variable, the "evidence" derived may contribute to policy and practice that focuses once again solely on the individual, suggesting in effect that cultural difference accounts for variations in the experience of health and illness. In the process, the scientific use of these social categories inadvertently reinscribes the predominant social approach to racializing groups of people by color or ethnic affiliation.[52] Instead, the nature of evidence needed is that which makes visible the *social* pathways that lead to health disparities.

Future research enterprise, thus, must seek a new level of rigor in conceptualization, expanding research to incorporate the role of power in knowledge development through theoretical frameworks that carry the capacity to uncover injustice and marginalization.[46]

The Limitations of Standardization in the Applications of Evidence-Based Practice

At the level of the pragmatic, a PCF lens also draws our attention to some potential shortcomings stemming from EBP's move toward standardization of patient care, in effect extending the general critique of acontextual application of research findings. By strictly or uncritically adhering to the tools that bring EBP into practice (clinical pathways, best practice guidelines), rich contextual issues that influence patients' experiences as they move through the healthcare system may be stripped away (eg, important factors that may influence a patient's ability to successfully recover from an acute episode may be overlooked). Thus, while tools such as care maps provide a beginning point for guiding practice, their usefulness is dependent to a large degree upon the nurse's professional judgment based on knowledge of science and the social context of people's lives.

One of the challenges of these tools is the tension between supporting standardization of practice and the corporate agenda versus supporting critical thinking regarding practice decisions.[4,8,19,53] Standardization can support and strengthen a profession's claim to legitimacy as indicated earlier, but it also lays the groundwork for external controls, the imposition of which, suggest Timmerman and Berg,[19] are the very antithesis of professional autonomy and power. Approaching this issue from another vantage point, a PCF lens prompts consideration of the embeddedness of EBP in current organizational discourses, and envisions ways to resist the associated *colonizing* possibilities. Organizational theory has been acknowledged, indeed promoted, as being distinctly Western, with its bent toward expansionism, managerialism, and rationalism.[54] In efforts to foster the development of organizational theory as legitimate "science," proponents have drawn on Enlightenment assumptions of universalism to establish management practices that would apply in all contexts, not unlike "natural law." Building on gender analyses that have unveiled the masculinist propensities of organizational theory, and the falsity of representing organizations as gender and race neutral,[55] a PCF lens offers unique analytic leverage in making visible the influence of *empire* on contemporary ways of knowing and being in the arena of organizational practices. PCF scholars have gone as far as to typify today's organizational practices as "colonial regimes."[56] The deconstructive imperative of postcolonial critique, thus, provides an angle of analysis from the margins as to how managerial concepts such as EBP tend to be taken up as neutral uncontested categories in organizational theory. To hold such concepts up for scrutiny becomes an important contribution, particularly as we ask "who is privileged or advantaged by management practices such as EBP?"

A PCF lens raises questions about when such standardization serves as a force for social justice (eg, in ensuring that all receive equitable care based on empirical knowledge for best practice), and when standardization becomes a force for inequities as its homogenizing bent writes out group histories and individual identities. On the one hand, several authors have argued on behalf of EBP as a mechanism to ensure equitable

healthcare for all by the merit of an objective application of "best practices" to all clients, regardless of group affiliation and a healthcare provider's potential propensity to discrimination.[57] On the other hand, the contingencies and particularities, all imbued with relations of power, exposed by postcolonial feminist and other critical theories stand in contrast to the standardization of EBP.[53] To treat all as equals risks the real chance of inequitable treatment where the unique qualities and life circumstances of certain people continue to be overlooked. A postcolonial feminist analysis of EBP, then, while not debunking the notion of EPB, would advocate critical reflection on the concept of "evidence" and the context of people's lives in which such evidence would be used. From a PCF perspective, we bring into focus multiple forms of evidence from different paradigms of inquiry.

To counter the epistemic violence that results from generic applications of incomplete knowledge, a shift is needed as to how evidence itself is established, the types of evidence valued within the clinical setting, and subsequently how evidence is applied. Our concern then lies with a culture of standardized clinical decisions based on a larger healthcare environment of managerialism—particularly where EBP becomes a routinized recipe approach to decision making without attentiveness to context, or a management-imposed method of clinical decision making that diminishes nurses' clinical decision-making processes. In this way, the PCF lens picks up cogent critiques of EBP and extends the analyses more specifically to consider *for whom* the standardization might not "fit."

The Obfuscation of Everyday Realities Such as Racism, Sexism, and Classism

The two proceeding concerns regarding incomplete knowledge development and uncritically applied standardization work in tandem to obscure a world of racialized, gendered, ageist, and classed relations within healthcare. To illustrate, our research has uncovered how a politics of belonging is created as the dynamics of racialization and gender oppressions are negotiated in today's healthcare settings,[10] and how the mechanisms of health reform have disproportionately disadvantaged those in minority positions.[9,58] Commonplace racialized assumptions drawn upon within healthcare (eg, that families from certain ethnocultural groups will care for their elderly) result in overlooking the needs of individuals made vulnerable by the mediating circumstances of their lives, and who often do not speak the languages of healthcare (English; medicalized discourse).[9] Societal discourses—typically taken-for-granted—regarding culture, aboriginally and egalitarianism as professional mandate similarly shape nurses' encounters with First Nations patients to the detriment of respectful care.[59] Women have been the "workhorses" of healthcare as nurses, care aides, frontline managers, rehabilitative specialists, nutritionists, kitchen staff, and cleaners, yet remain underrepresented in current management decisions and structures. White women, in particular, are in ambivalent positions, as they themselves have lost voice in the corporate discourses of today's healthcare management, but have also been complicit in longstanding patterns of racializing practices.

Through a PCF analysis of the EBP movement, we question whether the priorities and practice environments created by EBP foster critical reflection that acknowledges such everyday realities of privilege and disadvantage, oppression and resistance, within healthcare. Clearly, if we want to create spaces for addressing these relations of power, we must carefully consider the types of practice environments created by the agendas of EBP. Likewise, as far as EBP assumes a "standardized patient" in a homogeneous or universalist sense to whom evidence can predictably be applied, a PCF framing alerts us to the possibility of erasure of individual differences and imposition of dominant mainstream ways. For example, where clinical practice guidelines are invaluable in the case management of HIV/AIDS, experiences of urban First Nations women living with HIV/AIDS speak to the profound shortcomings of existing healthcare services and programs in meeting their needs, given the intersecting realities of poverty, gender positioning, and racialization.[60] Without making visible the context of their everyday lives, healthcare services fall short of

addressing their particular needs. Such situations require thoughtful practitioners who bring together evidence from a range of knowledge to apply in patient-oriented and context-specific ways. A PCF approach then draws attention to the pragmatics of the everyday and supports the inclusion of transformative knowledge in order to support nursing practice in the current context of healthcare delivery.

Transforming Practice Through Knowledge Development and Translation: Insights and Opportunities from a Postcolonial Feminist Perspective

In this final section, we consider in further detail the implications of the insights derived through a PCF reading of EBP for knowledge development and knowledge translation, both of which are foundational to transforming nursing practice. What are the lessons we might take from a PCF critique of the current EBP movement for application to knowledge translation efforts? Can the divergent epistemologies of EBP and PCF be brought together in a complementary alignment to expand our sources of evidence upon which to base practice? Some nurse scholars who critique EBP distance themselves from its applications. Given the widespread adoption of EBP, we look for ways to constructively engage with the evidence-based movement, with the assertion that PCF offers another angle by which to understand evidence, thereby enriching the possibilities for knowledge development and translation that open spaces for transformative practice. In this way, we hope to contribute to the EBP discourses in a manner that encourages critical engagement with the notion of evidence, pushing for an expanded understanding of the types of knowledge needed for clinical decision making.

Anderson explains that transformative knowledge is "under girded by critical consciousness on the part of healthcare providers, and . . . unmasks unequal relations of power and issues of domination and subordination, based on assumptions about 'race,' 'gender,' and class relations."[61(p205)] We take as a starting point that transformative knowledge for practice is dependent upon the interrelated processes of knowledge development and knowledge translation. In the arena of knowledge development, insights from a postcolonial feminist perspective have brought to light the common claims of representative research-derived generalizable knowledge that is, in reality, based on selective populations that often exclude marginalized populations. Great caution must thus be taken in applying this knowledge in a universalizing sense. In response, a PCF lens calls for the inclusion of subjugated knowledge in our knowledge development processes. In addition, the need for empirical evidence to provide a better understanding of the mechanisms of health disparities is also emphasized through a postcolonial feminist analysis of EBP, such that the broader intersecting forces impinging on life opportunities necessary for health—including access to education, housing, income, social networks, and healthcare resources—are identified and addressed. Expanded research agendas will be necessary to fill these gaps.

At its heart, the evidence-based movement draws on a view of science that holds to a hierarchy of evidence that profiles the purported objective, quantifiable outcomes of RCTs, and other measurement-based methods as superior to narrative-based "subjective" methods. Our PCF reading suggests the importance of recognizing the limitations of this trend, and seeking complementary sources of knowledge that bring to light both large-scale phenomena as well as the contingencies and particularities of situated knowledge. We call for what Lather articulates as "a more capacious scientificity of disciplined inquiry."[62(p28)] Such science does not "divest experience of its rich ambiguity because it stays close to the complexities and contradictions of existence."[62(p23)] Notably, an insistence on a broad range of inquiry methods is driven not by allegiance to any methods for the sake of method per se, but rather by recognition of the breadth and depth of knowledge required for transformative practice. That is, a PCF commitment might see research conducted via a range of

methodologies, across a range of quantitative and qualitative methods, with the goal of generating knowledge that supports practice in today's complex environments while illuminating the broader social forces (historical, economic, political) that shape how healthcare services are structured and delivered with ultimate implications for health outcomes. Importantly, the call for multiple sources of evidence accumulated in part (giving credence to practice-based and personal knowledge) through a range of disciplined scientific approaches takes a remarkably different stance to knowledge translation, seeing it as an *effort to foster understanding, reflection, and action,* instead of a narrow translation of research into practice.[62]

A postcolonial feminist framing makes clear that narrow applications of procedural knowledge without the incorporation of other ways of knowing and knowledge about the social context of health/illness for the individual healthcare recipient will continue to fall short of providing humanistic, effective, and efficient healthcare. As explained, the EBP movement has largely been taken up in practice through the tools of clinical pathways, best practice guidelines, and care maps. The orthodoxy of EBP suggests a linear approach to clinical decision making; however this is just one way of viewing the applications of professional knowledge. Although some aspects of clinical practice may well be predictable, the complexities of the clinical environment, along with the heterogeneity of people seeking healthcare services, point to the need for a thoughtful practitioner who draws on a variety of knowledge, with the clinical judgment to know *when* and *how* to integrate this knowledge. Moreover, as the feminist perspective cautions against viewing research participants as "objects of study" so too the warning can be taken not to construct the recipients of healthcare as "objects of evidence-based practice." Any efforts at transformative knowledge translation must grapple with this challenge of enhancing nursing practice for individualized, client-appropriate, contextualized care based on the latest knowledge and skill. To illustrate how PCF interpretation of EBP might support transformative nursing practice, we conclude with an example of a knowledge translation project.

Contextualizing Our Position: Reframing Cultural Safety

Providing the impetus for this article and its rereading of the EBP movement is a recently initiated knowledge translation pilot project, *Cultural Safety and Knowledge Uptake in Clinical Settings: A Model for Practice for Culturally Diverse Populations** (nominated principal investigator, J. Anderson funding Canadian Institutes of Health Research), that synthesizes knowledge from the programs of research of a team of investigators in the Culture, Gender, and Health Research Unit at the University of British Columbia (http://www.cghru.nursing.ubc.ca/) and, in a collaborative effort with clinicians, translates this knowledge into practice. Shared themes of these programs of research are culture, social justice, gender, and health, with substantive foci including inequities in access to health and healthcare services; vulnerabilities as structured by various socially constructed classifications (eg, racializing categories and stigmatizing labels) and by certain life transitions and circumstances (eg, poverty, aging, violence, migration, hospitalization, and transition to home); and strategies to reduce inequities and vulnerabilities through innovative approaches to knowledge translation that engage key stakeholders.

Specifically, our exemplar here draws on our experiences in developing and implementing a collaborative approach to knowledge translation (J. Baumbusch et al. unpublished data), grounded in the dialectic between research and practice, in which the integration of transformative knowledge—the reflexive knowledge that makes visible and critiques relations of power operating through social relations and structures, and envisions actions that shift these power relations—leads to transformations in practice. In clinical environments where

the language of clinical pathways, best practice guidelines, and care maps predominate, we are exploring how to best incorporate knowledge from this established program of research that has drawn extensively on postcolonial and feminist theories.

The concept of cultural safety, originating in the Maori context of New Zealand, has served as a starting point for several of our projects.[9,63] Conceptualized by Irihapeti Ramsden and incorporated into New Zealand's Nursing Council guidelines in 1992, *cultural safety* is defined as

> The effective nursing of a person/family from another culture by a nurse who has undertaken a process of reflection on own cultural identity and recognizes the impact of the nurse's culture on own nursing practice. Unsafe cultural practice is any action which diminishes, demeans, or disempowers the cultural identity and wellbeing of an individual, (cited in Clarke[64(pv)])

Cultural safety underscores the importance of acknowledging the historical sociopolitical context that shapes people's health and healthcare encounters, and in this way aligns with a postcolonial feminist framework. Yet, even within this framing, the types of knowledge or evidence that may be invoked when the concept of cultural safety is employed are not unproblematic.

Our initial steps to translate this concept into practice highlight the complexities of both the concept itself and some of the challenges of knowledge translation from a postcolonial feminist stance. In our earlier empirical work, we set out to establish what cultural safety looks like in practice.[9,63] However, rather than coming up with a practice guideline (eg, a neat framework of values, attitudes and/or practices characteristic of cultural safety), we concluded that cultural safety can best be understood as an interpretive lens brought to the healthcare encounter by the provider, in which the provider reflects upon his or her own sociocultural positioning with accompanying values and assumptions, and seeks to understand what each patient brings to the healthcare encounter. Clearly, cultural safety then becomes not the *subject* of a clinical pathway but rather a *way* of approaching professional practice. Moreover,

* This knowledge translation study is funded by the Canadian Institutes of Health Research (2005–2008). Principal Investigator: Dr J. Anderson; Coprincipal investigators: Dr M. Judith Lynam, Dr Sheryl Reimer Kirkham, Dr Annette Browne; Coinvestigators: Dr Paddy Rodney, Dr Colleen Varcoe; Dr Sabrina Wong). For more information, see the project Web site at: http://www.cghru.nursing.ubc.ca/.

"culture" itself is problematized to reveal the widespread tendencies to generalize and/or stereotype on the basis of presumed group affiliations when the nature of culture is itself socially constructed. Indeed, our research has impressed upon us the limitations of the languaging of cultural safety, where the very use of the term "culture" may reinscribe the notion of discrete cultural groups with the all too common accompanying propensities toward stereotyping. To reflect the shifting and contextual nature of how subject identities are enacted and perceived, and the empirical observations that anyone, regardless of social status, ethnic affiliations, gender, and so forth, may face a convergence of events such that they are particularly vulnerable,[9] we have coined the phrase "situated vulnerability" that does not essentialize groups as "vulnerable populations." Rather, we examine the contexts and conditions under which people are made vulnerable. This is not to undermine the suffering of those who have been disadvantaged, but rather, to acknowledge that vulnerability is a social construct, created through the social conditions of people's lives, and not a fixed state of being, or "ethnic trait."

The promotion of reflective practice through the use of transformative knowledge is an important avenue, while less tangible than a clinical pathway, in supporting nurses to provide individualized, client-appropriate care that is attuned to these situated vulnerabilities. Nurses require tools to support not only their objective/technological dimensions of practice but also the relational, contextual, and historical dimensions to assist professional nursing practice. Therefore, while the mechanisms of EBP (ie, clinical pathways, best practice guidelines, care maps) offer one route to clinical decision making applied to a relatively narrow range of clinical phenomena, we advocate for the incorporation of sociological, qualitative, and humanities-based knowledge into the frontline of nursing practice to foster the "critical consciousness"[61] necessary for reflexive thinking and transformative practice.

However, *how* to best translate this type of knowledge into clinical practice poses considerable challenge. We have found that translation of this type of transformative knowledge requires a much more intense relationship between research and practice where researchers embrace a more active role in the process of knowledge translation. In our current knowledge translation efforts, we are exploring more organic ways to facilitate the uptake of a wide range of knowledge, keeping in mind the goal of fostering "understanding, reflection, and action."[62(p23)] Although our initial work with managers and other administrative healthcare decision makers saw a preference for managerial discourses (particularly the language of "numbers") in the communication of research findings, we are now embarking on an exploration of the type of engagement required to facilitate the uptake of transformative knowledge for frontline nurses.

In this more active engagement, our team has been exploring how to translate research-based knowledge from the language of the academy into the language of practice, simultaneously engaging with different discourses in the clinic. We are delving into ways to prepare knowledge in such a way that is accessible to practitioners, resonates with their experiences of the realities of everyday practice, creates a space of openness to the uptake of transformative knowledge, and, ultimately, to transformations in practice. For example, we have taken as starting point practice tools that have been developed for discharge planning (ie, discharge planning guidelines) and used case examples to exemplify how individuals experiencing a vulnerable period in their lives—hospitalization—may not fit within the narrow constructs of the tool. Rather than viewing these individuals as outliers, we then engage practitioners in the process of critical reflection on how this individual's care could have been approached differently, and how guidelines around discharge planning could be written in a way that lead nurses to take up transformative knowledge and translate it into practice within the complex and demanding environments in which they work. Our experiences to date with translation of transformative knowledge has underscored for us the new terrain that this effort represents, particularly as we bring knowledge derived from critical inquiry to the mainstreamed enterprise of knowledge translation and EBP.

Conclusion

Over the past several decades, the discipline of nursing has struggled with the uptake of research-based knowledge at the point of care. EBP has been adapted from medicine and applied to nursing, although not without wide-ranging critique of this approach to knowledge uptake. To these critiques, we have added the perspectives of PCF regarding the shortcomings of EBP, and have recommended an expansion to EBP, in the form of translation of transformative knowledge, as a viable approach to knowledge uptake in clinical settings. This transformative knowledge draws not just on narrow notions of evidence, but seeks inclusive epistemologies that represent the realities of multiple sources of knowledge, including previously marginalized knowledge. The translation of transformative knowledge also guards against discourses of standardization associated with EBP, striving instead to understand the particularities of each situation; and how these particularities are structured by larger historically embedded systems of social classification such as racialization, class, and gender. When employed in this way, knowledge translation has the potential to enhance nursing practice through understanding, reflection, and action.

REFERENCES

1. Dawes M. Evidence-based practice. In: Dawes M, Davies P, Gray A, Mant J, Seers K, Snowball R, eds. *Evidence-Based Practice: A Primer for Health Care Professionals.* London: Churchill Livingstone; 1999:1–8.
2. Meleskie J, Wilson K. Developing regional clinical pathways in rural health. *Can Nurs.* 2003;99(8):25–28.
3. Canadian Nurses Association. *Nursing Now Issues and Trends in Canadian Nursing: Cultural Diversity—Changes and Challenges.* Ottawa, Ontario: Canadian Nurses Association; 2000.
4. Barnes L. The social production of an enterprise clinic: nurses, clinical pathway guidelines and contemporary healthcare practices. *Nurs Inq.* 2000;7(3):200–208.
5. Estabrooks C. Will evidence-based nursing practice make practice perfect? *Can J Nurs Res.* 1998;30(1):15–36.
6. Traynor M. The oil crisis, risk and evidence-based practice. *Nurs Inq.* 2002;9(3):162–169.
7. Walker K. Why evidence-based practice now? A polemic. *Nurs Inq.* 2003;10(3):145–155.
8. Winch S, Greedy D, Chaboyer W Governing nursing conduct: the rise of evidence-based practice. *Nurs Inq.* 2002;9(3):156–161.
9. Anderson J, Perry J, Blue C, et al. "Rewriting" cultural safety within the postcolonial and postnational feminist project: toward new epistemologies of healing. *ANS Adv Nurs Sci.* 2003;26(3):196–214.
10. Reimer Kirkham S. The politics of belonging and intercultural health care provision. *West J Nurs Res.* 2003;25(7):762–780.
11. Rogers W. Evidence based medicine and justice: a framework for looking at the impact of EBN upon vulnerable or disadvantaged groups. *J Med Ethics.* 2004;30:141–145.
12. Sackett D, Rosenerg W, Gray JAM, Haynes RB, Richardson WS. Evidence-based medicine: what it is and what it isn't. *BMJ.* 1996;312:71–72.
13. DiCensa A, Ciliska D, Guyatt G. Introduction to evidence-based nursing. In: DiCensa A, Guyatt DG, Ciliska D, eds. *Evidence-Based Nursing: A Guide to Clinical Practice.* St. Louis: Mosby Elsevier; 2005:3–19.
14. Fawcett J, Wilson J, Neuman B, Hinton WP, Fitzpatrick JJ. On nursing theories and evidence. *J Nurs Scholarsh.* 2001;33(2):115–119.
15. The Joanna Briggs Institute. *Evidence Based Practice Information Sheets for Health Professionals: Identification and Nursing Management of Dysphasia in Adults With Neurological Impairment.* Adelaide, Australia: Joanna Briggs Institute; 2000.
16. Thorne S, Sawatzky R. Particularizing the general: challenges in teaching the structure of evidence-based nursing practice. In: Drummond J, Standish P, eds. *The Philosophy of Nursing Education.* New York: Palgrave Macmillan. In press.
17. Carper B. Fundamental ways of knowing in nursing. *ANS Adv Nurs Sci.* 1978; 1(1):13–23.
18. McSherry M, Simmons M, Pearce P *Evidence-Informed Nursing: A Guide for Clinical Nursing.* London: Routledge; 2000.
19. Timmermans S, Berg M. *Gold Standard: The Challenge of Evidence-Based Medicine and Standardization in Health Care.* Philadelphia: Temple University Press; 2003.
20. Fanon F. *The Wretched of the Earth.* Harmondsworth, England: Penguin; 1963.
21. Said EW. *Orientalism.* New York: Vintage Books; 1978.
22. Collins PH. *Black Feminist Thought: Knowledge, Consciousness, and the Politics of Empowerment.* New York: Routledge; 1990.
23. Hooks B. *Black Looks: Race and Representation.* New York: Routledge; 1992.
24. Morrison T. *Playing in the Dark: Whiteness and the Literary Imagination.* Cambridge: Harvard University Press; 1992.
25. Brewer R. Theorizing race, class and gender: the new scholarship of black feminist intellectuals and black women's labour. In: James SM, Busia APA, eds. *Theorizing Black Feminisms: The Visionary Pragmatism of Black Women.* London: Routledge; 2006:13–30.
26. Anderson JM. Writing in subjugated knowledges: towards a transformative agenda in nursing research and practice. *Nurs Inq.* 2000;7(3):145.

27. Anderson JM. Toward a post-colonial feminist methodology in nursing research: exploring the convergence of post-colonial and black feminist scholarship. *Nurs Res.* 2002;9(3):7–27.
28. Anderson JM. Lessons from a postcolonial-feminist perspective: suffering and a path to healing. *Nurs Inq.* 2004;11(4):238–246.
29. Blackford J. Cultural frameworks of nursing practice: exposing an exclusionary healthcare culture. *Nurs Inq.* 2003;10(4):236–244.
30. Browne AJ, Smye V, Varcoe C. The relevance of postcolonial theoretical perspectives to research in aboriginal health. *Can J Nurs Res.* 2005; 37(4):16–37.
31. Mohammed S. Moving beyond the "exotic": applying postcolonial theory in health research. *ANS Adv Nurs Sci.* 2006;29(2): 98–109.
32. Racine L. Implementing a postcolonial feminist perspective in nursing research related to non-Western populations. *Nurs Inq.* 2003;10(2):91–102.
33. Reimer Kirkham S, Anderson JM. Postcolonial nursing scholarship: from epistemology to method. *ANS Adv Nurs Sci.* 2002; 25(1):1–17.
34. Street A, Blackford J. Cultural conflict: the impact of western feminism(s) on nurses caring for women of non-English speaking background. *J Clin Nurs.* 2002;11:664–671.
35. Ahmad W. *"Race" and Health in Contemporary Britain.* Buckingham, England: Open University Press; 1994.
36. Allen D, Benner P, Diekelmann N. Three paradigms for nursing research: methodological implications. In: Chinn PL, ed. *Nursing Research Methodology: Issues and Implications.* Rockville, Md: Aspen; 1986:23–38.
37. Barbee E. Racism in US nursing. *Med Anthropol Q.* 1993; 3(4):346–362.
38. Campbell J, Bunting S. Voices and paradigms? Perspectives on critical and feminist theory in nursing. *ANS Adv Nurs Sci.* 1991;13(3):1–15.
39. Webb C. Feminist methodology in nursing research. *J Adv Nurs.* 1984;9:249–256.
40. Allen D. Whiteness and difference in nursing. *Nurs Phil.* 2006;7:65–78.
41. Canales M. Toward an understanding of difference. *ANS Adv Nurs Sci.* 2000;22(4):16–31.
42. Drevdahl D, Phillips D, Taylor J. Uncontested categories: the use of race and ethnicity variables in nursing research. *Nurs Inq.* 2006;13(l):52–63.
43. Kendall J, Hatton D, Beckett A, Leo M. Racism as a source of health disparity in children with attention-deflcit/hyperactivity disorder. *ANS Adv Nurs Sci.* 2002;26(2):114–130.
44. Phillips D, Drevdahl D. "Race" and the difficulties of language. *ANS Adv Nurs Sci.* 2003;26(1):17–29.
45. McConaghy C. *Rethinking Indigenous Education: Culturalism, Colonialism, and the Politics of Knowing.* Brisbane, Australia: Post Pressed; 2000.
46. Meleis A, Im E. Transcending marginalization in knowledge development. *Nurs Inq.* 1999;6:94–102.
47. Horton R. Medical journals: evidence of bias against the diseases of poverty. *Lancet.* 2003;36l:712–713.
48. Whitehead M, Dahlgren G, Gilson L. Developing the policy response to inequities in health: a global perspective. In: Evans T, Whitehead M, Diderichsen F, Bhuiya A, Wirth M, eds. *Challenging Inequities in Health: From Ethics to Action.* New York: Oxford University Press; 2001:308–323.
49. Kemm J. The limitations of "evidence-based'" public health. *J Eval Clin Pract.* 2006;12(3):319–324.
50. Estroff S, Henderson G. Social and cultural contributions to health, difference, and inequality. In: Henderson G, Estroff S, Churchill L, King N, Oberlander J, Strauss R, eds. *The Social Medicine Reader: Social and Cultural Contributions to Health, Difference, and Inequality.* Durham, NC: Duke University Press; 2005:4–26.
51. Browne AJ, Smye V. A critical analysis of the relevance of collecting "ethnicity data" in health care contexts. Paper presented at: the Society for Applied Anthropology Conference; April 28, 2006; Vancouver, British Columbia.
52. Bhopal R, Donaldson L. White, European, Western, Caucasian, or what? Inappropriate labeling in research on race, ethnicity, and health. In: Henderson G, Estroff S, Churchill L, King N, Oberlander J, Strauss R, eds. *The Social Medicine Reader: Social and Cultural Contributions to Health, Difference, and Inequality.* Durham, NC: Duke University Press; 2005:252–262.
53. Georges JM, McGuire S. Deconstructing clinical pathways: mapping the landscape of health care. *ANS Adv Nurs Sci.* 2004; 27(1):2–11.
54. Frenkel M, Shenhav Y. From binarism back to hybridity: a postcolonial reading of management and organization studies. *Org Stud.* 2006;27(5):855–876.
55. Acker J. The future of "gender and organizations": connections and boundaries. *Gend Work Organ.* 1998;5(4):195–206.
56. Prasad A, Machel G. *Postcolonial Theory and Organizational Analysis: A Critical Engagement.* New York: Palgrave Macmillan; 2003.
57. Henley E, Peters K. 10 steps for avoiding health disparities in your practice. *J Fam Pract.* 2006;53(3):193–196.
58. Lynam J, Henderson A, Browne A, et al. Healthcare restructuring with a view to equity and efficiency: reflections on unintended consequences. *Can J Nurs Leadersh.* 2003;16(1): 112–140.
59. Browne A. Discourses influencing nurses perceptions of First Nations patients. *Can J Nurs Res.* 2005;37(4):62–87.
60. McCall J. *"I Chose to Fight": The Lives and Experiences of Women Who are Living With HIV/AIDS* [unpublished master's thesis]. Vancouver, British Columbia: University of British Columbia; 2006.
61. Anderson JM. Speaking of illness: issues of first generation Canadian women—implications for patient education and counseling. *Patient Educ Couns.* 1998;33:197–207.
62. Lather P. This is your father's paradigm? Government intrusion and the case of qualitative research in education. *Qual Inq.* 2004;10(1):15–34.
63. Reimer Kirkham S, Smye V, Tang S, et al. Rethinking cultural safety while waiting to do fieldwork: methodological implications for nursing research. *Res Nurs Health.* 2002;25:222–232.
64. Clarke M. Preface. In: Wepa D, ed. *Cultural Safety in Aotearoa New Zealand.* Auckland: Pearson Education New Zealand; 2005:v–vii.

The Authors Comment

Knowledge Development and Evidence-Based Practice: Insights and Opportunities from a Postcolonial Feminist Perspective for Transformative Nursing Practice

This article had its genesis in a seminar aimed at discussing the relevance of postcolonial feminist theories for nursing and healthcare scholarship, made possible by support from the Elizabeth Kenny McCann (EKM) Professorship held by Dr. Joan Anderson (2001–2005) at the University of British Columbia, and the EKM Doctoral Award held by J. Baumbusch. We dedicate this article to the late Professor McCann, whose vision of the connectedness between nursing education and practice inspired the direction of this article. The article signals the challenges facing the profession in regard to how nursing knowledge—particularly that which is framed as "evidence"—is generated and translated in practice, and offers insight into how theoretical perspectives in the critical traditions of postcolonial feminist scholarship might be drawn upon in response to these challenges.

—Sheryl Reimer Kirkham
—Jennifer Baumbusch
—Annette S.H. Schultz
—Joan M. Anderson

CHAPTER 37

Mediating the Meaning of Evidence Through Epistemological Diversity

Denise Tarlier

Nursing's disciplinary recognition of 'multiple ways of knowing' reflects an epistemological diversity that supports nursing praxis. Nursing as praxis offers a conceptual way to explore what it is about the interface of practice, knowledge and evidence in nursing that distinguishes us as a discipline. I suggest that the relationship between evidence and knowledge is defined and mediated by the same epistemological diversity that supports nursing as praxis. Just as the meaning and truth-value of evidence is evaluated from within the body of existing disciplinary knowledge, new evidence may prompt an evaluation of the meaning and truth-value of extant nursing knowledge. Nursing practice that relies on scientific evidence as a singular basis of practice knowledge is susceptible to exploitation by the diverse agendas operating within an ideology of evidence-based practice and the healthcare system. Mediating the meaning of evidence for nursing practice through acknowledgement of the diverse epistemologies that underpin nursing knowledge will contribute to a disciplinary-specific definition of what constitutes evidence for nursing, and will better direct how evidence is integrated into a disciplinary body of knowledge.

A disciplinary existential angst amongst nurses drives us to identify, define, rationalize and sometimes defend what nursing is and what nurses do. As a discipline, nurses are adamant that nursing—in theory—offers a unique perspective on health-care. In practice, nurses *know* that what they do for patients 'makes a difference', but have difficulty articulating *how* they know what they 'do'. That is, a fundamental disconnect exists

About the Author

DENISE TARLIER was born and grew up on the West Coast of Canada, in North Vancouver, British Columbia. She completed a diploma in general nursing in 1982 at the British Columbia Institute of Technology, followed by a certificate program in Operating Room Nursing in 1986, and a BSN from the University of British Columbia in 1992. She was drawn to working with Canada's remote northern Aboriginal populations. To better prepare for the demands of this complex clinical nursing role, she completed the diploma program in Outpost and Community Health Nursing at Dalhousie University in 1996, and subsequently, successfully challenged the American Academy of Nurse Practitioners (AANP) Family Nurse Practitioner certification examination in 1998, a time when nurse practitioner roles were just beginning to be recognized and formalized in Canada. After practicing in remote communities for several years, she returned to school (yet again) and completed an MSN (2001) and a PhD (2006) at the University of British Columbia. Dr. Tarlier is currently an Assistant Professor in the School of Nursing at Thompson Rivers University in Kamloops, British Columbia, where the focus of her scholarship continues to be guided by a strong clinical practice orientation to primary health care, rural and remote health services, Aboriginal health issues, and primary care and nurse practitioner nursing roles.

between knowing what nursing is and being able to explicate the source of nursing knowledge. This disconnect has implications for understanding what constitutes evidence for nursing practice. Nursing as praxis offers a conceptual way to explore what it is about the interface of practice, knowledge and evidence in nursing that distinguishes us as a discipline.

Nursing's disciplinary recognition of 'multiple ways of knowing' reflects an epistemological diversity that supports nursing praxis. Evidence, in the traditional positivist scientific sense that underpins modern health science (Scott-Findlay and Pollock 2004), is merely one source of nursing knowledge and not necessarily privileged over other ways. It is fundamental to the development of nursing knowledge, but is not in itself a sufficient basis for all practice knowledge. Epistemological diversity is necessary to define, evaluate and value what constitutes evidence for nursing practice. Examining how nursing's epistemological diversity sustains praxis will explicate how nursing as a discipline mediates the meaning of evidence in a healthcare system where evidence may have different meanings for different disciplines, and where the term 'evidence-based practice' has taken on ideological proportions.

Epistemological Diversity: A Nursing Tradition?

Nursing as a discipline has always embraced multiple and diverse epistemologies. Historically, acknowledgement of our diverse epistemological bases has been expressed in a variety of ways, but explicit recognition of nursing's diverse epistemologies has not taken place. Carper (1978) is credited as the first nursing scholar to describe what has since become commonly referred to as nursing's multiple ways of knowing (Fawcett et al. 2001), which she originally described as four fundamental patterns of knowing in nursing: empirical, ethical, aesthetic and personal knowing. Many others have built on Carper's seminal work, conceptualizing and writing about nursing's multiple ways of knowing in varying ways but with essentially the same two theses: (a) nursing practice is complex and holistic, thus nursing knowledge relies on more than a singular source of knowing (Jennings and Loan 2001); and (b) the singular source of knowledge represented by empirics is insufficient to account for all nursing knowledge (Nagle and Mitchell 1991).

The concept of multiple ways of knowing in nursing is patently the same concept as epistemological diversity.

Examining how various scholars, both in nursing and in related social sciences, have written about the concept of epistemological diversity substantiates this claim. The review presented here is brief and by no means inclusive, as comprehensive historical reviews already exist in the literature (e.g. Johnson and Ratner 1997; Meleis 1997).

In 1988, Jacobs-Kramer and Chinn extended Carper's (1978) work by presenting a model integrating the four patterns of knowing identified by Carper. These scholars later expanded on and further refined the model they proposed (Chinn and Kramer 1999). In the epilogue to their 1999 textbook, Chinn and Kramer described how their thinking about knowledge development had shifted over the years to better accommodate patterns of knowing—or epistemologies—that could not be accommodated appropriately within the empirical pattern, demonstrating a deliberate rebuttal of empirics as a singular epistemology for nursing knowledge. Most recently, Fawcett et al. (2001) used Carper's original work as the basis of a critical treatise on the interface of nursing theories and evidence-based practice, which once again affirmed 'the diverse patterns of knowing [that] constitute the ontological and epistemological foundations of the discipline of nursing' (117).

Nursing scholars Nagle and Mitchell (1991) approached epistemological issues in terms of theoretical and paradigmatic diversity. These authors concluded, 'it is myopic and naïve to suggest that a single-paradigm approach can adequately fulfill nursing's mandate' (22). Their conclusion was remarkably similar to that offered by Schwandt (1990). Schwandt, a social scientist, addressed epistemological diversity in terms of ontologies and methodologies. He concluded that any one particular epistemological-methodological coupling is insufficient on its own to represent the nature of truth in the context of the social sciences, and recognized the complex contextual issues that influence disciplinary epistemologies.

Wolfer (1993), another nursing scholar, used an 'aspects of "reality"' (141) framework based on a philosophy of mind/body/spirit to illustrate how different types of problems require different epistemologies, and also different ontologies. He characterized the different epistemologies in terms of body, mind and transcendental ways of knowing. While this approach is evocative of the traditional reductionist approach based on Cartesian dualism (Capra 1982), Wolfer asserted that all three ways of knowing are needed to provide holistic care. He claimed that his framework offered 'a way of looking at the reality of nursing which "sees" different types of knowledge, theory and research as complementary rather than competitive or exclusionary' (145).

In 1995, White suggested modifying Jacob-Kramer and Chinn's (1988) model of Carper's (1978) work to be inclusive of interpretive and critical ontologies and epistemologies. White added sociopolitical knowing as a fifth pattern to accommodate her modifications, recognizing that Carper's original definition of the empirical pattern excluded the relativist positions White proposed. Sociopolitical knowing was presented as an integrating pattern 'essential to understanding all the others' (83). The basis of White's claim was that sociopolitical knowing represented the contextual knowledge within which all other nursing knowledge was situated.

Johnson and Ratner (1997) described the nature of nursing knowledge in terms of ontology, epistemology and practical utility. Empirical and interpretive epistemologies are equally privileged in these scholars' conceptualizations of knowledge, thus furthering the claims made by earlier nursing scholars. Johnson and Ratner concluded that nursing practice knowledge is highly complex and 'multifarious' (19).

Most recently, physicians Upshur, VanDenKerkhof and Goel (2001) proposed a conceptual model of evidence that has patent similarities to both Carper's (1978) work and the conceptualizations of knowledge presented by Johnson and Ratner (1997). Upshur, VanDenKerkhof and Goel's (2001) model privileges information derived through both quantitative and qualitative methods of inquiry. Evidence is recognized as being mediated between context and method. While Upshur, VanDenKerkhof and Goel addressed the concept of evidence rather than knowledge, it is clear that the model they proposed is founded on diverse epistemologies and a radically broad conceptualization of empiricism that encompasses interpretive methods, philosophy and political theory. Whether or not this conceptualization of empiricism ultimately withstands critique, the model itself represents a notable break with the status quo in medicine; a discipline traditionally grounded in a biomedical, empirical epistemology.

The short review presented here illustrates some of the different ways in which scholars in the social science and health disciplines have characterized the epistemological underpinnings of practice knowledge. The differences between the characterizations may be largely explained by the temporal context at the time of writing: the presented works span two decades during which the dominant postpositivist view was continually challenged by emerging paradigms such as constructivism and critical theory. Through this evolutionary process, scholars first recognized and then worked toward situating and refining diverse epistemologies relative to existing and emerging philosophies.

Nursing Praxis

Despite the different approaches taken by various scholars, each article presented in the preceding review explored essentially the same concept: the complexities of holistic practice call for multiple and diverse ways of knowing. That is, multiple and diverse sources of knowledge necessarily underpin nursing practice knowledge. Defining 'epistemology' as a 'theory of knowledge' (Mautner 1996, 174), it is reasonable to think of and refer to these ways of knowing as diverse epistemologies. Nurse scholars have—over at least the past 20 years—recognized nursing's diverse epistemologies as fundamental to nursing as a complex and holistic practice. Moreover, a reciprocal, conscious, reflective bond between epistemology and practice is the basis of nursing as praxis (Jones 1997; Thorne 1997).

Praxis articulates nursing practice that is complex, holistic, reflective, and both grounded in and supportive of dynamically integrated knowledge, theory and practice (Jones 1997; Thorne 1997; Chinn and Kramer

1999). 'Praxis is theory and practice that are interrelated, integrated, and dialectical in nature. Inherent within praxis is reflection both on and in practice' (Jones 1997, 126). Holmes and Warelow (2000) claim that nurses must 'critically reflect upon their practices in order to elaborate the implicit and often complex theories and attitudes, by which it is established, developed and sustained' (179–80). Praxis describes practice that is continuously infused by nurses' critical reflection on and integration of diverse elements of practice. Thus, praxis implies practice that transcends what knowledge alone would support. The reciprocal integration of knowledge with practice in itself adds a dimension that elevates the whole of practice beyond the mere sum of its parts.

There has been a tendency in the nursing literature to reflect upon nursing practice as dualistic in nature: is nursing an art or a science? (Bishop and Scudder 1997). Dichotomizing nursing practice in this way is based in and reflects a positivistic, biomedical, reductionist ontology in that practice is being reduced to discrete parts. Such a dichotomy fails to represent the holistic and complex nature of nursing as praxis and is problematic because it fosters the possibility of viewing practice in 'either/or' terms, that is, practice as either a science or an art (Jones 2001). Some nursing scholars have recognized the inherent dangers of subscribing to this dichotomy and have suggested various alternative ways of conceptualizing practice: as a practical science (Johnson 1991), as practice (Bishop and Scudder 1997), as phronesis (Benner 2000; Flaming 2001), and even as pragmatism (Warms and Schroeder 1999).

I suggest that despite these alternative conceptualizations, the notion of practice as dichotomous persists; not merely within nursing but in how other health disciplines and society view nursing. For example, the tendency to dichotomize practice is at the root of what nursing scholars discuss as visible vs. invisible nursing practice (e.g. Rafael 1999). The persistence of such a dichotomous conceptualization of practice reflects just how deeply ingrained a biomedical, reductionist ontology and epistemology are in western society and within nursing (Jones 2001). This dominant paradigm has made it difficult for a discipline that aspires to recognition as a science (as nursing does) to openly admit to holding diverse other epistemologies. Thus, although nursing has recognized 'multiple ways of knowing' for almost 25 years, acknowledgement of these has remained within nursing and in these somewhat nebulous terms, rarely claimed outright as being diverse epistemologies.

Dichotomizing nursing practice (and thereby creating the 'either/or' dilemma) allows the possibility that the practice of nursing is purely a science.[1] Viewing practice as a science in turn supports the possibility that scientific evidence alone may be sufficient for practice knowledge. That is, that evidence derived through a singular, positivistic epistemology provides an adequate evidence base for nursing practice. Scott-Findlay and Pollock (2004) claim,

> Within the evidence-based practice paradigm, the implication of giving the authority for practice to the scientific evidence, in other words, the research findings (an inherently narrow implicit definition of evidence), is that other influences in the decision-making process (e.g. clinical practice knowledge) get lower value or priority' (95).

Thus, evidence or knowledge arising through other epistemologies, or ways of knowing, are less valued, and by implication, the 'art' of nursing is devalued (Wolfer 1993; Mitchell 1999; Flaming 2001; Rycroft-Malone et al. 2004). Some nursing scholars have adamantly decried the implicit devaluation of the art of nursing: 'Neither science of a basic nature nor the "creative use" of basic scientific knowledge will provide the tools necessary for the art of nursing' (Johnson 1991, 11). Without the art, the integrated, synchronous character of praxis is lost, and nursing practice is indeed at risk of becoming merely that part of practice that can be supported by scientific knowledge alone.

The diverse epistemologies privileged by nursing as a discipline are central to Johnson and Ratner (1997) and enable praxis. Paradoxically, praxis demands epistemologies that are sufficiently broad (Flaming 2001) to support all of its complexities. The foregoing review of scholarly works suggests that empirical ways of knowing alone are insufficiently broad to support nursing praxis. However, the positivist scientific tradition that dominates western approaches to healthcare (Harman 1996; Scott-Findlay and Pollock 2004) continues to privilege empirical epistemologies as the singular means to acquire, evaluate and determine the evidence that constitutes knowledge.

Issues of Evidence

Issues of what is considered evidence and how evidence is related to knowledge have become a focus of controversy in nursing, reflecting debate in the health disciplines generally (Madjar and Walton 2001; Dobrow, Goel and Upshur 2004). The controversy has been bitter at times and has led to polarization within disciplines (Greenhalgh and Worrall 1997, e.g. Charlton 1997; Shahar 1998; Mitchell 1999). Debate is based in the way evidence was formally defined by the Evidence-Based Medicine Working Group in their landmark 1992 paper. This group of medical practitioners and academics proposed what they referred to as an evidence-based approach to the practice of medicine, defining the primary sources of evidence as randomized controlled trials (RCTs) and meta-analyses of RCTs. Despite a later effort to partially ameliorate this definition (Sackett et al. 1996), the original definition eventually grew into the hierarchy of levels of evidence that underpin the concept of evidence-based medicine (EBM).

Evidence, according to the proponents of EBM, is judged in relation to a hierarchy of evidence that is based on study design and rigor (Centre for Evidence-Based Medicine 2001; Madjar and Walton 2001; Upshur 2001; Dobrow, Goel and Upshur 2004), and grounded in a positivist, reductionist ontology and epistemology (Upshur, VanDenKerkhof and Goel 2001). While at least four different hierarchies of evidence have

---

[1] Practice as a science is to be differentiated from practice that is based in part on science, which implies that practice is also based in part on something other than science (such as the art of practice) and nursing science, which implies that nursing creates its own science.

been developed (Upshur 2003), each of these clearly places a higher value on quantitative research findings from RCTs and systematic reviews of RCTs (Madjar and Walton 2001; Upshur 2003; Scott-Findlay and Pollock 2004; Dobrow, Goel and Upshur 2004), and information derived from other sources is accordingly assigned lesser value (Rycroft-Malone et al. 2004). Findings from qualitative studies do not qualify as evidence in this schema. Moreover, not only are qualitative findings excluded from the hierarchy of evidence, but there is also an implicit suggestion that such excluded findings represent a challenge or threat to 'real' evidence.

In contrast, many nursing scholars have recognized that the definition of evidence espoused by the proponents of EBM is too narrow and exclusive to support the complexities of nursing practice (Estabrooks 1998; Kitson, Harvey and McCormack 1998; Fawcett et al. 2001; Madjar and Walton 2001; Rycroft-Malone et al. 2004). These scholars have been adamant in their insistence that nursing as a discipline adopt a broader definition of evidence, one that recognizes the influence of context on the application of evidence in practice (Scott-Findlay and Pollock 2004) and considers qualitative research findings.

The call within nursing for a more inclusive understanding of evidence has begun to echo in the recent literature of other health disciplines. For example, the model of the taxonomy of evidence presented by physicians Upshur, VanDenKerkhof and Goel (2001) recognizes qualitative research findings as a form of evidence. In a study that investigated the utilization of social science research knowledge, Landry, Amara and Lamari (2001) found that behavioral and contextual factors were the most significant influences on research knowledge, suggesting that the existence of evidence alone was insufficient cause for uptake and use.

However, an inclusive definition of evidence is problematic. As the definition of evidence expands, the issue of what constitutes evidence becomes more ambiguous (Scott-Findlay and Pollock 2004). Where does one draw the line as to what one is willing to consider as evidence? Some scholars have expressed a willingness to push the meaning of evidence beyond research findings

altogether, and have proposed that clinical judgment and experience are forms of evidence (Estabrooks 1998; Rycroft-Malone et al. 2004). For example, Kitson, Harvey and McCormack (1998) define evidence as 'the combination of research, clinical expertise and patient choice' (150). But is a definition of evidence this broad any more useful to nursing practice than a too-restrictive definition? Are all knowledge and all experience to be privileged as evidence?

The Relationship Between Evidence and Knowledge

Upshur, VanDenKerkhof and Goel (2001) recently defined evidence as 'an observation, fact, or organized body of information offered to support or justify inferences or beliefs in the demonstration of some proposition or matter at issue' (93). These writers thus refer to the reality that research findings are seldom presented in research reports as neutral information or facts, but are pre-assigned some degree of truth-value by researchers, who present their work as an argument in favor of their conclusions—i.e. 'based on the *evidence.*' Additionally, while Upshur, VanDenKerkhof and Goel (2001) claim that their model of evidence is epistemologically 'rooted in empiricism' (93), they recognize management and political theory, social philosophy and Bayesian reasoning as methods of producing evidence, thus expanding the notion of evidence beyond the purely empirical. These writers conclude that their model of evidence integrates various disciplinary epistemologies, thus ultimately 'enabling a more holistic approach to evidence' (95). However, it is unclear where the boundaries between evidence and knowledge lie in this inclusive model of evidence.

I argue that the ambiguity about what constitutes evidence for nursing practice is based in a fundamental lack of conceptual clarity regarding the language of evidence-based practice (EBP), a problem that has also recently been recognized by other writers (i.e. Scott-Findlay and Pollock 2004). The margins between evidence and knowledge are elusive and overlapping. Scott-Findlay and Pollock have identified the pressing need to address the confusion that exists about the conceptual definitions of evidence and knowledge, in order to break the stalemate that has developed in scholarly debate regarding the nature of EBP for nursing, and allow a way forward.

The definitions offered by Scott-Findlay and Pollock (2004) represent an explicit way to consider the relationship between knowledge and evidence. These scholars make a strong case for differentiating between evidence as a particular form of knowledge (i.e. research findings) and other forms of knowledge (i.e. personal and experiential knowledge) that, while not considered evidence, are critically important influences on the uptake, integration and application of research findings within the context of the broader body of extant knowledge. To maintain this distinction, Scott-Findlay and Pollock propose that *evidence* be defined as exclusively research findings, arguing that this term offers greater clarity and specificity. Notably, these writers do not distinguish between quantitative and qualitative research findings, which is consistent with the diverse epistemological basis of nursing praxis.

Research findings are a tangible form of knowledge that may be shared or transferred among individuals. *Knowledge* implies individuals' broader or more general knowledge, and is defined as being intangible and personal: 'Information in the public domain must first be integrated, transferred, transmitted, or incorporated into the private (or personal) domain before it becomes knowledge' (Scott-Findlay and Pollock 2004, 93). Thus, research findings, as information, are taken up into an individual's more generalized body of knowledge through an integrative process. Disciplinary knowledge is therefore by implication structured as an aggregated form of knowledge rather than being a discrete entity unto itself.

I suggest that the relationship between evidence, or research findings and knowledge is defined and mediated by the same epistemological diversity that supports nursing as praxis. Research findings are adapted into a dynamic body of extant knowledge through a selective process that may also imply modification or rejection. The diverse epistemologies that underpin knowledge for

nursing praxis are necessary to define, evaluate, contextualize and value research findings from the perspective of nursing and through a disciplinary-specific lens (Thorne 2001).

Johnson and Ratner (1997) offer the following definition of knowledge: 'things perceived or held in consciousness, justified in some way, and therefore regarded as "true"' (4, citing Angeles 1981). The lay understanding of the word *evidence* similarly associates evidence with truth or validity (*Oxford dictionary of current English* 1998). Yet Upshur, VanDenKerkhof and Goel (2001) warn against equating evidence with the truth, saying that it is the defeasible nature of evidence that enables new information to be accommodated in the context of existing beliefs. That is, it is knowledge that imbues evidence (i.e. research findings) with meaning, and thus by extension, nursing disciplinary knowledge that imbues research findings with meaning and truth-value for nursing. To be readily accepted as true, new evidence must exhibit some congruency with what nurses already hold to be true within their existing disciplinary knowledge (Rycroft-Malone et al. 2004).

I suggest that what a discipline might accept as truth and knowledge are also defeasible (McCain 1998), and that defeasibility is the basis of the dynamic nature of knowledge. Thus, knowledge is not a static, manifest body, but a body more in the sense of a body of water: fluid and reactive. Just as the meaning and truth-value of research findings are evaluated from within the body of existing disciplinary knowledge, new research findings may prompt a re-evaluation of the meaning and truth-value of existing knowledge.

This process of reciprocal defeasibility addresses the transition in which information, such as research findings, becomes knowledge, or in other words, the process of evaluating the truth-value of new information from a disciplinary perspective. I propose that much of the ambiguity about evidence arises in how we think about this transition. Do we really consider 'information offered' to be evidence? Or is it more likely that by evidence, we mean information that has already been judged as having some truth-value? For instance, evidence as defined by proponents of EBM (Centre for

Evidence-Based Medicine 2001) is unquestioningly presented as having truth-value. The truth-value of this evidence is apparent and acceptable to those individuals or disciplines that subscribe to the same ontological and epistemological perspectives in which EBP is grounded; that is, a positivist western scientific perspective. While individuals within nursing may subscribe to such a perspective, it may be (and has been) problematic for nursing as a discipline that subscribes to diverse epistemologies to accept such evidence (i.e. research findings) as sufficient basis for nursing practice.

I will push both Scott-Findlay and Pollock's (2004) and Upshur, VanDenKerkhof and Goel's (2001) definitions of evidence further, and claim that research findings, observations, facts or information are just that, and do not constitute evidence until they have been judged by an individual as being 'true' or 'possibly true.' Information at this stage may more appropriately be conceptualized as 'appeals to evidence' (McCain 1998). Once an appeal to evidence has been evaluated as having truth-value, it becomes evidence, and as evidence, is integrated with existing knowledge. The diverse epistemologies that underpin nursing knowledge provide direction, helping nurses to navigate the process of evaluating the truth-value of information and its subsequent integration into nursing's knowledge base. Upshur, VanDenKerkhof and Goel (2001) claimed that personal belief is the term of measurement of evidence. I propose that disciplinary belief, or the extant body of disciplinary knowledge, is also a term of measurement. The key implication of defining evidence in this way is that the issue of what constitutes evidence becomes subject to (and thus specific to) disciplinary knowledge, rather than the one-size-fits-all definitions of evidence such as the Levels of Evidence (Centre for Evidence-Based Medicine).

While not explicitly recognizing the process of evaluation in their definition of evidence, Upshur, VanDen Kerkhof and Goel (2001) imply in their discussion that a process of evaluation occurs, framing the process in terms of analysis, interpretation and mediation of evidence. Other scholars have implicitly addressed the process of evaluating and valuing evidence relative to existing disciplinary knowledge. White (1995) touched on this notion when she stated, 'the remaining process for ascertaining credibility is the "fit" of the new knowledge with the extant knowledge in the area' (76). Fawcett et al. (2001) modified Carper's (1978) ways of knowing by labeling these as theories; they then claimed the theories to be 'diverse ontological and epistemological lenses through which evidence is interpreted and critiqued' (117). Madjar and Walton (2001) discussed the need for clinicians to 'recontextualize such findings and reassess their relevance in a particular situation' (39). Upshur (2001) refers to a conceptually similar process when he states, 'the weighing of evidence is contingent on context' (6), that is, on broader knowledge of the situation.

By defining evidence as research findings that are evaluated as having truth-value according to disciplinary epistemologies, it becomes possible to differentiate between evidence and knowledge. I claim that knowledge represents the sum of what is known and understood through diverse ways of knowing, is regarded as 'true' and therefore holds value. Research findings represent one source of knowledge within a larger body of knowledge. Research data are evaluated in accordance with existing knowledge and judged to be (a) consistent with existing knowledge and having truth-value, therefore accepted as evidence and incorporated into knowledge; (b) inconsistent with existing knowledge but convincingly 'true' and of sufficient value that existing knowledge shifts to allow the new knowledge to be incorporated within existing knowledge (e.g. when research demonstrated that the tradition of preoperative shaving of operative sites was in fact associated with higher rates of postoperative infections); or (c) inconsistent with existing knowledge and having insignificant truth-value, therefore refuted and not accepted as evidence. Thus, existing knowledge, which is based on diverse epistemologies, influences the uptake of research findings and the process though which it is evaluated, reflected upon, valued and recontextualized as evidence; that is, useful nursing knowledge, or knowledge that supports praxis.

The Ideology of Evidence-Based Healthcare

The concept of evidence-based medicine originated within the discipline of medicine just over a decade ago. It is ironic that while 'evidence' itself often takes decades to be accepted into and change healthcare practice (i.e. the research–practice gap), it has taken only 10 years for the concept of evidence-based practice to become firmly entrenched within the healthcare system. Estabrooks (1998) observed that EBM had 'taken on the qualities of a social movement' (18). The entrenchment of EBM and its spread into other disciplines as EBP has occurred despite ongoing controversy within medicine (Dobrow, Goel and Upshur 2004), as well as in disciplines such as nursing (Estabrooks 1998; Mitchell 1999), of the utility of what has been characterized as a 'cookbook' approach to practice. That is to say, the assertion that EBP is a better way to practice has been challenged, both on the premise that EBP itself lacks a convincing body of supporting evidence (Upshur 2003; Dobrow, Goel and Upshur 2004), and also on the grounds that EBP represents prescriptive service based on guidelines and protocols, rather than practice based on disciplinary and professional knowledge and clinical reasoning. Moreover, such prescriptive service lacks relevance when applied to the particularities of practice with individuals (Jones and Higgs 2000). In short, practice is reduced to a science: the 'art' of practice is lost.

So, if not unequivocal evidence, what is driving the uptake of EBP? To find the answer to this question, it is necessary to look beyond the practice of any of the health disciplines and consider the bigger picture of health-care. Stakeholders in health-care include more than practitioners and patients. Non-practitioner, non-patient stakeholders such as policy-makers, politicians, insurance companies, researchers, pharmaceutical corporations and other suppliers of healthcare products, all have a vested interest (i.e. financial or power) in defining what happens between practitioners and patients. EBP provides a structure that allows these system stakeholders to influence what happens at the practice level (i.e. between patients and practitioners), by influencing disciplinary under-

standings of what constitutes evidence for practice. The key question in defining EBP becomes not 'what constitutes evidence?' but 'what constitutes evidence for whom and why? Alleged agendas of EBP as a structure of the larger healthcare system include control over clinical decision-making between practitioners and patients (Mitchell 1999), redistribution of power (Estabrooks 1998), and control over resource allocation (Jennings and Loan 2001). Other implications of EBP have been identified as loss of autonomous practice and loss of practitioner-client accountability (Mitchell 1999). Within nursing, critics of EBP have pointed out that this approach to healthcare delivery may conflict with other approaches such as patient-centred care (Mitchell 1999; Rycroft-Malone et al. 2004). One basis of this conflict is recognition that the narrow definition of evidence supported by EBP fails to accommodate the inclusive definition of evidence and the range of disciplinary knowledge that influences clinical practice in nursing (Estabrooks 1998; Mitchell 1999; Madjar and Walton 2001).

Paradoxically, research-based evidence is fundamental to the process of uptake and integration of new knowledge into the existing body of knowledge that supports nursing practice. Both the science and the art of nursing benefit when new research-based information is admitted as evidence to nursing's knowledge base. The conflict that surrounds the issue of evidence for nursing is at best superficial and at worst counterproductive to the task of expanding nursing's body of disciplinary knowledge. I claim that the paradox derives from the degree to which the concept of EBP has taken on ideological proportions. Despite Estabrooks's (1998) caution against allowing EBP to 'develop into an ideology' (31), EBP has in fact become an ideology in health-care, driven by health system stakeholders for the purposes described above.

Sustaining Nursing Praxis by Mediating the Meaning of Evidence

I have proposed that epistemological diversity supports nursing praxis, or nursing as a complex and holistic practice. I have shown that a singular epistemology, such as that represented by the prevailing ideological construction of EBP supports, in contrast, a dichotomized conceptualization of nursing as a science. Nursing viewed as a science rather than as praxis would, by definition, privilege scientific evidence in the positivist, western scientific tradition as a singular way of knowing.

Nursing practice that relies on scientific evidence as a singular basis of practice knowledge is susceptible to exploitation by the diverse agendas operating within an ideology of EBP and the healthcare system. Extra-disciplinary definitions of evidence, as well as extra-disciplinary understandings of what constitutes 'best care' or 'best practice', could be imposed on nursing through the use of EBP as an ideological tool, because nursing, without diverse epistemologies, would have no means of defining, evaluating and valuing research findings in a way that supports and develops nursing knowledge for praxis. Thus, epistemological diversity is both the means by which nursing mediates a disciplinary definition of research-based evidence that serves to sustain praxis, and the basis that enables nurses to critically evaluate alternative sources of knowledge (i.e. non-research-based information).

The mediation of evidence from a disciplinary perspective suggests that it may be difficult to achieve an interdisciplinary consensus concerning the question of what constitutes evidence for health-care. Is consensus necessary or even possible in an interdisciplinary health-care system? Consensus has implications for interdisciplinary communication and shared meanings in regard to EBP, as well as to other terms such as 'best practice,' that are becoming catch-phrases in health-care.

The lack of epistemological and conceptual clarity around evidence (Estabrooks 1998; Scott-Findlay and Pollock 2004) suggests there is still a long ways to go before interdisciplinary consensus is realized. Thorne (2001) suggests that interdisciplinary consensus may not be possible, and urges nursing to define evidence and knowledge in ways that are coherent within nursing's unique disciplinary philosophy. I suggest that the critical first steps in defining evidence and knowledge for nursing are to work toward clarifying the language of EBP (Scott-Findlay and Pollock 2004), to affirm nursing practice as praxis, and to acknowledge the epistemological

diversity that sustains praxis. Mediating the meaning of evidence for nursing praxis through diverse epistemologies will contribute to a disciplinary-specific definition of what constitutes evidence for nursing praxis and will explicate how evidence is integrated into a disciplinary body of knowledge.

Nurses need to have faith in how praxis directs us to know the world, and to look first and foremost to developing knowledge in ways that are consistent with the diverse ways in which we know the world (Jones 1997). The soundest strategy for mediating an interdisciplinary understanding of evidence in health-care—and how evidence is used in health-care—is for nurses to clearly articulate what constitutes evidence for nursing. Understanding and appreciating disciplinary differences is possible if the differences are articulated. Interdisciplinary respect may be more valuable over the long-term than interdisciplinary consensus.

Interdisciplinary consensus on what constitutes evidence may not be possible, as the health disciplines tend to subscribe to different epistemologies and therefore different 'truths'. From this perspective, health-care itself, understood as a collective entity, is based on the diverse epistemologies represented by not only the various health disciplines, but also other stakeholders, including the consumers of health-care. Perhaps health-care itself may ultimately be recognized as a form of praxis.

Acknowledgments I am indebted to Dr Sally Thorne and Dr Angela Henderson at the School of Nursing, University of British Columbia, for their support and guidance in the development of this paper. I would also like to acknowledge the valuable suggestions made by Shannon Scott-Findlay, PhD (c), particularly in reviewing the content pertaining to evidence-based practice and knowledge translation.

REFERENCES

Angeles PA. 1981. *Dictionary of philosophy.* New York: Barnes and Noble.

Benner P. 2000. The roles of embodiment, emotion and lifeworld for rationality and agency in nursing practice. *Nursing Philosophy* 1:5–19.

Bishop AH, and JR Scudder. 1997. Nursing as a practice rather than an art or a science. *Nursing Outlook* 45:82–5.

Capra F. 1982. *The turning point: Science, society, and the rising culture.* Toronto: Bantam.

Carper BA. 1978. Fundamental patterns of knowing in nursing. *Advances in Nursing Science* 1:13–23.

Centre for Evidence-Based Medicine, Oxford. 2001. Levels of evidence and grades of recommendations, http:// cebmjr2.ox.ac.uk/docs/levels.html (cited November 2003)

Charlton BG. 1997. Restoring the balance: Evidence-based medicine put in its place. *Journal of Evaluation in Clinical Practice* 3: 87–98.

Chinn PL and MK Kramer. 1999. *Theory and nursing. Integrated knowledge development,* 5th edn. St Louis: Mosby.

Dobrow MJ, V Goel and REG Upshur. 2004. Evidence-based health policy: Context and utilisation. *Social Science and Medicine* 58:207–17.

Estabrooks CA. 1998. Will evidence-based nursing practice make practice perfect? *Canadian Journal of Nursing Research* 30: 15–36.

Evidence-Based Medicine Working Group. 1992. Evidence-based medicine. A new approach to teaching the practice of medicine. *Journal of the American Medical Association* 268: 2420–5.

Fawcett J, J Watson, B Neuman, PH Walker and JJ Fitzpatrick. 2001. On nursing theories and evidence. *Journal of Nursing Scholarship* 33:115–19.

Flaming D. 2001. Using phronesis instead of 'research-based practice' as the guiding light for nursing practice. *Nursing Philosophy* 2:251–8.

Greenhalgh T and JG Worrall. 1997. From EBM to GSM: The evolution of context-sensitive *medicine. Journal of Evaluation in Clinical Practice* 3:105–8.

Harman WW. 1996. The shortcomings of Western science. *Qualitative Inquiry* 2:30–8.

Holmes C and P Warelow. 2000. Nursing as normative praxis. *Nursing Inquiry* 7:175–81.

Jacobs-Kramer MK and PL Chinn. 1988. Perspectives on knowing: A model of nursing knowledge. *Scholarly Inquiry for Nursing Practice* 2:129–39.

Jennings BM and LA Loan. 2001. Misconceptions among nurses about evidence-based practice. *Journal of Nursing Scholarship* 33:121–7.

Johnson JL. 1991. Nursing science: Basic, applied, or practical? Implications for the art of nursing. *Advances in Nursing Science* 14: 7–16.

Johnson JL and PA Ratner. 1997. The nature of knowledge used in nursing practice. In *Nursing praxis: Knowledge and action,* eds SE Thorne and V Hayes, 3–22. Thousand Oaks, CA: Sage.

Jones M. 1997. Thinking nursing. In *Nursing praxis: Knowledge and action,* eds SE Thorne and V Hayes, 125–39. Thousand Oaks, CA: Sage.

Jones M and J Higgs. 2000. Will evidenced-based practice take the reasoning out of practice? *Clinical Reasoning in the Health Professions,* eds J Higgs and M Jones, 307–15. Boston: Butterworth Heinemann.

Kitson A, G Harvey and B McCormack. 1998. Enabling the implementation of evidence-based practice: A conceptual framework. *Quality in Health Care* 7:149–58.

Landry R, N Amara and M Lamari. 2001. Utilization of social science research knowledge in Canada. *Research Policy* 30:333–49.

Madjar I and J Walton. 2001. What is problematic about evidence? In *The nature of qualitative evidence,* eds JM Morse, JM Swanson and AJ Kuzel, 28–45. Thousand Oaks, CA: Sage.

Mautner T. 1996. *The Penguin dictionary of philosophy.* London: Penguin.

McCain RA. 1998. Economic efficiency: A 'reasonable dialog' in economics: Part I, defeasible reasoning. In *Essential principles of economics: A hypermedia text,* williamking. www.drexel.edu/top/prin/txt/EcoToC.html (cited November 2003).

Meleis AI. 1997. *Theoretical nursing: Development and progress,* 3rd edn. Philadelphia: Lippincott.

Mitchell GJ. 1999. Evidence-based practice: Critique and alternative view. *Nursing Science Quarterly* 12:30–5.

Nagle LM and GJ Mitchell. 1991. Theoretic diversity: Evolving paradigmatic issues in research and practice. *Advances in Nursing Science* 14:17–25.

Oxford dictionary of current English. 1998. ed. D Thompson. Oxford: Oxford University Press.

Rafael ARF. 1999. From rhetoric to reality: The changing face of public health nursing in southern Ontario. *Public Health Nursing* 16:50–9.

Rycroft-Malone J, K Seers, A Titchen, G Harvey, A Kitson and B McCormack. 2004. What counts as evidence in evidence-based practice? *Journal of Advanced Nursing* 47:81–90.

Sackett DL, WM Rosenberg, JA Gray, RB Haynes and WS Richardson. 1996. Evidence-based medicine: What it is and what it isn't. *British Medical Journal* 312:71–2.

Schwandt TR. 1990. Paths to inquiry in the social sciences: Scientific, constructivist, and critical theory methodologies. In *The paradigm dialog,* ed. EG Guba, 258–76. Newbury Park, CA: Sage.

Scott-Findlay S and C Pollock. 2004. Evidence, research, knowledge: A call for conceptual clarity. *Worldviews on Evidence-Based Nursing,* Second Quarter: 92–7.

Shahar E. 1998. Evidence-based medicine: A new paradigm or the emperor's new clothes? *Journal of Evaluation in Clinical Practice* 4:277–82.

Thorne SE. 1997. Introduction: Praxis in the con text of nursing's developing inquiry. In *Nursing praxis: Knowledge and action,* eds SE Thorne and V Hayes, ix–xxi. Thousand Oaks, CA: Sage.

Thorne SE. 2001. The implications of disciplinary agenda on quality criteria for qualitative research. In *The nature of qualitative evidence,* eds JM Morse, JM Swanson and AJ Kuzel, 141–59. Thousand Oaks, CA: Sage.

Upshur REG. 2001. The status of qualitative research as evidence. In *The nature of qualitative evidence,* eds JM Morse, JM Swanson and AJ Kuzel, 5–26. Thousand Oaks, CA: Sage.

Upshur REG. 2003. Are all evidence-based practices alike? Problems in the ranking of evidence. *Canadian Medical Association Journal* 169:672–3.

Upshur REG, EG VanDenKerkhof and V Goel. 2001. Meaning and measurement: An inclusive model of evidence in health care. *Journal of Evaluation in Clinical Practice* 7:91–6.

Warms CA and CA Schroeder. 1999. Bridging the gulf between science and action: The 'new fuzzies' of neopragmatism. *Advances in Nursing Science* 22:1–10.

White J. 1995. Patterns of knowing: Review, critique, and update. *Advances in Nursing Science* 17:73–86.

Wolfer J. 1993. Aspects of 'reality' and ways of knowing in nursing: In search of an integrating paradigm. *IMAGE: Journal of Nursing Scholarship* 25:141–6.

The Author Comments

Mediating the Meaning of Evidence Through Epistemological Diversity

The interdisciplinary perspectives I was exposed to in a first-year PhD course, Topics in Knowledge Utilization, offered by Dr. Carole Estabrooks at the University of Alberta, along with my clinical practice background in primary health care, challenged me to better understand how population-based "best" evidence (i.e., evidence according to the hierarchical Levels of Evidence models) could be made relevant to the contexts of the small, remote, unique Aboriginal populations I faced in my practice. I speculated that similar understandings, grounded in clinical practice experience, were also the basis of the apparent disconnect between how researchers and clinicians each understood the uptake and utilization of evidence in practice, and I began writing about the meaning of evidence from a primary health care perspective. My understanding of these issues continued to evolve through lively discussions and debate with nursing colleagues in the doctoral student philosophy seminars offered by Dr. Sally Thorne and Dr. Angela Henderson at the University of British Columbia. The article, *Mediating the Meaning of Evidence Through Epistemological Diversity,* took shape in response to my efforts to understand how nurses might best contribute to the development of evidence-based knowledge for nursing practice, within the interdisciplinary team models that increasingly bring together the "disciplines" of research and practice, as well as the traditional different practice disciplines.

—DENISE TARLIER

CHAPTER 38

Fundamental Patterns of Knowing in Nursing

Barbara A. Carper

It is the general conception of any field of inquiry that ultimately determines the kind of knowledge the field aims to develop as well as the manner in which that knowledge is to be organized, tested and applied. The body of knowledge that serves as the rationale for nursing practice has patterns, forms and structure that serve as horizons of expectations and exemplify characteristic ways of thinking about phenomena. Understanding these patterns is essential for the teaching and learning of nursing. Such an understanding does not extend the range of knowledge, but rather involves critical attention to the question of what it means to know and what kinds of knowledge are held to be of most value in the discipline of nursing.

Identifying Patterns of Knowing

Four fundamental patterns of knowing have been identified from an analysis of the conceptual and syntactical structure of nursing knowledge (Carper, 1975). The four patterns are distinguished according to logical type of meaning and designated as: (a) empirics, the science of nursing; (b) esthetics, the art of nursing; (c) the component of a personal knowledge in nursing; and (d) ethics, the component of moral knowledge in nursing.

Empirics: The Science of Nursing

The term *nursing science* was rarely used in the literature until the late 1950s. However, since that time there

expressive rather than merely formal or descriptive," according to Rader, "is about as well established as any fact in the whole field of esthetics" (Rader, 1960, p. xvi). An aesthetic experience involves the creation and/or appreciation of a singular, particular, subjective expression of imagined possibilities or equivalent realities which "resists projection into the discursive form of language" (Langer, 1957). Knowledge gained by empirical description is discursively formulated and publicly verifiable. The knowledge gained by subjective acquaintance, the direct feeling of experience, defines discursive formulation. Although an esthetic expression requires abstraction, it remains specific and unique rather than exemplary and leads us to acknowledge that "knowledge—genuine knowledge, understanding—is considerably wider than our discourse" (Langer, 1957, p. 23).

For Wiedenbach (1964), the art of nursing is made visible through the action taken to provide whatever the patient requires to restore or extend his ability to cope with the demands of his situation. But the action taken, to have an esthetic quality, requires the active transformation of the immediate object—the patient's behavior—into a direct, nonmediated perception of what is significant in it—that is, what need is actually being expressed by the behavior. This perception of the need expressed is not only responsible for the action taken by the nurse but reflected in it.

The esthetic process described by Wiedenbach resembles what Dewey (1958) refers to as the difference between recognition and perception. According to Dewey, recognition serves the purpose of identification and is satisfied when a name tag or label is attached according to some stereotype or previously formed scheme of classification. Perception, however, goes beyond recognition in that it includes an active gathering together of details and scattered particulars into an experienced whole for the purpose of seeing what is there. It is perception rather than mere recognition that results in a unity of ends and means which gives the action taken an aesthetic quality.

Orem speaks of the art of nursing as being "expressed by the individual nurse through her creativity and style in designing and providing nursing that is effective and satisfying" (Orem, 1971, p. 155). The art of nursing is creative in that it requires development of the ability to "envision valid modes of helping in relation to 'results' which are appropriate" (Orem, 1971, p. 69). This again invokes Dewey's (1958) sense of a perceived unity between an action taken and its result—a perception of the means and the end as an organic whole. The experience of helping must be perceived and designed as an integral component of its desired result rather than conceived separately as an independent action imposed on an independent subject. Perhaps this is what is meant by the concept of nursing the whole patient or total patient care. If so, what are the qualities that enable the creation of a design for nursing care that eliminate or would minimize the fragmentation of means and ends?

Esthetic Pattern of Knowing

Empathy—that is, the capacity for participating in or vicariously experiencing another's feelings—is an important mode in the esthetic pattern of knowing. One gains knowledge of another person's singular, particular, felt experience through empathic acquaintance (Lee, 1960; Lippo, 1960). Empathy is controlled or moderated by psychic distance or detachment in order to apprehend and abstract what we are attending to, and in this sense is objective. The more skilled the nurse becomes in perceiving and empathizing with the lives of others, the more knowledge or understanding will be gained of alternate modes of perceiving reality. The nurse will thereby have available a larger repertoire of choices in designing and providing nursing care that is effective and satisfying. At the same time, increased awareness of the variety of subjective experiences will heighten the complexity and difficulty of the decision making involved.

The design of nursing care must be accompanied by what Langer refers to as sense of form, the sense of "structure, articulation, a whole resulting from the relation of mutually dependent factors, or more precisely, the way the whole is put together" (Langer, 1957, p. 16). The design, if it is to be esthetic, must be controlled by the perception of the balance, rhythm, proportion and unity of what is done in relation to the dynamic integration and articulation of the whole. "The doing may be energetic, and the undergoing may be acute and intense," Dewey (1958) says, but "unless they are related to each other to form a whole," what is done becomes merely a matter of mechanical routine or of caprice.

The esthetic pattern of knowing in nursing involves the perception of abstracted particulars as distinguished from the recognition of abstracted universals. It is the knowing of a unique particular rather than an exemplary class.

The Component of Personal Knowledge

Personal knowledge as a fundamental pattern of knowing in nursing is the most problematic, the most difficult to master and to teach. At the same time, it is perhaps the pattern most essential to understanding the meaning of health in terms of individual well-being. Nursing considered as an interpersonal process involves interactions, relationships and transactions between the nurse and the patient-client. Mitchell points out that "there is growing evidence that the quality of interpersonal contacts has an influence on a person's becoming ill, coping with illness and becoming well" (Mitchell, 1973, p. 49–50). Certainly the phrase "therapeutic use of self" which has become increasingly prominent in the literature implies that the way in which nurses view their own selves and the client is of primary concern in any therapeutic relationship.

Personal knowledge is concerned with the knowing, encountering and actualizing of the concrete, individual self. One does not know *about* the self; one strives simply to *know* the self. This knowing is a standing in relation to another human being and confronting that human being as a person. This "I-Thou" encounter is unmediated by conceptual categories or particulars abstracted from complex organic wholes (Buber, 1970). The relation is one of reciprocity, a state of being that cannot be described or even experienced—it can only be actualized. Such personal knowing extends not only to other selves but also to relations with one's own self.

It requires what Buber (1970) refers to as the sacrifice of form—i.e., categories or classifications—for a knowing of infinite possibilities, as well as the risk of total commitment.

> Even as a melody is not composed of tones, nor a verse of words, nor a statue of lines—one must pull and tear to turn a unity into a multiplicity—so it is with the human being to whom I say You . . . . I have to do this again and again; but immediately he is no longer You. (Buber, 1970, p. 59)

Maslow (1956) refers to this sacrifice of form as embodying a more efficient perception of reality in that reality is not generalized nor predetermined by a complex of concepts, expectations, beliefs and stereotypes. This results in a greater willingness to accept ambiguity, vagueness and discrepancy of oneself and others. The risk of commitment involved in personal knowledge is what Polyani calls the "passionate participation in the act of knowing" (Polyani, 1964, p. 17).

The nurse in the therapeutic use of self rejects approaching the patient-client as an object and strives instead to actualize an authentic personal relationship between two persons. The individual is considered as an integrated, open system incorporating movement toward growth and fulfillment of human potential. An authentic personal relation requires the acceptance of others in their freedom to create themselves and the recognition that each person is not a fixed entity, but constantly engaged in the process of becoming. How then should the nurse reconcile this with the social and/or professional responsibility to control and manipulate the environmental variables and even the behavior of the person who is a patient in order to maintain or restore a steady state? If a human being is assumed to be free to choose and chooses behavior outside of accepted norms, how will this affect the action taken in the therapeutic use of self by the nurse? What choices must the nurse make in order to know another self in an authentic relation apart from the category of patient, even when categorizing for the purpose of treatment is essential to the process of nursing?

Assumptions regarding human nature, McKay observes, "range from the existentialist to the cybernetic, from the idea of an information processing machine to one of a many splendored being" (McKay, 1969, p. 399). Many of these assumptions incorporate in one form or another the notion that there is, for all individuals, a characteristic state which they, by virtue of membership in the species, must strive to assume or achieve. Empirical descriptions and classifications reflect the assumption that being human allows for prediction of basic biological, psychological and social behaviors that will be encountered in any given individual.

Certainly empirical knowledge is essential to the purposes of nursing. But nursing also requires that we be alert to the fact that models of human nature and their abstract and generalized categories refer to and describe behaviors and traits that groups have in common. However, none of these categories can ever encompass or express the uniqueness of the individual encountered as a person, as a "self." These and many other similar considerations are involved in the realm of personal knowledge, which can be broadly characterized as subjective, concrete and existential. It is concerned with the kind of knowing that promotes wholeness and integrity in the personal encounter, the achievement of engagement rather than detachment; and it denies the manipulative, impersonal orientation.

Ethics: The Moral Component

Teachers and individual practitioners are becoming increasingly sensitive to the difficult personal choices that must be made within the complex context of modern health care. These choices raise fundamental questions about morally right and wrong action in connection with the care and treatment of illness and the promotion of health. Moral dilemmas arise in situations of ambiguity and uncertainty, when the consequences of one's actions are difficult to predict and traditional principles and ethical codes offer no help or seem to result in contradiction. The moral code which guides the ethical conduct of nurses is based on the primary principle of obligation embodied in the concepts of service to people and respect for human life. The discipline of nursing is held to be a valuable and essential social service responsible for conserving life, alleviating suffering and promoting health. But appeal to the ethical "rule book" fails to provide answers in terms of difficult individual moral choices which must be made in the teaching and practice of nursing.

The fundamental pattern of knowing identified here as the ethical component of nursing is focused on matters of obligation or what ought to be done. Knowledge of morality goes beyond simply knowing the norms or ethical codes of the discipline. It includes all voluntary actions that are deliberate and subject to the judgment of right and wrong—including judgments of moral value in relation to motives, intentions and traits of character. Nursing is deliberate action, or a series of actions, planned and implemented to accomplish defined goals. But goals and actions involve choices made, in part, on the basis of normative judgments, both particular and general. On occasion, the principles and norms by which such choices are made may be in conflict.

According to Berthold, "goals are, of course, value judgments not amenable to scientific inquiry and validation" (Berthold, 1968, p. 196). Dickoff, James and Wiedenbach also call attention to the need to be aware that the specification of goals serves as "a norm or standard by which to evaluate activity . . . [and] . . . entails taking them as values—that is, signifies conceiving these goal contents as situations worthy to be brought about" (James & Weidenbach, 1968, p. 422).

For example, a common goal of nursing care in relation to the maintenance or restoration of health is to assist patients to achieve a state in which they are independent. Much of the current practice reflects an attitude of value attached to the goal of independence, and indicates nursing actions to assist patients in assuming full responsibility for themselves at the earliest possible moment or to enable them to retain responsibility to the last possible moment. However, valuing independence and attempting to maintain it may be at the expense of the patient's learning how to live with physical or social dependence when necessary; e.g., in instances when prognosis indicates that independence cannot be regained.

Differences in normative judgments may have more to do with disagreements as to what constitutes a "healthy" state of being than lack of empirical evidence or ambiguity in the application of the term. Slote suggests that the persistence of disputes, or lack of uniformity in the application of cluster terms, such as health, is due to "the difficulty of decisively resolving certain sorts of value questions about what is and is not important." This leads him to conclude "that value judgment is far more involved in the making of what are commonly thought to be factual statements than has been imagined" (Slote, 1966, p. 220).

The ethical pattern of knowing in nursing requires an understanding of different philosophical positions regarding what is good, what ought to be desired, what is right; of different ethical frameworks devised for dealing with the complexities of moral judgments; and of various orientations to the notion of obligation. Moral choices to be made must then be considered in terms of specific action to be taken in specific, concrete situations. The examination of the standards, codes and values by which we decide what is morally right should result in a greater awareness of what is involved in making moral choices and being responsible for the choices made. The knowledge of ethical codes will not provide answers to the moral questions involved in nursing, nor will it eliminate the necessity for having to make moral choices. But it can be hoped that:

> The more sensitive teachers and practitioners are to the demands of the process of justification, the more explicit they are about the norms that govern their actions, the more personally engaged they are in assessing surrounding circumstances and potential consequences, the more "ethical" they will be; and we cannot ask much more (Greene, 1973, p. 221).

Using Patterns of Knowing

A philosophical discussion of patterns of knowing may appear to some as a somewhat idle, if not arbitrary and artificial, undertaking having little or no connection with the practical concerns and difficulties encountered in the day-to-day doing and teaching of nursing. But it represents a personal conviction that there is a need to examine the kinds of knowing that provide the disci-

pline with its particular perspectives and significance. Understanding four fundamental patterns of knowing makes possible an increased awareness of the complexity and diversity of nursing knowledge.

Each pattern may be conceived as necessary for achieving mastery in the discipline, but none of them alone should be considered sufficient. Neither are they mutually exclusive. The teaching and learning of one pattern do not require the rejection or neglect of any of the others. Caring for another requires the achievements of nursing science, that is, the knowledge of empirical facts systematically organized into theoretical explanations regarding the phenomena of health and illness. But creative imagination also plays its part in the syntax of discovery in science, as well as in developing the ability to imagine the consequences of alternate moral choices.

Personal knowledge is essential for ethical choices in that moral action presupposes personal maturity and freedom. If the goals of nursing are to be more than conformance to unexamined norms, if the "ought" is not to be determined simply on the basis of what is possible, then the obligation to care for another human being involves becoming a certain kind of person—and not merely doing certain kinds of things. If the design of nursing care is to be more than habitual or mechanical, the capacity to perceive and interpret the subjective experiences of others and to imaginatively project the effects of nursing actions on their lives becomes a necessary skill.

Nursing thus depends on the specific knowledge of human behavior in health and in illness, the esthetic perception of significant human experiences, a personal understanding of the unique individuality of the self and the capacity to make choices within concrete situations involving particular moral judgments. Each of these separate but interrelated and interdependent fundamental patterns of knowing should be taught and understood according to its distinctive logic, the restricted circumstances in which it is valid, the kinds of data it subsumes and the methods by which each particular kind of truth is distinguished and warranted.

The major significances to the discipline of nursing in distinguishing patterns of knowing are summarized as: (a) the conclusions of the discipline conceived as subject matter cannot be taught or learned without reference to the structure of the discipline—the representative concepts and methods of inquiry that determine the kind of knowledge gained and limit its meaning, scope and validity; (b) each of the fundamental patterns of knowing represents a necessary but not complete approach to the problems and questions in the discipline; and (c) all knowledge is subject to change and revision. Every solution of an existing problem raises new and unsolved questions. These new and as yet unsolved problems require, at times, new methods of inquiry and different conceptual structures; they change the shape and patterns of knowing. With each change in the shape of knowledge, teaching and learning require looking for different points of contact and connection among ideas and things. This clarifies the effect of each new thing known on other things known and the discovery of new patterns by which each connection modifies the whole.

REFERENCES

Berthold, J. S. (1968). Symposium on theory development in nursing: Prologue. *Nursing Research, 17,* 196–197.

Buber, M. (1970). *I and thou.* (W. Kaufman, Trans.). New York: Scribner.

Carper, B. A. (1975). Fundamental patterns of knowing in nursing. (Doctoral dissertation, Columbia University Teachers College). *Dissertation Abstract International, 36,* 4941B. (University Microfilms No. 76–7772).

Dewey, J. (1958). *Art as experience.* New York: Capricorn.

Dickoff, J., James, P., & Wiedenbach, E. (1968). Theory in a practice discipline: Part I, Practice-oriented theory. *Nursing Research, 17,* 415–435.

Greene, M. (1973). *Teacher as stronger.* Belmont, CA: Wadsworth.

Kuhn, T. (1962). *The structure of scientific revolutions.* Chicago: University of Chicago Press.

Langer, S. K. (1957). *Problems of art.* New York: Scribner.

Lee, V. (1960). Empathy. In M. Rader (Ed.), *A modern book of esthetics* (3rd ed.). New York: Holt, Rinehart and Winston.

Lippo, T. (1960). Empathy, inner imitation and sense-feeling. In M. Rader (Ed.), *A modern book of esthetics* (3rd ed.). New York: Holt, Rinehart and Winston.

Maslow, A. H. (1956). Self-actualizing people: A study of psychological health. In C. E. Moustakas (Ed.), *The self.* New York: Harper and Row.

McKay, R. (1969). Theories, models and systems for nursing. *Nursing Research, 18,* 393–399.

Mitchell, P. H. (1973). *Concepts basic to nursing.* New York: McGraw-Hill.

Nagel, E. (1961). *The structure of science.* New York: Harcourt, Brace and World.

Northrop, F. S. C. (1959). *The logic of the sciences and the humanities.* New York: World.

Orem, D. E. (1971). *Nursing: Concepts of practice.* New York: McGraw-Hill.

Polanyi, M. (1964). *Personal knowledge.* New York: Harper and Row.

Rader, M. (1960). Introduction: The meaning of art. In M. Rader (Ed.), *A modern book of esthetics* (3rd ed.). New York: Holt, Rinehart and Winston.

Slote, M. A. (1966). The theory of important criteria. *Journal of Philosophy, 63,* 211–224.

Weitz, M. (1960). The role of theory in aesthetics. In M. Rader (Ed.), *A modern book of esthetics* (3rd ed.). New York: Holt, Rinehart and Winston.

Wiedenbach, E. (1964). *Clinical nursing:* A helping art. New York: Springer.

The Author Comments

Fundamental Patterns of Knowing in Nursing

The genesis for this article, which was part of my doctoral dissertation, was my perplexity and confusion as an inexperienced teacher regarding what should be included in the nursing curriculum. Both student and teacher became disoriented in a maze of seemingly disparate disarticulated facts. My search for some meaningful guide to a sense of the whole to counteract this fragmentation led me to design a study to qualitatively analyze the types of knowledge that exemplified nursing. The resulting dissertation and article allowed nurses the freedom to begin asking questions about nursing and move beyond the assumptions about the essence of nursing and stimulate new thinking about the discipline. I never anticipated how popular the article would become!

—Barbara A. Carper

CHAPTER 39

Nursing Epistemology: Traditions, Insights, Questions

Phyllis R. Schultz
Afaf I. Meleis

Epistemology is the study of what human beings know, how they come to know what they think they know and what the criteria are for evaluating knowledge claims. Nursing epistemology is the study of knowledge shared among the members of the discipline, the patterns of knowing and knowledge that develops from them, and the criteria for accepting knowledge claims. Three types of knowledge specific to nursing as a discipline are described here: clinical knowledge, conceptual knowledge and empirical knowledge. Different criteria for evaluating each type are suggested.

Nursing epistemology is the study of the origins of nursing knowledge, its structure and methods, the patterns of knowing of its members, and the criteria for validating its knowledge claims. Just as women are aware increasingly that their perceptions, observations and reasoning about the world contribute understandings that are unique, so too nurses, as members of a discipline and profession made up mostly of women, are changing in consciousness as knowledge for and from the practice of nursing continues to grow. This paper explores the epistemology of nursing; it grows out of the belief that, as nurses, our ways of knowing have not yet been fully articulated but that they will emerge if we allow ourselves to see the world through the eyes of practicing nurses and their clients.

The term "epistemology" comes from philosophy, where it is defined as the study of knowledge, or theory of knowledge (Flew, 1984). As a practice discipline and

*From P. R. Schultz and A. I. Meleis, Nursing epistemology: Traditions, insights, questions, Journal of Nursing Scholarship, 1998, 20(4), 217–221.
Copyright 1998 by Blackwell. Reprinted with permission by Blackwell Publishing.*

About the Authors

PHYLLIS SCHULTZ was born on March 9, 1938. She holds BSN, MN, MA, and PhD degrees from colleges and universities in North Dakota, Georgia, and Colorado and completed postdoctoral studies at the University of California, San Francisco. Her 40-year nursing career included 19 years in various clinical positions, including intensive care, primary care, and community health, coupled with 21 years in higher education at the University of Colorado Health Sciences Center and the University of Washington. Her scholarship focused on examining the theoretical, empirical, and clinical foundations of community nursing and administration as unique practice fields within the nursing domain. She considers her 1987 article "When the client is more than one" key to advancing nursing knowledge in these fields, and she is coauthor of several review chapters and articles since then that have contributed to the literature in the discipline. Currently, she is learning how to be a long-distance grandmother as well as exploring ways of "being" after a lifetime of "doing."

AFAF I. MELEIS, a nurse and medical sociologist, is currently the Margaret Bond Simon Dean of Nursing at the University of Pennsylvania School of Nursing. She completed her undergraduate nursing education at the University of Alexandria, Egypt (1961), and came to the United States as a Rockefeller Fellow (1962) to pursue her graduate education. She earned an MS in nursing (1964), an MA in sociology (1966), and a PhD in medical and social psychology (1968) from the University of California, Los Angeles. Her scholarship focuses on theory and knowledge development, including her theory on living with transitions, immigrant and international health, and women's role integration and health. She is the author of more than 150 articles and 40 chapters and numerous monographs, proceedings, and books, including the widely used book, *Theoretical Nursing: Development and Progress*. Currently, Dr. Meleis serves as President of the International Council on Women's Health Issues. She has received several national and international awards and honorary doctorates, including the 1990 Medal of Excellence for professional and scholarly achievements, presented by Egyptian President Hosni Mubarak, and an Honorary Professorship from the Department of Health Sciences, the Hong Kong Polytechnic University.

profession, nursing is often described as both an "art" and a "science." Articulating its epistemology is therefore a complex task: The study of nursing knowledge must range from the seemingly intuitive "knowing" of the experienced and expert nurses to the systematically verified knowledge of empirical researchers.

The epistemology of any field of inquiry depends on the nature of the phenomena studied and on the propensities of the inquirers who are developing knowledge in the field. Nursing epistemology, then, is the study of how nurses come to know what they think they know, what exactly nurses do know, how nursing knowledge is structured and on what basis knowledge claims are made.

What Is Knowing/ What Is Known?

For any person, knowing begins with the processes of observation, perception and experience in encountering the world and being in the world. These processes give rise to describing and interpreting phenomena, including anticipating, with some degree of accuracy, what is likely to happen at some future time. It is helpful to think of "knowing" as a process and the knowledge that comes from that process as the product (Benoliel, 1987; Chinn & Jacobs, 1987).

According to Benoliel, "Knowing can be viewed as an individual's perceptual awareness of the complexities of a particular situation and draws on inner knowledge resources that have been garnered through experience in living" (p. 151). It rarely can be expressed through discourse but is experienced through the acts of persons (Benner, 1983; Chinn & Jacobs, 1987). By contrast, knowledge as product is often expressed in some form of communication such as informal conversations, formal oral presentations, written articles and texts or art forms such as paintings, poetry, novels or music.

In a practice discipline, knowing is also working on solutions to problems that are important for the welfare of clients. It includes the ability to identify the questions at the forefront of inquiry in the field, the issues involved in answering these questions, the ways to go about answering the answerable questions and the ways to handle the unanswerable questions. Knowing is also having the wisdom to recognize which questions have top priority, which are secondary and which are trivial; it is recognizing which questions can be answered in the near future and which have to be deferred.

In epistemology, Chisholm (1982) formulated the questions about knowing:

1. "What do we know? What is the extent of our knowledge?"
2. "How are we to decide whether we know? What are the criteria of knowledge?" (p. 50) Chisholm identified three epistemological positions as possible answers to these questions: skepticism, methodism and particularism. Skeptics say that these are unanswerable questions because we cannot answer either set without presupposing an answer to the other. This position is untenable for a practice discipline because we have to take care of real people with real health problems.

By "methodism," Chisholm (1982) meant that to have knowledge is to have a preferred method of inquiry and procedures for recognizing reliable or credible knowledge (i.e., one begins by answering the second set of questions (set 2). Chisholm explicitly identified empiricism as a "type of 'methodism'" (p. 67). Recent debates in nursing about qualitative and quantitative data collection with their corresponding metaphysical and epistemological foundations reflect a type of methodism in nursing (Schultz, 1987). This methodism has led some nurse inquirers to subscribe to science in general and to empiricist science in particular as the preferable epistemological position in nursing.

The allegiance to empiricism can explain some of the sense of separation that has arisen among nurse inquirers who hold different epistemological positions and use different methods of inquiry. Some rely on reflection and reasoning; others elect structured observation and hypothesis testing; still others prefer phenomenological dialogue and reflective interpretation. Academicians tend to insist on knowledge that is formal, orderly, validated and communicable. Practitioners trust knowledge that results in appropriate actions with clients in specific situations. To espouse the methodist's epistemological position is to fail to recognize the legitimacy of these multiple ways of knowing; it is to resist accepting the complexity and holistic character of nursing (Benoliel, 1987; Chinn & Jacobs, 1987; Visintainer, 1986).

By "particularism," Chisholm (1982) meant "We can know and know that we know some particular thing at a particular point in time" (p. 74). This position starts from the premise that there are some things we know, whether or not we agree on the methods and procedures for knowing (Chisholm, 1982; Schultz, 1987). Philosophers begin with rather ordinary, everyday cases of knowledge such as "I know how to drive a car" and "I know that seven plus five equals twelve." Similarly, "I know that the sentence, Some mushrooms are poisonous, is true" (Lehrer, 1974). These three statements can be classified as (a) recounting a practical skill, (b) communicating a conceptual insight and (c) articulating an empirical hypothesis.

As nurses, we begin with particular cases of knowledge from (a) our practice, (b) our theories, or (c) our research. Statements about what we "know" are reflected implicitly or explicitly in the writings of our clinicians, theorists and researchers, for example:

1. The experiences of persons in health and illness are revealed in characteristic patterns. These patterns tend to be repetitive, orderly, predictable, and unified; they reflect organization.

2. Some individuals have health and illness experiences that do not fit the general pattern. Thus another case of what we "know" in nursing is that it is predictable that individuals may be unpredictable in their health and illness experiences.
3. Human health and illness can be perceived and understood through uncovering the meanings that individuals, groups and societies derive from their experiences.
4. The health and illness of persons are interactive with environments.
5. Nursing acts influence the responses of persons in health and illness; nursing and the experiences of persons with health and illness are interactive.

Statements such as these about what we "know" in nursing are what we want to begin with in formulating the criteria of knowledge in our discipline. But before we explore such criteria, we will discuss patterns of knowing revealed in the nursing literature, and those from a study of women (Belenky et al., 1986), which may contribute to our understanding of the types of knowledge in present-day nursing.

Patterns of Knowing in Nursing

The complexity of nursing's epistemology was clearly demonstrated by Carper's (1978) delineation of four fundamental patterns of knowing in nursing: empirics, ethics, esthetics and personal knowledge. Each of these four patterns has recently been specified epistemologically by Chinn and Jacobs (1987). Here we will elaborate only on personal knowledge, because of our belief in the importance of the practitioner as the knower in nursing's development of knowledge.

Personal knowledge was described by Carper (1978) as self-knowledge, or awareness of the self. This description seems to leave out the knowledge from practice that Benner (1983) termed "practical knowledge," following the reasoning of Polanyi (1964) in his *Personal Knowledge*. For Polanyi, "personal" referred to a characteristic of the knower; "knowledge," to a mental process:

I regard knowing as an active comprehension of the things known, an action that requires skill . . .

Comprehension is neither an arbitrary act nor a passive experience, but a responsible act claiming universal validity. (p. xiii)

Thus to know the self is part of comprehending "the things known." Knowing what one knows is also part of comprehending.

Polanyi (1964) distinguished between knowledge as theory and knowledge as practical skill. He termed knowledge that may not be articulated through language as "tacit knowing"; knowledge that is communicable through discourse he termed "explicit knowing." Another way to phrase this distinction is "knowing how" and "knowing that," which Benner (1983) found useful in explaining what expert nurses know. Expert nurses may enter a caring encounter with awareness of the self as therapeutic agent (Carper, 1978) and with a foundation of formal concepts, theories, facts and skills learned in their education (the knowing that). According to Benner (1983), as the encounter, or event, unfolds, they refine, elaborate or disconfirm this "foreknowledge"; the encounter then deserves to be termed "experience" and contributes to the knowing how. These three aspects of personal knowledge—knowing the self, knowing that and knowing how—are the sum of what one knows. All three are brought to the caring situation and are used to identify and solve the problems of the discipline.

Unfortunately, we know very little about personal knowing, especially about knowing the self and knowing how, in part because they can only be articulated retrospectively (Chinn & Jacobs, 1987). The knowing how from practice may, however, be brought to consciousness and made communicable through innovative methods of inquiry such as interpretive, grounded theory or phenomenological research (Benner, 1983; 1985; Pyles & Stern, 1983; Ray, 1987). For example, using a grounded theory approach, Pyles and Stern described the "nursing gestalt," by which expert critical care nurses identify impending cardiogenic shock and prevent untimely death. They learned that novice nurses must work with expert critical care nurses (the Gray Gorilla concept) to acquire their know how for practice. Their findings corroborated those of Benner's

(1983) study of the knowledge embedded in clinical practice.

Also, in a study of critical care nursing using phenomenology as method, Ray (1987) discovered that the essence of nursing in critical care involves technological and ethical caring; it is an experiential dialectic between technical competence (doing no harm) and compassion (in response to suffering), which are mediated through ethical choice (preserving autonomy and ensuring justice).

Efforts to bring to consciousness the self-knowledge and knowing how of nursing practice may be aided by examination of women's ways of knowing identified by Belenky et al. (1986). The patterns they discovered were not supposed to be hierarchical, although unfortunately their descriptions appear to be so. In applying their framework to nurses, we will assume that different patterns of knowing exist simultaneously. The five patterns of women's knowing that Belenky et al. identified are silence, received knowledge, subjective knowledge, procedural knowledge and constructed knowledge. Each of the five patterns is explained in the following:

Silence. Persons "experience themselves as mindless and voiceless and subject to the whims of external authority" (p. 16). Belenky et al. add that silent women know at the "gut level" but have not cultivated their capacity for abstract thought; nor do they attempt to articulate why they do what they do. They accept the voices of authority for direction in their work and life because of others' power, not necessarily expertise. Others are "right"; the silent one is "wrong" and "dumb."

According to Colliere (1986) silent nurses may not know how to conceptualize their daily experiences; they follow the voices of others because of fear of others' power. They do not have the language to generalize from what they know so that their knowledge can be communicated. They have learned to be silent. Their work, their patterns of knowing and their knowledge are invisible.

Received knowledge. Persons "perceive themselves as capable of receiving, even reproducing, knowledge from all-knowing external authorities but not capable of creating knowledge on their own" (p. 15). Individuals who use this way of knowing rely on others for the words to communicate what they know. For this type of knower, knowledge is observable; there is no ambiguity in it, and it depends on the expertise of others.

Many nurses have contented themselves with using the words of others to express and guide their knowing. American nurses have used medical knowledge, psychological and sociological knowledge, philosophical knowledge and administrative knowledge to communicate what they know. Following the same pattern, nurses in other countries have used nursing theories developed in the United States to communicate the nature of their practice.

Subjective knowledge. Knowledge is "conceived of as personal, private, and subjectively known and intuited" (p. 15). The subjective pattern of women's knowing reminds us of the debates in nursing today about the usefulness and reliability of experiential knowing (i.e., knowledge from practice). Knowers such as this in nursing offer us their subjective wisdom from their own inner voices, which may enhance our understanding of complex situations, but their knowledge is transient, and not cumulative. Such knowers may find it difficult to articulate the processes that they have gone through in knowing because knowing for them is intuitive, experienced, not thought out and something felt rather than cognitively appraised or constructed.

Procedural knowledge. These knowers depend on careful observation, structured procedures and systematic analyses. In short, they are rationalists. They use objectivity as a measure of what can be known as well as repeated observations under controlled situations for corroboration. They distance themselves from experience in order to know. Though they use subjective awareness to provide insights, they adhere to the idea that objectivity yields the knowledge that is most reliable.

Nurse researchers and academicians are the strongest adherents of this way of knowing. Following strict procedures for inquiry is considered the way to secure reliable knowledge for teaching the principles and practices of nursing and for further inquiry. As we emphasize increasingly research-based practice, clinicians are joining the ranks of the rational, procedural knowers in nursing.

Constructed knowledge. A pattern of knowing in which persons "view all knowledge as contextual, experience themselves as creators of knowledge, and value both subjective and objective strategies of knowing" (p. 15). These knowers integrate the different ways of knowing and the different voices (including the silent voice). To them, "all knowledge is constructed, and the knower is an intimate part of the known" (p. 37).

Nurses who subscribe to this view of knowing see theories as approximations of reality that are ongoing and always in process; their frames of reference are constructed and reconstructed (Visintainer, 1986), and posing questions is as important as attempting to answer questions. These nurses believe that knowing is achieved as much through openness and curiosity and through examination of the assumptions and context within which questions are posed as through adherence to procedures or systematic observation and replication.

For nurses who subscribe to this view of knowing, the development of knowledge is a never-ending process. There are glimmers of certain knowledge if one understands the whole of a situation including formal knowledge of the phenomenon. Experts (i.e., experienced knowers) develop a connected knowing through conversing with each other and through identifying patterns, consistencies and order in the evidence provided by the various ways of knowing (Benoliel, 1987; Schultz, 1987). Their knowledge is corroborated by knowledge from other disciplines.

Types of Nursing Knowledge and Criteria of Credibility

From our reflections on the traditional patterns of knowing in nursing and on women's ways of knowing, we have identified three types of knowledge specific to nursing as a discipline: clinical knowledge, conceptual knowledge and empirical knowledge. Discussed below are their relationships to the different patterns of knowing and possible criteria of credibility for each type.

Clinical Knowledge

Clinical knowledge results from engaging in the gestalt of caring, from bringing to bear multiple ways of knowing in order to solve the problems of patient care. Florence Nightingale knew the needs of the soldiers who fought in the Crimean War because she worked with them day and night; she was able to see the results of limited resources and exposure to the unhygienic environment. She realized that not only were diseases afflicting the soldiers, but the care they failed to receive affected their recovery.

Clinical knowledge is manifested primarily in the acts of practicing nurses; it is individual and personal. Historically, it has often been voiceless except in descriptions of the art of nursing, which have come to be viewed as less important and credible since nursing has been developing formal empirical foundations for practice. Clinicians experience patients' situations and "do" (i.e., they act based on these experiences).

Historically, clinical knowledge has been the product of a combination of personal knowing and empirics. It has usually involved intuition and subjective knowing, although these have tended to be ignored, denigrated or denied (Rew & Barrow, 1987). In the past, the empirical base was often "received empirics" from medicine or the social and behavioral sciences. Increasingly, however, empirical studies by nurses inform clinical practice. Further, intuition and subjective knowing are regaining their legitimacy as necessary components of humane care (Watson, 1985). The aesthetic and ethical patterns of knowing are also contributing to the development of clinical knowledge in response to the changing needs of persons interacting with technological and organizational environments.

Traditionally, clinical knowledge has been communicated retrospectively, through the publication of articles on specific client problems. These accounts, in national journals of nursing and increasingly in international journals, report individual case descriptions or summaries of multiple cases that provide answers for questions and problems in practice. These published accounts often reflect received knowledge and procedural knowledge and are characterized by prescriptions for practice.

The credibility of clinical knowledge has been based on the usefulness of its communicated wisdom—"It works." This criterion meets the requirement of purposefulness of a practice discipline (Chinn & Jacobs, 1987). Do we need other modes of corroboration? Can the art of nursing yield as reliable and reproducible knowledge as does the "science" of nursing? Should it? Perhaps models of practice, the discovery of patterns within and across clients and testimonials of subjective knowledge might be appropriate criteria for the credibility of clinical knowledge. These are unanswered questions.

Conceptual Knowledge

Conceptual knowledge is abstracted and generalized beyond personal experiences; it explicates the patterns revealed in multiple client experiences in multiple situations and articulates them as models or theories. Concepts are defined, and statements about the relationships among them are formulated. These propositions are supported by empirical and/or anecdotal evidence or defended by inferences and logical reasoning. This type of knowledge is manifested in the works of nurse theorists who seek answers to questions such as, Who is our client? What is it that nurses do that influences persons' health (Meleis, 1985)? These theorists develop comprehensive formulations of the nursing world. They use knowledge from other disciplines but through reflection and imagination evolve perspectives on that knowledge that are unique to nursing. They are influenced by procedures followed in the development of other fields but adhere to procedures supportive of the values and purpose of nursing.

Conceptual knowledge is the product of reflection on nursing phenomena. It emanates from curiosity and evolves from innovation and imagination in inquiry, along with persistence and commitment to the accumulation of facts and reliable generalizations. This type of nursing knowledge requires logical reasoning and comes primarily from individuals who take the position that knowledge is constructed within a context, and its development is a never-ending process.

Empirical knowing has influenced the development of conceptual knowledge in nursing through a dynamic interplay between systematic observation (empirics) and theorizing (reflecting, describing, synthesizing) (Weekes, 1986). The results of an inquirer's own research and that of others are used to support the propositional structure of frameworks or theories. But imagination and risk taking are important in their origination.

Will aesthetic knowing lead to formal conceptualizations of nursing that reflect its art? Will conceptual frameworks and models emerge from ethics as a pattern of knowing to describe this dimension of nursing? The answers to these questions depend on the degree to which nurse inquirers can view multiple ways of knowing as equally valuable in contributing to the mission of nursing.

The credibility of conceptual knowledge rests, in part, on the extent to which nurses find useful models and theories in communicating what they know. Whether or not a particular conceptual formulation holds up to critical appraisal depends also on its coherence and logical integrity—two criteria for evaluating theories (Meleis, 1985; Chinn & Jacobs, 1987).

Conceptual knowledge is often communicated in the form of propositional sentences. Thus it is the propositions and their relationships to each other that are evaluated for credibility. Chisholm's six levels of epistemic preferability illustrate the criteria for evaluating propositional credibility. Schultz (1987) explicated these levels with a proposition exemplifying a nursing knowledge claim:

> Nursing acts influence persons' energy exchange for healing and health. For the person who believes this claim the statement is (1) self presenting to him or her at a particular point in time; (2) the claim has some presumption in its favor because it is not contradicted by other beliefs; (3) the claim is judged to be acceptable because it is not disconfirmed by the set of propositions having some presumption in their favor; (4) the claim is epistemically in the

clear because it is not disconfirmed by the set of acceptable propositions and therefore (5) the claim is beyond reasonable doubt. Having met these conditions, the claim is judged to be (6) evident or certain (p. 141).

These are stringent criteria. Since nurses attend to individual experiences as well as to general patterns of experience, we may need to formulate different criteria of credibility for the conceptualization of nursing phenomena.

Empirical Knowledge

Empirical knowledge results from research. By research, we do not mean simply the empiricist approach per se but also historical, phenomenological, interpretive and critical theory approaches (Chinn, 1986). Empirical knowledge is manifest in published reports and is often used to justify actions and procedures in practice. It forms the basis for new studies and thereby contributes to the cumulative body of knowledge of a discipline. It often stimulates theoretical conceptualizations.

Researchers rely, in part, on received and procedural knowledge to inform their inquiries, but the hypotheses they test may originate in subjective knowledge; that is, their experiences with and reflections on nursing phenomena may give rise to hunches that lead to innovative methods or approaches to inquiry. If the empirical inquirer is also a practitioner, self-knowledge and practical knowledge may be brought to bear on the methods of inquiry. It is less clear how the aesthetic or ethical patterns of knowing contribute to the development of empirical knowledge except that usually (a) researchers adhere to ethical precepts in the conduct of their studies and (b) nurse inquirers are turning to the arts and humanities for approaches to systematic inquiry.

Advocates of different types of research approaches and methods have carved out criteria to validate their findings that are congruent with the particular designs and epistemological orientations that they follow (Gortner, 1984; Sandelowski, 1986). For all, however, the credibility of empirical knowledge rests on the degree to which the researcher has followed procedures

accepted by the community of researchers and on the logical derivation of conclusions from the evidence without bias or prejudice (Schultz, 1987; Gortner & Schultz, 1987). Of particular importance is whether or not the researcher is cognizant of previous research findings, knowledgeable about the procedures by which they were discovered, and dedicated to basing new research efforts on previous knowledge (Benoliel, 1987).

In addition to the procedural criteria accompanying various research designs and methods, the credibility of empirical knowledge is assessed by the systematic review and critique of research published in annual reviews (Werley & Fitzpatrick, 1983-1986; Fitzpatrick & Taunton, 1987), by consensus conferences focused on corroborating what is known about specific phenomena (e.g., pain) (National Institute of Health, 1987), and by invitational conferences to clarify the state-of-the-art on a topic and suggest new directions to be taken (Duffy & Pender, 1987). The epistemic preferability criteria enumerated above for conceptual knowledge claims may also be useful for assessing the credibility of empirical knowledge claims.

Ultimately credibility criteria must be consistent with nurses' various ways of knowing and types of knowledge. Can criteria be developed to accommodate the epistemological plurality of nursing, its complexity and holism? Is there one set of criteria or are there several? These are unanswered questions, but let us consider the possibility that the criteria for accepting knowledge vary for each type of knowledge.

Conclusion

Throughout this paper, we have deliberately avoided using the concept of "truth." Unfortunately inquirers from differing and contradictory perspectives have a propensity to put forth the view that their way of knowing yields *the* truth rather than *a* truth. Perhaps it is inappropriate to use the language of truth in nursing or in any practice discipline that deals with complex human experiences. Perhaps comprehending the context and patterns of human experiences, adjusted for individual differences, is more appropriate for claiming universal validity (Polanyi, 1964; Visintainer, 1986). Perhaps it is not sufficient to speak of facts alone, rather we should speak of experiences, intuition *and* facts. Perhaps it is not enough to rely on research as the medium for knowledge development; conceptualization and expert knowledge from clinical practice may be equally powerful and credible.

If we agree that there are different ways of knowing, different unknowns to be known, different propensities of knowers for knowing and different aspects to be known about the same phenomenon, then perhaps we can develop appropriate criteria for knowing from what we do know and, then, for knowing what we want to know.

REFERENCES

Belenky, M. F., Clinchy, B. M., Goldberger, N. R., & Tarule, J. M. (1986). *Women's ways of knowing*. New York: Basic Books.

Benner, P. (1983). Uncovering the knowledge embedded in clinical practice. *Image: The Journal of Nursing Scholarship, 15*(2), 36–41.

Benner, P. (1985). Quality of life: A phenomenological perspective on explanation, prediction, and understanding in nursing science. *Advances in Nursing Science, 8*(1), 1–14.

Benoliel, J. Q. (1987). Response to "Toward holistic inquiry in nursing: A proposal for synthesis of patterns and methods." *Scholarly Inquiry for Nursing Practice: An International Journal, 1*(2), 147–152.

Carper, B. A. (1978). Fundamental patterns of knowing in nursing. *Advances in Nursing Science, 1*(1), 13–23.

Chinn, P. L. (1986). *Nursing Research Methodology*. Rockville, MD: Aspen Publications.

Chinn, P. L., & Jacobs, M. K. (1987). *Theory and nursing: A systematic approach* (2d ed.). St. Louis: The C. V. Mosby Company.

Chisholm, R. M. (1982). *The foundations of knowing*. Minneapolis: University of Minnesota Press.

Colliere, M. F. (1986). Invisible care and invisible women as health care-providers. *International Journal of Nursing Studies, 23*(2), 95–112.

Duffy, M. E., & Pender, N. J. (1987). *Conceptual issues in health promotion research*. Indianapolis: Sigma Theta Tau Publications.

Fitzpatrick, J. J., & Taunton, R. L. (1987). Annual Review of Nursing Research (Vol. 5). New York: Springer Publishers.

Flew, A. (1984). *A dictionary of philosophy* (2d Ed.). New York: St. Martin's Press.

Gortner, S. R. (1984). Knowledge in a practice discipline: Philosophy and pragmatics. In C. Williams (Ed.), *Nursing research and policy formation: The case of prospective payment* (pp. 5–16). Kansas City, MO: American Academy of Nursing.

Gortner, S. R., & Schultz, P. R. (1987). Approaches to nursing science methods, *IMAGE: Journal of Nursing Scholarship, 20*(1), 22–24.

Lehrer, K. (1974). *Knowledge*. London: Oxford University Press.

Meleis, A. I. (1985). *Theoretical nursing*. Philadelphia: J. B. Lippincott Co.

National Institute of Health Consensus Development Conference (1987). The integrated approach to the management of pain. *Journal of Pain and Symptom Management, 2*(1), 35–44.

Polanyi, M. (1964). *Personal knowledge: Towards a post-critical philosophy*. New York: Harper Torchbooks.

Pyles, S. H., & Stern, P. N. (1983). Discovery of nursing gestalt in critical care nursing: The importance of the gray gorilla syndrome. *Image: The Journal of Nursing Scholarship, 15*(3), 51–57.

Ray, M. A. (1987). Technological caring: A new model in critical care. *Dimensions of Critical Care Nursing, 6*(3), 166–173.

Rew, L., & Barrow, E. M. (1987). Intuition: A neglected hallmark of nursing knowledge. *Advances in Nursing Science, 10*(1), 49–62.

Sandelowski, M. (1986). The problem of rigor in qualitative research. *Advances in Nursing Science, 8*(3), 27–37.

Schultz, P. R. (1987). Toward holistic inquiry in nursing: A proposal for synthesis of patterns and methods. *Scholarly Inquiry for Nursing Practice: An International Journal, 1*(2), 135–146.

Visintainer, M. A. (1986). The nature of knowledge and theory in nursing. *IMAGE: Journal of Nursing Scholarship, 18*(2), 32–38.

Watson, J. (1985). *Nursing: Human science and human care*. Norwalk, CT: Appleton-Century-Crofts.

Weekes, D. P. (1986). Theory-free observation: Fact or fantasy. In P. L. Chinn, (Ed.). *Nursing Research Methodology*. Rockville, MD: Aspen Publications, 11–22.

Werley, H. H., & Fitzpatrick, J. J. (1983–1986). *Annual Review of Nursing Research* (Vols. 1–4).

About the Author

JILL WHITE was born in Wagga Wagga, a country town in southeast Australia. She grew up viewing health care, particularly the hospital, as central to the well-being of the community. However, it was also clear that in the 1950s, the power over illness rested firmly with the doctors and, to a lesser extent, with the nurses, with the virtual exclusion of anyone personally significant to the patient. This, even as a junior Red Cross member, made no sense to her. Making sense of how nurses work together with people in health and illness has become her passion. This led her into nursing, nursing education, and the politics of nursing and health care. Her life has been significantly enriched by her husband Richard and two terrific stroppy wonderful teenaged children.

to this, however, was the work of Jacobs-Kramer and Chinn[2] a decade after Carper's article first appeared. Jacobs-Kramer and Chinn extended Carper's framework by producing a model that elucidated their understanding of the creation and development, the expression and transmission, and the assessment of each of Carper's patterns of knowing. Their intention was for such an elucidation to facilitate the integration of these patterns of knowing in nursing into clinical practice.

The lack of recent dialogue about the patterns themselves or about the model may reflect the decreased interest in the use of models generally in nursing, part of a move from reductionist thinking. The continued citation of both Carper and Jacobs-Kramer and Chinn, however, suggests their work is still being used in teaching.

The "patterns" of Carper[1] and "model" of Jacobs-Kramer and Chinn[2] do provide convenient conceptual organizers for introducing students to different ways of knowing in nursing. The patterns and model can be used to facilitate exploration of nursing practice and to enhance understanding of the rich history of modern nursing writing. They enable the contributions of nurses from the past to be analyzed in terms of the dominant social, political, and philosophical contexts of their time and enable nurses to trace with understanding the cumulative and disparate knowledge development that contributes to the discipline of nursing.

Given that the patterns and the model are still being used in education, it is appropriate that they be reviewed and critiqued within the context of nursing knowledge

development in the mid-1990s. This article offers such a review, critique, and update.

In her seminal article "Fundamental Patterns of Knowing in Nursing," Carper[1] identified the following patterns:

- empirics, or the science of nursing;
- ethics, or the moral component;
- the component of personal knowledge; and
- esthetics, or the art of nursing.

In this article the author explores each of these patterns in turn, looking first at what Carper had to say, then at the extension of this pattern within the Jacobs-Kramer and Chinn model, and finally at questions that arise with reference to the current literature and each particular pattern. Table 40-1 summarizes the essential elements of Jacobs-Kramer and Chinn's model of nursing knowledge.

Empirics: The Science of Nursing

Carper described empirics as

knowledge that is systematically organized into general laws and theories for the purpose of describing, explaining and predicting phenomena of special concern to the discipline of nursing . . . . The first fundamental pattern of knowing in nursing is empirical, factual, descriptive, and ultimately aimed at developing abstract theoretical explanations. It is exemplary, discursively formulated, and publicly verifiable.[1(pp14–15)]

Table 40-1
Summary of Essential Elements: Model of Nursing Knowledge

Dimension	Empirics	Ethics	Personal	Esthetics
Creative	Describing Explaining Predicting	Valuing Clarifying Advocating	Encountering Focusing Realizing	Engaging Interpreting Envisioning
Expressive	Facts	Codes	Self: authentic and disclosed	Art-act
	Theories	Standards		
	Models	Normative-ethical theories		

	Descriptions to impart
	  understanding
		Descriptions of ethical
		  decision making		

Assessment: critical question	What does this represent? How is this representative?	Is this right? Is this just?	Do I know what I do? Do I do what I know?	What does this mean?
Process-context	Replication	Dialogue	Response and reflection	Criticism
Credibility index	Validity	Justness	Congruity	Consensual meaning

Source: Jacobs-Kramer M., Chinn P. Perspectives on knowing: a model of nursing knowledge. *Schol Inq Nurs Pract.* 1988;2(2):129–139.

The key element here is that the "ultimate aim" of this knowing is "theory" development. Inherent in theory development is the ontological position that nature has a single or dominant reality commonly experienced and about which one can draw generalizable abstract explanations. This clearly encompasses the traditional view of scientific knowledge with its stance of objectivity and context-free replicability. This view was the dominant one in the nursing research and writing at the time of Carper's doctoral work. However, it is debatable at this time whether this pattern encompasses all research-based knowing, which Jacobs-Kramer and Chinn expressed as "facts, theories, models and descriptions that impart understanding."[2(p132)]

The realist ontological position, whose assumptions allow generalization, may also be seen as including grounded theory and ethnographic research, which generate generalizable abstractions. However, the relativist position of the interpretive paradigm as represented by phenomenology, for example, also seeks to provide "descriptions that impart understanding" but would not be consistent with Carper's definition of having an ultimate aim of developing abstract theoretical explanations that could be "systematically organized into general laws and theories."[1(p14)]

It is therefore suggested that the definition of the empirical pattern of knowing needs to be modified to accommodate the relativist ontological positions of knowledge development using methodologies such as phenomenology. If not modified, nursing needs to acknowledge the limitations of this definition in encompassing empirical knowing that seeks not to generalize, but rather through interpretation or description to put before the reader context-embedded stories whose purpose is to enrich understanding.

The inclusion of the word "understanding" by Jacobs-Kramer and Chinn[2] within the aim of the empirical pattern of knowing may be confusing; "understanding" is more commonly associated with the aim of research within the interpretive paradigm. The ontological position of the interpretive paradigm embraces the notion of multiple realities that cannot be generalized and puts this paradigm outside Carper's definition of this pattern of knowing. As discussed later, interpretive and critical research is encompassed more appropriately elsewhere.

Table 40-3
Ethics: Essential Elements

Dimension	Original Model[2]	Modifications
Creative	Valuing Clarifying Advocating	Valuing the moral idea of caring Critically appraising values Existential advocacy[23] Sensitizing to other value positions Fostering articulation of everyday notions of good[6]
Expressive	Codes, standards Normative theories Descriptions of decision making	Codes, standards Normative theories Observation Storytelling to explore embedded notions of good
Assessment: critical question	Is it right? Is it just?	Is it good? Is it just? Is it right? Does it embody caring?
Process-context	Dialogue	Dialogue Critical reflection Collaborative values elaboration
Credibility index	Justness	Justness Goodness Caring Congruence with personal values of patient

one strives simply to *know* the self. This knowing is a standing in relation to another human being and confronting that human being as a person."[1(p18)] The pattern of personal knowing develops when the nurse approaches the patient not as an object or category of illness, but strives instead "to actualize an authentic personal relationship between two persons."[1(p19)] This pattern requires the nurse to allow the person who is the patient-client to "matter." It involves engagement as opposed to detachment.

Mayeroff, whom Carper[1] cited as a source for her notion of personal knowing, saw a special feature of caring for a person as being "able to understand [the person] and his world as if I were inside it."[24(p42)] For Mayeroff relationship is about reciprocity, about helping the other "grow" and through this, growing oneself. However, Mayeroff's words harbor subtle paternalism: "I want it to grow in its own right . . . and I feel the other's growth as bound up with my own sense of well-

being."[24(p8)] Such a position mitigates against genuine reciprocity.

Mayeroff's reciprocity was elaborated on and refined in the works of Watson[12] in describing her concept of "transcendental moment," by Taylor[25] in her exposition of the "ordinariness" of nursing, in Morse's[26] work on nurse-patient relationships, and in Moch[27] in her exploration of "personal knowing," and probably most well known within nursing is Benner's[5] seminal work *From Novice to Expert.* Benner's notion of involvement and engagement was further developed collaboratively with Tanner[28] on intuition and with Wrubel[7] on the primacy of caring.

The idea of "being-with," of presence, of letting the person matter and being open to help that person make meaning out of his or her experience, is an essential feature of nursing practice. Without this knowing of self that allows an openness to the knowing of another person, nursing is only technical assistance, not involved care. In Carper's words, "It is concerned with the kind of knowing that promotes wholeness and integrity in the personal encounter, the achievement of engagement rather than detachment, and it denies the manipulative, impersonal orientation."[1(p20)]

In the model of nursing knowledge described by Jacobs-Kramer and Chinn,[2] the pattern of personal knowing is seen as being created by "experiencing the self—encountering and focusing on self while realizing the realities and potentialities."[2(p135)] It also involves "experiencing, encountering and focusing."[2(p135)] These are not easy concepts to grasp. Carper herself said of this pattern that it "is the most problematic, the most difficult to master and to teach. At the same time, it is perhaps the pattern most essential to understanding the meaning of health in terms of individual well-being."[1(p18)]

The creation of personal knowing may be enhanced through the use of art, poetry, literature, and storytelling in an endeavor to more truly "understand [the person] and his world as if I were inside it."[24(p42)] An example of this is poetry about childbirth that helps the midwife "see" inside the patient's world; poems such as Sharon Doubiago's "South American Mi Hija" (in Chester[29]) show the intensity that can allow the soul to grow, whereas stories such as Anais Nin's "Birth" (in Chester[29]) illuminate the potential for the soul to shrivel if a woman is not supported by the right kind of caring. Poems such as "Sunshine Across Living Centre" in Krysl and Watson[30] help nurses "see" the humanity of nurse and patient in interaction. The expressive dimension is the self as authentic (privately known) and disclosed (revealed to others): "Personal knowledge is expressed as ourselves, through the self."[2(p135)]

The assessment of this pattern comes through the "focus on the self as privately known and expressed to others. Assessment of self is a process carried out by the self through a rich inner life."[2(p135)] The critical questions involve exploration for congruence between knowing what we do and doing what we know, between the authentic and disclosed self. The process through which this assessment is made is the reflection and response of others to us, which we reflect on in turn. Agan put it succinctly by suggesting that "credibility of this type of knowing is determined through *individual reflection that is informed by the responses of others* [italics added]."[31(p70)] The credibility index is therefore congruence with the authentic and disclosed self.

Although the volume of literature in this area has provided much clarification and extension of the notion of personal knowing, the "essential elements" identified by Jacobs-Kramer and Chinn[2] are still pertinent. An elaboration could include, within the creative dimension, some examples of the means by which "encountering, focusing and realizing" might be facilitated (eg, poetry, art, literature, and storytelling) and within the process-context dimension, reflection informed by the response of others (see Table 40-4).

Table 40-4
Personal Knowing: Essential Elements

Dimension	Original Model[2]	Modifications
Creative	Encountering Focusing Realizing	Encountering, focusing, and realizing through practice and through art, literature, poetry, and storytelling
Expressive	Self: authentic and disclosed	Self: authentic and disclosed
Assessment: critical question	Do I know what I do? Do I do what I know?	Do I know what I do? Do I do what I know?
Process-context	Response and reflection	Reflection informed by the response of others and our reflection on our response to the life-world of other
Credibility index	Congruity	Congruity

Esthetics: The Art of Nursing

Carper suggested that the delay in explicating the esthetic pattern of knowing is associated with nursing's attempt to see itself as scientific and to "exorcise the image of the apprentice-type education system."[1(p16)] This delay has certainly been overcome, and there has been intense interest in this pattern recently. The pattern had its beginnings in the works of many early nursing writers. Wiedenbach[32] suggested that esthetic practice is making "visible through action" the nurse's perception of what the patient needs. Orem[33] spoke of the "creativity and style in design" of the provision of care. Orem also mentioned as necessary in artful practice the ability to "envision" models of helping with regard to the appropriate outcomes. Benner[5] was foremost in the development of the notion of perceiving the whole of a situation, without reference to rational processes, in her work on expert nursing practice. The concept of "intuitive" knowing developed by Benner and Tanner,[28] Rew,[34] and Agan[31] (and mentioned earlier as part of personal knowing) is an important component of perceiving and envisioning.

The design of the art-act combines all patterns of knowing in its esthetic form—it is all of and more than the other patterns: "The design, if it is to be esthetic, must be controlled by the perception of balance, rhythm, proportion and unity of what is done in relation to the dynamic integration and articulation of the whole."[1(p18)]

Carper named "empathy" as an important mode in the esthetic pattern of knowing; however, there is currently debate in the nursing literature over the appropriateness of this concept for nursing. Morse, Bottorff, Anderson, O'Brien, and Solberg suggested that "empathy was uncritically adopted from psychology and is actually a poor fit for the clinical reality of nursing practice."[35(p273)] They recommended exploration of other communication strategies that have been devalued, such as sympathy, pity, consolation, compassion, and commiseration. To these Taylor[25] might add affiliation, fun, and friendship.

Whatever the definitional outcome, the basic requirement of effective and authentic interpersonal engagement remains. This is highlighted in the recent Australian work of Taylor[25] and in the innovative work of Lumby[36] in her development of a critical feminist methodology for exploring nursing.

According to Jacobs-Kramer and Chinn,

> Esthetic knowledge finds expression in the art-act of nursing. Like personal knowledge, the expression of esthetic knowledge is not in language. We can unfold our art and retrospectively recollect and write about its features, and we can record it using electronic media, but the knowledge form itself is not what we write or record. The knowledge form *is* the art-act [italics added].[2(p137)]

They then proceeded to raise an important issue, albeit indirectly, that experience is an important component of esthetic knowing:

> As practice contexts are encountered, processes within the creative dimension of esthetics are initiated. Through the process of engagement, interpreting, and envisioning, "past" knowledge is enfolded into esthetics, and clients are uniquely cared for. As caring processes continue, new knowledge merges.[2(pp137–138)]

In putting forward experience as a necessary condition to esthetic practice, it may be necessary to include this context-specific experience as part of the creative and generative dimension, suggested by Jacobs-Kramer and Chinn as including "engaging, interpreting and envisioning." The addition of experience, particularly context-specific experience, suggests that these acts are cumulative, aligning with Benner's[5] position that expertise is context specific and not a transferable skill.

In exploring the assessment dimension within Carper's model of knowledge, Jacobs-Kramer and Chinn followed her inclusion of notions of esthetic appreciation from other art forms. They suggested that the critical question is, "What does this mean?"

> Criticism requires empathy and an intent to fully appreciate what the actors meant to convey. As the art-act is criticized, credibility is discerned by reaching

Table 40-5
Esthetics: Essential Elements

Dimension	Original Model[2]	Modifications
Creative	Engaging Interpreting Envisioning	Cumulative experience by engaging, interpreting and envisioning and including the "artful enfoldment" of all other patterns
Expressive	Art-act	Art-act
Assessment: critical question	What does this mean?	What does this mean?
Process-context	Criticism	Exhibition and criticism Recognition as authentic to other nurses
Credibility index	Consensual meaning	Consensual meaning

for consensus—a full and rich understanding of the art-act that brings together the perspectives of a community of co-askers who construct and confer meanings.[2(p137)]

Table 40-5 presents the essential elements for the esthetic pattern.

The major point of Jacobs-Kramer and Chinn's model development appears to be the unfolding of a story that suggests that each pattern may be seen by "examination of the art-act that integrates all knowledge patterns as expressed in practice . . . [as it] provides a comprehensive, context-sensitive means for enfolding multiple knowledge patterns."[2(p138)] This, they suggested, leads nursing away from "a quest for structural truth and towards a search for dynamic meaning."[2(p138)]

The model and its exposition of essential elements provide critical questions that may structure our process of inquiry, processes by which the inquiry might take place, and credibility indices to which claims of rigor may be addressed. If it is to be useful in the process of our practice-based inquiry, the model must adequately account for all patterns of knowing and their appropriate processes of inquiry.

Sociopolitical Knowing: Context of Nursing

The patterns and inquiry processes in Jacobs-Kramer and Chinn's[2] model appear adequate to the description of the nurse-patient relationship and the persons of the nurse and the patient. What appears to be missing is the context—the sociopolitical environment of the persons and their interaction. This represents a fifth pattern of knowing essential to an understanding of all the others.

The other patterns address the "who," the "how," and the "what" of nursing practice. The pattern of sociopolitical knowing addresses the "wherein." It lifts the gaze of the nurse from the introspective nurse-patient relationship and situates it within the broader context in which nursing and health care take place. It causes the nurse to question the taken-for-granted assumptions about practice, the profession, and health policies.

Sociopolitical knowing may be conceptualized as including understandings on two levels: (1) the sociopolitical context of the persons (nurse and patient), and (2) the sociopolitical context of nursing as a practice profession, including both society's understanding of nursing and nursing's understanding of society and its politics.

The sociopolitical context of the persons of the nurse-patient relationship fundamentally concerns cultural identity, for it is in culture that "self" is intrinsically located. This cultural location influences each person's understanding of health and disease causation, language, identity, and connection to the land. Such understanding goes well beyond Carper's[1] or Mayeroff's[24] notion of personal knowing. It is related to deeply embedded historical issues of connection to and dislocation from land and heritage.

Chopoorian suggested that "nursing ideas lack an archaeology of the social, political, and economic worlds that influence both client states and nursing roles."[37(p41)] She claimed that unequal class structure, power relationships, and political and economic power produce sexism, racism, ageism, and classism, which in turn affect health and result in illness. Chopoorian continued, "Nursing practitioners continually confront the human responses to the underlying social dynamics of poverty, unemployment, undernutrition, isolation and alienation precipitated through the structures of society."[37(pp40–41)]

Violence, drug dependence, and diabetes are examples of responses to what are inherently political rather than simply personal problems, and nurses' efforts to deal with them require nurses to articulate what they see resulting from societies' structures. Stevens suggested that nurses must provide a "critique of domination within fundamental social, political and economic structures and the analysis of how domination affects the health of persons and communities."[38(p58)] This effect includes the position and visibility of nursing in policy planning and decision making about health issues.

To have a voice in these decisions, nurses must both be articulate about what they know and do and be recognized by others as having something to contribute to debate. Nurses must have an understanding of the gatekeeping mechanisms within the political arena and their function. It is a paradox that when people are involved with nurses and nursing as patients or as concerned friends, the contribution of nurses is prized. Why then is it so quickly forgotten when these same people are influencing health care decisions? Diers and Fagin[39] suggested that the reason is visible in the metaphors the public associates with nursing, which include nurturance, dependence, and intimacy. These images are often reminders of personal pain and vulnerability, the natural reaction to which is suppression. To resurface an understanding of nursing is to resurface the context and all that is associated with it. Nurses must find a way of helping people remember, when they are well and politically able, what they knew of nursing when in crisis. Nurses must find the intersections between the health-related interests of the public and nursing and must become involved and active participants in these interests.

A sociopolitical understanding in which to frame all other patterns of knowing is an essential part of nursing's future in an increasingly economically driven world. Nurses must explore and expose alternative constructions of health and health care, find means of enabling all concerned to have a voice in this care provision, and develop processes of shared governance for the future. Table 40-6 illustrates how the sociopolitical dimension might be added to the model of knowing.

As Chinn said of nursing in the next century, "it is time to construct critical analyses of our present that are informed by the ethical and political ideals that we seek. It is time to begin to envision what our future nursing might be like and to create knowledge and skills that we need to begin to make it happen."[40(p56)] Understanding the context of nursing practice is fundamental to this endeavor. Appreciation and exploration of all the patterns of knowing in nursing and their interactions can contribute to the future articulation and development of nursing practice and nurses' place in determining the future of nursing practice and of health care.

Table 40-6
Sociopolitical Knowing:
Essential Elements

Dimension	Characteristics
Creative	Exposing and exploring alternate constructions of reality
Expressive	Transformation Critique
Assessment: critical question	Whose voice is heard? Whose voice is silenced?
Process-context	Critique and hearing all voices
Credibility index	Shared governance, enlightenment Movement toward equity

REFERENCES

1. Carper B. Fundamental patterns of knowing in nursing. *ANS.* 1978;1(1):13–23. Reprinted with permission from Aspen Publishers, Inc. (c) Copyright 1978.
2. Jacobs-Kramer M, Chinn P. Perspectives on knowing: a model of nursing knowledge. *Schol Inq Nurs Pract.* 1988;2(2):129–139. Used by permission of Springer Publishing Company, Inc., New York 10012.
3. Kuhn T. *The Structure of Scientific Revolutions.* Chicago, Ill: University of Chicago Press; 1970.
4. Sandelowski M. Rigor or rigor mortis: the problem of rigor in qualitative research revisited. *ANS.* 1993;16(2):1–8.
5. Benner P. *From Novice to Expert: Excellence and Power in Clinical Nursing Practice.* Menlo Park, Calif: Addison-Wesley; 1984.
6. Benner P. The role of experience, narrative, and community in skilled ethical comportment. *ANS.* 1991;14(2):1–21.
7. Benner P, Wrubel J. *The Primacy of Caring: Stress and Coping in Health and Illness.* Menlo Park, Calif: Addison-Wesley; 1989.
8. Bishop A, Scudder J, eds. *Caring, Curing, Coping.* University, Ala: University of Alabama Press; 1985.
9. Bishop A, Scudder J. *The Practical, Moral and Personal Sense of Nursing.* Albany, NY: State University of New York Press; 1990.
10. Cooper M. Reconceptualizing nursing ethics. *Schol Inq Nurs Pract.* 1990;4(3):209–218.
11. Cooper M. Principle-oriented ethics and the ethic of care: creative tension. *ANS.* 1991;14(2):22–31.
12. Watson J. *Nursing: Human Science and Human Care.* Norwalk, Conn: Appleton-Century-Crofts; 1985.
13. Watson J. The moral failure of the patriarchy. *Nurs Outlook.* 1990;28(2):62–66.
14. Gilligan C. In a different voice: women's conception of self and morality. *Harvard Educ Rev.* 1979;47:481–517.
15. Gilligan C. *In a Different Voice.* Cambridge, Mass: Harvard University Press; 1982.
16. Noddings N. *Caring—A Feminine Approach to Ethics and Moral Education.* Berkeley, Calif: University of California Press; 1984.
17. Pellegrino E. Being ill and being healed. In: Kestenbaum V, ed. *The Humanity of the Ill.* Knoxville, Tenn: University of Tennessee Press; 1982.
18. Pellegrino E. The caring ethic. In: Bishop A, Scudder J, eds. *Caring, Curing, Coping.* University, Ala: University of Alabama Press; 1985.
19. Zaner R. How the hell did I get here? In: Bishop A, Scudder J, eds. *Caring, Curing, Coping.* University, Ala: University of Alabama Press; 1985.
20. Zaner R. *Ethics and the Clinical Encounter.* Englewood Cliffs, NJ: Prentice Hall; 1988.
21. Kohlberg L. *The Philosophy of Moral Development.* San Francisco, Calif: Harper & Row; 1981.
22. Moss C. Has Gilligan's "Different Voice" made a difference? In: *Nursing Research: Scholarship for Practice.* Geelong, Victoria, Australia: Deakin Institute of Nursing Research, Deakin University; 1992.
23. Gadow S. Existential advocacy: philosophical foundation of nursing. In: Spicker S, Gadow S, eds. *Nursing: Images and Ideals: Opening Dialogue with the Humanities.* New York, NY: Springer; 1980.
24. Mayeroff M. *On Caring.* New York, NY: Harper & Row; 1971.
25. Taylor B. Enhancement of the nursing encounter through a shared humanity. In: *Nursing Research: Scholarship for Practice.* Geelong, Victoria, Australia: Deakin Institute of Nursing Research, Deakin University; 1992.
26. Morse J. Negotiating commitment and involvement in the nurse-patient relationship. *J Adv Nurs.* 1991;16:455–468.
27. Moch S. Personal knowing: Evolving research and practice. *Schol Inq Nurs Pract.* 1990;4(2):155–165.
28. Benner P, Tanner C. Clinical judgment: how expert nurses use intuition. *Am J Nurs.* 1987;87:23–31.
29. Chester L, ed. *Cradle and All.* Boston, Mass: Faber & Faber; 1989.
30. Krysl M, Watson J. Existential moments of caring: facets of nursing and social support. *ANS.* 1988;10(2):12–17.
31. Agan RD. Intuitive knowing as a dimension of nursing. *ANS.* 1987;10(1):64–70.
32. Wiedenbach E. *Clinical Nursing: A Helping Out.* New York, NY: Springer-Verlag; 1985.
33. Orem D. *Nursing: Concepts of Practice.* New York, NY: McGraw-Hill; 1971.
34. Rew L. Intuition and decision-making. *Image J Nurs Schol.* 1988;20(3):150–154.
35. Morse J, Bottorff J, Anderson G, O'Brien B, Solberg S. Beyond empathy: expanding expressions of caring. *Adv Nurs.* 1992;17:809–821.
36. Lumby J. *A Woman's Experience of Illness: The Emergence of a Feminist Method for Nursing.* Geelong, Victoria, Australia: Deakin University; 1993.
37. Chopoorian T. Reconceptualizing the environment. In: Moccia P, ed. *New Approaches in Theory Development.* New York, NY: National League for Nursing; 1986.
38. Stevens P. A critical social reconstruction of environment in nursing: implications for methodology. *ANS.* 1989;11(4):56–68.
39. Diers D, Fagin C. Nursing as a metaphor. *N Engl J Med.* 1981;309(2):116–117.
40. Chinn P. Looking into the crystal ball: positioning ourselves for the year 2000. *Nurs Outlook.* 1991;39(6):251–256.

About the Authors

JACQUELINE FAWCETT received her Bachelor of Science degree from Boston University in 1964, her master's in Parent–Child Nursing from New York University in 1970; and her PhD in Nursing, also from New York University, in 1976. Dr. Fawcett currently is Professor, College of Nursing and Health Sciences, University of Massachusetts, Boston. She is Professor Emerita at the University of Pennsylvania. Starting with her dissertation, Dr. Fawcett conducted a program of research dealing with wives' and husbands' pregnancy-related experiences that was derived from Martha Rogers' conceptual system. Subsequently, she undertook a program of research dealing with responses to caesarean birth derived from the Roy Adaptation Model of Nursing. A third program of research, also derived from the Roy Adaptation Model, focuses on function during normal life transitions and serious illness. Dr. Fawcett is perhaps best known for her meta-theoretical work, including many journal articles and several books. Since 1996, Dr. Fawcett has lived in the mid-coast region of Maine with her husband John and a now-tame feral cat, Lydia Dasher. She and her husband own Fawcett's Art, Antiques, and Toy Museum. She swims laps and walks on a treadmill at a fitness center for exercise and relaxation and sails on a windjammer off the Maine coast during the summer.

JEAN WATSON is Distinguished Professor of Nursing and holds the Murchinson-Scolville Chair in Caring Science at the University of Colorado Health Sciences Center (HSC). She is founder of the original Center for Human Caring and previously served as Dean of the University of Colorado HSC School of Nursing. She is a Past President of the National League for Nursing. Born in West Virginia, July 21, 1940, Dr. Watson earned undergraduate and graduate degrees in nursing and psychiatric-mental health nursing and holds her PhD in educational psychology and counseling. Dr. Watson is known for her theoretical work on the art and science of human caring. Her latest books and articles address empirical measurements of caring and new postmodern philosophies of caring and healing that bridge paradigms and point toward transformative models for the 21st century. Dr. Watson is the recipient of many awards and honors, including an international Kellogg Fellowship in Australia, a Fulbright Research Award in Sweden, five honorary doctoral degrees, the National League for Nursing's Martha E. Rogers Award, New York University's Distinguished Nurse Scholar Award, and the Fetzer Institute's Norman Cousins Award. Her hobbies include international travel, skiing, hiking, biking, and writing.

BETTY M. NEUMAN was born September 11, 1924, on a 100-acre farm near Lowell, OH. She received her nursing diploma in 1947 from what is now the Akron General Hospital; her BSN in 1957 and MS (major in mental health and community health) in 1966, both from University of California, Los Angeles. In 1985, she obtained her PhD degree in Clinical Psychology from the Pacific Western University School of Psychology in Los Angeles. Her most significant contribution is her theoretical model, the Neuman Systems Model, first published in 1972. Despite its widespread significance and application, Dr. Neuman regards her model as a work in progress. Her model has helped enhance the scientific perspective and basis of nursing and provides theoretic grounding for nursing education, research, and practice throughout the world. Dr. Neuman's hobbies include participating in the holistic health movement through her own primary prevention health regimen of walking and weight training. She is also a licensed real estate agent and continues to travel for consultations and speaking engagements.

PATRICIA HINTON WALKER is Professor of the Graduate School of Nursing at the Uniformed Services University of the Health Sciences in Bethesda, MD. Born in Kansas, she graduated with a BSN from the University of Kansas and subsequently received her master's and doctorate degrees from the University of Mississippi. Dr. Walker is a recognized scholar who has continually tried to integrate education, practice, and research through faculty practice and practice-based research. She influenced the development of faculty practices as a business and nationally focused many of her presentations and publications on the link between practice and research, particularly cost and quality outcomes research. Her focus on outcomes is exemplified through the promotion of cost and quality outcomes research linked to the practice environment and her leadership with faculties nationally and internationally for competency-based education. For recreation and fulfillment outside nursing, she plays golf, plays the piano, and enjoys creative cooking.

JOYCE J. FITZPATRICK is the Elizabeth Brooks Ford Professor of Nursing, Case Western Reserve University, Frances Payne Bolton School of Nursing, where she served as Dean from 1982 to1997. Her educational background includes a BSN from Georgetown University, an MS from The Ohio State University (psychiatric nursing), a PhD from New York University, an MBA from Case Western Reserve University, and an honorary doctorate (Doctor of Humane Letters) from Georgetown University. She has a strong and continuing interest in nursing science development, including both theory and research. She is author of more than 250 scholarly publications and author/editor of more than 30 books (having won the *American Journal of Nursing* Book of the Year award 18 times in the past 20 years), editor of the *Annual Review of Nursing Research* series, and editor of the journal that she launched in 1989, *Applied Nursing Research*.

on theory-guided practice (Walker & Redmond, 1999). More specifically, as Ingersoll (2000) pointed out, almost all discussions of evidence-based practice are focused on the primacy of the randomized clinical trial as the only legitimate source of evidence. Furthermore, most discussions of evidence-based practice treat evidence as an atheoretical entity, which only widens the theory-practice gap (Upton, 1999). Moreover, although multiple patterns of knowing in nursing have been acknowledged at least since the publication of Carper's work in 1978, nurses have ignored this disciplinary perspective and reverted to a medical perspective of evidence when discussing evidence-based nursing practice.

The purpose of this paper is to invite readers to join in a dialogue about what constitutes the evidence for theory-guided, evidence-based nursing practice. We are initiating the dialogue by offering a comprehensive description of theoretical evidence that encompasses diverse patterns of knowing in nursing. We advance the argument that each pattern of knowing can be considered a type of theory and that the different forms of inquiry used to develop the diverse kinds of theories

yield different kinds of evidence, all of which are needed for evidence-based nursing practice.

On Nursing Theories

Diverse patterns of knowing were identified by Carper (1978), who expanded the historical view of nursing as an art and a science in her classic paper, "Fundamental Patterns of Knowing in Nursing." She identified four ways or patterns of knowing in nursing: empirics, ethics, personal, and aesthetics. Carper's work is significant in that it "not only highlighted the centrality of empirically derived theoretical knowledge, but [also] recognized with equal importance and weight, knowledge gained through clinical practice" (Stein, Corte, Colling, & Whall, 1998, p. 43). Chinn and Kramer (1999) expanded Carper's work by identifying processes associated with each pattern of knowing. Their work has enhanced understanding of each pattern of knowing and has brought Carper's ideas to the attention of a wide audience of nurses.

The pattern of empirical knowing (Table 41-1) encompasses publicly verifiable, factual descriptions,

Table 41-1
Patterns of Knowing: Types of Nursing Theories, Modes of Inquiry, and Evidence

Pattern of Knowing: Type of Nursing Theory	Description	Mode of Inquiry	Examples of Evidence
Empirics	Publicly verifiable, factual descriptions, explanations, or predictions based on subjective or objective group data; the science of nursing	Empirical research	Scientific data
Ethics	Descriptions of moral obligations, moral and nonmoral values, and desired ends; the ethics of nursing	Identification, analysis, and clarification of beliefs and values; dialogue about and justification of beliefs and values	Standards of practice, codes of ethics, philosophies of nursing
Personal	Expressions of the quality and authenticity of the interpersonal process between each nurse and each patient; the interpersonal relationships of nursing	Opening, centering, thinking, listening, and reflecting	Autobiographical stories
Aesthetics	Expressions of the nurse's perception of what is significant in an individual patient's behavior; the art and act of nursing	Envisioning possibilities, rehearsing nursing art and acts	Aesthetic criticism and works of art

explanations, and predictions based on subjective or objective group data. In other words, empirical knowing is about "averages." This pattern of knowing, which constitutes the science of nursing, is well established in nursing epistemology and methods. Empirical knowing is generated and tested by means of empirical research. The next section of this paper extends the common focus on empirics as the primary focus of evidence, and offers a new lens for considering theory-guided evidence and diverse ways of knowing that can and should be integrated into nurses' evidence-based practice initiatives.

Diverse Patterns of Knowing

In contrast to empirics, the other patterns of knowing are less established, but they are of increasing interest for the discipline of nursing in particular and for science in general. Ethical knowing, personal knowing, and aesthetic

knowing are required for moral, humane, and personalized nursing practice (Stein et al., 1998). The pattern of ethical knowing (Table 41-1) encompasses descriptions of moral obligations, moral and nonmoral values, and desired ends. Ethical knowing, which constitutes the ethics of nursing, is generated by means of ethical inquiries that are focused on identification and analysis of the beliefs and values held by individuals and groups and the clarification of those beliefs and values. Ethical knowing is tested by means of ethical inquiries that focus on dialogue about beliefs and values and establishing justification for those beliefs and values.

The pattern of personal knowing refers to the quality and authenticity of the interpersonal process between each nurse and each patient (Table 41-1). This pattern is concerned with the knowing, encountering, and actualizing of the authentic self; it is focused on how nurses come to know how to be authentic in relationships with patients, and how nurses come to know how to express their concern and caring for other people. Personal knowing is not "knowing one's self" but rather knowing how to be authentic with others, knowing one's own "personal style" of "being with" another person. Personal knowing is what is meant by "therapeutic nurse-patient relationships." Personal knowing is developed by means of opening and centering the self to thinking about how one is or can be authentic, by listening to responses from others, and by reflecting on those thoughts and responses.

The pattern of aesthetic knowing shows the nurse's perception of what is significant in the individual patient's behavior (Table 41-1). Thus, this pattern is focused on particulars rather than universals. Aesthetic knowing also addresses the "artful" performance of manual and technical skills. Aesthetic knowing is developed by envisioning possibilities and rehearsing the art and acts of nursing, with emphasis on developing appreciation of aesthetic meanings in practice and inspiration for developing the art of nursing.

Carper (1978) and Chinn and Kramer (1999) pointed out that each pattern of knowing is an essential component of the integrated knowledge base for professional practice, and that no one pattern of knowing should be used in isolation from the others. Carper (1978) maintained that "Nursing . . . depends on the scientific knowledge of human behavior in health and in illness, the aesthetic perception of significant human experiences, a personal understanding of the unique individuality of the self and the capacity to make choices within concrete situations involving particular moral judgments" (p. 22). Elaborating, Chinn and Kramer (1999) pointed out the danger of using any one pattern exclusively. They said:

> When knowledge within any one pattern is not critically examined and integrated with the whole of knowing, distortion instead of understanding is produced. Failure to develop knowledge integrated within all of the patterns of knowing leads to uncritical acceptance, narrow interpretation, and partial utilization of knowledge. We call this "the patterns gone wild." When this occurs, the patterns are used

in isolation from one another, and the potential for synthesis of the whole is lost. (p. 12)

The current emphasis on empirical knowing as the only basis for evidence-based nursing practice is an outstanding example of a "pattern gone wild."

Patterns of Knowing as Theories

The question arises as to whether the multiple, diverse patterns of knowing can be considered sets of theories. The answer to that question depends, in part, on one's view of a pattern of knowing and a theory. A pattern of knowing can be thought of as a way of seeing a phenomenon. The English word "theory" comes from the Greek word, "theoria," which means "to see," that is, to reveal phenomena previously hidden from our awareness and attention (Watson, 1999). For the purposes of this paper, a theory is defined as a way of seeing through "a set of relatively concrete and specific concepts and the propositions that describe or link those concepts" (Fawcett, 1999, p. 4). Theories constitute much of the knowledge of a discipline. Moreover, theory and inquiry are inextricably linked. That is, theories of various phenomena are the lenses through which inquiry is conducted. The results of inquiry constitute the evidence that determines whether the theory is adequate or must be refined.

Collectively, the diverse patterns of knowing constitute the ontological and epistemological foundations of the discipline of nursing. Inasmuch as both patterns of knowing and theories represent knowledge, and are generated and tested by means of congruent, yet diverse processes of inquiry (Table 41-1), we maintain that each pattern of knowing may be regarded as a type of theory. These four types of theories are subject to different types of inquiry. Henceforth, then, we will refer to the patterns of knowing as empirical theories, ethical theories, personal theories, and aesthetic theories. Our decision to regard the patterns of knowing as types of theories is supported by Chinn and Kramer's (1999) reference to ethical theories and Chinn's (2001) articulation of a theory of the art of nursing. Other global perspectives indicate the direction of diverse patterns of knowing as types of theories. For example, Scandinavian nurses view nursing within a caring science model, and they acknowledge personal knowing, personal characteristics, and moral and aesthetic knowing of caring practices as theoretical ways of knowing that elicit diverse forms of evidence (Dahlberg, 1995, Fagerstrom & Bergdom Engberg, 1998; Kyle, 1995; Snyder, Brandt, & Tseng, 2000; von Post & Eriksson, 2000).

Furthermore, we, like some of our international colleagues, maintain that the content of ethical, personal, and aesthetic theories can be formalized as sets of concepts and propositions, just as the content of many empirical theories has been so formalized (Fawcett, 1999; von Post & Eriksson, 2000). Moreover, regarding all four patterns of knowing as types of theories reintroduces the notions of uncertainty and tentativeness that typically are associated with empirical theories (Fagerstrom & Bergdom Engberg, 1998; Morse, 1996; Polit & Hungler, 1995).

The four types of theories constitute much, if not all, of the knowledge needed for nursing practice. A potentially informative analysis, which follows from the conclusion that the patterns of knowing can be regarded as sets of theories, is the examination of extant theories to determine in which pattern of knowing each is located. That analysis is, however, beyond the scope of this paper and will not be pursued here. Rather, we are attempting to make connections between the four types of theories, representing the four patterns of knowing, and what constitutes evidence for nursing practice.

On Evidence

These four types of theories underlie all methodological decisions, and they are the basis for generating multiple forms of evidence. The question of what constitutes evidence depends, in part, on what one regards as the basis of the evidence. We maintain that theory is the reason for and the value of the evidence. In other words, evidence itself refers to evidence about theories. Similarly, theory determines what counts as evidence. Thus, theory and evidence become inextricably linked, just as theory and inquiry are inextricably linked.

Any form of evidence has to be interpreted and critiqued by each person who is considering whether the theory can be applied in a particular practice situation. This view indicates acknowledgement of diverse forms of knowing as inherent in any global or cultural interpretation of knowledge or theory (Zoucha & Reeves, 1999). The four types of theories are diverse ontological and epistemological lenses through which evidence is both interpreted and critiqued. The current emphasis on the technical-rational model of empirical evidence denies or ignores the existence of a theory lens. In contrast, our theory-guided model of evidence requires and acknowledges interpretation and critique of diverse forms of evidence. As shown in the Table, we regard the scientific data produced by empirical research as the evidence for empirical theories. We count as scientific both qualitative and quantitative data and we support the call for qualitative outcome analysis (Kyle, 1995; Morse, Penrod, & Hupcey, 2000; Snyder et al., 2000). The evidence for ethical theories is illustrated in formalized statements of nurses' values, such as standards of practice, codes of ethics, and philosophies of nursing. The evidence for personal theories is found in autobiographical stories about the genuine, authentic self. The evidence for aesthetic theories is manifested or expressed as aesthetic criticism of the art and act of nursing and through works of art, such as paintings, drawings, sculpture, poetry, fiction and nonfiction, dance, and others.

Our view of the reason for evidence differs from the prevailing discussion in the literature. In current literature, typically a procedure or intervention is presented in isolation from the theory that undergirds that procedure or intervention, and in isolation from the value of the evidence. Hence the term, "evidence-based practice." We maintain that the more appropriate term is "theory-guided, evidence-based practice" (Walker & Redmond, 1999). Given the diversity of kinds of theories needed for nursing practice (See Table 41-1), evidence must extend beyond the current emphasis on empirical research and randomized clinical trials, to the kinds of evidence also generated from ethical theories, personal theories, and aesthetic theories.

Our view of the diversity of types of theories and the type of evidence needed for each type of theory addresses, at least in part, current criticisms of the evidence-based practice movement. We agree with Mitchell (1999) that the "proponents of evidence-based practice have . . . grossly oversimplified and misrepresented the process of nursing" (p. 34). Mitchell was particularly concerned that "The notion of evidence-based practice is not only a barren possibility but also that evidence-based practice obstructs nursing process, human care, and professional accountability" (p. 30). We respond to Mitchell's concern by including evidence about personal theories, which include authenticity in nurse-patient interpersonal relationships. Moreover, Mitchell (1999) maintained that "Evidence-based practice does not support the shift to patient-centered care, and it is inconsistent with the values and interests of consumers" (p. 34). Here, we respond to Mitchell's concerns by including evidence about ethical theories, which include the values of nurses. Mitchell (1999) also was concerned that "Evidence-based practice, if taken seriously, may restrain some nurses from defining the values and theories that guide the nurse-person process" (p. 31) and relationship. This point relates to our view that the art of nursing is expressed through the nurse-person process and the evidence derived from interpretations of tests of aesthetic theories and ethical theories.

Furthermore, our view of the diversity of types of theories and corresponding types of evidence needed for theory-guided, evidence-based nursing practice elaborates Ingersoll's (2000) definition of evidence-based nursing practice. Her definition is as follows: "Evidence-based nursing practice is the conscientious, explicit, and judicious use of theory-derived, research-based information in making decisions about care delivery to individuals or groups of patients and in consideration of individual needs and preferences" (p. 152). Our view makes explicit the multiple kinds of theories—ethical, personal, aesthetic, and empirical—whereas Ingersoll's reference to theory could easily be construed to mean only empirical theory or, perhaps because of the reference to individual needs and preferences, to include empirical and aesthetic theories.

We maintain the appropriateness of recognizing and appreciating empirical, ethical, personal, and aesthetic theories and the corresponding critique and

interpretation of the evidence about each kind of theory. Such critique and interpretation of evidence is crucial for nursing practice because it is embedded in the values and phenomena located within a broad array of nursing theories. Moreover, by recognizing the four types of theories, more nurses and other health professionals may appreciate and use theories. They may agree with us that theories and values are the starting point for the critique and interpretation of any evidence needed to support clinical practices that may enhance the quality of life of the public we serve.

Conclusions

We invite readers to expand the dialogue about theory-guided, evidence-based practice. We urge nurses everywhere to consider the implications and consequences of the current virtually exclusive emphasis on empirical theories and empirical evidence-based nursing practice. We urge our nurse colleagues throughout the world to join us and those who have accurately pointed to the limitations of viewing nursing as a strictly empirical endeavor (Bolton, 2000; Dahlberg, 1995; Fagerstrom & Bergdom Engberg, 1998; Hall, 1997; Zocha & Reeves, 1999) to consider what might be gained by recognition and development of ethical, personal, and aesthetic theories and by formalization of those kinds of theories. Accordingly, we encourage all nurses to actualize their claim of a holistic approach to practice by adopting a more comprehensive description of evidence-based nursing practice, a descriptive that allows for critique and interpretation of evidence obtained from inquiry guided by ethical, personal, aesthetic, and empirical theories, as well as by any other kinds theories that may emerge from new understandings of nursing as a human science and a professional practice discipline.

REFERENCES

Bolton, S. C. (2000). Who cares? Offering emotional work as a "gift" in the nursing labor process. *Journal of Advanced Nursing, 32,* 580–586.

Carper, B. A. (1978). Fundamental patterns of knowing in nursing. *Advances in Nursing Science, 1*(1), 13–23.

Scientific Inquiry in Nursing: A Model for a New Age

Holly A. DeGroot

Despite the acknowledged need for widespread and rapid scientific advancement in nursing, little systematic attention has been paid to the progenitor of research, the individual investigator. The nature of scientific problem solving as the fundamental process of research practice is explored, and a model of scientific inquiry is proposed. Variables in the model are discussed in relation to their potential effect on the inquiry process, and strategies that facilitate the practice of research are identified.

Concern with the growth of nursing science has received full attention from nursing scholars over the past decade. The need for nursing as a foundation for nursing science and professional growth has been repeatedly acknowledged by contemporary nursing authors (Donaldson & Crowley, 1978; Hardy, 1983). Roy (1983) considers theory development as the number one priority for this decade. Current economic pressures have added unprecedented urgency to this scientific quest as health care policy makers and administra-

tors demand research verification of nursing's disciplinary contribution.

Theory development literature in nursing has largely focused on theory construction (Dickoff, James, & Weidenbach, 1968; Jacox, 1984; Meleis, 1985), the nature of nursing's scientific advancement (Hardy, 1983; Newman, 1983), and the identification of conceptual and methodological deficiencies (Batey, 1977; Gortner, 1977; Jacobsen & Meininger, 1985). Despite agreement that creative strategies are required to

From H. A. DeGroot, Scientific inquiry in nursing: A model for a new age. Advances in Nursing Science, April 1998, 10(3), 1–21.
Copyright © 1998. Reproduced with permission of Lippincott Williams & Wilkins.

About the Author

HOLLY A. DEGROOT is currently Chief Executive Officer of Catalyst Systems, LLC, Novato, CA, a nurse-owned and nurse-operated firm dedicated to evidence-based staffing decisions in health care. As founder of Catalyst 15 years ago, Dr. DeGroot has developed the largest objective database of its type on nursing workload and staff utilization patterns. In addition, she has created a family of patient classification measures and staffing methodologies for virtually every inpatient and outpatient clinical area where patient care is provided. She has been closely involved in regulatory and legislative issues involving nurse staffing throughout the United States, frequently providing expert testimony and advice on related topics. Dr. DeGroot has worked in several administrative, faculty, and research positions throughout her career and also serves as faculty in the graduate program in Nursing Administration and Informatics at the University of California, San Francisco. Born in Pittsburgh, PA, Dr. DeGroot has spent the majority of her life in northern California, where she enjoys swimming, reading, traveling, and writing.

resolve these theoretical inadequacies (Caper, 1978; Oiler, 1982), surprisingly little attention has been paid to the process and practice of scientific inquiry with the individual investigator as the unit of analysis. An understanding of the nature of scientific activity and the factors that influence individual inquiry and research practice is essential if nursing is to exercise its fullest intellectual power for theory development.

The Nature of Scientific Activity

Science has been characterized as a "creative and imaginative human activity" (Goldstein & Goldstein, 1978, p. 4) and as a form of contemplative wisdom (Weiskopf, 1973). Bronowski observes that "all science is the search for unity and hidden likenesses" (Bronowski, 1965, p. 14). As the method of inquiry employed in this quest, the research process is virtually indistinguishable from what Bigge (1982) calls reflective thinking. This is "a reflective process within which persons either develop new or change existing tested generalized insights or understanding. So construed, reflective thinking combines both inductive—fact gathering—and deductive processes in such a way as to find, elaborate and test hypotheses" (Bigge, 1982, p. 105).

It is clear that the research process and the reflective thinking process constitute parallel attempts directed toward problem solving. Polanyi (1962) distinguishes between two phases of problem solving: an initial stage of perplexity and a subsequent stage of taking action directed toward dispelling the perplexity. Polanyi summarizes the four well-known stages of discovery in problem solving: (a) stage of preparation, during which a problem is initially recognized; (b) stage of incubation, which is an unconscious preoccupation with the problem; (c) stage of illumination, characterized by the tentative discovery of a possible solution; and (d) stage of verification, during which the solution withstands tests of practical reality. Implicit in this notion of scientific activity as a process of reflective thinking and of problem solving is the fundamental relationship of both to creativity. Bronowski (1965) asserts that while science is involved in a search for hidden likenesses, creativity is the discovery of hidden likeness.

Creativity can be viewed as a five-step process that is triggered by identifying or sensing a problem (Mackinnon, 1979). The first stage is called the period of preparation, during which experience, cognitive skills, and problem-solving techniques are acquired. The second stage, or period of concentrated effort, is often accompanied by frustration that results from unsuccessful attempts to solve the problem. Next comes a period of withdrawal, which is akin to the incubation stage of problem solving. In this stage the problem and its possible solutions are considered on a conscious as well as subconscious level. This stage is characterized by what Worthy (1975) has termed "fruitful obsession." The fourth stage, or moment of insight, is accompanied by a feeling of exhilaration that comes from the sudden discovery of a solution to the problem. Worthy calls this "aha thinking," which results in intuitive leaps and sudden insights related to problem solution. The last step in the creative process, the period of verification, is characterized by the elaboration of the newly created insight or solution and its subsequent testing, refinement, extension, and evaluation. The attainment of this fifth and final step in the creative process forms the foundation and the starting point for further creative activities. That this creative process bears a striking resemblance to the problem-solving and reflective thinking processes of scientific activity, as outlined earlier, is central to the discussion of scientific inquiry.

Since scientific problem solving necessarily involves an individual's contribution to the creative process, characteristics of creative persons and their work are also important to consider. Creativity in individuals has been associated with divergent thinking, intelligence, commitment or involvement, and a preference for complexity from which simplicity and order may be derived (Nicholls, 1983). The willingness to take risks (Albert, 1983) and to use imagination and intuition (Yukawa, 1973) are other fundamental characteristics of creative individuals. Introversion, playfulness, and a well-developed sense of humor also figure heavily with these individuals (Worthy, 1975).

Characteristics of the outcomes or products of creative problem solving (e.g., research findings and theories) have also been identified (MacKinnon, 1979). Originality and the ability of the solution to actually solve an existing problem are key characteristics. In addition, the solution must be "produced," which implies development, refinement, and communication of the problem solution. Additional criteria have relevance if nursing theory is considered to be the creative "product." These criteria are that the creative outcome or theory contains truth and beauty and that it contributes to the quality of human existence. It has also been observed that creativity can be generated as much by the nature of the problem as by the person attempting to solve it (Albert, 1983; Yukawa, 1973). Creative problem solving has beneficial psychological effects on others who are exposed to the process by encouraging and engaging them in more imaginative and creative activity. Although creativity alone does not ensure successful problem solving, it is a vital ingredient for the theoretical complexity of knowledge generation in human sciences. It should be remembered that less than successful problem solving can be equally rich in stimulating creative scientific problem solving because it forces the consideration of alternative possibilities (Yukawa, 1973).

Phases of Inquiry

It is clear from this discussion that the quintessence of scientific inquiry is creative problem solving conducted through the research process. Scientific inquiry thus comprises at least four interrelated phases: (a) formulation of the research problem, (b) method selection, (c) method implementation, and (d) communication of findings. Each of these phases shares common characteristics that have implications for a model of scientific inquiry. Although these phases are typically presented as the orderly and normative approach to inquiry, it has been pointed out that the actual research process has little resemblance to such a rational model (Martin, 1982). The inquiry process has been aptly described as a series of dilemmas that can be neither solved nor avoided (McGrath, 1982).

Problem Formulation

The pivotal point for a system of scientific inquiry is the research problem, question, or hypothesis, for it reflects all that came before and directs all research activity that will follow. Kerlinger goes a step further, calling the research problem or hypothesis the "working instrument of theory" (Kerlinger, 1973, p. 20). The research problem (a term to be used alternatively with "research question" or "research hypothesis," denoting the same or similar entity) is a highly subjective construction. As such, it is an intensely personal and intimate creation because of its contextual and historical proximity to the very essence of its creator. Not surprisingly, Polanyi calls research problems "intellectual desires" (Polanyi, 1962, p. 152), noting that in any scientific controversy personal attacks rather than scientific arguments are the norm because intellectual passions, not reason, are truly at odds.

Since the formulation of a research question is a creative effort based on imagination, ingenuity, and insight (Polit & Hungler, 1983), the research results stemming from it ultimately reflect the intellectual power of the question and, undeniably, the researcher. Research problem selection is closely related to personal values (Kaplan, 1964; Tucker, 1979) and actually discloses the direction of human will and intuition (Noddings & Shore, 1984). Runkel and McGrath observe that as a researcher attempts to formulate the research problem, "he begins with his own previous way of thinking about things; he seeks help in organizing his complexities from literature and colleagues; finally, he is inevitably affected by his own personal experience as he interacts with the world" (Runkel & McGrath, 1972, p. 13). Not surprisingly, this characteristic of subjectivity is inherent in the other phases of inquiry as well.

Selection of Methods

Although Kaplan (1964) acknowledges at least four distinct usages of the term "methodology," only the fourth is inclusive enough for a discussion of the process of scientific inquiry. This definition incorporates specific techniques and procedures as well as abstract philosophical imperatives. Kaplan asserts that the use of this expanded meaning allows for the inclusion of a wide range of activities, including concept delineation, hypothesis formation, observation and measurement, and model and theory construction, as well as explanation and prediction. The advantage of such a definition is that it treats all tools that a researcher has at his or her disposal (including the conceptual and the concrete) and the research implementation phases, such as data collection and analysis, as interrelated components of inquiry. Conceived in this way, factors influencing problem formulation directly or indirectly influence all phases of inquiry.

The implications of this expanded and integrated view of research methodology are not universally appreciated. At the very least, authors agree that the methods are dictated by the research question (Kerlinger, 1973; Kaplan, 1964; Runkel & McGrath, 1972; Wilson, 1985). However, there seems to be tacit endorsement of a greater rationality and objectively of method selection than actually exists. For example, some authors (Polit & Hungler, 1983) subscribe to a design selection hierarchy, usually with experimental designs at the top and nonexperimental approaches clearly at the bottom. This view implies that the selection of design methodology is based primarily on whether the research can meet the three requirements for a true experiment, namely, the ability for manipulation, control, and randomization. If these requirements can be met by the proposed study, the choice of methods is clear. If researchers are somehow unable to meet these requirements for experimentation, they are at once relegated to the realm of nonexperimental methodology. Kerlinger (1973) goes as far as to categorize nonexperimental methods as "compromise designs," consigning them rather casually to the bottom of the design hierarchy. Unfortunately this stance serves to create a methodological double bind: Methods are purportedly dictated by the question, but it is less desirable to ask questions that must be answered by "lower-order" designs and methods.

Brink and Wood (1983) propose a similarly straightforward and deductive approach to method selection based on the level of the research question. These levels are a function of existing amounts of knowledge related to the phenomena of interest. These authors also suggest that selection of methods may be based primarily on the existence of valid and reliable measures. Little attention is given to other factors that may influence the selection of research methods.

Method Implementation and Communication of Findings

How methods are implemented through the use of data collection techniques and analytical strategies is affected by the same subjective considerations inherent in problem formulation and method selection phases of inquiry. There is a wide range of methodological possibilities open to experimental and non-experimental approaches, with choices to be made at each juncture. Whether one decides to use open-ended interview *v* standardized questionnaire, grounded theory *v* hermeneutic interpretation, analysis of covariance (ANCOVA) techniques *v* multiple regression correlation (MRC), or a convenience *v* a stratified random sample is influenced by a combination of interrelated factors. Even the communication of research findings is similarly influenced as choices are made about which journal to submit the results to, what information should be included in the report, how conservative or liberal the interpretations will be, and what the theoretical implications of the findings are.

Despite the rigorous assertions that method selection and implementation are primarily rational processes, some authors concede the influence of subjective factors on these phases of inquiry (Martin, 1982; Kuhn, 1970; Luria, 1973; Polkinghorne, 1983). These include factors such as disciplinary norms, personal research style, fund-

ing realities, and other value-laden considerations. Tucker (1979) points out that scientific activity is essentially a process involving a series of value decisions to be made by the researcher and that perhaps the largest number of these decisions is made in relation to methodological issues. Polkinghorne goes one step further, asserting that "particular methods do not operate independently of a system of inquiry" and in fact "the use of a method changes only as a researcher uses it in different systems of inquiry" (Polkinghorne, 1983, p. 6). This perhaps is the most important point of all, for it posits the inextricable relationship between each phase of inquiry and the subjective factors that necessarily influence each phase.

A Model of Scientific Inquiry

The model proposed here is fundamentally a systems/process model applied to a human system of inquiry (see Figure 42-1). As such, the system comprises six interrelated

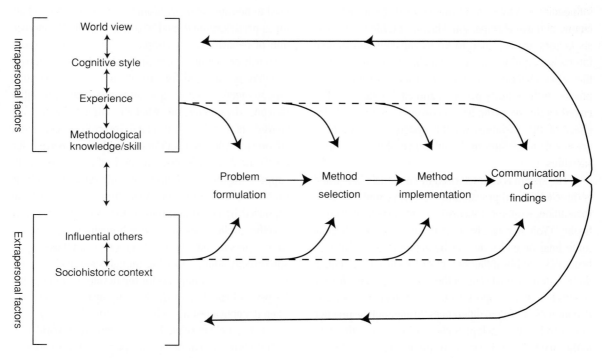

Figure 42-1   *A model of scientific inquiry.*

Table 42-1
Major Factors Influencing Scientific Inquiry in Nursing

Intrapersonal Factors
World view
    Nature of human beings
    Nature of knowledge and truth
    Nature of nursing science
Cognitive style
Experience
    Life experience
    Professional nursing experience
    Research experience
    Theoretical experience
Methodological knowledge and skill

Extrapersonal Factors
Influential others
    Individual
    Institutional
Sociohistorical context

influencing variables, subdivided into four intrapersonal factors and two extrapersonal factors (Table 42-1). The six factors are assumed to be in constant and mutual interaction, and when there is a change in one variable the other variables are affected. There are four basic phases to the inquiry process, and each phase is influenced by the six variables. Accordingly, the cumulative effect of the variables on the system as a whole is greater than the sum of the influence of the individual variables.

The system is characterized by continual change and is directed toward growth and increasing sophistication. In addition, it operates according to the principal of equifinality (Von Bertalanffy, 1968), which asserts that the same final or end state can be achieved from different beginnings and by different paths or routes. Even though there is never a final state in the research process for the researcher, this proposed inquiry system accepts and encourages individual differences throughout the practice of research, since each path chosen can get equally close to the "truth." The six factors or influencing variables are not intended to represent all intrapersonal or extraper-

sonal possibilities. Rather they should be viewed as a major class of variables that operate in addition to other factors such as personality, intelligence, or other values and beliefs. In addition, individual investigators vary in their awareness of the existence and nature of these variables as well as in the relative degree of influence any one factor may exert on the inquiry process.

Intrapersonal Factors

World View

The first personal variable that influences the process of inquiry is called world view, which consists of the researcher's general philosophical orientation, or world view, of the nature of human beings, the nature of knowledge and truth, and the nature of nursing science. Beliefs about human nature are fundamental to the development of the researcher's theoretical learnings, to the delineation of appropriate research questions, and, ultimately to the selection of research methodology. Relevant beliefs about human nature include such considerations as whether human beings are considered to be rational or irrational, whether human behavior is predetermined, and what the basis is for motivation of behavior. For example, are human motivations primarily conscious or unconscious? Is human behavior dictated by the need for growth or by the deprivation humans feel? Research questions generated will differ sharply, depending on whether human beings are viewed as highly self-directed individuals constantly striving for self-actualization v individuals who are at the mercy of their subconscious and who are constantly suppressing the primal urges the subconscious seeks to satisfy. Tucker points out that these latter beliefs as espoused by Freud and others, for example, have very specific implications for research methodology as well. He reminds us that the belief that one cannot ask a person directly about his or her thoughts and feelings provided the primary impetus for the development of popular psychological methods that employ unobtrusive and often deceptive testing techniques (Tucker, 1978).

Other beliefs related to a researcher's world view include how human beings are perceived in relation to their environment. For example, are people viewed as primarily passive reactors to events that impinge on them, or are they seen as proactive or mutually interactive with the environment? Does the human boundary end at the skin, or does the human field extend, as Rogers (1970) insists, beyond the skin to actually merge with the environmental field? Other perceptions that contribute to a researcher's world view relate to the multidimensionality of human beings. Are people seen as the popularized "biopsychosocial" beings, or are they seen as "biopsychosocial-spiritual-cultural" being? The very nature of the research questions would be altered by these two alternative views in that they would contain a very different constellation of variables and possible methodological implications.

These beliefs form the basis for establishing theoretical congruence, or the degree to which prevailing theories comfortably conform to one's world view. For example, if one believed that human beings were passive reactors to their environment and that behavior is motivated by the desire to avoid discomfort, it is unlikely that a systems perspective or symbolic interaction-based method would be very appealing. In this way beliefs about human nature delimit the realm of theoretical possibility in the practice of research.

Beliefs about the *nature of knowledge and truth* also affect a researcher's world view and thus the process of inquiry. Two major competing schools of thought best illustrate the diversity of these beliefs. Logical positivism, later known as the received view, asserts that objective, axiomatic truth exists that is discoverable and able to be verified by hypotheticodeductive methods (Suppe, 1977). Only certain methods that are objective and produce sense data can appropriately demonstrate this truth with any certainty, and only that knowledge derived in this manner counts as true scientific knowledge. The received view, as the dominant contemporary conception of science, conflicts sharply with what Polkinghorne (1983) calls the postpositivist view. A postpositivist conception of scientific knowledge and truth has evolved in reaction to the rather obvious limitations of the received view, especially for the human sciences. This view holds that the pursuit of knowledge and truth is necessarily historical, contextual, and theory laden. It claims no access to certain truth or knowledge but rather accepts certain knowledge to be "true" if it withstands practical tests of reason and utility. In this way, although knowledge may be useful, it is still fallible. Postpositivism does not cling to any one method of science and in fact encourages the use of the most appropriate method for the particular research question. Polkinghorne notes that "those methods are acceptable which produce results that convince the community that the new understanding is deeper, fuller, and more useful than the previous understanding" (Polkinghorne, 1983, p. 3).

The received view, or logical positivist approach to science, conforms closely to the correspondence norms of truth (Kaplan, 1964). What constitutes truth is the degree of correspondence between facts and their related theories and the degree to which propositions can be verified or shown to be false. Truth can be achieved only when it is shown that a proposition cannot be falsified. The received view also relies, in part, on the coherence theory of truth and its appreciation of theoretical aesthetics and logical simplicity in content and form. The postpositivist view, on the other hand, aligns itself with the pragmatic theory of truth, which emphasizes practical utility in problem solving and the degree of community consensus about that utility.

In the conduct of research positivism lends itself to reductionistic observables that must be quantified and verified, while postpositive concerns can be deductive or inductive in nature and can use either quantitative or qualitative strategies. It is clear that whether a researcher has positivist or postpositivist leanings and consciously or unconsciously subscribes to one theory of truth over another, these beliefs have a major effect on the formulation of the research question and the methodological strategy chosen. Thus it is unlikely that a researcher steeped in positivistic principles would ever ask a research question requiring the existential research methods of hermeneutic analysis.

A researcher's world view is also shaped by his or her beliefs about the *nature of nursing science.* Whether or not one believes that nursing is a "science of human health and behavior across the life span" (Gortner, 1983, p. 5) and is specifically concerned with "the diagnosis and treatment of human responses to actual or potential health problems" (American Nurses' Association, 1980, p. 9) has ultimate implications for the types of events, states, and situations perceived to be problematic. Although client, nursing, environment, and health have all been considered phenomena central to nursing (Fawcett, 1978), one might disagree as to the emphasis that one component has in relation to another or on whether some or all of these concepts must be included in a theoretical formulation for nursing. For example, Stevens (1979) deemphasizes the environmental aspects, while Fawcett (1978) states that at least one or more of the four concepts must be present if the theory is to be called a nursing theory. Flaskerud and Halloran (1980) insist that the concept of nursing must always be included in any theoretical formulation for it to be considered nursing theory, while Conway (1985) believes the inclusion of nursing is inappropriate.

Whether nursing science is believed to conform more to a human science model (postpositivist) or to a natural science model (positivist) also has implications for the formulation of research problems. As a human science nursing must take into account various characteristics of the human realm. For example, the systemic character of human phenomena and the unclear nature of their boundaries are important to consider (Polkinghorne, 1983). The former necessitates investigating the whole rather than its individual parts, while the latter implies acceptance of indistinct conceptual boundaries. The process nature of the human realm must also be taken into consideration, as it signifies continual growth and repatterning over time. This implies the use of longitudinal or time series designs to fully explicate our phenomena of interest (Metzger & Schultz, 1982).

Fundamental to human sciences is the additional awareness that our perceptions about human phenomena are limited by our perceptions as human being. Total objectivity is an unattainable ideal because "there is no absolute point outside phenomena from which to investigate. Moreover, the knowledge gained in the investigation changes the character of what has been investigated" (Polkinghorne, 1983, p. 263). It also is not possible to directly access the human realm by direct observation. Rather, it must be observed indirectly through our interpretation of human behavioral expressions. This is an important point, since one of the major forms of human expression is through language. This implies that access to human phenomena is rightly obtained from written or oral expressions, for example. Credibility is thus established for subjective data collection methods that include interviews and questionnaires. A natural science mode, however, dictates a hypotheticodeductive approach to research with reliance on objective quantitative methods.

This notion of nursing as a human science—one modeled after a natural science—also has implications for expectations regarding nursing's scientific advancement. Some authors (Hardy, 1983; Newman, 1983) propose carte blanche acceptance of Kuhn's model for scientific growth, even though Kuhn clearly indicates that the model was developed for natural sciences (Kuhn, 1970). Expecting periods of normal science that will be periodically interrupted by scientific revolutions is perhaps unrealistic for nursing as a human science (Meleis, 1985). It may, in fact, lead to erroneous conclusions about scientific progress and, worse yet, hopelessly distort nursing's future direction. Kuhn points out that the rigid pattern of education for normal activity in the natural sciences "is not well designed to produce the man who will easily discover a fresh approach" (Kuhn, 1970, p. 166). It might well be that alleged patterns of revolution in natural science exist only because there is no other way for creative change to occur or for discoveries to be incorporated in such severely structured disciplines. It is clear that an investigator's fundamental beliefs about the nature of human beings, the nature of knowledge and truth, and the nature of nursing science contribute mightily to the definition of a research problem and ultimately to its solution.

Cognitive Style

It has long been observed that individuals have a preferred style of problem solving (Bloom & Broder, 1950) and that this style is a major factor in successful problem solving (Shouksmith, 1970). These cognitive styles "represent a person's typical modes of perceiving, remembering, thinking and problem solving" (Messick, 1970, p. 188). As such, cognitive styles exert a major influence on both the identification of a research problem and the ultimate approach to a solution.

In his theory of experiential learning, Kolb (1981) conceives of learning as a fourstage cycle that includes observations and reflections, formation of abstract concepts and generalizations, testing of implications of concepts and new situations, and concrete experience. Four kinds of abilities are required if this process is to be effective. Concrete experience (CE) is characterized by open, unbiased involvement, while the second ability, reflective observation (RO) involves considering experiences from many perspectives. Abstract conceptualization (AC) involves formulation and integration of concepts into logical and sound theories, and active experimentation (AE) reflects the ability to apply these theories in decision making and problem solving. These abilities can be considered polar opposites on two bisecting dimensions with CE and AC on either end of one continuum and AE and RO as opposites on the other. Kolb points out that the most sophisticated and highly evolved ability, that of creative insight, actually involves synthetic interaction between these abstract and concrete dimensions. In addition, individuals appear to develop cognitive styles that generally emphasize some abilities over others, and those abilities remain remarkably stable over time. It can be demonstrated, however, that styles tend to become somewhat more reflective and analytical as an individual gets older.

Through his research Kolb identifies four cognitive styles. *Convergers* operate predominantly between abstract conceptualization and active experimentation, with an aptitude toward practical application of ideas. These persons approach problems in a hypotheticodeductive way, focusing on a single solution to a problem, often preferring to deal with nonhuman entities. The opposite of convergers are *divergers,* whose abilities lie in concrete experience and reflective observation. These people are "idea generators" who have strong and active imaginations and who are able to connect many unrelated but specific instances into a meaningful whole. Divergers are social and aesthetic in orientation and are often drawn to the humanities and the liberal arts. *Assimilators* operate predominantly in the abstract conceptualization and reflective observation modes and thus show great strength in inductive reasoning and theory formulation. These people are drawn to the logical and the abstract, with little attention to the need for practical application. *Accommodators,* operating on the opposite dimension from assimilators, are adept at concrete experience and active experimentation. These are action-oriented, risk-taking individuals who are often involved in implementation of an idea or a study. Accommodators are highly adaptive to changing situations and use the trial and error approach to problem solving.

These cognitive styles provide a useful way to conceive of general learning and problem-solving styles in individuals. Kolb (1981) warns against strict stereotyping, however, noting that research on cognitive style has consistently demonstrated how diverse and complex these processes actually are in real life. For example, cognitive function will vary in an individual according to the cognitive domain or situational demand.

The four cognitive styles described by Kolb (1981) can be related to inquiry norms in an academic discipline as well. Natural sciences and mathematics generally fall into the abstract-reflective quadrant; science-based professions are abstract-active; and social professions are more concrete-active. The concrete-reflective quadrant is characteristic of humanities and social sciences. Interestingly, in one study of a single university setting described by Kolb (1981), nursing fell into the abstract-active quadrant (converger), while in a much larger study nursing students and faculty fell into the concrete-reflective (diverger) category.

Kolb also proposes a typology of knowledge structures and inquiry processes in academic disciplines, suggesting that "forms of knowledge in different fields can be differentially attractive and meaningful to individuals with different learning styles" (Kolb, 1981, p. 245). That convergers would be drawn to or flourish in science-based empirical disciplines devoted to discrete analysis and conformance to correspondence norms is not surprising, nor is the attraction that the humanities and social science hold for divergers who profess to humanism, norms of coherence, and the conduct of research by historical analysis, field study, or clinical observation. That individuals with various cognitive styles would be attracted to nursing is also not surprising given the acknowledged complex and multifaceted nature of nursing's domain of interest. Certain cognitive styles are undoubtedly drawn to some scientific inquiry strategies more than others. For instance, the assimilator style might prefer theory generation using grounded theory methodology (Glaser & Strauss, 1967), while the accommodator style might choose involvement in clinical trials or intervention studies. A researcher whose predominant style is that of a converger might choose to be involved in theory-testing physiological research with animal subjects, while divergers might be drawn to phenomenological studies. Cognitive style appears to be a variable with major influence in a model of scientific inquiry.

Experience

The role of personal experience in scientific inquiry should not be underestimated. Both *life experience and professional nursing experience* provide fertile ground for problem awareness to grow. Problem identification and formulation of the research question become the fruit of that experience. Evidence of the verification or refutation of theories in the real world is also provided by this experience. Theories that work well are easily identified, while theories that fall short can be revised, extended, or discarded. Anomalous cases become readily apparent, as do continuing perplexities that remain unexplained by existing theories. One's sense of substantive significance stems from this experience, and intuition serves as a guide to the problems that have the most personal and professional meaning.

Prior *research experience* is also an important aspect of this variable, for it is through this experience that investigators learn which questions are able to be answered by current methods, which research approaches have worked in the past, and which ones

have not. Experience also teaches what research needs to be conducted in the future and how it might best be accomplished. It also tells researchers whether prior research endeavors fit well enough with what Luria (1973) calls their research style. If prior research experience has been satisfactory and successful, an attempt will be made to replicate aspects contributing to that success, whether substantive or methodological in nature. While research success teaches investigators to utilize similar problem-solving strategies in the future, less than successful research is often as instructive because of the demand for increasingly novel and creative approaches in subsequent studies.

Theoretical experience is another type of experience that affects the process of inquiry. One aspect of this experience relies upon the existing knowledge base in a substantive area and the researcher's individual perception of that knowledge base. Theoretical experience allows the researcher to identify the existing gaps in knowledge and the significant areas that remain unexplored or unexplained. Individual researcher perception is important in this type of experience, for it is that perception that drives interest in unexplored domains. Scientific advancement depends on theoretical experience over time because of the necessarily progressive nature of research questions based on prior studies. Insight gained from longstanding familiarity with theoretical issues is of inestimable value and contributes to the overall level of understanding about the phenomenon of interest. This level of understanding in turn affects the content and level of subsequent research questions.

A second aspect of theoretical experience relates to the degree to which the researcher has been open to various theoretical approaches and intellectual strategies related to the exploration of the research problem area. If the researcher remains intellectually open to diverging and opposing views, the quality of theoretical understanding will be affected even though initial theoretical orientation may be maintained. Obviously the greater the clarity of understanding of the problem area the greater the possibility of significant answers. This type of intellectual exploration also allows for greater problem tension to exist, which in turn results in greater efforts to resolve the problems (Polyani, 1962). Bruner (1966) points out that it is precisely this dialectical tension between the concrete and the abstract that allows for creativity in problem solving.

Methodological Knowledge and Skill

The level and type of methodological knowledge and skill possessed by a researcher have a major influence on the process and product of scientific inquiry. Since the seeds of the answer lie in every research question (Mackinnon, 1979) and it is asserted that researchers have a preferred style of problem solving (Kolb, 1981), it is natural that researchers pose research questions that they will be able to answer. Kaplan calls this the "law of the instrument" and observes that "it comes as no particular surprise to discover that a scientist formulates problems in a way which requires for their solution just those techniques in which he himself is especially skilled" (Kaplan, 1964, p. 28). He also points out that the cost of becoming an expert in any one research area results in what can be called a "trained incapacity." That is, the more expert one becomes in something the harder it is to solve a problem any other way. Maslow agrees, asserting that "it is tempting, if the only tool you have is a hammer, to treat everything as if it were a nail" (Maslow, 1966, pp. 15–16).

It would seem that the relationship of methodological skills to the formulation of the research question and the process of inquiry for a single investigator study is closer than is often admitted. This limitation may be easier to overcome in larger studies with more than one investigator or over many studies, each conducted by different investigators. Capitalizing on the methodological strengths of multiple investigators to study complex nursing phenomena allows for greater theoretical possibilities through the use of multiple research methods. Polkinghorne points out that multiple methods allow more to be learned about a research problem than could be discovered from any one procedure or method alone (Polkinghorne, 1983).

Extrapersonal Factors

Two classes of extrapersonal variables are proposed to relate to the process and practice of scientific inquiry: influential others and the sociohistoric context.

Influential Others

Two major types of influence on scientific inquiry are inherent in the variable of influential others: individual and institutional. Individual influences are initially conveyed primarily by mentors and other professors in graduate school, the primary wellspring of research values and training for the budding nursing scientist (Tinkle & Beaton, 1983). Here, individual faculty methodological preferences and research values are made known implicitly or explicitly, and disciplinary norms are passed on (Kuhn, 1970). Expectations regarding appropriate methods of scientific inquiry are embedded in each experience and are reinforced at every juncture. It is the prevailing "faculty view" that determines the ultimate breadth and depth of curricular exposure to various research strategies, and it is faculty expertise that delimits actual research opportunities for students. It is here in graduate research training that a nursing scientist's individual research style is born (Luria, 1973).

While the acquisition of disciplinary norms is unquestionably important, the notion implies existing disciplinary consensus on what those norms actually are. Nursing has not quite come to such a conscious consensus, although there is no evidence of the consistent use of diverse research methods to study nursing's complex phenomena (Jacobsen & Meininger, 1985). When disciplinary research norms are not collectively shared, Toulmin points out that "theoretical debate in the field becomes largely—and unintentionally—methodological and philosophical; it is directed less at interpreting particular empirical findings than at debating the general acceptability (or unacceptability) of rival approaches, patterns of explanation and standards of judgment." (Toulmin, 1972, p. 380). The result is, of course, adamant assertions about one method over another, and the student scientist may be forced early on to align with one camp or another. Thus the norms that sense of professional pride will prevail and nursing's scientific competence will be rightly judged by the ability to solve the discipline's most significant problems.

REFERENCES

Albert, R. S. (Ed.). (1983). *Genius and eminence: The social psychology of creativity and exceptional achievement.* Oxford, England: Pergamon Press.

American Nurses' Association (1980). *Nursing: A social policy statement.* Kansas City: Author.

Batey, M. V. (1977). Conceptualization: Knowledge and logic guiding empirical research. *Nursing Research, 26*(5), 324–329.

Bigge, M. (1982). *Learning theories for teachers* (4th ed.). New York: Harper & Row.

Bloom, B., & Broder, C. (1950). *The problem solving process of college students.* Chicago: University of Chicago Press.

Brink, P., & Wood, M. (1983). *Basic steps in planning nursing research, from question to proposal* (2nd ed.). Monterey, CA: Wadsworth.

Bronowski, J. (1965). *Science and human values.* New York: Harper & Row.

Bruner, J. (1966). *The process of education.* New York: Atheneum.

Carper, B. A. (1978). Fundamental patterns of knowing in nursing. *Advances in Nursing Science, 1*(1), 13–23.

Claxton, C., & Ralston, Y. (1978). *Learning styles: Their impact on teaching and administration.* Washington, DC: The American Association for Higher Education.

Conway, M. (1985). Toward greater specificity in defining nursing's metaparadigm. *Advances in Nursing Science, 7*(4), 73–81.

Dickoff, J., James, P., & Weidenbach, E. (1968). Theory in a practice discipline: Part I—practice oriented theory. *Nursing Research, 17*(5), 415–435.

Donaldson, S. K., & Crowley, D. M. (1978). The discipline of nursing. *Nursing Outlook, 26*(2), 113–120.

Fawcett, J. (1978). The relationship between theory and research: A double helix. *Advances in Nursing Science, 1*(1), 49–62.

Feyerabend, P. (1981). How to defend society against science. In I. Hacking (Ed.), *Scientific revolutions.* London: Oxford University Press.

Flaskerud, J. H., & Halloran, E. J. (1980). Areas of agreement in nursing theory development. *Advances in Nursing Science, 3*(1),1–7.

Glaser, B., & Strauss, A. (1967). *The discovery of grounded theory: Strategies of qualitative research.* New York: Aldine.

Goldstein, M., & Goldstein, I. (1978). *How we know: An exploration of the scientific process.* New York: Plenum Press.

Gortner, S., & Nahm, H. (1977). An overview of nursing research in the United States. *Nursing Research, 26,* 10–33.

Gortner, S. (1983). The history and philosophy of nursing science and research. *Advances in Nursing Science, 5*(2), 1–8.

Hardy, M. (1983). Metaparadigms and theory development. In N. L. Chaska (Ed.), *The nursing profession: A time to speak* (pp. 427–435). New York: McGraw-Hill.

Jacobsen, B., & Meininger, J. (1985). The design and methods of published nursing research: 1956–1983. *Nursing Research, 34,* 306–311.

Jacox, A. (1974). Theory construction in nursing: An overview. *Nursing Research, 23*(1), 4–13.

Jacox, A. (1981, June). *Competing theories of science.* Paper presented at the 1981 Forum on Doctoral Education in Nursing, Seattle, WA, June 1981.

Kaplan, A. (1964). *The conduct of inquiry.* New York: Harper & Row.

Kerlinger, F. (1973). *Foundations of behavioral research* (2nd ed.). New York: Holt, Rinehart & Winston.

Kolb, D. (1981). Learning styles and disciplinary differences. In A. Chickering (Ed.), *The modern American college* (pp. 232–255). San Francisco: Jossey-Bass.

Kuhn, T. S. (1970). *The structure of scientific revolutions* (2nd ed.). Chicago: University of Chicago Press.

Luria, S. E. (1973). On research styles and allied matters. *Daedalus, 102*(2), 75–84.

Mackinnon, D. (1979). Creativity: A multifaceted phenomenon. In J. D. Roslansky (Ed.), *Creativity* (pp. 19–32). Amsterdam: North-Holland.

Martin, J. (1982). A garbage can model of the research process. In J. McGrath, J. Martin, & R. Kulka (Eds.), *Judgment calls in research* (pp. 17–39). Beverly Hills, CA: Sage.

Maslow, A. H. (1966). *The psychology of science: A reconnaissance.* South Bend, IN: Gateway Editions.

McGrath, J. E. (1982). Dilemmatics: The study of research choices and dilemmas. In J. McGrath, J. Martin, & R. Kulka (Eds.), *Judgment calls in research* (pp. 69–102). Beverly Hills, CA: Sage.

Meleis, A. I. (1985). *Theoretical nursing: Development and progress.* Philadelphia: J.B. Lippincott.

Messick, S. (1970). The criterion problem in the evaluation of instruction: Assessing possible, not just intended extremes. In M. Wittrock & D. Riley (Eds.), *Evaluation of instruction: Issues and problems.* New York: Holt, Rinehart & Winston.

Metzger, B., & Schultz, S. (1982). Time series analysis: An alternative for nursing. *Nursing Research, 31*(6), 375–378.

Newman, M. A. (1983). The continuing revolution: A history of nursing science. In N. L. Chaska (Ed.), *The nursing profession: A time to speak* (pp. 385–393). New York: McGraw-Hill.

Nicholls, J. G. (1983). Creativity in the person who will never produce anything original or useful. In R. S. Albert (Ed.), *Genius and eminence: The social psychology of creativity and exceptional achievement* (pp. 265–279). Oxford, England: Pergamon Press.

Noddings, N., & Shore, P. (1984). *Awakening the inner eye intuition in education.* New York: Teachers College Press.

Oiler, C. (1982). The phenomenological approach in nursing research. *Nursing Research, 31*(3), 178–181.

Polanyi, M. (1962). *Personal knowledge.* Chicago: University of Chicago Press.

Polit, D., & Hungler, B. (1983). *Nursing research: Principles and methods* (2nd ed.). Philadelphia, J.B. Lippincott.

Polkinghorne, D. (1983). *Methodology for the human science systems of inquiry.* Albany, NY: State University of New York Press.

Rogers, M. E. (1970). *A theoretical basis for nursing.* Philadelphia: F.A. Davis.

Roy, S. C. (1983). Theory development in nursing: Proposal for direction. In N. L. Chaska (Ed.), *The nursing profession: A time to speak* (pp. 453–465). New York: McGraw-Hill.

Runkel, P., & McGrath, J. (1972). *Research on human behavior: A systematic guide to method.* New York: Holt, Rinehart & Winston.

Shouksmith, G. (1970). *Intelligence, creativity and cognitive style.* New York: Wiley Interscience.

Stevens, B. (1979). *Nursing theory: Analysis, application, evaluation.* Boston: Little, Brown.

Suppe, F. (1977). *The structure of scientific theories* (2nd ed.). Chicago: University of Illinois Press.

Thompson, J. (1985). Practical discourse in nursing: Going beyond empiricism and historicism. *Advances in Nursing Science, 7*(4), 59–71.

Tinkle, M. B., & Beaton, J. L. (1983). Toward a new view of science: Implications for nursing research. *Advances in Nursing Science, 5*(2), 27–36.

Tucker, R. (1979). The value decisions we know as science. *Advances in Nursing Science, 1*(2), 1–12.

Toulmin, S. (1972). *Human understanding* (Vol. 1). Oxford, England: Clarendon Press.

Von Bertalanffy, L. (1968). *General system theory.* New York: George Braziller.

Weiskopf, V. (1973). Introduction. In H. Yukawa (Ed.), *Creativity and intuition: A physicist looks east and west* (J. Bester, trans.). Tokyo: Kodansha International.

Wilson, H. S. (1985). *Research in nursing.* Menlo Park, CA: Addison-Wesley.

Worthy, M. (1975). *Aha! A puzzle approach to creative thinking.* Chicago: Nelson Hall.

Yukawa, H. (1973). *Creativity and intuition: A physicist looks at east and west* (J. Bester, trans.). Tokyo: Kodansha International.

The Author Comments

Scientific Inquiry in Nursing: A Model for a New Age

This work arose from an intensely passionate intellectual process that kept me in its grips for the first 2 years of doctoral study at the University of California, San Francisco. Coursework in theory development, the philosophy of science, and research methods challenged my assumptions about the research process, forcing a reflective process unlike any I had ever experienced. To understand my role as a budding nurse scientist and how I might best contribute to nursing's knowledge base, I struggled with the question, "How does science really happen?" and, more to the point, "What factors truly affect the conduct of research?" It seemed reasonable that insight into the many influences and pressures I was facing in defining my own research interests would be crucial to the resolution of these issues in my career. Fortunately, the new understanding I gained led to the creation of the model for scientific inquiry in nursing and a sense of peace about my career decisions.

—HOLLY A. DEGROOT

But there is an important differentiation of concepts that is critical to this discussion. Ordinary or everyday concepts are not the same as scientific concepts (for this discussion, see Mitcham, 1999; Morse, 2000; Rodgers, 2000a). Ordinary concepts are those used by people in everyday life. They have a common meaning, which may be implicit but is understandable within that cultural unit. Ordinary definitions of concepts are found in the dictionary. They change over time to reflect common usage, for example, "soccer mom" or "globalization" now carry conceptual meanings that have evolved through usage. Twenty or 30 years ago, these concepts would have been meaningless.

Scientific concepts are a different entity in that a degree of precision is required in order for the conceptual label to encompass a unit of meaning that is used consistently within a scientific discipline. These concepts require a more specific or narrow definition so that those using the conceptual unit in scientific endeavors are clearly using it in the same way, with the same meaning, so that findings are meaningfully understood (Morse, 2000). The concern of science with specification of concept usage is reflected in the issues of construct validity. Conceptual clarity is necessary for solid theoretical integration (Knafl & Deatrick, 2000). Therefore, scientific concepts are more precise meaning units that when linked together propositionally form a theoretical representation of reality.

This difference in types of concepts (ordinary vs. scientific) is important to concept analysis techniques. Scientific endeavors rely on more precisely defined concepts (Mitcham, 1999; Morse, 2000). When ordinary or implied meanings of concepts are used to build theory in scientific enterprises, the waters are muddied (e.g., see Hupcey, Penrod, Morse, & Mitcham, 2001). For example, when considering trust in nurse-patient relationships, is *my* conceptualization of trust the same as the next reader's? Is trust different from *reliance?* If so, how? It is important for conceptual units of scientific theory to be explicit in their representation of a precise meaning of an element of human experience. In this article, we assert that the *scientific* understanding of a concept is the concern of concept analysis, not ordinary conceptual meaning. This is not to say that ordinary meaning has no merit in scientific work, rather this form of data is relevant to concept advancement techniques, not concept analysis.

Concepts-Theory Linkages

Often, as scientific units of meaning, concepts are described as building blocks of theory (Fawcett, 1978), triggering images of a brick and mortar wall. Using this analogy, theory is built block by block as a process of stacking and securing concepts together. This view is problematic in that the linkages between concepts are presented as linear, a rather simplistic approach. For example, a "block" (concept) on the first course of the "wall" (theory) may be integrally linked with a "block" on the third course—yet the two don't touch or link in any way except to support the "wall" (theory). Thus, this representation is inadequate in illustrating the complex integration of concepts important to nursing and other sciences concerned with human experiences or behaviors.

Hempel (1966) offers a different concept-theory analogy in his work in natural science, describing concepts as the "knots in a network of systematic interrelationships" (p. 94). Extending this analogy, theory could be represented as a tapestry of interwoven, knotted conceptual threads (Penrod & Hupcey, 2005). Thus, no single strand (i.e., concept) in the tapestry (i.e., theory) stands apart from the others in a meaningful way. To pull one conceptual thread from the tapestry produces a piece of string or thread (i.e., the concept) that no longer reveals its accent or color within the larger pattern (i.e., conceptual meaning).

The tapestry analogy is useful to emphasize the importance of strong, well-integrated concepts for supporting theory. However, there is a deeper implication in this analogy that warrants some consideration: concepts are assigned meaning through placement within the context of theory. If we were to examine only red threads pulled from different tapestries, we could analyze the characteristics of threads themselves; however, the contribution of these threads to each tapestry lies in the contrast and intricacies developed when the red thread is knotted and woven with other strands in the larger work. That is, concepts cannot be analyzed irrespective of their theoretical frame. Paley (1996) has argued that concepts must be examined within the niches created in specific theories integrating those concepts. He asserts that the most meaningful way to clarify concepts is to examine the theories in which the concepts are embedded. We agree with Paley and have further asserted that the power of concept analysis (and subsequently, methods of advancing the concept) is to identify the existing theoretical strands and, ultimately, to tie and retie the conceptual knots to form a stronger, more coherent tapestry of nursing theory (Penrod & Hupcey, 2005).

Concepts that are of concern to the caring sciences, including nursing, are embedded in complex tapestries of behavioral, cognitive and emotive meaning (e.g., theories). It is difficult, if not impossible, to untangle the discrete thread of a concept from this tapestry of meaning. Therefore, attempts to isolate a concept in the process of analysis become an artificial endeavor. We cannot isolate concepts that are inherently linked in abstract meaning without in some way limiting the utility of analysis for understanding complex human experiences. From a practical perspective, this means that the scientific literature that precisely orders or interprets ordinary conceptual meaning, must be analyzed for explicit and implicit meaning during the analytic process. Implicit meaning may be derived through an analysis of the positioning of concepts in a theoretical frame or by linguistic cues. We assert that scientific concepts cannot be critically analyzed if pulled from or isolated from the broader theoretical landscape without seriously compromising the value of the analytic product. In other words, processes of concept analysis must examine multiple theoretical frames to derive insights regarding conceptual meaning that transcend specific theoretical bounds and ring true to the human construction of meaning with the degree of precision required in scientific endeavors.

Far too often, manuscripts related to concept analyses describe the literature surrounding a word label without ever addressing the scientific meaning of the concept in any depth. In these papers, there is an obvious lack of conceptual thinking as the author processes mounds of literature from a narrow and restricted perspective. Available methods of concept analysis may be easily misconstrued to permit such superficial analysis, especially those that prescribe the concoction of contrived cases to support the analysis. Often, these model cases suffer an obvious lack of depth and the derived conceptualization is unable to capture the meanings inherent to complex human experiences (for further discussion, see Hupcey, Morse, Lenz, & Tasón, 1996). Such endeavors fall short of truly determining scientific meaning in a way that permits an understanding of the state of the science surrounding the concept.

Concept-Truth Linkages

We believe that the power of concept analysis lies in identifying how a concept works within existing theories in order to derive a theoretical definition of the mean-ing ascribed to that concept. This definition of meaning derived from the contextual basis of the science (that is, theories) represents the "state of the science." This assertion is rooted in our metaphysical perspectives of truth or reality, primarily ontology. On one hand, truth could be conceived as an absolute value that can be discovered through precise scientific endeavors. On the other hand, truth can be conceived as a construction of those who experience a given phenomenon at a given point in time. Somewhere between these two endpoints of a continuum, there is a middle ground—a stance that accepts the power of the human experience in formu-lating conceptual meaning that is subsequently clarified through language expounding that meaning within a specific theoretical context for scientific use.

Kikuchi's (2003) interpretation of moderate realism embraces a quest for understanding reality focusing on *probable* truth rather than *absolute* truth. Concepts are abstracted through a cognitive process that is based on percepts (formed through perceptions along with memory and imagination). Concepts are, therefore, "grounded in reality or empirically derived" (p. 12).

Context becomes critical as the individual is situated in a set of circumstances that influences percepts and the abstraction of concepts. Yet the convergence of what is known through a rigorous examination of these multiple contextually based conceptions reveals the *probable* truth that is embraced by moderate realists. Moderate realism asserts, "reality exists independent of the human mind" (p. 12), supporting a notion that probable truth transcends individual experience.

Using the tapestry analogy, concept analysis centers on following and pulling selected conceptual threads in multiple tapestries of meaning. The insights gleaned through each examination (now new threads of meaning) are then rewoven or reknotted and tie into a new tapestry of meaning for that concept. The theoretical tapestry represents the probable truth revealed through an examination of multiple, and often, divergent contextual conceptualizations of concepts grounded in empirical, human experiences.

This is the position that we adopt in this series of papers. Through techniques of concept analysis, conceptual insights are isolated and examined. These insights are then integrated into a summative view of the state of the science surrounding the concept of interest. Since concepts are the backbone of theory *in practice* (that is, concepts help nurses to organize meaning to understand complex human experiences and behaviors in ways that influence the practice of nursing) such work is a critically important scientific endeavor.

Given this perspective, we propose that it is time to clarify methodological approaches to concept analysis and concept advancement. Concept analysis is a means for identifying scholars' best efforts at establishing the probable truth as reflected in the scientific literature. In this case, the label "scientific literature" refers to scholarly works pertaining to the concept of interest, including empirical, theoretical, and philosophical writings. The goal of concept analysis is to establish the state of the science. As such, concept analysis has the potential to serve as an essential method of inquiry in a progressive nursing science, not merely as an academic exercise. We believe that the findings of a critical concept analysis provide evidence for determining the most appropriate means for subsequently advancing the concept. In essence, concept advancement techniques progressively build the concept by explicating implicit meaning into more abstract theoretical formulations that transcend contextual conceptions. Such a clarification of methods supports an evolutionary turn toward praxis by uniting nursing research, theory, and practice in a way that, we believe, could advance the science of nursing significantly.

Traditional Approaches to Concept Analysis

A number of approaches are used to guide the process of "concept analysis" in nursing. It is important to note, however, that the terms describing the overarching analytic processes, purposes for using such techniques, and the nature of the findings produced by each method differ. Ultimately these factors affect the critical examination of the concept, and may result in analytic findings that do not truly reflect the state of the science. Others have critiqued common techniques of concept analysis (for example, see Hupcey, Morse, Lenz, & Tasón, 1996). For clarity, we provide a brief overview of the approaches described by: Wilson (1963), Walker and Avant (1995), Chinn and Kramer (1995), Rodgers (2000b), and Schwartz-Barcott and Kim (2000) (further delineated by Schwartz-Barcott, Patterson, Lusardi, & Farmer, 2002). Our focus in this review centers on the purpose, process, and products of these methods.

Wilson (1963) introduced a method of examining concepts that involved discussion of 11 considerations: questions of concept; 'right answers'; model cases; contrary cases; related cases; borderline cases; invented cases; social context; underlying anxiety (of the researcher); practical results; and results in language. This ambitious discourse endures as a classic reference in concept analysis literature. While Wilson's intent was not to delineate a method of concept analysis, this analytic process serves as the basis for many methods of concept analysis in nursing.

Although Wilson (1963) described the purpose of his work as, "set[ting] forth a framework through which one can build understanding of the essential meaning of a concept in varied contexts" (p. 93), he also stated that "the analysis of concepts is essentially an imaginative process; certainly it is more of an art than a science" (p. 33). This emphasis on process or the art of exploring concepts overshadows the notion of a product. A Wilsonian analysis enhances critical thinking processes, but does not necessarily produce documentation of a scientific examination of a concept (i.e., a product). Herein arises the difficulty in applying this method to scientific endeavors; while the art of the imagination contributes to the derivation of the scientific conceptualization, the influence of imaginative processes often precludes the "evidence" found in the literature that reflects the essential meaning of the concept within a scientific context (especially complex behavioral concepts, like trust or uncertainty). The difficulty with Wilson's text is that, while insightful and very comprehensive, it fails to prepare one to embark on a methodological analysis of the state of the concept in the science (reflected soundly in the literature).

Walker and Avant (1983, 1988, 1995) describe concept analysis as a technique of concept development that is used when the concept is unclear, outmoded, or unhelpful. This method adapts Wilson's work into an eight-step process: select a concept; determine aims or purposes of analysis; identify uses; determine defining attributes; construct a model case; construct borderline/related/contrary/invented/and illegitimate cases; identify antecedents and consequences; and define empirical referents. Both qualitative and quantitative techniques are prescribed within this process. The purpose of this technique is described as theory development. The products of the process include clear and precise theoretical and operational definitions for use in research (1995, p. 46), thus supporting the achievement of the purpose. Concepts are defined as evolving ("change over time," 1995, p. 37) within a constructivist perspective. "The best one can hope for from a concept analysis is to capture the critical elements of it at the current moment in time" (1995, p. 37). While this approach to concept analysis is perhaps, in our experience, the most commonly used in nursing, this method often fails to produce an analysis of the concept that reaches the degree of insight implied by the authors. Of primary concern, how does the researcher come to know that the concept is unclear, outmoded, or unhelpful without a full analytic review of the state of the science?

Chinn and Kramer's (1991, 1995; Chinn & Jacobs, 1983, 1987) approach to concept analysis is an adaptation of the work of Wilson and Walker and Avant. They assert that the primary purpose of concept analysis is the development of theory. Their technique focuses on five steps: select a concept; clarify the purpose; identify data sources; explore context and values; and formulate criteria. It is interesting to note their emphasis on constructed exemplary cases and the inclusion of diverse data sources including popular literature, visual images, and people. The purpose of the analytic process described by these scholars is to identify, clarify, and examine the word label, the phenomenon represented by the label, and the values, feelings, and attitudes that are associated with both the symbol and the phenomenon. The product of this process is considered to be tentative in nature and subject to alteration and change as new evidence becomes available. This method extends analysis beyond the state of the science into the personal and societal realms. While we agree that such conceptualizations (the personal and the societal) are critical to advancing a concept to capture the empirical essence of the human experience, we do not believe that these realms of meaning are appropriate to discerning the probable truth exposed in the scientific literature.

Rodgers (1993, 2000b) described an 'Evolutionary View' of concept analysis that is embedded in the cycle of concept development. The purpose of concept analysis is "clarification of the concept and its current use, and uncovering the attributes of the concept as a basis for further development" (2000b, p. 83). In this method, Rodgers attempted to move beyond the essential features of a concept to capture "the dynamic nature of concepts, changing with both time and context" (2000b, p. 99). The process in this form of concept analysis was designed around the dynamic (not static) perspective of a concept: identifying the concept;

choosing the setting and sample (literature); collecting and managing the data; analyzing the data; identifying a model case; interpreting the results; and identifying implications. The product of analysis (or results) is described as a heuristic device to provide "the clarity necessary to create a foundation for further inquiry and development" (2000b, p. 84). Emphasizing the cyclic nature of concept development even further, Rodgers (1993) said,

> I do not consider the attributes of a concept to be a fixed set of necessary and sufficient conditions, or an *essence*. Consequently, . . . this cluster of attributes may change, by convention or by purposeful redefinition, over time to maintain a useful, applicable, and effective concept. (p. 75)

The evolutionary approach challenges an essentialist position on concepts. This method of concept analysis is based in a complex, intellectually rigorous integration of more contemporary philosophical positions. Such complexity makes it difficult to disentangle the process of concept analysis as separate and discrete from concept development. Application of this method has been more limited than more traditional forms of concept analysis (e.g., Walker & Avant), perhaps because it challenges our philosophical interpretation of concepts or perhaps because it depicts concepts as such dynamic entities that are difficult to grasp for scientific examination and use.

Schwartz-Barcott and Kim (1986, 1993, 2000) described their "Hybrid Model," which was originally developed in a doctoral course to merge philosophy of science, sociology, and field research into a three-phase approach to concept analysis: theoretical work (based in the literature); field work (based on empirical data); and analytical work (integrating the final product). Schwartz-Barcott and Kim (2000) described this process in terms of concept development and analysis with the implicit purpose of fortifying the "building blocks of a theory" (2000, p. 130) for ultimate integration. This method moves concept analysis from an academic mental exercise into the realm of clinically based fieldwork, thus making an important contribution

methodologically. However, the basis of the fieldwork (i.e., the theoretical work) remains underdeveloped. The method does not formulate a strong analysis of the state of the science from which to launch appropriate and well-focused fieldwork. Recently, Schwartz-Barcott and colleagues (2002) clarified their fieldwork strategies into three distinct pathways for clarifying and establishing theoretical congruence between a concept and clinical settings: theoretical selectivity; theoretical integration; and theory creation. The resultant products of the procedural application of the refined pathways are yet to be seen.

Emergent Perspectives on Concept Analysis

Despite the fact that the aforementioned methods of concept analysis were available and used in nursing, their application to phenomena of concern to nursing had varying degrees of success (Morse, Hupcey, Mitcham, & Lenz, 1996). In critical response to these methods, a series of papers on concept analysis published by Morse and colleagues (Hupcey et al., 1996; Morse, 1995; Morse, Hupcey, et al., 1996; Morse, Mitcham, Hupcey, & Tasón, 1996) presented new perspectives on concept analysis. One of the insightful notions regarding concept analysis was the need to establish "criteria for the evaluation of the level of maturity of concepts" (Morse, Mitcham, et al., p. 387). Maturity was defined as a concept which "is well-defined, has clearly described characteristics, delineated boundaries, and documented preconditions and outcomes" (Morse, Mitcham, et al., 1996, p. 387). The evaluation of conceptual maturity was based on four broad philosophical principles, epistemological, pragmatic, linguistic, and logical (Morse, Hupcey, et al., 1996). The epistemological principle sets criteria for conceptual definitions and differentiation. The pragmatic principle addresses criteria surrounding utility and fit of conceptualizations. The linguistic principle centers on consistency and appropriateness of use. And finally, the logical principle develops criteria for examination of theoretical integration with other concepts.

Thus, this series of papers provides an analytic lens through which the truth-value of current conceptualizations may be examined.

We believe that the principles described by Morse and colleagues (Hupcey et al., 1996; Morse, 1995; Morse, Hupcey, et al., 1996; Morse, Mitcham, et al., 1996) reveals the best estimate of probable truth evident in the scientific literature. The application of these analytic criteria has the potential to produce a principle-based examination of the concept as it appears in the scientific literature; however, use to date has been limited. From our experience, we have come to discover that the entanglement of analysis and advancement techniques muddles analytic processes, resulting in novice analysts wallowing in data and wondering when, or if, they will ever be finished with the project. Further, in order to address operational difficulties, we have clarified strategies for applying these principles in a concept analysis (Penrod & Hupcey, 2005). Yet, one thing is clear: principle-based concept analysis is a complex method and demands that the researcher *analyzes* scientific meaning (not everyday notions) and *thinks critically* (not imaginatively).

Discussion

Given these diverse approaches to concept analysis, it is not surprising that the potential contribution of concept analyses on the evolution of nursing science has been constrained. We believe that some of the limitations in the utility of the product of concept analyses are related to how nurse researchers and educators *think* about concept analysis. For example, while all of the approaches discussed above are somehow related (and taught) under the rubric of *concept analysis,* analytic terms are confused and entangled within broader concept-based research techniques, including concept development, creating conceptual meaning, and theory building. Data collection/field work appears to be premature in some approaches: how can the researcher proceed with fieldwork strategically until a thorough understanding of the state of the science is fully established? Therefore, clarifying the principles underlying concept analysis is a logical first step in addressing these methodological limitations.

First, we assert that the purpose of concept analysis is to determine the state of the science (or best estimate of probable truth) surrounding a concept of interest. Thus, concept analyses are concerned with scientific literature, not creative imagination, art forms, fiction, interview data, or any other form of representation. Second, the process of concept analysis is primarily at the level of integration, not synthesis. The researcher must engage in a thorough and thoughtful analysis of what is known by examining the implicit and explicit assumptions cited in the scientific literature (i.e., scholarly works pertaining to the concept of interest, including empirical, theoretical, and philosophical writings). Concept analysis is more than an organization of findings; the integrated perspective produces a higher level understanding of the concept of interest. In other words, when theoretical frameworks are examined for meaning and contextual boundaries are transcended, the evidence of probable truth is revealed. Therefore, the product of concept analysis is some form of a summary of the state of the science that reveals the scientific community's best estimate of probable truth, given the evidence portrayed in the extant literature. While this product certainly contributes to the science of nursing, it is not a form of concept advancement; it is an analysis of what is known.

In our view, principle-based concept analysis (Penrod & Hupcey, 2005) provides a useful and meaningful framework for determining the global state of the science (or probable truth) surrounding a concept. However, the real value of this emergent method lies in the evidence culled to support the summative conclusions (truth-value) related to each principle rather than on an assigned word label that denotes the degree of maturity (e.g., immature vs. partially mature). The notion of conceptual maturity is a significant contribution to understanding concepts, but the label that connotes level of maturity is insufficient for determining the most appropriate techniques for concept advancement.

This is an important methodological distinction. Concept analysis is an integration of what is known, not an evaluation of quality or maturity of the concept. Concept advancement is not driven by the label denoting level of maturity; rather, gaps in understanding identified through comprehensive principle-based concept analysis are the most significant findings that direct subsequent concept-based inquiries.

Principle-based concept analysis requires the researcher to focus on evidence found in the scientific literature, not constructed cases, imaginative exploration, or hypothetical exemplars. Through the integration of insights derived from a principle-based examination of the scientific literature, the researcher should be able to derive a summative paragraph (or theoretical definition) on what is known in order to expose gaps or inconsistencies in current thinking. This enables the researcher to strategically progress toward a deeper examination of divergent views to advance a better explication of probable truth.

Principle-based concept analysis appears to provide the most comprehensive examination of the concept within theoretical frames of reference documented in the scientific literature. By applying the overarching principles based in the philosophy of science, the analyst is forced to take a much broader stance in an examination of theory, research, and philosophy papers; but most importantly, the analysis is based in the scientific literature (not lay literature or other forms of representation). This analysis reveals the state of the science, and must be based in the literature of the selected disciplines.

Yet, even the application of such a comprehensive analytic technique will only provide us with a perspective of the state of the science, that is, the baseline understanding that enables the researcher to determine how to strategically advance the concept of interest by addressing identified gaps or inconsistencies. Concept analysis is the initial step in concept advancement; analysis must precede efforts at advancement. Analysis of a concept clarifies what is known of the concept at that time. As such, concept analysis can be used to estimate the probable truth revealed in the scientific literature as a first step in enhancing the knowledge base of the discipline. Such delimitation of analytic processes focuses the researcher on scientific perspectives of reality that can then be further developed through processes of concept advancement.

REFERENCES

Chinn, P. L., & Jacobs, M. K. (1983). *Theory and nursing: A systematic approach.* St. Louis: Mosby.

Chinn, P. L., & Jacobs, M. K. (1987). *Theory and nursing: A systematic approach* (2nd ed.). St. Louis: Mosby.

Chinn, P. L., & Kramer, M. K. (1991). *Theory and nursing: A systematic approach* (3rd ed). St. Louis: Mosby.

Chinn, P. L, & Kramer, M. K. (1995). *Theory and nursing: A systematic approach* (4th ed.). St. Louis: Mosby.

Fawcett, J. (1978). The relationship between theory and research: A double helix. *Advances in Nursing Science, 1*(1), 49–62.

Hempel, C. G. (1966). *Philosophy of natural science.* Englewood Cliffs, NJ: Prentice-Hall.

Hupcey, J. E., Morse, J. M., Lenz, E., & Tasón, M. C. (1996). Wilsonian methods of concept analysis: A critique. *Scholarly Inquiry for Nursing Practice, 10,* 185–210.

Hupcey, J. E., Penrod, J., Morse, J. M., & Mitcham, C. (2001). An exploration and advancement of the concept of trust. *Journal of Advanced Nursing, 36,* 282–293.

Kikuchi, J. (2003). Nursing knowledge and the problem of worldviews. *Research and Theory for Nursing Practice: An International Journal, 17*(1), 7–11.

King, I. M. (1988). Concepts: Essential elements of theories. *Nursing Science Quarterly, 7*(1), 22–25.

Knafl, K. A., & Deatrick, J. A. (2000). Knowledge synthesis and concept development in nursing. In B. L. Rodgers & K. A. Knafl (Eds.), *Concept development in nursing: Foundations, techniques, and applications* (2nd ed., pp. 39–54). Philadelphia: W. B. Saunders.

Merleau-Ponty, M. (1998). *Phenomenology of perception* (C. Smith, Trans.). New York: Routledge. (Original work published 1962).

Mitcham, C. (1999, February). Concepts of concepts: Philosophical perspectives. In J. M. Morse (Chair), *Issues in concept and theory development.* Symposium conducted at the Advances in Qualitative Methodology Conference, Edmonton, Canada.

Morse, J. M. (1995). Exploring the theoretical basis of nursing using advanced techniques of concept analysis. *Advances in Nursing Science, 17*(3), 31–46.

Morse, J. M. (2000). Exploring pragmatic utility: Concept analysis by critically appraising the literature. In B. L. Rodgers & K. A. Knafl (Eds.), *Concept development in nursing: Foundations, techniques, and applications* (2nd ed., pp. 333–352). Philadelphia: W. B. Saunders.

Morse, J. M., Hupcey, J., Mitcham, C., & Lenz, E. (1996). Concept analysis in nursing research: A critical appraisal. *Scholarly Inquiry for Nursing Practice, 10,* 257–281.

Morse, J. M., Mitcham, C., Hupcey, J. E., & Tasón, M. C. (1996). Criteria for concept evaluation. *Journal of Advanced Nursing, 24,* 385–390.

Paley, J. (1996). How not to clarify concepts in nursing. *Journal of Advanced Nursing, 24,* 572–577.

Penrod, J., & Hupcey, J. E. (2005). Enhancing methodological clarity: Principle-based concept analysis. *Journal of Advanced Nursing, 50*(4), 403–409.

Rodgers, B. L. (1993). Concept analysis: An evolutionary view. In B. L. Rodgers & K. A. Knafl (Eds.), *Concept development in nursing: Foundations, techniques, and applications* (2nd ed., pp. 73–92). Philadelphia: W. B. Saunders.

Rodgers, B. L. (2000a). Philosophical foundations of concept development. In B. L. Rodgers & K. A. Knafl (Eds.), *Concept development in nursing: Foundations, techniques, and appli-cations* (2nd ed., pp. 7–38). Philadelphia: W. B. Saunders.

Rodgers, B. L. (2000b). Concept analysis: An evolutionary view. In B. L. Rodgers & K. A. Knafl (Eds.), *Concept development in nursing: Foundations, techniques, and applications* (2nd ed., pp. 77–102). Philadelphia: W. B. Saunders.

Schwartz-Barcott, D., & Kim, H. S. (1986). A hybrid model for concept development. In P. L. Chinn (Ed.), *Nursing research methodology: Issues and implementation* (2nd ed., pp. 91–101). Rockville, MD: Aspen.

Schwartz-Barcott, D., & Kim, H. S. (1993). An expansion and elaboration of the hybrid model of concept development. In B. L. Rodgers & K. A. Knafl (Eds.), *Concept development in nursing: Foundations, techniques, and applications* (pp. 107–133). Philadelphia: W. B. Saunders.

Schwartz-Barcott, D., & Kim, H. S. (2000). An expansion and elaboration of the hybrid model of concept development. In B. L. Rodgers & K. A. Knafl (Eds.), *Concept development in nursing: Foundations, techniques, and applications* (2nd ed., pp. 129–160). Philadelphia: W. B. Saunders.

Schwartz-Barcott, D., Patterson, B. J., Lusardi, P., & Farmer, B. C. (2002). From practice to theory: Tightening the link via three fieldwork strategies. *Journal of Advanced Nursing, 39,* 281–289.

Walker, L. O., & Avant, K. C. (1983). *Strategies for theory construction in nursing.* Norwalk, CT: Appleton Century-Crofts.

Walker, L. O., & Avant, K. C. (1988). *Strategies for theory construction in nursing* (2nd ed.). Norwalk, CT: Appleton & Lange.

Walker, L. O., & Avant, K. C. (1995). *Strategies for theory construction in nursing* (3rd ed.). Norwalk, CT: Appleton & Lange.

Wilson, J. (1963). *Thinking with concepts.* Cambridge, England: Cambridge University Press.

The Authors Comment

Concept Analysis: Examining the State of the Science

Immersed in our work involving concept analysis, qualitative methodology, and theory building, we found the earlier writings on methods and the products of concept-driven work to be confusing or poorly integrated. Despite the potential power of this endeavor, it appeared that concept analyses were drifting toward becoming academic exercises, partly because the methods were not fully explicated. We launched this work in an effort to refocus thinking by stimulating discussion of a new interpretive framework. This and the accompanying article on concept advancement are benchmarks in the evolution in our thinking as we tried to assemble a coherent and meaningful framework for concept advancement that was useful to nurse scientists. We are indebted to our colleagues, especially the expert reviewers at *Research and Theory for Nursing Practice* who guided revisions with both enthusiastic encouragement and sharp critique.

—Judith Hupcey
—Janice Penrod

CHAPTER 44

Concept Advancement: Extending Science Through Concept-Driven Research

Janice Penrod
Judith E. Hupcey

As methods for concept analysis have evolved, scholars have confounded the initial exploration of a concept with techniques for developing the conceptual unit, extending nursing theory, and establishing nursing knowledge. We argue that nursing is at a critical juncture in the methodological development of concept-driven research. In order to maximize the potential contribution of this type of research, approaches to concept analysis must be held separate and distinct from approaches to concept advancement. We advocate the use of principle-based concept analysis to determine appropriate techniques for advancing a concept. Concept advancement refers to strategic concept-driven inquiries that incrementally build the specification of conceptual meaning to a more precisely defined unit of meaning that has greater utility for research application. Examples of a project that employed strategic techniques for concept advancement are used to illustrate the flow of serial small projects.

Methods of concept analysis used in nursing have evolved over the last several decades producing a plethora of techniques for examining concepts and enhancing their potential contribution to a scientific endeavor. Yet through this evolution, a serious methodological flaw has arisen.

Nursing scholars have confounded the initial exploration of a concept with techniques for developing the conceptual unit, extending nursing theory, and establishing nursing knowledge. We believe that an important juncture faces nursing science: distinguishing techniques for

From Research and Theory for Nursing Practice: An International Journal, *19(3), Penrod, J. and Hupcey J, Concept advancement: Extending science through concept-driven research, pp. 231–241. Copyright © 2005, Springer Publishing Company. Used with permission.*

About the Authors

Janice Penrod was born and raised in central Pennsylvania. She studied nursing at the University of Pittsburgh (BSN 1976) and then continued her graduate education at the Pennsylvania State University (MS 1996; PhD 2001). Dr. Penrod held varied positions in nursing education and practice before joining the faculty at the Penn State School of Nursing, where she is an Associate Professor of Nursing (College of Health and Human Development) and of Humanities (College of Medicine) and serves as the Professor in Charge of Graduate Programs in Nursing. The foci of her scholarship are family caregiving, end-of-life care, and geriatric nursing. She unwinds by spending time with her family and simply enjoying life at her rural home along a river.

Judith Hupcey was raised in New York and attended college and worked in New York City. She received her BS and MS in nursing from Columbia University and a Master's and Doctoral degree in Nursing Education from Teachers College, Columbia University. Dr. Hupcey held numerous clinical positions at St. Luke's-Roosevelt Hospital Center including working as an Adult Nurse Practitioner in a medical clinic that specialized in the care of underserved adolescents and adults. After joining the faculty at the Penn State School of Nursing, Dr. Hupcey was awarded a Nursing Research Service Award (NRSA) postdoctoral fellowship focusing on qualitative method and concept development. She is now an Associate Professor of Nursing (College of Health and Human Development) and of Humanities (College of Medicine). Her research interests include family caregiving, in particular spousal caregivers, palliative care, and heart failure. She spends her summers with her husband, three children, and dogs in New Hampshire, where she enjoys racing sailboats and trailoring kids' boats to sailing regattas throughout New England.

concept analysis (that is, examining the state of the science or what is currently known of the concept) from techniques for concept advancement; that is, strategically and systematically expanding the knowledge base surrounding the concept of interest through a serial approach to concept-driven research.

This article sets forth considerations to guide concept advancement based on gaps in understanding identified through principle-based concept analysis. First, concept analysis is differentiated from concept advancement. Principle-based concept analysis is briefly discussed to provide a basis for understanding advancement strategies. Concept advancement is discussed in terms of guiding considerations, theory building, and methodological considerations. An example of a conceptually driven research project that employed strategic techniques for concept advancement is used to illustrate the flow of serial small projects.

Differentiation of Concept Analysis from Concept Advancement

Rodgers and Knafl (2000) cogently address the need for new or refined methods for advancing conceptually based research. While their seminal work has opened the issue of concept development in nursing and has made significant inroads to addressing methodological concerns, an overriding concern continues: Many methods of concept development subsume techniques for concept analysis. Lack of differentiation of these two very distinct processes has contributed to researchers' confusion regarding how to strategically advance conceptual understanding to a level that promotes greater precision in research and ultimately affects nursing practice. We agree that "the full potential of concept analysis, as well as other means to develop concepts, has yet to be tapped by nurse scholars" (p. 4) and respond to their call for "additional work to develop new methods or to expand on the ones presented in this text" (p. 3).

To present this work under the rubric of concept *development* or concept *analysis* would only further the current state of confusion. We assert that the first step in achieving some degree of clarity in concept-driven research is to clearly explicate means for determining the state of the science, as it currently exists, as separate and distinct from specific strategies for advancing the concept by establishing new science. Therefore, we have adopted the terminology concept analysis and concept advancement to describe these processes. Together, these processes do contribute to concept development; however, this distinction offers new insights into strategies for advancing concept-driven research that have previously eluded nurse scholars.

Through the use of a principle-based method of concept analysis (see Hupcey & Penrod, 2005; Penrod & Hupcey, 2005), the researcher is able to determine the current state of understanding of a selected concept as reflected in the scientific literature (defined as including empirical, theoretical, and philosophical writings pertaining to the concept of interest). A methodical analysis of the state of science provides a *basis* for knowing how to strategically advance a concept beyond the current state of the science. Advancement refers to the incremental specification of the conceptual unit of meaning to enhance the precision of the conceptual label. Methodologically, advancement is typically achieved through a series of well-focused, concept-driven inquiries that systematically address identified gaps in understanding. From this perspective, concept analysis focuses on the integration of what is known. Concept advancement techniques actually move the state of the science forward through synthesis of new insights.

We purport that concept analysis is just what the term implies—an analysis of what is known to reveal the state of the science surrounding the concept. But, understanding the state of the science does not necessarily move science forward. We often tell our students, "You can only reshuffle the deck so many ways"—meaning that the depth of understanding a scientific conceptualiza-

tion at any point in time is limited by the state of the science supporting that understanding. This notion does not diminish the power of a well-done concept analysis. Concept analyses can make a significant contribution to the science by integrating both explicit and implied meaning to promote a clearer understanding of the concept, yet the primary focus of concept analysis remains at the level of integration. In order to advance science, we must strategically address persistent gaps or inconsistencies in understanding that are revealed through concept analysis. This is where techniques for concept advancement come in. Here we are no longer reshuffling the deck; we are adding new cards of understanding.

Advancement is an iterative process of refining a concept to enhance its scientific precision through research that is driven by the concept, not by a phenomenon. While concept analysis serves as a useful tool for enhancing the researcher's understanding and interpretation of a phenomenon of interest, concept-driven research focuses on the nature of the concept itself. For example, a researcher studying the phenomenon of placing an older adult into nursing home care may be interested in the concept of uncertainty as it pertains to making placement decisions; however, this form of inquiry stands in sharp contrast to the researcher who studies the concept of uncertainty across a number of contexts with the purpose of advancing conceptual meaning. Concept-driven research is challenging in that the researcher moves across phenomena, contexts, and methods to derive a more precise understanding of the concept for the ultimate purpose of deriving theory with greater scope and utility. This perspective of concept advancement clarifies considerations that are useful for guiding a strategic progression of inquiries to enhance conceptual precision.

Principle-Based Concept Analysis: Examining the State of the Science

Principle-based concept analysis is the critical examination of the scientific literature guided by the application of four philosophic principles. These principles were initially described by Morse and colleagues (Hupcey,

Morse, Lenz, & Tasón, 1996; Morse, 1995; Morse, Hupcey, Mitcham, & Lenz, 1996; Morse, Mitcham, Hupcey, Tasón, 1996) and subsequently operationalized by Penrod and Hupcey (2005). Prior to beginning the actual analysis, the concept of interest is identified and scientific literature from relevant disciplines is collected. Then, this literature is examined according to principles based in the philosophy of science: epistemologic, linguistic, pragmatic, and logical. The products of this form of concept analysis are of two types: summative statements of the degree to which the literature addresses each principle and the integration of insights into a theoretical definition that integrates what is known of the concept, or the state of the science.

As defined by Morse, Hupcey, Penrod, and Mitcham (2002) the epistemological principle reflects the science surrounding the nature of knowledge asking "Is the concept clearly defined and well-differentiated from other concepts?" (p. 8). Pragmatic perspectives of the science have to do with utility and fit. Questions here are "Does the concept fit with the phenomena common to the discipline? Is it useful to the discipline?" (p. 8). The linguistic principle is rooted in language, posing the question, "Is the concept used consistently and appropriately within context? Is it decontextualized?" (p. 8). Finally, the logical principle is based in the science of logic. "Does the concept hold its boundaries through theoretical integration with other concepts?" (p. 8). Though complex, we believe this approach is one of the most thorough and comprehensive methods available for analyzing the state of science. (For a more detailed discussion of the application of principle-based concept analysis, see Penrod & Hupcey, 2005 and Hupcey & Penrod, 2005.)

Concept Advancement: Guiding Considerations

Results of a concept analysis bring the researcher to ask the next question: "How can these findings best be used to advance the concept?" As one considers methods for advancing concept-driven research, the evidence organized through concept analysis and the evaluation of that evidence leads to identification of unanswered questions about the concept itself and to subsequent research approaches that can address limitations in its development for scientific purposes. Concept advancement is a strategic exploration of the concept to build the knowledge base supporting a clear explication of precise conceptual meaning.

The following discussion about concept advancement presents useful consideration when evaluating the findings of a concept analysis in order to identify gaps in understanding that serve as primary determinants for subsequent inquiries to advance the concept. While concept advancement typically progresses through a series of small discrete projects, strategies for advancement are not directed by a single principle. Since the principles used in concept analysis are in essence multiple philosophical perspectives of the state of the science, it is critical that the researcher step back to examine these layers of understanding as a unified whole. The findings of a concept analysis present the researcher an opportunity to examine a more comprehensive view of the concept from multiple perspectives in order to determine the most promising paths for advancement, as demonstrated by a research program on the concept of uncertainty discussed below.

First, the summary statements derived for each of the principles used in the analysis are carefully reviewed, starting with the epistemological principle. The epistemological principle is essential to the other principles because a concept must be clearly defined in order to be logical, pragmatic, or linguistically intact. Reliance on everyday meaning is not adequate for scientific endeavors; concepts used in science must be clearly and precisely defined in order to ensure that the meaning assumed by readers is consistent. While principle-based concept analysis does acknowledge both explicit and implicit meaning as valid forms of evidence, implicit meaning must rely on some form of supportive evidence, not conjecture. Implicit meaning is that which can be logically deduced given the evidence presented. For example, the selection and use of a certain measurement tool implies a certain conceptual meaning was employed in the study. Conversely, simply using a word label and relying on the reader's interpretation without any referents or evidence is not adequate to meet the epistemological principle, for there is no evidence to support the implied meaning.

Yet definition alone is not enough. The pragmatic principle requires that the fit with phenomena of interest to the discipline is evident and supported. In turn, the issue of contextualization is further addressed by the linguistic principle, which requires examination of the degree of decontextualization of the concept. The notion of decontextualization means that patterns of meaning (explicated in the definition) extend beyond a narrow contextual frame into multiple contexts in which the concept is manifest. Beyond the scope of the concept's application across contexts (i.e., the linguistic principle), the systematic linking of the concept with other related or co-occurring concepts in a theory is further addressed in the logical principle.

Consider the literature available to support the analysis: How much literature is available? What is the quality of that literature? Despite the potential significance of a single, seminal work, the volume of literature surrounding a concept of interest is critically important in relation to how well the conceptualization addresses each of the principles. We do not know of any single work that is comprehensive enough to adequately address all four principles. This requires multiple inquiries. The closest examples are typically articles that refer to either multiple parts of a large study or a series of small studies in one area; yet even in these cases, a review of the cited literature often reveals previous or related work that should be included in the analytic phase.

These considerations provide a lens for examining the findings culled through principle-based concept analysis. Typically, this analytic review of findings generates several avenues for advancing the concept in subsequent projects. In our work, we have found it useful to identify gaps in understanding generated by the principles addressed in analysis by first generating lists of questions or statements of limitations related to each area of inquiry.

Then, step back from the specific principle-based conclusions to examine the gaps in understanding from a broader perspective. Recall that these principles are varied perspectives of examining what is known or the state of the science. As such, the principles do not yield prescriptive avenues for advancing the science based on deficiencies. Specific conceptual issues generated by each principle are often highly related in a manner that permeates the whole of what is known. Thus this phase of determining the route for concept advancement through subsequent concept-driven research depends on a holistic perspective of the conceptual gaps to identify research questions that would produce findings that could "fill the gaps." Concept maps or other forms of modeling what is known and what is not known are often helpful. Selection of the path for subsequent inquiries is highly related to issues of theory building.

Concept Advancement as Theory Building

Recall that the process of concept advancement is incremental. Serial advancement of the concept depends on the researcher's agenda, but the potential of the process is to develop a concept toward a more precise scientific definition that permits integration into conceptual frameworks that enhance research or informs or directs practice. As a concept is advanced theoretically, linkages with co-occurring or related concepts become evident. These linkages are the essence of emergent theory, which remains focused on the concept of interest, yet clearly extends understanding beyond a single concept. Therefore, as concept advancement work progresses, the research moves toward theory building.

Seminal work in theory building by Dickoff and James (1968) and later Diers (1979) support this notion of using concept advancement to build higher-level theory. In this enduring schema of levels of theory in the practice discipline of nursing, the most basic level of theory is factor isolating or naming theory. The driving question is, "what *is* this?" (Diers, p. 36). The purpose of this level of theory is to describe, or to "tak[e] empirical reality to the level of 'idea'" (Diers, p. 37).

When the evidence culled from the scientific literature through principle-based concept analysis is insufficient to support a conclusion that the concept is clearly defined and differentiated from other concepts, the researcher is guided toward a descriptive question: "What is it?" In describing this lowest level of theory, Diers (1979) has defined concept-driven research as aimed primarily at advancing a concept epistemologically and secondarily at the pragmatic principle. When the concept is epistemologically adequate, the "what is it" question has been answered. Pragmatic adequacy reveals that the derived conceptualization is useful for understanding phenomena of concern to the discipline; or in other words, the answer to the "what is it" question works for issues of concern to the discipline.

The second level of theory, factor-relating (situation depicting or situation describing), addresses relation-searching questions, such as: "What's happening here?" (Diers, 1979, p. 38). This level subsumes adequate naming and explores the nature of relationships among factors (or concepts). In concept advancement terms, this level of theoretical work addresses issues or gaps centered primarily around logical concerns, as the concept holds its boundaries of meaning as it is integrated with other concepts.

The research questions guiding these initial forms of inquiry are concept-driven and focus on discovery. This is the nature of concept advancement work: the discovery of new knowledge that enhances conceptual understanding (through synthesis) to build a solid foundation for the explication of higher level theory that has more direct practice implications. These two basic levels of theory are the foundation for higher levels of theory, including situation-relating (or predictive) and situation-producing (or prescriptive) theory.

Concept Advancement: Methodological Considerations

Principle-based concept analysis provides the analytic insights necessary for directing the researcher's selection of methods in the course of subsequent concept advancement projects. The principles (i.e., epistemological, linguistic, logical, and pragmatic) guide the researcher's critical review of the literature across broad domains of the philosophy of science to enhance a comprehensive, multifaceted analysis of the state of the science. This analysis reveals gaps in understanding through a systematic critique of the evidence that demonstrates the degree to which a principle is supported.

Methods used in the discovery phases of concept-driven research (i.e., factor-naming and factor-isolating research) explore specific qualities or gaps in understanding that are identified through a thorough analysis of the literature. These gaps are formulated as research questions. The questions lead the researcher in the selection of the research method that is best suited for a focused inquiry that will provide the evidence necessary to advance conceptual understanding in particular areas of weakness. The discovery of new knowledge to build conceptual understanding is primarily a qualitative endeavor. Each focused inquiry builds the body of evidence by synthesizing new knowledge related to the concept that supports the continued specification of conceptual meaning, or, in other words, concept advancement.

Concept Advancement: Uncertainty

In this section, we highlight a program of research that illustrates how principle-based concept analysis was used to identify gaps and research questions that launched a series of conceptually driven inquiries to advance the concept of uncertainty. Subsequently, the refined conceptualization was integrated within the theoretical context of end-of-life caregiving in a form of theory building. This discussion demonstrates how a holistic view of the evidence culled through principle-based concept analysis was used to guide successive inquiries in a progressive strategic fashion.

This program of research began with an investigation of family caregivers' experiences during the placement of their older adult charge into nursing home care (Penrod, 1996; Penrod & Dellasega, 1998). Uncertainty arose as a primary theme in the caregivers' experience. In another study in which methods for linking the concepts of enduring and suffering were explored, the concept of uncertainty again arose as a significant behavioral state that occurred in response to a significant threat to health (Morse & Penrod, 1999). As the first author began dissertation work, the concept of uncertainty was selected as the concept of interest (Penrod, 2001a). Conceptually driven research to further explore this emergent concept was driven by a principle-based concept analysis (Penrod, 2001b).

During this analysis, it was apparent that the anthropological literature was replete with use of the everyday concept uncertainty (for complete discussion see Penrod, 2001a). In these cases, the concept (uncertainty) was used without definition; rather, the word label was associated with the description of states or circumstances that were more powerful in relating meaning than the more narrowly defined scientific definitions that were offered in other literatures. Characteristics of the states or circumstances in which the everyday concept was used were congruent with the evolving conceptual insights, but there were inadequate data in the literature to support a valid analysis of the depth of implied meaning appreciated through these readings.

In this case, derivation of implied meaning would have relied on the reader's evoked interpretation, not on data. While such insights are important to the pursuit of concept advancement projects, such interpretation is not a valid finding of a concept analysis. Subsequently, this analysis produced an integrated theoretical definition that was found to be narrowly probabilistic, with an emphasis on cognitive processing of the appraisal of threat posed by a situation (Penrod, 2001b).

The reliance on everyday or ordinary meaning in the scientific literature indicated weakness in the epistemological development of the concept. Insights derived through analysis of the anthropological literature led the researcher to consider the pragmatic principle more closely. Clinical experience and documented evidence did not support the emphasis on cognitive processing of probabilities—there were times of uncertainty in which a more basic way of knowing dominated and times when no probabilities could be ascertained. The question that arose in this phase of the research was: "What is it?" Or more specifically, what meaning is embedded in the lived experience of uncertainty that is not captured in the integrated scientific definition?

Given this inquiry, concept advancement proceeded through a phenomenological study of states of uncertainty experienced by family caregivers. The phenomenology revealed the essences of the lived experience of uncertainty. Most importantly, the phenomenology permitted a deeper understanding of the importance of precognitive ways of knowing during experiences of uncertainty, types of uncertainty that arose as patterns of dominance in the essences shifted, and modes of uncertainty that emerged in response to perceived situational or existential evidence acknowledged by the caregivers. These findings were then reintegrated to produce a more comprehensive theoretical definition of uncertainty (inaptly referred to as a concept correction, Penrod, 2001a).

While the phenomenological inquiry provided an understanding of varied forms of uncertainty, it was not clear how these forms evolved, shifted, and changed during situations that were fraught with opportunities to experience uncertainty. Such understanding is critical to developing interventions to support caregivers through uncertain times. Therefore, the preliminary concept-driven studies were used to build a proposal highlighting newly identified gaps in understanding states of uncertainty and the continued refinement of the theoretical understanding of the states through incremental concept advancement work.

Funding was received for continued exploration of states of uncertainty, now in the context of caregivers providing end-of-life care [1 R03 NR08538-02 PI: Penrod, J.; in progress]. Under this funding, a grounded theory study was conducted to further delineate experiences of uncertainty during end-of-life care, the prominence of varied forms of uncertainty across the trajectory of caregiving, and strategies that caregivers found helpful in successfully managing uncertainty. In the second phase of the funded project, the focus of the research program shifts toward theory building, integrating the refined concept of uncertainty in factor-isolating theory that positions the concept within the broader theoretical context of end-of-life caregiving. The primary thrust of this work remains focused on concept advancement, as the researchers continue to focus efforts on the concept of uncertainty through the context of end-of-life caregiving.

The logical progression of this work is continued advancement of the concept to support the development of higher level theory (i.e., predictive and prescriptive theory) that integrates the concept into meaningful schemas for clinical intervention. This is the nature of concept advancement work: the specification of conceptual meaning to a more precisely defined unit of meaning that has greater utility for research application.

Discussion

Concept analysis tells us "what is" in the current state of the science. The question that arises is to how best use these findings to advance the concept. From our perspective, the importance of principle-based concept analysis is the identification of gaps and inconsistencies in the scientific understanding of a concept that supports the determination of appropriate avenues to advance the concept toward greater utility. We do not believe that labeling the summative conclusions of the analysis as the level of maturity (as suggested by Morse et al., 1996) is sufficient for determining precise strategies for incrementally enhancing conceptual understanding.

It should be noted that as this scheme of concept advancement has evolved over the past several years, we have worked with a variety of terms to describe particular techniques for advancing concepts. Concept refinement, clarification, delineation, comparison, and correction have all been used to indicate specific purposes for advancement of a concept; however, these terms are poorly differentiated. We have purposefully avoided the used of these terms and have attempted to redirect the focus of concept advancement on the identified gaps, related research questions, and most suitable methods of inquiry. We believe that concept advancement is a much more suitable rubric for this type of research.

There are significant methodological issues that must be addressed as researchers work to incrementally advance a concept through a series of studies. The temptation for the researchers to prematurely slip into a mode of deductive reasoning in serial studies presents a serious threat to validity that must be consciously addressed as each study is designed and implemented. Another methodological issue surrounds how to actually use the findings to advance the concept. While techniques to enhance inductive validity (see Hupcey, 2002; Hupcey & Penrod, 2003; Morse & Mitcham, 2002; Penrod, 2002) and the integration of findings using template comparison (Hupcey & Penrod, 2003) have been described elsewhere; further work is needed to refine these methods for conceptually driven research to enhance the utility of the methods for researchers.

The significance of serial small, discrete projects surrounding the advancement of a concept of interest should not be underestimated. Dissemination of these studies builds the knowledge base incrementally; these studies contribute to advancement of nursing science. But these projects are also critical to the evolution of nurse scholars as research scientists, since the progressive projects surrounding concept advancement often culminate in the identification of programs of research. Considering the limitations in funding available for more junior researchers and the need to develop a focused area of research for most tenure review boards, we believe that this incremental approach to the theoretical development of a concept of interest paves the way for larger, more sustainable projects with clinical importance. Given this significance, we anticipate further development of techniques for concept advancement research that culminates in theory to guide sensitive evidence-based nursing care.

REFERENCES

Dickoff, J., & James, P. (1968). A theory of theories: A position paper. *Nursing Research, 17,* 197–203.

Diers, D. (1979). *Research in nursing practice.* Philadelphia: J. B. Lippincott.

Hupcey, J. E. (2002). Maintaining validity: The development of the concept of trust [Electronic version]. *International Journal of Qualitative Methods, 1*(4), 31–43. Retrieved January 21, 2005 from http://www.ualberta.ca/~ijqm/english/engframeset.html

Hupcey, J. E., Morse, J. M., Lenz, E. R., & Tasón, M. C. (1996). Wilsonian methods of concept analysis: A critique. *Scholarly Inquiry for Nursing Practice, 10,* 185–210.

Hupcey. J. E., & Penrod, J. (2003). Concept advancement: Enhancing inductive validity. Research *and Theory for Nursing Practice: An International Journal, 17*(1), 19–30.

Hupcey, J. E., & Penrod, J. (2005). Concept analysis: Establishing the state of the science. *Research and Theory for Nursing Practice: An International Journal, 19*(2), 197–208.

Morse, J. M. (1995). Exploring the theoretical basis of nursing using advanced techniques of concept analysis. *Advances in Nursing Science, 17,* 31–46.

Morse, J. M., Hupcey, J., Mitcham, C. & Lenz, E. R. (1996). Concept analysis in nursing research: A critical appraisal. *Scholarly Inquiry for Nursing Practice, 10,* 257–281.

Morse, J. M., Hupcey, J. E., Penrod, J., & Mitcham, C. (2002). Developing qualitatively derived theory using techniques of concept integration. *Research and Theory for Nursing Practice: An International Journal, 16*(1), 5–18.

Morse, J. M., & Mitcham, C. (2002). Exploring qualitatively-derived concepts: Inductive-deductive pitfalls [Electronic version]. *International Journal of Qualitative Methods, 1*(4), 3–15. Retrieved February 9, 2005 from http://www.ualberta.ca/~ijqm/english/engframeset.html

Morse, J. M., Mitcham, C., Hupcey, J. E., & Tason, M. C. (1996). Criteria for concept evaluation. *Journal of Advanced Nursing, 24,* 385–390.

Morse, J. M., & Penrod, J. (1999). Linking concepts of enduring, suffering, and hope. *Image: Journal of Nursing Scholarship, 31*(2), 145–150.

Penrod, J. (1996). *Caregivers' perspectives of placement decisions* (Unpublished master's thesis). University Park, PA: The Pennsylvania State University.

Penrod, J. (2001a). *The advancement of the concept of uncertainty using phenomenological methods.* (Unpublished doctoral dissertation). University Park, PA: The Pennsylvania State University.

Penrod, J. (2001b). Refinement of the concept of uncertainty. *Journal of Advanced Nursing, 34,* 238–245.

Penrod, J. (2002). Advancing uncertainty: Untangling and discerning related concept [Electronic version]. *International Journal of Qualitative Methods, 7*(4), 44–58. Retrieved February 9, 2005 from http://www.ualberta.ca/~ijqm/english/engframeset.html

Penrod, J., & Dellasega, C. (1998). Caregivers' perspectives of placement decisions. *Western Journal of Nursing Research, 20,* 706–722.

Penrod, J., & Hupcey, J. E. (2005). Enhancing methodological clarity: Principle-based concept analysis. *Journal of Advanced Nursing, 50*(4), 403–409.

Rodgers, B. L., & Knafl, K. A. (2000). Introduction to concept development in nursing. In B. L. Rodgers & K. A. Knafl (Eds.), *Concept development in nursing: Foundations, techniques, and applications* (2nd ed., pp. 1–6). Philadelphia: W. B. Saunders.

The Authors Comment

Concept Advancement: Extending Science Through Concept-Driven Research

We wrote this article, along with the article on concept analysis, to address a problem whereby the techniques or methods described as concept analysis or development were beginning to blur a critical juncture in concept-driven research: identifying gaps in the state of the science that inform the next inquiry. We hope that the distinction drawn by positing analysis as separate and distinct from advancement would clarify the importance of this strategic decision point. The term "advancement" emerged throughout the ongoing discussions with students and colleagues that culminated in these publications. The beauty of this label is that it captures the essence of the process without encumbering pre-existing notions associated with other terms. We have been astounded with the positive response to this work and look forward to continued involvement in this critically important area of nursing science.

—Janice Penrod
—Judith E. Hupcey

CHAPTER 45

Empowerment: Reformulation of a Non-Rogerian Concept

Nelma B. Crawford Shearer
Pamela G. Reed

The authors present a reformulation of empowerment based upon historical and current perspectives of empowerment and a synthesis of existing literature and Rogerian thought. Reformulation of non-Rogerian concepts familiar to nurses is proposed as a strategy to accelerate the mainstreaming of Rogerian thought into nursing practice and research. The reformulation of empowerment as a participatory process of well-being inherent among human beings may provide nurses with new insights for practice. This paper may also serve as a model for reformulating other non-Rogerian concepts and theories for wider dissemination across the discipline.

I listened to the audio-tapes recorded for my research project while the nurses participating in the telephone intervention study talked and listened to the participants. Listening to the tapes has been an education in itself. While reviewing the tapes, it became apparent that one of the nurses making the telephone calls does not listen to the participant although I am sure she would strongly disagree with me. She is bent on getting the study participant to exercise and drink water. One participant in particular refers to listening to her body and states, "I know when something is wrong." The nurse responds by telling her she should instead talk with her doctor.

—Notes Recorded by a Rogerian Research Nurse,
March 18, 2002

From N. B. Crawford Shearer and P. G. Reed, Research and Nursing Science Quarterly, *2004; 17(3):253–259.*
Copyright © 2004 SAGE Publications. Reprinted with permission by SAGE Publications, Inc.

About the Authors

NELMA B. CRAWFORD SHEARER is Associate Professor at Arizona State University College of Nursing & Healthcare Innovation in Phoenix. She received her BS in nursing from South Dakota State University in 1972, an MEd from the University of Missouri-St. Louis in 1977, an MS in nursing from Southern Illinois University-Edwardsville in 1987, and a PhD with a major in nursing from the University of Arizona in 2000. Dr. Shearer is an American Nurse Foundation Scholar and a John A. Hartford Foundation Institute of Geriatric Nursing Research Scholar. In 2006, she received the Geriatric Nursing Research award from the Western Institute of Nursing in partnership with the Hartford Institute for Geriatric Nursing. Dr. Shearer conducts research in promoting health empowerment in adults, and is currently funded by The National Institutes of Health/(NINR) for the study "Health Empowerment Intervention with Homebound Older Adults." In her spare time, Dr. Shearer enjoys her family, entertaining friends, antiquing, gardening, and going for long bike rides.

PAMELA G. REED is a Professor at the University of Arizona College of Nursing in Tucson, where she also served as Associate Dean for Academic Affairs for seven years. She is a three-time graduate of Wayne State University in Detroit, receiving a BSN in 1974, an MSN in 1976 (with a double major in child–adolescent psychiatric mental health nursing and teaching), and her PhD with a major in nursing (focused on life-span development and aging) in 1982. Dr. Reed pioneered research into spirituality and well-being with her doctoral research with terminally ill patients. She also developed a theory of self-transcendence and two widely used research instruments, the *Spiritual Perspective Scale* and the *Self-Transcendence Scale*. Her publications and funded research reflect a dual scholarly focus: spirituality and other facilitators of well-being and decision-making in end-of-life transitions; and nursing metatheory and knowledge development. Dr. Reed also enjoys time with her family, reading, classical music, swimming, and hiking in the mountains and canyons of Arizona.

The misuse of power in healthcare by the nurse in this audio-tape not only rendered her unable to foster the patient's power to participate in the health process but also effectively diminished her own power as a facilitator of healthcare. This excerpt is an example of the still far too prevalent practice among 21st-century nurses of authoritarian and paternalistic approaches to helping patients change their health patterns. Despite advances in Rogerian theory and unitary nursing practice as well as the shift from positivism to more critical philosophic perspectives, the presence of Rogerian thought in mainstream nursing is seriously lacking. We have a sense of urgency in finding ways to promote Rogerian thought and action in nursing. Toward this end, we present the reformulation of a non-Rogerian concept, namely, empowerment, as a strategy for mainstreaming Rogerian

thought into nursing practice. Our intent is also to articulate a process of reformulation that can be used in regard to other non-Rogerian concepts.

Nurse theoretician Whall (1980), drawing from philosopher of science Kaplan's (1964) ideas on the autonomy of inquiry, instructed scholars that concepts and theories are not owned by any one discipline and may be reformulated according to their own disciplinary perspective and purposes. It may be wise to reformulate rather than eradicate concepts and theories that are incongruent with a disciplinary perspective. As others (Barrett, Caroselli, Smith, & Smith, 1997) have aptly pointed out, the term empowerment, traditionally defined as to *put power into* an individual, can reflect a mechanistic and authoritative view of the nurse-client relationship that is incongruent with Rogerian science. The prefix *em* means, "to cause to be," "to put into," "to provide with" *(Merriam-Webster's Collegiate Dictionary,* 1993, p. 379). Chinn (2000) also implied that there was a better term to be found, but she suggested that nurses use the term as is until an alternate is identified.

Barrett's (1990) classic concept of *power as knowing participation in change* offers nursing a significant and enduring concept that is similar to, but still qualitatively different from, the concept of empowerment. Barrett's underlying assumption about participation in ongoing change renders her concept as unique, and not merely a substitute for the authoritarian applications of empowerment.

Barrett's (1990) unique concept of power as knowing participation in change notwithstanding, it is also strategic to communicate Rogerian ideas through carefully reformulated concepts familiar to nursing that can create new meaning for clinicians and researchers. Empowerment is a ubiquitous concept not only in the healthcare literature but across many social disciplines. Discarding this concept as non-Rogerian can diminish the fund of knowledge upon which nursing may draw in developing its own knowledge base. With reformulation, which may not be possible with all non-Rogerian concepts, the concept of empowerment has the potential to help nurses transform their practice with patients.

This reformulation is based upon a complex but rather straightforward metatheoretical process (Reed, 1986). It involves a review of basic definitions of the concept, historical perspectives, and paradigmatic views from various disciplines that influence current thought on empowerment. A full review of the research literature and a concept analysis may also be conducted early on in the reformulation. Next, the assumptions and principles of the major nursing theoretical perspective that guide the reformulation are explicated. It is also an important step to critically address the nursing practice paradigms that may influence translation of the concept into action. Highlights of the reformulation of empowerment are presented here, as based upon a synthesis of existing literature and classic Rogerian thought related to this concept.

Definitions and Descriptions

Dictionary definitions of empowerment are: "(1) to give official authority or legal power to; (2) to enable; (3) to promote self-actualization or influence of" *(Merriam-Webster's Collegiate Dictionary,* 1993, p. 379). Varying perspectives notwithstanding, empowerment generally is a desired goal in nursing. It connotes active participation in one's own healthcare. Further, moral views and behaviors, personal integrity, and a sense of personal and social responsibility have been found to be qualities of empowerment (Kuokkanen, Leino-Kilpi, & Katajisto, 2002).

Empowerment is generally associated with increased self-esteem and self-worth, inner-confidence, and well-being (for example, Gibson, 1991; Kieffer, 1984; Nyatanga & Dann, 2002). However, the nurse's practice paradigm may bring a less desirable translation of the concept into practice.

History and Current Paradigms

According to Minkler and Wallerstein (1997), the word *empowerment* first appeared in the literature during the 1950s, a time of social action organization in which the emphasis was on addressing power imbalances. Empowerment rooted in social action became more influential throughout the 1960s and 1970s within the contexts of civil rights, the women's movement, gay rights, the disability rights movement, and other community-based action. During the 1980s in the psychology literature empowerment was viewed as a participatory process through which individuals take control over their lives and environment (Rappaport, 1984). It was not until the 1990s, when healthcare providers' and consumers' focus turned to health promotion, that the concept appeared on a regular basis in the nursing and health education literature. In the context of health education, empowerment has been viewed as a process and an outcome; as a process, empowerment involves relationships and the transfer of the power base from one group to another, with the outcome of "liberation, emancipation, energy and sharing power" (Leyshon, 2002, p. 467). Empowerment can be understood from various broad perspectives. The social and the contextual developmental comprise two major perspectives.

Social Paradigm

As a social process, empowerment is linked with external social forces that act on the individual and affect one's sense of control and feelings of power. For example, social support as an external feedback mechanism has been studied as a process that can provide needed reinforcement, resources, assistance, and motivation (Ellis-Stoll & Popkess-Vawter, 1998) and enable the individual (Hawks, 1992). Other external social forces have been studied from the perspective of emancipation from oppression. Several authors have suggested that promoting empowerment could be accomplished through addressing political constraints (Gutierrez, 1995; Labonte, 1994), environmental constraints (Ryles, 1999), and social constraints (Fulton, 1997). Two theories addressing these constraints are critical social theory and feminist theory, which offer perspectives about power applicable in nursing.

Critical social theory evolved from Marxism during the postmodern era and from the revolutionary thinking of Paulo Freire (1968/1981) in Brazil. Freire's basic assumption is that human being's "ontological vocation is to be a Subject who acts upon and transforms one's world" (Richard Shaull, as cited in Freire, 1968/1981, p. 12). The goals of critical social theory are to make people aware of the social constraints under which they may be consciously or unconsciously living, free people's thinking, and establish unconstrained communication.

Feminist thought of the 1960s extended the suffragists' cause of the late 19th–early 20th century to address the educational, occupational, professional, and role-related constraints experienced by women. While diverse views on feminism exist, a unifying theme is the elimination of patriarchal social constraints and the oppression of women (Kirkley, 2000). Feminist theory acknowledges basic human potential in all human beings, and incorporates interactions and life experiences that contribute to human transformation; this transformation of oppressive situations facilitates empowerment (Kane & Thomas, 2000). Empowerment from a feminist perspective draws from the ideology of equality by emphasizing the choices and freedom of women (Caroselli, 1995).

More recently, postmodern feminism has introduced a multicultural and global focus in which differences in race, class, national origin, and gender are regarded as relevant in the discourse on constraints upon women's freedom and well-being (Tong, 2001). Postcolonial feminist theory has shifted away from the earlier emphasis on achieving a unified notion of women toward developing an appreciation of differences while holding a collective goal of equal opportunity. There is less of a stance of victimization and a more creative, proactive approach to one's social environment that develops the human potential of all (Ramphele, 1997).

Developmental Paradigm

Empowerment may also be understood in reference to the lifespan developmental perspective that emerged in the late 1970s (Lerner, 1997). Lifespan development is an orientation to the study of human beings as continuously innovative, embedded in a dynamic environment, and possessing inherent potential. The lifespan developmental perspective emphasizes both systematic patterns of change such as biologically based influences and non-normative patterns of change across the lifespan such as life events that cannot be predicted by time and do not occur for everyone. Development is no longer viewed as a linear process as it was until the late 20th century. Rather, developmental change is now understood to derive unpredictably from mutual influences between person and environmental contexts. Person-environment processes, including those involving human relationships, are central to developmental progress and well-being.

Treatment approaches from a life-span view focus on maximizing client strengths and minimizing weaknesses (Baltes, Lindenberger, & Staudinger, 1998) rather than on predetermined interventions designed to change client behaviors. The client is regarded as possessing a repertoire of developmentally based abilities that can be deduced through the nurse-client relationship to address healthcare needs. From this perspective, the client is a resource and active partner in healthcare.

Nursing care is directed less toward changing the client and more toward optimizing human potential.

The Rogerian Perspective

Given nursing's basic assumptions about the importance of human potential and development, connectedness, and the social context in health and well-being, both the social and developmental paradigms offer elements that are useful in reformulating the concept empowerment. However, a nursing theoretical perspective is needed to cull ideas from the various non-nursing paradigms and synthesize a coherent and philosophically relevant description of the concept. Rogers' (1980, 1992) science of unitary human beings provides such a perspective.

Rogers (1980, 1990, 1992) defined nursing's focus as the study of human beings in mutual process with the environment. Rogers proposed three principles of homeodynamics, which outlined her assumptions about the nature of the human-environment process as well as functioned to guide the practice of nursing. The principle of helicy describes the nature of human change as continuous, innovative, unpredictable, and reflective of the diversity of human and environmental field patterns. The principle of integrality proposes how this change occurs, that is through a continuous mutual process of human and environmental energy fields. The principle of resonancy emphasizes the existence of patterns inherent in the process of change and unique to each human system. Knowledge about this pattern is acquired through research and careful assessment of various human indicators, which can then be used to facilitate health (Reed, 1997a).

Related Theories

Several theoretical frameworks support the Rogerian postulate that human beings desire to participate knowingly in change and in their patterning. This idea has a central place in Barrett et al.'s (1997) power enhancement, Newman's (1997) expanding consciousness, and Reed's (1997a) participatory nursing process. Synthesis of ideas from these frameworks supports a reformulation of the concept of empowerment.

Barrett

Basic to Barrett's (1990, 1994) theory of power is the assumption of ongoing change, and the client's awareness of and belief in one's ability to fully participate in the changes involved in health and healthcare. The partnership between client and nurse facilitates the client's participation in healthcare. During the health-seeking event, the participatory nurse-client relationship evolves. The nurse uses various methods that enhance the client's knowing participation in change. One such approach centers on finding out what is happening with the client, directing attention away from the nurse as the initiator of nursing care and toward a participatory relationship in which both the nurse and client facilitate the change process. The nursing goal is "power enhancement through changing the environment" (Barrett et al., 1997, p. 34).

Newman

Newman's (1997) theory of health as expanding consciousness proposes a mutual process between client and nurse by which meaning and understanding of the client's health patterns are recognized and insight is gained. The nurse does not attempt to control the interaction and change the client. Instead, the nurse facilitates pattern recognition and health choices faced by the client (Newman, 1990). This process of pattern recognition expands the client's developing insight and facilitates potential action.

Reed

Reed's (1997a) treatise on the ontology of nursing describes nursing as a "participatory process that transcends the boundary between patient and nurse" (p. 77). She defined nursing as an inherent process of well-being that functions within and among human systems. Nursing, in its most basic meaning, is not an external process of 19th century invention; rather it is a resource that has existed among human beings since the beginning of human history. Empowerment is an expression and indicator of this inherent nursing process. Like nursing, empowerment is relational not external. Emerging from this participatory mutual process is the recognition of one's pattern of well-being and awareness of natural resources for healing self (Reed, 1997b).

From this participatory perspective of empowerment, there is an awareness of the mutual process of power that is inherent in the nurse-client system itself, rather than located in either the nurse or client alone. The process promotes well-being through the power inherent in this integrality of client and nurse.

Nursing Practice Paradigms

It is not uncommon for healthcare providers to think that they can empower their clients and in so doing expect clients will comply with the health plan (for example, Hawks, 1992; Holmes & Saleebey, 1993). Empowerment as it is often implicitly if not explicitly linked to the concept of compliance in practice, neither appeals to the informed consumer nor reflects contemporary nursing philosophy of practice. Clinical practice and anecdotal experiences consistently indicate that clients do not always follow through with the nurse's prescribed plan of care (Hess, 1996). The uninformed nurse, thinking that the client has been amply empowered, may be puzzled as to why the person does not *comply* with the healthcare plan.

Confounding empowerment with compliance is insidious and prevails even in very recent literature appearing to advance understandings of empowerment beyond authoritarian assumptions, for example, "non-compliance demonstrated the patient's need to exercise their empowerment" (Nyatanga & Dann, 2002, p. 238), as though non-compliance really exists in patients and is linked to empowerment. The authors go on to explain that the nursing discipline should cease using the term *patients,* come around to the true philosophy of empowerment, and relinquish the discipline's authoritarian approach. However, the problem is not so much the lack of the correct understanding of empowerment as it is the nurse's choice of practice paradigm that influences applications of empowerment.

Parse (1987, 1992) identified two nursing paradigms, totality and simultaneity, that guide thinking about empowerment in nursing practice. Employing a Rogerian view of empowerment, however, involves a shift in thinking from the totality paradigm to the simultaneity paradigm of nursing practice.

Totality

According to the totality paradigm, humans are bio-psycho-social-spiritual beings interacting with and in response to the internal and external environment (Parse, 1992). Human change is considered predictable, controllable, reversible, and occurring primarily in response to environmental stimuli. Health is viewed as achieving equilibrium in physical, mental, social, spiritual, cultural, and other aspects of human experience. Within this paradigm, the nurse knows what is best for the client and shares knowledge that may or may not be empowering. The nurse-client relationship is designed to influence change in the client. Empowerment is accomplished through the efforts of the nurse as data collector, assessor of the disease state, care planner, and change agent for the client. In this relationship, the nurse as the authority shares knowledge as power to enable the client to make informed yet appropriate and compliant choices in health activities.

The totality paradigm is evident in empowerment approaches that emphasize external agents and forces that affect or constrain individuals. Compliance is often a goal. Interactions between person and environmental influences are acknowledged within this paradigm, but the inherent mutual process and resources among person and environment are neither acknowledged nor exploited.

Simultaneity

Within the simultaneity paradigm (Parse, 1992), human beings are recognized through pattern rather than through parts that can be independently manipulated, changed, and studied. Change is creative and innovative and occurs as part of the person-environment process. Health involves the client's purposeful participation in developing self-awareness and choosing health patterns. Clients exercise their power by participating in their healthcare and healthcare decisions. The nurse's approach is to inspire, not dictate this process, to be facilitative, not authoritative.

Empowerment Reformulated

Rogers did not specifically address empowerment in publications on her science of unitary human beings. Nonetheless, a Rogerian view of empowerment can be proposed, as one synthesized from social and developmental paradigms, and guided by Rogerian theory and practice paradigms. From Rogers (1992) it is understood that there is an emphasis on participating knowingly in the process of change rather than on submission and lack of power, control, or choice. Attention to external agents of power and victimization are inconsistent with these assumptions. The nurse is not one who empowers (or disempowers) but rather one who facilitates empowerment in clients, with actions deriving from an understanding of the client's relational nature, relevant social context, and developmental potential.

This new view of empowerment is based upon four assumptions derived from Rogerian theory and related theories: (a) Empowerment is neither a resource that is external to the person nor bestowed by others, power is inherent and ongoing (Labonte, 1989); (b) empowerment is a relational process, expressive of the mutuality of person and environment; (c) empowerment is an ongoing process of change that is continuously innovative; and (d) empowerment is expressive of a human health pattern of well-being, and can be assessed and enhanced through nursing knowledge, including practice and science-based inquiry.

Empowerment as reformulated, then, is defined as *a health patterning of well-being in which the client optimizes the ability to transform self through the relational process of nursing*. It may necessarily involve identifying and transcending sources of oppression that constrain human potential and limit self-understanding of personal resources. And the client's success in this process further strengthens the nursing process of empowerment.

The Rogerian ideas of Barrett et al.'s (1997) power enhancement, Newman's (1997) expanding consciousness and Reed's (1997a) participatory process of well-being, together provide for a reformulated view of empowerment—one that extends the possibilities of change for all participants (Cowling, 2001) as a dynamic human health process. Empowerment can then be understood as a complex and participatory process of changing oneself and one's environment, recognizing patterns, and engaging inner resources for well-being. It is a process greater than any one theory can represent. It is a process that is central to a unitary perspective of human beings (Cowling, 2001).

A Case Study

The following story illustrates the experience of empowerment and offers an example of the mutual process of power that is inherent in the nurse-client system. In this participatory human health process Susan, a community health nurse, focuses on patterning the environment with Ida to promote Ida's sense of power to participate in healthcare and healthcare decisions. In talking with Ida, Susan focuses on Ida's strengths, facilitates a supportive relational process, and provides empowering education that promotes Ida's health.

Several years ago, Susan met Ida during a home visit. Ida was in her late 70s, diagnosed with chronic obstructive pulmonary disease (COPD), osteoporosis, and heart failure. She was on many medications, including nebulizer treatments, inhalers, continuous oxygen, and pills. Ida had been in the hospital frequently for COPD exacerbations. She told Susan that she didn't like going to the hospital: "They didn't do much for me other than increasing my breathing treatments and giving me IV steroids," and "I can do that at home."

Ida lived with her son, daughter-in-law, and their two children. She had an upstairs bedroom and stayed there except for meals, which she would take down in the kitchen if her breathing would allow it. She said the family did not provide her with much support, and often she would go for days without anyone coming in to say "hi." Ida was lonely. She filled her time with crafts including crocheting and making items with beads plus she liked to read and watch video movies. She told

About the Author

ANN L. WHALL is a native Michiganian and three-time graduate of Wayne State University in Detroit. She is an Advanced Nurse Practitioner in Michigan and was a Fulbright Distinguished Scholar in the United Kingdom, examining expert nurses' use of implicit memory in dementia care. The focus of her scholarship is gero-mental health, especially improving and/or maintaining the function of person with dementia. Throughout her career Dr. Whall has been "driven by the desire to explicate the depth and exquisite nature of nursing knowledge which has historically been unrecognized exterior to nursing." As a diploma graduate, she was denied admittance to graduate programs exterior to nursing on the basis of a belief that nursing was "manual art, not a science." Among her most significant accomplishment is as Recipient of the John A. Hartford Doris Schwartz Award in 2003 for "visionary and exemplary" contributions advancing the field of gerontologic nursing research and American Nurses' Association Book of the Year awards for her theory development textbooks. Dr. Whall has published widely, held several visiting professorships, and completed multiple research studies and related publications, often with an identifiable emphasis upon the metatheoretical nature nursing knowledge. Dr. Whall enjoys classical music, golfing, interacting with her three children, and developing international connections within nursing.

Within these disciplines, family theories form a substantive knowledge base that is viewed from the context of each discipline. The discipline of nursing has largely adopted the existing theories of family functioning from sociology and psychology. The use of this theoretical base takes place across clinical areas of nursing.[5–7] In general, these theories have not been viewed from the syntax of nursing theory.

This discussion is premised on the assumption that the discipline of nursing considers family functioning a proper subject of inquiry or a substantive knowledge base for nursing. Nursing conceptual frameworks, or theories, with their broad level of applicability, can be used as the theoretical umbrella or syntax by which existing theories of family functioning may be examined for adequacy as well as weakness, for the purposes of reformulation and revision. The consideration of existing theories from a discipline other than nursing in light of nursing knowledge is supported by nursing theorists.

According to Fawcett, for an existing theoretical structure to be viewed as a nursing theory, that theory must first be evaluated and reformulated in terms of congruence and consistency with the central concepts of nursing theory (person, environment, health, and nursing).[8] This is consistent with Hardy's position that because nursing draws upon biopsychosocial knowledge, it is free to draw upon knowledge developed by these disciplines; but nursing has an obligation to alter theories it draws upon to fit the problems associated with nursing.[9] Ellis also addressed this issue when she discussed theories of, in, and for nursing.[10] Existing theories used in nursing are to be examined in light of current nursing knowledge. Fawcett also makes the point that once reformulation of the major concepts of an existing theory has occurred, along with evaluation of the relational statements, the resultant formulations can be designated as nursing theory.[8]

The major nursing theories are mostly at the conceptual framework level in terms of theory development; nursing theories are not, therefore, generally situation-producing or -prescriptive. According to Fawcett, it is crucial that prescriptive theories borrowed from other fields be carefully scrutinized in terms of the basic concepts of nursing theory. The discussion here attempts to address this issue and move forward the scrutiny of borrowed family theory.

Family Functioning Theory

Theories of family functioning from the discipline of psychology appear to have the most applicability to nursing practice. Most sociological theories are deductive and midrange; in contrast, some psychological theories of family functioning are inductive and situation-prescribing. Psychological theories of family functioning thus tend to be more useful to nursing practice. Rather than discussing what is, psychological theories tend to prescribe what will be of assistance to a particular family. Because nursing as a discipline is concerned with caring, helping, and nurturing, lack of specificity in many a priori midrange sociological formulations leads to delay or impasse in utilization. Duffey and Muhlenkamp point out that the usefulness of theoretical structures is of prime importance in the evaluation of theories.[11] The psychologically based theories referred to here are those of the family theorists considered somewhat psychoanalytic in approach, such as Framo[12] and Boszormenyi-Nagy;[13] those considered communicationist in approach, such as Haley,[14] Satir,[15] and Jackson;[16] and those using a systems approach, such as Napier and Whitaker,[17] and Minuchin et al.[18] These theorists discuss specific approaches, interventions, and goals in dealing with family functioning.

Nursing Theory

All nursing theories deal somewhat with four central concepts: person, environment, health, and nursing. Because nursing theories are generally at the broad conceptual framework level of theory development, for the purposes of this discussion nursing theory is considered to be the syntax of nursing.[8,9] The nursing theories referred to are those of King, Peplau, and Rogers.[1–3]

The syntax of nursing theory indicates the way to handle the four central concepts; the existing theory or substantive knowledge area can thus be viewed in terms of congruence and consistency with person, environment, health, and nursing. Given that existing theories do not discuss nursing as such, aspects of the nursing process which are addressed, such as goal and mode of intervention, can also be evaluated. It is important to note that the nursing theories vary in the way in which the central concepts are handled.

Most nursing theories define *person* in some holistic fashion. However, the way in which the term *holistic* is interpreted by nursing theorists varies; some believe that aspects of a person may be addressed separately, while others insist upon terms that handle only the whole person. Nursing theorists also consider environment in various field-figure arrangements, either as separate, as a unified entity with person, or as a somewhat unified entity.

The term *health* is also discussed in different ways by the nursing theorists. Some describe the health-illness continuum; others discuss health in more holistic terms, such as optimum well-being. Both linear and holistic approaches to family health are represented in the existing theories of family functioning. Likewise, the concepts of person and environment are primarily handled in either a linear or holistic manner. The congruence between nursing theory and existing theories of family functioning forms the basis of the following discussion.

Holism and Linearity

Maslow states that if one is to perceive holistically, then it is necessary to assess holistically or in some manner that considers the total and not the parts.[19] In a discussion of reductionist tendencies, he says that "good knowers," or those who know not only through cognitive operations but also through the senses, do not split mind from body, but attempt to perceive the whole person.[19] Once the Cartesian position that mind and body may be considered separately is accepted, it follows that the parts may be assessed separately. Maslow explains that the latter approach leads to reductionism, or the belief that a sum of the parts equals the whole.

Linear conceptualizations place person, health, or environment on a plane. The health-illness continuum is a familiar linear conceptualization. If the person is seen as progressing through time and space in such a fashion that past problems may be returned to and addressed, then the whole of the person is not perceived. Obviously, because no one gets younger, all persons progress through time and space. For this linear conceptualization to remain consistent, the person is perceived separately from the environment of time and space. Therefore, the separatism of many linear models does not handle the concepts of person and environment as a whole.

When the conceptualization is such that problems may be returned to, addressed, and corrected, then for a while the time and space environment is ignored. The person is thus viewed as independent from the environmental field, and it is then possible to discuss the person adapting in a time-lag sequence to the environment. Problems of the environment can be addressed as separate from the person and vice versa.

The helper, who can be viewed as separate from the field, may "fix-up" the environment or the client separately, without joining the field. From this linear field-independent perspective, active participation of client with helper becomes questionable. In the world of strict linear formulations, the helper may be separate from the client, the client separate from the environment, and all on a continuum in which progression and retrogression are possible. This approach appears antithetical to Maslow's holistic approach. Because the whole person is generally considered the proper subject matter for nursing,[1–3,20] it is important to consider the implications of the use of linear concepts.

Congruence of Family Functioning and Nursing Theories

Existing theories of family functioning primarily use holistic or linear approaches, view environment as separate or as a whole with person, and address health as a linear continuum or as part of the whole of time and space. Minuchin et al classify theories of family functioning as primarily holistic or linear. Theories of family functioning are divided into three general types: psychoanalytic, communicationist, and systems.[18] The Minuchin et al classification system is used to organize the following discussion.

Psychoanalytic Approach

In the commonly held psychoanalytic view, each of the family architects, the parents, brings into the present family unit needs formulated via the heritage of their early life experiences.[12] The parents, as individuals, are thus the prime unit of consideration. Early events in the lives of the parents are of prime importance; these early events must be addressed for there to be a change in the present family unit.[13] This view considers personhood as deterministically foretold by prior events.

The type and magnitude of past events can determine the type of mate selected, the career chosen, and even the selection of friends. The psychoanalytic view is thus primarily a linear approach in which energy may be stopped (fixated), progress (be worked through), or even go backward (regression). The marriage partners are mostly seen as separate, in terms of influence from the present environmental field. The present family is clearly not the prime focus of intervention because resolution of present difficulties lies in the working through of past problems.

As in the classical psychoanalytic approach, theories of family functioning using this theory base consider the therapeutic relationship to be of prime importance. Because much of the problem is unconscious and therefore unavailable to the client, the client depends upon the helper to discover and work through past problems.

In this view the family is an aggregate of individuals with complementary needs. The question is not one of whole family unit versus individual interventions, but one of preeminence and a working out of symptoms of the most needy individual through the rest of the family members. Theories of family functioning that demonstrate this view begin with a working through of the "tension states" or underlying problems of the marital partners. Once these tensions are resolved, the family unit is expected to function well. Health is thus viewed as a working through of past difficulties so that it is no longer necessary to attempt to repetitively work through the past problems in to the present.

Nursing Theory

Nursing theories congruent with the psychoanalytic view would consider person, environment, and health in some composite fashion—person as a biopsychosocial being with the psychological portion preeminent. Health is seen as a continuum with the possibility of assisting the client back to health through the interpersonal relationship. Because of past experiences, the client is unable to clearly discern problems and thus depends upon the nurse for clarification; the client is therefore less active. The helper assists each client to work through present problems that reflect past deficits. The goal and focus of the intervention is insight developed via the interpersonal relationship.

Although there are some inconsistencies, Peplau's approach to nursing theory is generally congruent with the psychoanalytic approach to family functioning.[2] Peplau defines *person* as an organism that strives to reduce tension generated by needs and defines *nursing* as a significant interpersonal process. The person is viewed as a biopsychosocial being with emphasis upon the psychological aspects. This composite view of person is compatible with a linear view of tension reduction. The client responds to the nursing intervention, primarily the interpersonal relationship, with a reduction in tension. The tension is generated primarily from past needs. A notable incongruence between Peplau's approach and the psychoanalytic approach is that Peplau insists upon participation of the client in such things as mutual goal setting and action. The family is not addressed as a specific unit. This is considered consistent with Peplau's discussion of person as an individual striving to work through individual needs.

Communicationist Approach

Minuchin et al identify a second group of family theorists as communicationists, including Haley,[14] Bateson,[21] and Satir.[15] Due to the theorizing of Harry Stack Sullivan, a shift in thinking took place, with interest focusing upon the pattern of signals by which information is transferred within dyads and triads.[18] The communicationists emphasize present communication patterns in terms of pattern, sequence, and hierarchy, rather than the past nature of people.[13] The person is perceived as actively involved in the present, not the past and the cause-effect influence of early relationships. The communicationists stress the ways in which the person

interacts, not only in terms of parts but also the whole. The field within which the person functions becomes highlighted. The helper and client influence and become influenced by one another; the split between action and reaction becomes less with the concept that actions and reactions occur together in the same field. Persons interact with the environment in terms of patterns and cues. The unit of intervention thus changes from helper and individual client to helper uniting with the field, and in particular, the dyadic and triadic relationships in which the client is involved.[15]

The communicationist approach is viewed as an extension of the prior psychoanalytic view, from individual to interactional patterns among people. Double bind communication patterns, scape-goating processes, pseudomutualities and silencing strategies within the dyads or triads of the family are of prime importance. The locus of difficulty lies in transmission processes. Homeostasis considerations prevail as equilibrium concepts imply that equality of relationships is health. The goal becomes clarification of relationships among all people within the dyadic and triadic patterns. The helpers' authority is subject to challenge, for as part of the field, the helper is an active participant in the communication sequences. The communicationist approach, emphasizing mutual action and reaction among people, may imply a time lag, thus suggesting linearity. However, the linearity is much less clear than in the psychoanalytic approach. The field is emphasized and field and person are treated as one.

Nursing Theory

King's theory, which focuses on transactions within the dyad of nurse and client, is most consistent with the approach of the communicationists. King states that person (*man* in her terminology) is a reacting being with awareness of the environment.[1] The response or reaction is a comprehensive response of mind and body; the nurse and client work together toward a mutually acceptable goal. Health implies continuous adaptation to internal and external stresses. The relationship between nurse and client is prime. Although the environment is discussed as one with the individual, families are not specifically addressed. The therapeutic relationship is central and the person and nurse are viewed as part of the same field. Although King sometimes uses linear terms such as reaction and adaptation, the linearity of person is less clear than in psychoanalytic conceptualizations. As with the communicationists, King's model implies field dependence. The interpersonal orientation implies that the client and nurse are of the same field.

Systems Approach

The systems theories of family functioning emerged in the late 1950s and are considered extensions of the communicationist approach. The unit of intervention in systems theory is a dramatic departure from previous theory. Not only is the family unit perceived holistically, but it must be analyzed and approached holistically, not reductively. No longer are subsystem dyads considered primary and sometimes seen alternatively. In the pure systems approach, the family is always seen together. Sometimes three and four generations are included in the approach, and all problems are handled in total family sessions. According to a systems framework, the family is a type of unitary living organism.[18] The family is a living system relating to the systems of community, country, and universe. Just as one organ of the body relates to and is influenced by every other organ, the family system is influenced by internal subsystems as well as the larger community system. The family grows and changes, giving birth to new and different forms, just as an organism grows, changes, and reproduces. The family is a system in that it is a series of interrelated parts. Family rules govern the system and the individual's margin of choice. An important point is that family systems theorists generally imply a closed system perspective. Dysfunction or illness is defined as the closing down of the family system in much the same way as the closing down of the body's circulatory system is dysfunctional for the whole body. In terms of mode of intervention, the helper works with the system and becomes part of the system. By changing a key element of the system, not always the most negative portion, the total system changes and hopefully dysfunctions are alleviated.

Nursing Theory

In terms of a nursing conceptual framework, Rogers is perhaps closest to the family systems approach.[3] The greatest departure perhaps is that Rogers considers the person from an open rather than a closed systems perspective. The person is always open or in mutual, simultaneous interaction with the environment. As do family systems theorists, Rogers sees boundaries as more perceptual than real, everything is connected to everything else. According to both Rogers and the family systems theorists, pattern and organization characterize the system. Change in one portion of the system affects changes in the whole, and these changes create reverberations in the system in wavelike fashion.

The unit of intervention for both Rogers and family system theorists is the total *family system*. Both consider the fields of nurse and family environments as coextensive and infinite energy fields. There is also congruence between the approaches of Rogers and family systems theory in terms of working within the system as opposed to external manipulation in a psychoanalytic sense. Health in Rogers' terms is a value judgment, because disease conditions are not entities by themselves but manifestations of the total pattern of the family system. The goal of nursing is to promote a symphonic interaction between persons (subsystems of the family), the family system, and the environment. The focus is thus redirection of patterns and organization within the family.[22]

Behaviorist Approach

The behaviorist approach to family is not discussed at length here because it is not well developed. However, compatible positions might be found between the behaviorist approaches to family and nursing theorists such as Roy who discuss adaptation.[19] According to Minuchin et al, the behaviorist views the family as a unit to decondition individual behavior, producing certain signals that organize the patient's behavior. The person is considered as somewhat separate, not one with the field.[18] Thus the unit of intervention is the individual. The behaviorist helper appears separate from the system. The view is one of person interacting with the environment to bring about an adopted state on the health-illness continuum. The linear causality focus of the behaviorist does not appear compatible with the communications or systems theorists who view person as part of total system or field.

Importance of Theory Reformulation

Reformulation of the theories of family functioning so as to achieve consistency with nursing approaches is important. With some of the theories of family functioning, such as the systems approach, reformulation in terms of nursing theory may be readily achieved. The perspective, however, would be changed from a closed to an open systems perspective. In the case of the psychoanalytic approach, reformulation in terms of the nursing theory that requires client independence may not be as readily achieved. If nursing is to follow a holistic approach to person, environment, and health—and the major nursing theories would lead one to believe this is the direction with the most support—then linear conceptualizations in both existing theories and nursing theories need to be evaluated. Newman states the true holistic approach is not to be confused with the summing of many facts, but with factors reflective of the whole.[22] Reformulation of linear aspects may be necessary.

The important point is that the existing theory is to be examined for reformulation in terms of the nursing theory. In the past, the nursing approach was often reformulated for congruence with existing theories from other disciplines.

REFERENCES

1. King I: *Toward a Theory of Nursing: General Concepts of Human Behavior.* New York, John Wiley & Sons, 1971.

2. Peplau H: *Interpersonal Relations in Nursing.* New York, Putnam, 1952.

3. Rogers M: *The Theoretical Basis of Nursing.* Philadelphia, FA Davis, 1970.

4. Schwab J: Structure of the disciplines: Meanings and significances, in Ford G (ed): *The Structure of Knowledge and the Curriculum.* Chicago, Rand McNally & Co, 1964, pp 6–30.

5. Miller J, Janosik E: *Family Focused Care.* New York, McGraw-Hill, 1980.

6. Hymovich D, Barnard M: *Family Health Care.* New York, McGraw-Hill, 1979.

7. Smoyak S: *The Psychiatric Nurse as a Family Therapist.* New York, John Wiley & Sons, 1975.

8. Fawcett J: The what of theory development, in *What, Why and How of Theory Development.* New York, National League for Nursing, 1978.

9. Hardy M: Evaluating nursing theory, in *What, Why and How of Theory Development.* New York, National League for Nursing, 1978.

10. Ellis R: Characteristics of significant theories. *Nurs Res* 17: 217–222, May-June 1968.

11. Duffey M, Muhlenkamp A: A framework for theory analysis. *Nurs Outlook* 22:570–574, September 1974.

12. Framo J: Rationale and techniques of intensive family therapy, in Boszormenyi-Nagy I, Framo J (eds): *Intensive Family Therapy: Theoretical and Practical Aspects.* New York, Harper & Row, 1965.

13. Boszormenyi-Nagy I: Intensive family therapy as process, in Boszormenyi-Nagy I, Framo J (eds): *Intensive Family Therapy: Theoretical and Practical Aspects.* New York, Harper & Row, 1965.

14. Haley J: *Problem Solving Therapy.* San Francisco, Jossey-Bass, 1978.

15. Satir V: *Conjoint Family Therapy.* Palo Alto, Calif, Science & Behavior Books, 1967.

16. Jackson D: The question of family homeostasis. *Psychiatr Q Suppl* 31: 79–90, 1957.

17. Napier A, Whitaker C: *The Family Crucible.* New York, Harper & Row, 1978.

18. Minuchin S, Rosman B, Baker L: *Psychosomatic Families.* Cambridge, Mass, Harvard University Press, 1978.

19. Maslow A: *The Psychology of Science.* South Bend, Ind, Gateway, 1966.

20. Roy C: *Introduction to Nursing: An Adaptation Model.* Englewood Cliffs, NJ, Prentice-Hall, 1976.

21. Bateson G: The birth of a matrix or double bind and epistemology, in Berger M (ed): *Beyond the Double Bind.* New York, Brunner/Mazel, 1978.

22. Newman M: *Theory Development in Nursing.* Philadelphia, FA Davis, 1979.

The Author Comments

Congruence Between Existing Theories of Family Functioning and Nursing Theories

As a public health nurse, I was cognizant of the historical value placed upon the family as a unit of care within nursing. Yet, in the nursing literature in the late 1970s, there was little knowledge presented from a nursing perspective. Most was derived "as is" from nonpractice-oriented disciplines that were exterior to nursing. I wrote this article based on my dissertation research after being challenged by my dissertation chairperson, Dr. Joyce Fitzpatrick, to explicate the differences between the nursing perspective and that of others. The members of the Nursing Theory Think Tank also challenged the existence of a nursing perspective upon family. This article was also a response to that challenge.

—ANN L. WHALL

CHAPTER 47

Development of Situation-Specific Theories

An Integrative Approach

Eun-Ok Im

One type of "ready-to-wear" theories that can bring about better nursing care outcomes regardless of their philosophical bases is situation-specific theories proposed by Im and Meleis in 1999. In this paper, some propositions for an integrative approach to the development of situation-specific theories are made. First, situation-specific theories are described as practice theories while they are compared with middle-range theories. Then the integrative approach is detailed, which includes (a) checking assumptions for theory development; (b) exploring through multiple sources; (c) theorizing; and (d) reporting, sharing, and validating. Finally, the paper concludes with suggestions for further development of the integrative approach.

ACROSS disciplines, scholars can now sympathize with the epistemic pluralism that is the practical philosophy of most working scientists in general.[1] Until recently, scholars believed in the unity of scientific knowledge, and they accepted its fragmentation only as a pragmatic necessity. However, these days, scholars are quite happy to go along with philosophical plurality across many disciplines.[2]

Nursing history also shows the same changes toward epistemic pluralism in theoretical and philosophical thinking. In the 1950s, under the tremendous influences of logical positivism, grand theories were

From E-O Im, Development of situation-specific theories. An integrative approach. Advances in Nursing Science, 2005, 28(2), 137–151.
Copyright © 2005. Reproduced with permission of Lippincott Williams & Wilkins.

About the Author

EUN-OK IM was born in South Korea and moved to the United States her 20s. She received a PhD in nursing from the University of California, San Francisco, where she also held a postdoctoral position. She is currently Professor at The University of Texas at Austin. Professor Im has gained national and international recognition as a methodologist and theorist in international cross-cultural Internet research through more than 50 peer-reviewed publications and over 100 professional presentations. Her published articles on situation-specific theories, feminist critique, and Internet research methodologies are cited by many researchers around the world. Her hobbies are reading novels, knitting, and watching movies.

developed and used to answer questions on the nature, mission, and goals of nursing, and nursing scholars and theorists believed in the unity of nursing knowledge. In the 1960s–1980s, metatheoretical questions on the types and contents of theories were asked and argued, yet their philosophical basis was still empiricism.[3–6] From the middle of the 1980s onward, tremendous efforts in concept development were made with the introduction of qualitative philosophical thinking.[7–11] From the beginning of the 1990s, numerous middle-range theories were developed and published,[14–17] and philosophical pluralism in theoretical nursing became more prominent.[12–14] Through these historical changes, now, nursing scholars even envision and sympathize with epistemic pluralism, and seek ready-to-wear theories in nursing practice that may bring about better nursing care outcomes regardless of their philosophical bases.[15]

Nursing has struggled to develop "ready-to-wear" theories. "Ready to wear" refers to easy applicability to research and practice. One type of "ready-to-wear" theories is situation-specific theories, proposed by Im and Meleis in 1999.[16] *Situation-specific theories* are defined as theories that focus on specific nursing phenomena, that reflect clinical practice, and that are limited to specific populations or to particular fields of practice.[16,17] Situation-specific theories belong to a different level than grand theories and middle-range theories, which can incorporate diversities and complexities in nursing phenomenon, consider sociopolitical, cultural, and historical contexts of nursing encounters, and

be easily applicable to nursing practice.[17] In this paper, *middle-range theories* mean theories that have more limited scope and less abstraction than grand theories, address specific phenomena or concepts, reflect practice, and aim to be easily testable[18]; *grand theories* are systematic constructions of the nature of nursing, the mission of nursing, and the goals of nursing care.[17] Situation-specific theories are also intended not to be universal theories that can be applicable to any time, any socially constraining structures, or any politically limiting situations. Rather, they are intended to be more clinically specific, reflect a particular context, and include blueprints for action.[16,17] Philosophically, this new type of theory has roots in postempiricism, critical social theory, feminism, and hermeneutics,[16] all of which agree with current epistemic pluralism in nursing.

When situation-specific theories were proposed, an integrative approach was also proposed as a strategy for developing them. *The integrative approach* was originally proposed by Meleis[17] and has been extended through later work by Im and Meleis.[16] The integrative approach has some essential components, such as the clinical grounding that drives the basic or clinical questions as well as the questions themselves. Also essential are opportunities for clinical involvement and for conceptually thinking about the health/illness responses, the situations, and the environment.[17] However, the propositions of the integrative approach tended to be too abstract for novice theorists to utilize in actual theory development. Further development/refinement of the integrative approach is essential for the future development and practical use of situation-specific theories, which may ultimately result in a stronger link between theory and practice and subsequently produce better nursing care outcomes than other types of theories. In this paper, some propositions for the integrative approach to the development of situation-specific theories are made. First, situation-specific theories are described as practice theories while they are compared with other types of theories. Then the integrative approach is detailed. Finally, the paper concludes with suggestions for further development of the integrative approach.

Situation-Specific Theories, Practice Theories, and Middle-Range Theories

Figure 47-1 shows the relationships among practice theories, situation-specific theories, middle-range theories, and grand theories reported in the literature. In recent literature, situation-specific theories are sometimes labeled as *micro-theories* or *practice theories* (a term that is interchangeable with *micro-theories)*, or even as middle-range theories.[11,13,18] In a sense, situation-specific theories can be categorized as practice theories

because situation-specific theories certainly aim at functioning as practice theories. Jacox[6] proposed that *practice theories* be considered those theories that outline the actions that nurses must take to meet a nursing goal (producing some desired change or effect in the patient's condition). In these terms, situation-specific theories can be considered practice theories because one of the goals of situation-specific theories is to provide a blueprint for nursing practice.[16] Peterson[18] even categorized situation-specific theories and practice theories in the same category, noting that the literature included a confusing variety of terms to refer to the level of theory that is considered less abstract, more specific, and narrower in scope than middle-range theories.

Although practice theories have been welcome in nursing because nursing is inherently a practice-oriented discipline, they have often been criticized as well. The major criticism is that they are procedural and not based on a well-developed body of nursing science.[18] For this reason, some theorists have worked to blend middle-range theories with practice theories, and their hybrid efforts have been highly evaluated because they elevate the resulting practice above simple dictates or imperatives.[11] Since situation-specific theories, in nature, are practice theories, those blending efforts are

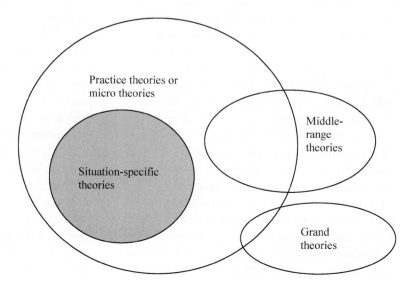

Figure 47-1. *Relationships among practice theories, middle-range theories, grand theories, and situation-specific theories.*

unnecessary for situation-specific theories. In addition, situation-specific theories can provide a basis for the development of the knowledge base for nursing practices through research and practice efforts in specific nursing situations because they are more than just guidelines or standardized procedures for nursing practice.[16]

Situation-specific theories, however, are different from middle-range theories because the former can be applicable only to specific nursing phenomenon or particular nursing clients while the latter can be applicable across nursing practice fields.[16,18] For example, the middle-range theory of transition proposed by Meleis and her colleagues[19] was developed based on several studies of ethnically diverse samples undergoing a wide range of transitions, including menopausal, maternal, and caregiving transition; subsequently, they aimed to cover all types of transitions in nursing situations. However, the situation-specific theory of the menopausal transition of Korean immigrant women by Im and Meleis[20] aimed at only the specific population of menopausal low-income Korean immigrant women in the United States.

Situation-specific theories are also different from middle-range theories in terms of their testability. Middle-range theories contain a limited number of variables and testable relationships.[21] In other words, middle-range theories are based on logical positivistic and/or postpositivistic ideas that assume the testability of a theory.[18] Grand theories are criticized as too abstract to be tested empirically. The basic assumption here is that the testability of theories is based on a logical positivistic idea.

Situation-specific theories do not always assume their testability.[16] Some situation-specific theories will certainly aim at the operationalization of central concepts for hypotheses testing in real settings. However, other situation-specific theories are not supposed to be testable because they are developed on philosophical foundations (e.g., hermeneutics, phenomenology, critical theory, postmodernism) in which positivistic apparatuses such as hypotheses do not have a place.[16] Rather, the situation-specific theories aim at helping researchers understand central concepts through qualitative fieldwork and/or participant observation. If a situation-

specific theory was developed based on postempiricism, it can aim at operationalization, measurements, and hypothesis testing. On the contrary, if a situation-specific theory originated with a phenomenological perspective, the theory may not be used to operationalize, measure, and/or test a hypothesis. Rather, the theory may aim at explaining and understanding the lived experience of human beings in the middle of the phenomenon.

In the discipline of nursing, many strategies for concept development and theory development have been proposed. The concept development strategies proposed and used in nursing include the Wilsonian method,[21,22] the Walker and Avant approach,[10,11] Rogers' evolutionary concept analysis method,[23] the Hybrid method,[9] and the simultaneous analysis method.[7,8] Many strategies for developing a theory have been also proposed, and used as well.[10,11,17,23,24] Rodgers and Knafl[23] asserted that these currently existing concept and theory development strategies for grand theories and middle-range theories do not adequately consider that the theory development process, specifically the concept development process, is evolutionary, and that there is no step-by-step recipe for developing a theory.

The view of Rodgers and Knafl assumes that concepts are formed by the identification of characteristics common to a class of objects or phenomena and the abstraction and clustering of these characteristics, which is influenced heavily by socialization and public interaction.[23,25] This view assumes that, because these contextual factors vary, there will be variations in concepts over time or across situations. Currently, most nursing theorists and scholars agree that the theory development process is a continuous, dynamic, and evolutionary process influenced by contexts surrounding the theory development process.[11,23] This is somewhat problematic in practical applications to nursing practice and research, however. It is easy to understand in an abstract way, but in reality, the assumption that theory development is evolutionary, not algorithmic and linear, poses a potential contradiction because a theory might evolve away from the specific time, place, and population for which it was originally conceived. Since situation-specific theories are limited to a specific population and a particular nursing phenomenon/situation, which, in turn, limits the contexts (eg, time, place, situation) for theory applications, the theory development process becomes more feasible and easily applicable to nursing practice and research even in light of the evolutionary nature of theory development.[16] Consequently, with the specificity and easy applicability of situation-specific theories, nurses may produce better nursing care outcomes than with other types of theories that do not limit the time, nursing situations, or nursing clients.

The Integrative Approach

In the integrative approach, the conceptualization and theorizing processes can happen all at once, or they might take years and never quite evolve into a useful integrated view of reality.[17] Yet, to provide a convenient guideline, in this section, the process of the integrative approach to the development of situation-specific theories is proposed step by step. This process may not happen subsequently or in a continuous way. Rather, some steps of the process would be skipped, while others could happen repetitively. The steps suggested in this paper are actually what nursing researchers and practitioners have frequently used in their research projects and practice without recognition. Based on an in-depth review of the literature published within the past 5 years, the steps used in the development of situation-specific theories in the literature are summarized and proposed as follows. The process of the integrative approach is also summarized in Figure 47-2.

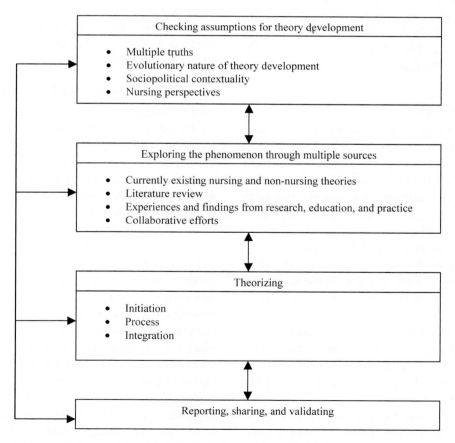

Figure 47-2. *An integrative approach to situation-specific theories.*

Checking Assumptions for Theory Development

A theorist who wants to develop a situation-specific theory needs to check her or his assumptions for theory development first. The assumptions for the development of situation-specific theories include (*a*) multiple truths; (*b*) evolutionary nature of theory development; (*c*) sociopolitical contextuality; and (*d*) nursing perspectives. These assumptions are the basis for the whole theory development process of situation-specific theories. If a theorist does not agree with these assumptions, she or he may need to reconsider if she or he really wants to develop a situation-specific theory. For example, if her or his assumption for theory development is based on the universality of health/illness experience, she or he might not aim at the development of a situation-specific theory because a situation-specific theory assumes multiple truths, which negates the universality of health/illness experience. Rather, she or he needs to aim at developing a grand theory or a middle-range theory.

Multiple Truths

Under the influences of positivism and scientism, nursing phenomena have been considered to be universal phenomena which can occur to any racial, cultural, and gender groups in the same way.[29,30] Thus, most nursing theories have also assumed that nursing phenomena are universal and homogeneous, and traditional approaches to knowledge development depend on the assumptions of universality, homogeneity, and normality.[29] Yet nursing phenomenon are becoming more complex and complicated by multiple factors, including the increasing diversity of nursing clients.[30] A consensus has developed among nurse scholars recently in which theoretical development must take into consideration the diversity and complexity of nursing phenomena.[30,31] Without doing so, the theoretical foundation of the nursing discipline cannot achieve the connections for which nursing has been striving.

As posited in the paper by Im and Meleis,[16] the development of situation-specific theories assumes philosophical, theoretical, and methodological plurality, which is more congruent with the nature and goals of nursing and which can incorporate the diversity and complexity of nursing phenomenon. The philosophical bases of the substance and syntax of nursing knowledge have been debated by many nursing scholars.[26–28] Meleis[17] divided the philosophical positions of nursing scholars into three: (*a*) the purist position; (*b*) the radical separationist position; and (*c*) the nonpurist position. The bona fide purist position claims that a philosophical viewpoint should guide and direct theory development, research strategy, and clinical practice.[17] The radical separationist position asserts that a discipline's theory and research are distinct entities and do not necessarily have to be congruent philosophically and methodologically.[17] The nonpurist position takes a philosophical, theoretical, and methodological pluralistic position.[17] The project to develop situation-specific theories assumes this nonpurist philosophical position as well as the existence of multiple truths, not one universal scientific truth.

Evolutionary Nature of Theory Development

Another assumption for the development of situation-specific theories is that the theory development process is cyclic and evolutionary. As discussed above, a concept which is currently regarded as a norm or a standard may not be a norm or a standard in the future.[23] In other words, the integrity or stability of that norm through time cannot be predicted or ensured. Concepts are formed by the identification of characteristics common to a class of objects or phenomena and the abstraction and clustering of these characteristics.[25] Therefore, as characteristics of nursing phenomena change, concepts also change. A concept which is not considered as important now can evolve into an important concept in future nursing. Consequently, a situation-specific theory which is developed for a particular population in a specific situation will not be appropriate for the same population in a different time or a different sociopolitical context. Thus, the situation-specific theory for the same population in the same situation also needs to be changed with changes in time and sociopolitical contexts.

Sociopolitical Contextuality

A third assumption for the development of situation-specific theories is the sociopolitical contextuality of nursing phenomena. The current theory development process involved in the development of grand theories and middle-range theories rarely considers the sociopolitical, cultural, and/or historic contexts inherent to each client-nurse encounter.[32] Rather than accounting for the contextuality of nursing phenomenon, they usually try to reduce the phenomenon into several central concepts; operationalize and measure the concepts; explore/test the concepts and constructs through quantitative and qualitative data collections; and refine the theories.[11,18] Consequently, they frequently aim at theories that can be applicable to all nursing fields and explain central concepts across the fields. Since situation-specific theories are limited to a specific population and/or a particular area of interest, the theories can easily incorporate the contextuality of the phenomenon.[16] Indeed, the development of situation-specific theories assumes that nursing phenomena or client-nurse encounters happen in sociopolitical contexts, that sociopolitical contexts need to be incorporated in the theory development process, and that the theories cannot be always applicable to any historical moment, any social structure, or any political situation.

Nursing Perspectives

An essential assumption for the development of situation-specific theories is that they are based on nursing perspectives. Nursing perspectives give a unique view on a phenomenon. When we view a same phenomenon with two different perspectives, the phenomenon described by each of the two different perspectives may be different from each other. For example, when we view Asian American cancer patients' lack of pain reporting using a biological perspective, we may focus on the physiological characteristics of Asian Americans without considering their whole beings in the contexts of their daily lives. Consequently, we may assume that Asian Americans' lack of pain reporting is a simple biological difference from other ethnic groups, which may lead us to look for basic biological difference between the ethnic groups.

When we view the same phenomenon (lack of pain reporting) from a nursing perspective, we may view the patients' bio-psycho-socio-cultural beings within the contexts of their daily lives. Rather than focusing on inter-ethnic biological differences, we may focus on how their psycho-socio-cultural contexts circumscribe their pain experience and how we could provide adequate pain management while considering their unique pain experience.

In the development of situation-specific theories, a nursing perspective is mandatory.[16] The theories developed without a nursing perspective might distort the descriptions of nursing phenomenon and mislead nursing research and/or practice. Yet more than one nursing perspective exists.[17] A nursing perspective may be based on biomedical models; it may also be based on feminist perspectives emphasizing sociopolitical environments and reflecting oppressed groups' interests (mostly women's). In either case, it should also reflect nurses' concerns, views, values, and attitudes.

Exploring Through Multiple Sources

After checking assumptions for her or his theory development, a theorist needs to explore her or his phenomenon of interest through multiple sources. The multiple sources may include: (*a*) currently existing nursing and non-nursing theories related to the phenomenon of interest; (*b*) literature reviews; (*c*) findings and experiences from research, education, and practice; and (*d*) collaborative efforts. Theorists usually use more than one of these sources for theory development at the same time. Each source is discussed in detail as follows.

Currently Existing Nursing and Non-nursing Theories

Nursing and non-nursing conceptual models, grand theories, and middle-range theories can serve as the foundation for the development of situation-specific theories. From the early days of nursing theory development, theory derivation has been prevalent in nursing.[11] Usually, theory derivation in nursing has been done by using analogy to obtain explanations or predictions about a phenomenon in nursing from the explanations or predictions in another field including medicine, psychology, sociology, and public health.[13] Recently, theories from nursing have been combined with those from other disciplines to create middle-range theories.[11,18] In the development of situation-specific theories, both nursing and/or non-nursing theories may provide the basis for analogy for explanations, understandings, or predictions of a particular situation of a specific population of interest as well.

An example is the above mentioned theory of menopausal transition of Korean immigrant women,[20] which was developed based on a middle-range theory of transition.[33] In the development of the situation-specific theory, major research questions were set based on the middle-range theory of transition. Then, each concept was explored through both quantitative and qualitative findings from a study on menopausal transition of Korean immigrant women. Based on the findings related to the concepts, the theory of transition was modified, and further developed as a situation-specific theory for menopausal transition of Korean immigrant women. Compared with the middle-range theory of transition, the situation-specific theory of menopausal transition of Korean immigrant women has increased specificity of the conceptualization and is easily applicable to the situation through the modifications based on actual study findings.

Literature Reviews

An extensive review of literature can provide a systematic analysis of currently existing knowledge about a nursing phenomenon and frequently provide an excellent source for theory development.[10,11] In this paper, the literature review means a review of previous research findings, theoretical work, and statistical governmental reports. Indeed, the literature review has been an essential basis for concept development and theory development. Walker and Avant[11] included literature synthesis as a method of concept synthesis and suggested that theory synthesis incorporate published research literature, direct statistical information, and qualitative research as the second step of three phases of theory development.

Many examples of theory development through literature review can be easily found in the nursing literature. An example would be the transition theory by Schumacher and Meleis[33] who conducted an extensive literature review on all types of transitions in nursing and proposed a theoretical framework of transitions. Based on the analysis of the literature, they proposed a set of major concepts related to transitions, which include types of transitions, properties of transitions, transition conditions, and nursing therapeutics. Although this example of the transition theory aims to be a middle-range theory, the review of the literature as a source of theory development can be easily incorporated into the integrative approach. In addition, a literature review frequently provides a starting point for theory development by giving us a picture of the state of the science in the area and initiating our theoretical thinking on the major and/or central concept(s) in the nursing phenomenon in question.[11] Hulme[34] provided an excellent example of an integrative literature review on currently existing grand, middle-range, and situation-specific theories related to health problems of adults who experienced childhood sexual abuse.

Findings and Experiences from Research, Education, and Practice

Findings and experiences from research projects, educational programs, and/or clinical practice in hospital and/or community settings can provide a source for theoretical development. Most nursing theories tend to be initiated by the theorists' experiences from their long clinical, academic, or research experience in nursing.[17] Theorists can easily raise theoretical questions from their own experience. Kirkevold[35] posited that integrative nursing research experience has great potential for clarifying the theoretical perspective and substance of the nursing discipline, as well as making research-based knowledge more accessible to clinical nurses. Lyons[36] argued that nursing can generate a knowledge base through reflecting on nurses' own experience. Reed[37] mentioned that her theory of self-transcendence was developed using clinical experience and empirical investigations.

Collaborative Efforts

International and interdisciplinary collaborative efforts may provide sources for the development of situation-specific theories as well. To be specific to a situation and/or a population, such a theory sometimes needs to incorporate a more detailed and exact source for theory development. Collaborative efforts allow comparisons of ideas, scholarly dialogues, and an integration of different and/or disperse opinions and findings.[38] Experts in different areas of nursing who are working on the same nursing phenomenon will give different and new views/visions on nursing phenomena which cannot be easily obtained by independent work by one person. For example, when a collaborative team is working together on midlife women's menopausal experience, a nurse whose expertise is physiology can provide a different view on menopausal experience from a nurse anthropologist or a nurse feminist. In terms of theoretical development, the theory will be a nursing theory, but it will be based on diverse views on menopause.

Collaborations between academics and clinicians can also provide a source for theory development, which will provide a strong link between theory and practice. Gassner et al.[39] proposed a model devised by the project team, including four academics and six clinicians, and concluded that the model was effective in facilitating the collaborative relationships necessary for successful development and implementation of reality-based learning for nursing students. Collaboration with research participants can also provide an excellent source of theory development.[40] Taking the lead in identifying areas of practice for action research is a natural extension of nurses' role as advocates for nursing clients, and it may provide a new view of the research participants.[40]

International collaborative efforts also can provide an excellent source for theory development, especially for situation-specific theories, because such theories need to provide blueprints for nursing practice with a specific population that can be usually categorized along ethnic/cultural lines. Walker and Avant[11] even envision that international efforts of nursing theory development will strengthen nursing knowledge and theory development by incorporating different perspectives/views from different cultural backgrounds. International collaboration can give a new view on everything from the philosophy of life, accepted behaviors, and human relations to the way in which people live.[41–42] Recent advances in computer and communication technologies may facilitate international collaboration through electronic networks more easily than in the past, and we will see more and more international collaborative works in theoretical nursing.[43]

Theorizing

Initiation

While exploring the phenomenon of interest through multiple sources, a theorist may initiate her or his theory development with a simple literature review on a specific nursing phenomenon of her or his interests, from her or his own research, and/or from her or his practice experiences even before the review of the literature. Theory development can start from a mother theory and result in a modified form of the theory, which is more specific to the population of her or his interest or to the nursing situation. Theory development can be initiated by a single person or a group of colleagues who have been involved in the same area of interests. Recently, some theories have been even developed through international or interdisciplinary collaboration.[11,41–42] Theory development in the integrative approach may be initiated from one source or multiple sources at a time or at separate time points.

Process

Developing a situation-specific theory can take place through a theorizing process in several different ways. Although few nursing theorists claim to have developed situation-specific theories, many theories in nursing meet the definition of situation-specific theories. The following examples show that the process involved in the development of situation-specific theories can be diverse. These examples were searched using the PUBMED database. For the PUBMED search, key words including *nursing, theory,* and *theory development* were used, and only the articles published in English

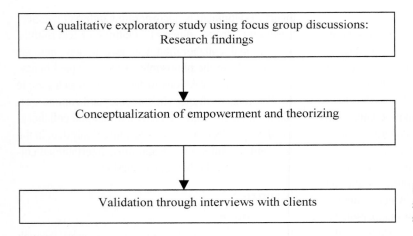

Figure 47-3. *The process involved in the development of the theoretical work by Falk-Rafael.*

during the past 5 years were searched in order to capture the current trends in nursing theory development. From the 215 articles retrieved through the search, tutorials, editorials, and literature review articles were excluded. Then, all the articles were reviewed in order to identify the process used in theory development. Among them, only the articles presenting situation-specific theories were selected for this paper.

One of the examples is the theoretical work by Falk-Rafael[44] (see Fig 47-3). Her theoretical work shows a unique type of process for theory development. She initiated her theoretical work through a qualitative exploratory study. She began the study by using a nominal group technique in a series of focus groups with public health nurses to identify their conceptualization of empowerment, the strategies they identified as empowering, and the outcomes of empowering strate-gies they observed in their practice. Based on the qualitative study, she then initiated the theorizing process and developed a model that conceptualized empowerment as a process of evolving consciousness in which increasing awareness, knowledge, and skills interacted with the clients' active participation to move toward actualizing potential. Finally, the developed model was shared and validated through interviews with clients whom nurses identified as having been empowered through their practice.

Recent nursing literature notes a type of theory development that integrates theory, research and practice. For example, LaCoursiere's theory of online social support (see Fig 47-4) was developed with an integrated framework that incorporates knowledge from multiple sources including (*a*) a conceptual literature review of existing frameworks and research findings related to social

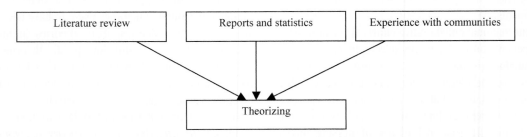

Figure 47-4. *The process involved in the development of the theoretical work by LaCoursiere.*

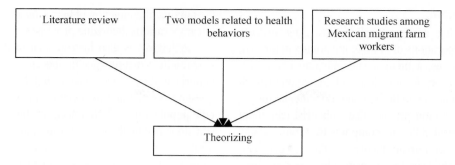

Figure 47-5. *The process involved in the development of the theoretical work by Poss.*

support, online communications, and the effect of the Internet or the Web; (*b*) reports and statistics from agencies and organizations focusing on the online health care experience; and (*c*) the author's experiences with online social support communities over a number of years. This type of theorizing can be easily found in nursing.

Another example of this type of theorizing is Poss's model for cross-cultural research among Mexican migrant workers in tuberculosis screening tests (see Fig 47-5).[46] In the theoretical work, the model was developed based on a literature review, two models that are often used to study health behaviors (the Health Belief Model and the Theory of Reasoned Action), and previous research studies

among Mexican migrant farm workers participating in a tuberculosis screening program.

The theory development process of situation-specific theories can also be found in the development of the integrative model for environmental health research by Dixon and Dixon (see Fig 47-6).[47] The theorists developed the theory based on their experiences in both academic and activist communities relative to environmental health and a review of the research literature. Then, a working hypothesis that may be useful in guiding investigations or suggesting needed policies was extracted and used in their research on the engagement in environmental health issues at the individual and community levels.

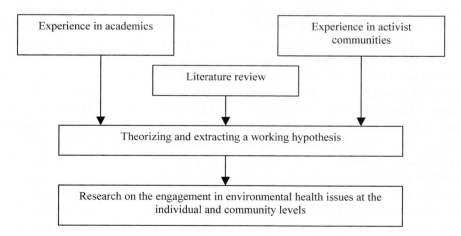

Figure 47-6. *The process involved in the development of the theoretical work by Dixon and Dixon.*

Integration

While initiating and proceeding theorizing process based on explorations of nursing phenomenon through multiple sources, a theorist can integrate her or his analysis, discovery, formulation, and evaluation through conceptual schemes, reflexivity, and documentation.

The integration process that a theorist can adopt includes several different components. From existing nursing and non-nursing theories, a theorist may start with broad established facts, principles, laws, or theories that are known and generally accepted as true and use them to address narrower yet related phenomena, concepts/variables, and propositions. A theorist may start from her or his experience in research, education, practice, research findings, or literature review with smaller, narrower concepts/variables and formulates new propositions that may ultimately lead to the development of new facts, principles, laws, and theories. A theorist may also formulate potential propositions based on personal and nursing knowledge, skills, values, meanings, and experience and not on empirically-based evidence or facts. Although distinctively different, these ways of integration may combine. Furthermore, these integration processes can happen for a long period of time, and a theorist might go through several waves of integration through her or his research projects and practice in clinical settings.

In these integration efforts, conceptual schemes with beginning hunches can be instrumental.[16] Conceptual schemes can be initiated, developed, and refined throughout the theory development process. The most important part of the conceptual schemes is internal and external dialogues.[16,17] Through conceptual thinking, memo-writing, and journal-writing, a theorist can initiate and maintain her or his internal dialogues so that her or his theorizing process can be further organized, refined, and integrated.[17] In addition, a theorist may initiate and maintain an external dialogue through discussions with colleagues, research members, students, and research participants and through participation in seminars, conferences, and/or panel discussions. In both ways, the theorist can develop and refine her or his conceptual schemes that are related to the nursing phenomenon of her or his interests and can integrate various theorizing processes.

Reflectivity is also instrumental in the process of integration. Situation-specific theories consider social, cultural, and historical contexts, but their scope and the questions are limited to specific situations and/or specific populations.[17,30] Therefore, in the development of situation-specific theories, considerations of social, cultural, and historical contexts should be incorporated from the beginning stage of the theory development process, which requires reflectivity of the theorists. Sufficient reflectivity to uncover what may be deep-seated but poorly recognized views on the specific situations and/or the specific populations central to the theory development and a full account of the theorists' views, thinking, and conduct can help the theorist's integration of her or his theorizing processes.[17]

The theorists also need to be reflective about their own values and meanings related to specific situations and/or specific populations. Values are enduring beliefs, attributes, or ideals that establish moral and ethical boundaries of what is right and wrong in thought, judgment, character, attitude, and behavior.[48] Thus, values form a foundation for correct thinking and decision making throughout the theorist's life; values develop over time and reflect individual, family, social, cultural, and religious influences as well as personal choice.[48] Thus, during the integration process, a theorist needs to be reflective on their own meanings attached to the specific situations and/or the specific populations.

Documentation of all stages involved in the theory development process can be instrumental in integration efforts. As situation-specific theories emphasize contextuality and reflectivity in the process of theory development, the theoretical and analytic decision trails created by the theorists during the development process need to be ascertained as well.[16] Theorists may continually question their conceptualization and theorizing, critiquing each step of the development process and the impact of the theories within their social and political environment. This process needs to be well documented through theoretical diaries and/or memos, so that the documentation supports the integration of the theory development process.[17] Systematically documenting the rationale, outcome, and evaluation of all actions related to theory development is an important component of the development of the situation-specific theories.[17] This documentation will result in well-grounded, cogent, justifiable, relevant, and meaningful theory development processes and outcomes.

Reporting, Sharing, and Validating

When the documenting of theorizing and integration takes the form of a manuscript, a model, or a research report, these need to be reported and shared with nursing communities. Nurse theorists have emphasized reporting and sharing of their work.[29] The criteria for theory evaluation that have been proposed and used in nursing usually include social utility and/or contagiousness as an important criterion.[17,50] Through reporting and sharing, theory development may be constructively critiqued by peers, and theoretical products can be further developed.

The validation of theories by nursing clients can also enhance the efforts to develop a theory. The relevance of an approach needs to be reflected from the very beginning of the process. Here, relevance means that a nursing theory can serve nursing clients' own issues and interests in improving their lives.[32] To ensure relevance, situation-specific theories may be checked with nursing clients in the specific situation and/or with the particular population through a member validation process, and theorists always need to be reflective about nursing clients' own views, needs, and interests throughout the theory development process. When nursing clients perceive a theory to be representative of their real experience, the theorized model is more easily applicable to the nursing phenomenon that the clients are experiencing, which subsequently improves understanding and nursing care outcomes.

Conclusions

In this article, an integrative approach to the development of situation-specific theories is proposed. This proposition is an extension of a suggested outline of the integrative approach previously drawn by Im and Meleis.[16] The proposed integrative approach describes the development process of situation-specific theories that aim to produce ready-to-wear-theories and that ultimately aim to link better nursing care outcomes through their specificity and diversity. None of the steps/stages in the proposed approach is entirely new to nurses, whether they are clinicians, theorists, or researchers.[17] Nurses may be involved in the theory development process in many ways, and we can see the growing acceptance of theory development as a significant aspect of knowledge development in nursing.

Theory development cannot grow in isolation.[17] The integrative approach proposed in this paper needs more discussion, constructive criticism, and feedback from researchers, practitioners, and theorists alike. The integrative approach should not be limited only to the proposed process. As knowledge and technology in nursing advance, we may see different types and processes of theory development in nursing in the near future.[11] As we keep in mind that theory development process is dynamic, cyclic, and changing over time, we need to continue to welcome the changes and remain open to the potential growth of theoretical nursing for better nursing care outcomes.

REFERENCES

1. Ziman J, Midgley M. Pluralism in science: a statement. *Interdisc Sci Rev.* 2001;26:153.
2. Ziman J. Emerging out of nature into history: the plurality of the sciences. *Phil Trans R Soc Lond.* 2003;361:1617–1633.
3. Chinn PL. Response: revision and passion. *Sch Inq Nurs Pract.* 1987;l:21–24.
4. Ellis R. Characteristics of significant theories. *Nurs Res.* 1968; 17:217–222.
5. Hardy ME. The nature of theories. In: Hardy ME, ed. *Theoretical Foundations for Nursing.* New York: MSS Information Corp; 1974.
6. Jacox A. Theory construction in nursing: an overview. *Nurs Res.* 1974;23:4–13.
7. Haase JE, Britt T, Coward DD, Leidy NK, Penn PE. Simultaneous concept analysis of spiritual perspective, hope, acceptance, and self transcendence. *Image J Nurs Sch.* 1992;24:l4l–147.
8. Haase JE, Leidy NK, Coward DD, Britt T, Penn PE. Simultaneous concept analysis: a strategy for developing multiple interrelated concepts. In: Rodgers B, Knafl K, eds. *Concept Development in Nursing.* Philadelphia: WB Saunders Co; 1993: 175–192.

9. Schwartz-Barcott D, Kim HS. An expansion and elaboration of the hybrid model of concept development. In: Rodgers BL, Knafl KA, eds. *Concept Development in Nursing: Foundations, Techniques, and Applications.* Philadelphia, PA: WB Saunders Co; 2000:129–160.

10. Walker LO, Avant KC. *Strategies for Theory Construction in Nursing.* 3rd ed.. Norwalk, CT: Appleton & Lange; 1995.

11. Walker LO, Avant KC. *Strategies for Theory Construction in Nursing.* 4th ed.. Norwalk, CT: Appleton & Lange; 2005.

12. Chinn PL. Why middle-range theory? *Adv Nurs Sci.* 1997;19(3): viii.

13. Peterson SJ, Bredow TS. *Middle Range Theories: Application to Nursing Research.* Philadelphia, PA: Lippinccott Williams & Wilkins; 2004.

14. Smith MJ, Liehr PR. *Middle Range Theory for Nursing.* New York: Springer Publishing Co; 2003.

15. Gortner SR. The history and philosophy of nursing science and research. In: Reed PG, Shearer NC, Nicoll LH, eds. *Perspectives on Nursing Theory.* Philadelphia: JB Lippincott; 2003: 105–112.

16. Im EO, Meleis AI. Situation-specific theories: philosophical roots, properties, and approach. *Adv Nurs Sci.* 1999;22(2): 11–24.

17. Meleis AI. *Theoretical Nursing: Development and Progress.* 3rd ed. Philadelphia: Lippincott; 1997.

18. Peterson SJ. Introduction to the nature of nursing knowledge. In: Peterson SJ, Bredow TS, eds. *Middle Range Theories: Application to Nursing Research.* Philadelphia, PA: Lippinccott Williams & Wilkins; 2004:3–41.

19. Meleis AI, Sawyer LM, Im EO, Messias DK, Schumacher K. Experiencing transitions: an emerging middle-range theory. *Adv Nurs Sci.* 2000;23(1):12–28.

20. Im EO, Meleis AI. A situation-specific theory of Korean immigrant women's menopausal transition. *Image.* 1999;31: 333–338.

21. Whittemore R, Roy SC. Adapting to diabetes mellitus: a theory synthesis. *Nurs Sci Q.* 2002;15(4):311–317.

22. Hupcey JE, Morse JM, Lenz ER, Tason MC. Wilsonian methods of concept analysis: a critique. *Sch Inq Nurs Pract.* 1996;10: 253–277.

23. Rodgers BL, Knafl KA. *Concept Development in Nursing: Foundations, Techniques, and Applications.* Philadelphia, PA: WB Saunders Co; 2000.

24. Chinn PL, Kramer MK. *Theory and Nursing: Integrated Knowledge Development.* St Louise: CV Mosby; 1999.

25. Rodgers BL. Philosophical foundations of concept development. In: Rodgers BL, Knafl KA, eds. *Concept Development in Nursing: Foundations, Techniques, and Applications.* Philadelphia, PA: WB Saunders Co; 2000:7–37.

26. Kim HS. Putting theory into practice: problems and prospects. *J Adv Nurs.* 1993;18(1):1632–1639.

27. Moccia PA. A critique of compromise: Beyond the methods debate. *Adv Nurs Sci.* 1988; 10:1–9.

28. Thompson JL. Practical discourse on nursing: going beyond empiricism and historicism. *Adv Nurs Sci.* 1985;7:59–71.

29. Hall JM, Stevens PE. Rigor in feminist research. *Adv Nurs Sci.* 1991;13:l6–29.

30. Meleis AI. A passion for making a difference: Revisions for empowerment. *Sch Inq Nurs Pract.* 1998;12:87–94.

31. Baker C. Cultural relativism and cultural diversity: implications for nursing practice. *Nurs Sci.* 1997;20:3–11.

32. Hall JM, Stevens PE, Meleis AI. Marginalization: a guiding concept or valuing diversity in nursing knowledge development. *Adv Nurs Sci.* 1994; 16(4):23–41.

33. Schumacher KL, Meleis AI. Transitions: a central concept in nursing. *Image.* 1994;26:119–127.

34. Hulme PA. Theoretical perspectives on the health problems of adults who experienced childhood sexual abuse. *Issues Mental Health Nurs.* 2004;25:339–361.

35. Kirkevold M. Integrative nursing research—an important strategy to further the development of nursing science and nursing practice. *J Adv Nurs.* 1997;25(5);977–984.

36. Lyons J. Reflective education for professional practice: discovering knowledge from experience. *Nurse Educ Today.* 1999; 19(1):29–34.

37. Reed PG. Toward a nursing theory of self-transcendence: deductive reformulation using developmental theories. *Adv Nurs Sci.* 1991;13(4):64–77.

38. Norbeck JS, Tilden VP International nursing research in social support: theoretical and methodological issues. *J Adv Nurs.* 1988; 13(2): 173–178.

39. Gassner LA, Wotton K, Clare J, Hofmeyer A, Buckman J. Evaluation of a model of collaboration: academic and clinician partnership in the development and implementation of undergraduate teaching. *Collegian.* 1999;6(3): 14–21.

40. Neill SJ. Developing children's nursing through action research. *J Child Health Care.* 1998;2:11–15.

41. Gennaro S. International nursing: the past 25 years and beyond. *MCN Am J Matern Child Nurs.* 2000;25(6):296–299.

42. Beunza I, Boulton N, Ferguson C, Serrano R. Diversity and commonality in international nursing. *Int Nurs Rev.* 1994;41(2):47–52.

43. Sparks SM. Electronic networking for nurses. *Image.* 1993; 25(3):245–248.

44. Falk-Rafael AR. Empowerment as a process of evolving consciousness: a model of empowered caring. *Adv Nurs Sci.* 2001; 24(1):1–16.

45. LaCoursiere SE A theory of online social support. *Adv Nurs Sci.* 2001;24(l):60–77.

46. Poss JE. Developing a new model for cross-cultural research: synthesizing the health belief model and the theory of reasoned action. *Adv Nurs Sci.* 2001;23(4): 1–15.

47. Dixon JK, Dixon JE An integrative model for environmental health research. *Adv Nurs Sci.* 2002;24(3):43–57.

48. Johnson BM, Webber EB. *An Introduction to Theory and Reasoning in Nursing.* Philadelphia, PA: Lippincott Williams & Wilkins; 2004.

49. Benner P, Tanner CA, Chesla CA. *Expertise in Nursing Practice: Caring, Clinical Judgment, and Ethics.* New York: Springer Publishing Co; 1996.

50. Fawcett J. Framework for analysis and evaluation of conceptual models of nursing. In: Reed PG, Shearer NB, Nicoll LH, eds. *Perspectives on Nursing Theory.* 4th ed. Philadelphia: Lippincott Williams & Wilkins; 2004:87–94.

The Author Comments

Development of Situation-Specific Theories: An Integrative Approach

When I taught doctoral theory classes, many students wanted clear directions for theory development, especially for development of situation-specific theories. Despite some philosophical conflicts and disagreement about the level of abstraction, I think that situation-specific theories are an innovative direction for nursing theory that could be easily linked to nursing research and practice, and that could incorporate diversities and complexities of nursing phenomena in our ever-changing twenty-first century.

—Eun-Ok Im

Middle Range Theory: Spinning Research and Practice to Create Knowledge for the New Millennium

Patricia Liehr
Mary Jane Smith

The foundation of middle range theory reported during the past decade was described and analyzed. A CINAHL search revealed 22 middle range theories that met selected criteria. This foundation is a firm base for new millennium theorizing. Recommendations for future theorizing include: clear articulation of theory names and approaches for generating theories; clarification of concept linkages with inclusion of diagrammed models; deliberate attention to research-practice connections of theories; creation of theories in concert with the disciplinary perspective; and, movement of middle range theories to the front lines of nursing research and practice for further analysis, critique, and development.

A spinner prepares wool by combing, to discard debris and align the strands of a matted mass in much the same way as content is sifted to tease central ideas out of extraneous ones. Just as the spinner twirls strands to compose a single thread; the nurse theorist spins central ideas into a synthesized thread for research and practice. Twisting single threads with each other enhances the strength of the product; as does the crafting of research-practice links in the creation of strong middle range theory. The beauty of any woven article is dependent on its warp and weft; likewise, the esthetics of the discipline is dependent on its theories. Spinning, like theorizing, is rigorous work aimed at creating esthetic, useful products. This article describes and analyzes a decade of middle range

About the Authors

PATRICIA LIEHR was born in Pittsburgh, PA, and received her first nursing education at Ohio Valley General Hospital, School of Nursing in Pittsburgh; her baccalaureate education at Villa Maria College in Erie, PA; and her master's in education at Duquesne University in Pittsburgh. Her doctorate in nursing was completed at the University of Maryland, and she did postdoctoral study as a Robert Wood Johnson Scholar at the University of Pennsylvania. She is now Professor and Associate Dean for Research & Scholarship at the Christine E. Lynn College of Nursing, Florida Altantic University in Boca Raton, FL. Over time, in her scholarly work, she has woven the threads of theory, practice, and research together to enhance her understanding of each. Interestingly, she is a weaver with little time for warp and weft these days . . . but still a weaver in her heart. Her scholarly endeavors focus on human language, including and extending beyond words and on the scientific structures, which guide nurse-person dialogue.

MARY JANE SMITH was born in Johnstown, PA, and earned a BSN and an MNEd from the University of Pittsburgh and a PhD from New York University. She has taught nursing theory to master's-level students for 25 years and, more recently, to doctoral students. She has been on the faculty at West Virginia University since 1981, during the past several years as Associate Dean for Graduate Academic Affairs. The focus of her scholarly work is gathering and analyzing the stories of becoming pregnant for teenaged high school students, time-pressured busyness for graduate students, and intervening in drinking/driving situations for rural youth. She likes to cook, garden, and dance.

theory products that establish a foundation for the new millennium. This foundation highlights the current structure of middle range theory and offers direction for 21st century spinning.

The Historical Context of Middle Range Theory

Modernism, postmodernism, and neomodernism are historical descriptors that represent change in the course of a developing discipline by influencing thinking and scholarship. Modernism espouses beliefs about human beings that affirm a unidimensional and stable existence, while post modernism adheres to views that affirm multidimensional, ever-changing, and complex human unfolding existence.[1] Watson[2] identified the postmodern for nursing as reconnecting with "the truths of unfoldment, an expansion and fusing of horizons of meaning, an attending to the authenticity, ethos, and ethic of caring relations, context, continu-ity, connections, aesthetics, interpretation and construction."[2(p63)] She concludes that these postmodern dimensions tie directly to developing the art and science of nursing as a caring-healing transformative praxis paradigm. Reed[3] moves beyond postmodernism to neomodernism and calls for a synthesis of modernism and postmodernism. She describes the synthesis as a metanarrative reflecting the human developmental potential, transformation, and self-transcendent capacity for health and healing, including a recognition of the developmental histories of persons and their contexts.[3] It is expected that theories that offer direction for the new millennium will emerge from the historical context that defines the time. The current context urges a focus on the human developmental potential of health and healing and supports a nursing knowledge base that synthesizes art and science; practice and research. Theories at the middle range level of discourse are in keeping with the historical context launching the new millennium.

Merton describes theories of the middle range as those that lie between the minor but necessary working hypotheses that evolve in abundance during day-to-day research and the all-inclusive systematic efforts to develop unified theory that will explain all the observed uniformities of social behavior, social organization and social change.[4(p39)]

He goes on to describe the principal ideas of middle range theory as relatively simple. Simple, in this sense, means rudimentary straightforward ideas that stem from the perspective of the discipline. An example of such an idea is that when individuals tell their story to one who truly listens, a change takes place. This idea is central to the middle range theory of attentively embracing story.[5] The ideas of middle range theory are simple yet general and are more than mere empirical generalizations.

In keeping with the views of Merton,[4] the following descriptions of middle range theory are found in the nursing literature: testable and intermediate in scope,[6] adequate in empirical foundations,[7] neither too broad nor too narrow,[8] circumscribed and substantively specific,[9] and more circumscribed than grand theory but not as concrete as practice theory.[10] In 1974, Jacox[11] described middle range theories as those including a limited number of variables and focused on a limited aspect of reality. Each of these descriptions highlights a scope somewhere in the middle, allowing for broad definitions. Lenz[12] addresses the issue of definitional clarity and believes that although the definitions of middle range theory are consistent, theories of varying scope have been labeled middle-range and the discipline may be well served by recognizing levels of theory within the middle range. She states the challenge for the discipline will be to not generate a plethora of middle range theories, but to develop a few that are empirically sound, coherent, meaningful, useful, and illuminating.[12] To meet the challenge set by Lenz in the next century, it is essential that middle range theories emerge from the twisting of research and practice threads by nurse scholars who are building on the work of others and creating the future direction of the discipline. The spinning of middle range theory in the next century will be guided by the existing middle range theory foundation.

The Existing Middle Range Theory Foundation

To assess the current foundation of middle range theory, a CINAHL search of the past 10 years of nursing literature was done entering middle range theory, mid-range theory, and nursing as search terms. The search was conducted independently in two institutions. All papers written in English that surfaced from the combined search were evaluated for inclusion in the foundation list of middle range theories (Table 48-1). Criteria for inclusion were

1. The theory was identified as middle range by its author;
2. The theory name was accessible in the paper;
3. Concepts of the theory were explicitly identified or implicitly identified in propositions; and
4. The development of the theory was the major focus of the paper.

These criteria represent an intent to be inclusive, providing the broadest view of available middle range nursing theory. However, some papers excluded were primarily methodological in focus.[13,14] These were identified in the literature search but did not meet the criteria. Table 48-1 describes the middle range theory foundation that has emerged during the past decade. Along with including identifying and locating information about the theory, it notes the inclusion of a diagrammed model and the approaches for theory generation identified by the author.

Analysis of the Middle Range Theory Foundation

The Middle Range Theories

There are 22 middle range theories proposed as the current foundation. Two theories, Unpleasant Symptoms[7,15] and Balance between Analgesia and Side Effects,[16,17] are accompanied by two citations. Unpleasant Symptoms is the only theory to have documented, ongoing development in the past decade. The second citation for Balance between Analgesia and Side Effects provides examples of use of the theory for research but does not alter its original structure. Powell-Cope,[18] using Swanson's[19] theory

Table 48-1
Middle Range Theories Over the Decade: 1988–1998

Year Published	Author(s), Journal	Name of Theory	Inclusion of Model		Theory Generating Approach
			Yes	No	
1988	Mishel *Image*	Uncertainty in Illness	X		Empirical research, literature synthesis from nursing and other disciplines
1989	Thompson, et al. *Journal of Nurse Midwifery*	Nurse Midwifery Care		X	Philosophy of nurse-midwifery profession, survey data, patient-nurse practice video-tapes, empirical research
1990	Kinney *Issues in Mental Health Nursing*	Facilitating Growth and Development		X	Middle range model from Erickson's Modeling and Role Modeling theory, practice
1991	Reed *ANS*	Self-Transcendence		X	Literature reviews, clinical experience, empirical research, deductive reformulation of life span theories from developmental psychology with Rogers Conceptual System
1991	Burke, Kauffmann, Costello, Dillon *Image*	Hazardous Secrets and Reluctantly Taking Charge	X		Grounded theory
1991	Thomas *Issues in Mental Health Nursing*	Women's Anger	X		Existential and cognitive-behavioral theories, literature review, clinical knowledge, intuition, logic
1991	Swanson *Nursing Research*	Caring		X	Phenomenological studies
1994	Powell-Cope *Nursing Research*	Negotiating Partnership		X	Extending Swanson's Caring theory using grounded theory
1995, 1997	Lenz, et al. *ANS*	Unpleasant Symptoms	X		Empirical research, clinical observation, concept analysis, collaboration
1995	Jezewski *ANS*	Cultural Brokering	X		Concept analysis, ethnography, grounded theory, practice experience, literature synthesis
1995	Tollett, Thomas *ANS*	Homelessness-Hopelessness	X		Testing Miller's Patient Power Resources Model using a quasi-experimental study
1996, 1998	Good, Moore, Good *Nursing Outlook*	Balance between Analgesia and Side Effects	X		Clinical practice guidelines; empirical research
1997	Auvil-Novak *Nursing Research*	Chronotherapeutic Intervention for Postsurgical Pain	X		*Chronobiologic theory, literature* synthesis, empirical research

(continued)

Table 48-1
Middle Range Theories Over the Decade: 1988–1998 (Continued)

Year Published	Author(s), Journal	Name of Theory	Inclusion of Model		Theory Generating Approach
			Yes	No	
1997	Olson, Hanchett *Image*	Nurse-Expressed Empathy and Patient Distress	X		Orlando's nursing model, empirical research
1997	Brooks, Thomas *ANS*	Interpersonal Perceptual Awareness	X		Concept analysis to extend King's Interacting System framework
1997	Polk *ANS*	Resilience	X		Concept synthesis using literature from other disciplines, Roger's *Science of Unitary Beings*
1997	Gerdner *Journal of American Psychiatric Nurses' Association*	Individualized Music Intervention for Agitation	X		Clinical practice, literature review, pilot study
1997	Acton *Journal of Holistic Nursing*	Affiliated Individuation as a Mediator of Stress	X		Middle range model from Erickson's Modeling and Role Modeling theory, Empirical research
1998	Eakes, Burke, Hainsworth *Image*	Chronic Sorrow	X		Concept analysis, literature review, qualitative research
1998	Huth, Moore *Journal of the Society of Pediatric Nurses*	Acute Pain Management	X		Clinical practice guidelines
1998	Levesque, et al. *Nursing Science Quarterly*	Psychological Adaptation	X		Middle range theories from other disciplines, empirical research, collaboration, Roy's Adaptation Model
1998	Ruland, Moore *Nursing Outlook*	Peaceful End of Life	X		Standards of care

of Caring—with the intent of extending it—derived yet another theory, Negotiating Partnerships. This was the only instance of one middle range nursing theory generating another. However, Levesque et al.[20] report that a foundation of middle range theories from other disciplines was the basis of their work.

Several theories that have been labeled middle range by persons who are not the primary author of the theory do not appear in the middle range foundation list. For instance, Fawcett[9] labels Orlando's Deliberative Nursing, Peplau's Interpersonal Relations, and Watson's Human Caring theory as middle range; however, none of these

came up in the literature search for middle range theory. Nolan and Grant[21] labeled Chenitz's theory of Entry into a Nursing Home as Status Passage as middle range and reported a test of the theory with a respite care sample. Review of Chenitz's theory[22] indicated that it was labeled practice theory by the author even though it may be at the middle range level of discourse. There are other theories that seem to be at the middle range level of discourse but have not been so identified by the primary author. One example is the work of Beck, who has developed a theory of postpartum depression that includes initial quantitative inquiry[23] followed by qualitative study.[24–26] Although this body of work is at the middle range level of discourse, Beck has not labeled it as middle range theory.

Based on the identified foundation of middle range theory, as the decade unfolded, there appeared to be increased willingness to label theory as middle range. Seven of the theories in Table 48-1 were proposed in the 4-year span between 1988 and 1992 and 15 were proposed in the most recent 4 years of the decade, since 1994, with six middle range theory papers published in 1997 alone. Some of the 1997 proliferation can be attributed to an issue of *Advances in Nursing Science* devoted to middle range theory. Three of the middle range theories listed in 1997 were published in this issue. In her editorial for the issue, Chinn[27] highlighted a shift in nurses' scholarly endeavors to create possibilities for healing science-art as evidenced by the issue's middle range theories, which, she noted, defy a single, limited perspective definition. The question about what constitutes theory at the middle range is not a black and white issue for which a precise and clear definition can be offered. Middle range theory holds to a given level of abstraction. It is not too broad nor too narrow, but somewhere in the middle. It is expected that finding the middle will come as theory in the middle range is spun in the next millennium.

Naming the Theory

Theory, especially at the middle range, is known to practitioners and researchers by the way it is named. It is essential that theories at the middle range be named in the context of the disciplinary perspective and at the appropriate level of discourse. Figuring out the name is a process of creative conceptualization that moves back and forth between putting together and pulling apart until the right name is found. Implicit in naming is a search for a conceptual structure as the theorist remembers and relives practice and research experiences, reflecting on proposed meaning in relation to the literature. This is a creative, energy-demanding process intended to uncover the heart of the theory. The central theory core is molded by the conceptual structure that exposes it and is articulated at the middle range level of abstraction as the name of the theory.

A theory name was accessible in each of the papers in Table 48-1, although some names were more accessible than others. A few theorists announced the presentation of a middle range theory and provided a name in the title of the paper,[7,15,28–31] while others embedded the name in the body of the paper. Facilitating Growth and Development[32] and Affiliated Individuation[33] both emerge from Modeling and Role-Modeling theory.[34] While each is described as a model at the middle range level of abstraction, distinguishing the unique name from the parent theory was difficult. The challenge of naming a middle range theory resides in determining the middle as sufficiently abstract to allow a breadth of application yet narrow enough to permit guidance in research and practice. Table 48-2

Table 48-2
Middle Range Nursing Theories by Level of Abstraction

High Middle	Middle	Low Middle
Caring	Uncertainty in Illness	Hazardous Secrets and Reluctantly Taking Charge
Facilitating Growth and Development	Unpleasant Symptoms	Affiliated Individuation as a Mediator of Stress
Interpersonal Perceptual Awareness	Chronic Sorrow	Women's Anger
Self-Transcendence	Peaceful End of Life	Nurse Midwifery Care
Resilience	Negotiating Partnerships	Acute Pain Management
Psychological Adaptation	Cultural Brokering	Balance between Analgesia and Side Effect
	Nurse-Expressed Empathy and Patient Distress	Homelessness-Helplessness
		Individualized Music Intervention for Agitation
		Chronotherapeutic Intervention for Post-Surgical Pain

organizes the existing middle range theories into the high-middle, middle, and low-middle level of abstraction, using the theory name. The theories were grouped, relative to each other, based on the generality or scope of the theory indicated by the name. Using the theory name to distinguish the level of abstraction has inherent limitations because the name may not reflect theory content. However, the theory name is its guiding label and this analysis highlights the importance of the theory name. It also highlights the existence of multiple levels of abstraction within the middle range, a fact introduced by Lenz,[12] for further recognition and development. To name a middle range theory is to locate it at an appropriate level of abstraction and to commit to a conceptual structure. Capturing a conceptual structure and expressing theory at the middle range level of abstraction will enable 21st century scholars to recognize, use, and critique the theory for practice and research applications.

Inclusion of a Model

Chinn and Kramer[35] define theory as "a creative and rigorous structuring of ideas that projects a tentative, purposeful, and systematic view of phenomena."[35(p106)] They include purpose, concepts, definitions, relationships, structure, and assumptions as components of theory suggested by their definition, noting that purpose and assumptions may be implicit rather than explicit. So, concepts with their definitions—and relationships expressed as structure—are the core components expected to be made explicit regardless of the theory's level of abstraction. One of the criteria for theories in the foundation list was the presentation of concepts. The relationship and structure components were evaluated by determining whether the theorist included a diagrammed model in the paper. Of the 22 theories in the foundation list, only 5 did not diagram a model.[18,19,32,36,37] Three[18,19,36] did not explicitly address relationships between concepts. One[37] specified relationships through propositions; one[32] described middle range relationships between concepts of a parent theory. All middle range theories since 1995 have included a diagrammed model.

Approaches for Generating Middle Range Theory

Lenz[12] has identified six approaches for generating middle range theory; these were used to categorize the methods used by the creators of the 22 theories identified in the foundation. The categories are not mutually exclusive because theorists often used more than one approach. Lenz's approaches are

1. Inductive theory building through research,
2. Deductive theory building from grand nursing theories,
3. Combining existing nursing and non-nursing theories,
4. Deriving theories from other disciplines,
5. Synthesizing theories from published research findings, and
6. Developing theories from clinical practice guidelines.

A review of the foundation theories indicates that fourteen* appeared to use inductive theory building through research. Three derived the theory from grand nursing theory,[20,29,43] two combined nursing and non-nursing theories,[30,37] four derived theories from those of other disciplines,[20,28,37,44] and two[16,45] developed theory from practice guidelines. The approach of synthesizing theories from published research identified by Lenz was difficult to determine when categorizing the theories. No middle range theory was cited that was generated only by published research. Even when not stated explicitly, there were implicit indications that every theory had referred to published research when generating the theory. Two theories[32,46] fit into none of the approaches described by Lenz. Ruland and Moore[46] recently have proposed using standards of care to generate middle range theory and Kinney[32] describes a practice example to demonstrate a middle range model. Including Kinney, seven theories[7,15,32,36,37,40,42,44] explicitly cited personal practice experiences as contributing to middle range theory development. Only four[7,15,36,40,42] of the seven also described research threads, thus enabling the spinning of research with practice in the building of middle range theory.

*References 7, 15, 18–20, 28, 29, 31, 33, 36, 38–42

The analysis of approaches for generating middle range theory suggests that Lenz's listing generally is comprehensive. The elimination of the approach noting synthesis from published research findings may be appropriate, and an expansion of "clinical practice guidelines" to "practice guidelines and standards" will cover the recent work by Ruland and Moore.[46] Inclusion of the practice thread is critical for 21st century spinning. Therefore, the following five approaches are proposed for middle range theory generation in the new millennium:

1. Induction through research and practice;
2. Deduction from research and practice applications of grand theories;
3. Combination of existing nursing and non-nursing middle range theories;
4. Derivation from theories of other disciplines that relate to nursing's disciplinary perspective; and
5. Derivation from practice guidelines and standards rooted in research.

It is unlikely that any of these theory generation approaches will stand alone as nursing moves into the next century. Each will need to be combined to most effectively guide the discipline. Guidance for the new millennium is most likely to emerge from theories that spin research and practice to focus on the human developmental potential of health and healing.

Juxtaposition With Grand Nursing Theory

As middle range theory is generated for the new millennium, it is essential that it move beyond the polarities often created between it and grand theories. The all-embracing grand theories were espoused by individuals who attempted to create a view of the whole of nursing. Groups have developed into small circles of schools of thought in which an all-or-nothing adherence to the perspective is advocated strongly. This approach has advanced the discipline through generation of scholarly pursuits and offers a grounding for middle range theory. It is not separate nor antithetical to middle range theory development. Merton[4] identifies the following criticisms

of middle range theory leveled by those who advocate grand approaches: (1) conceptualizing middle range theory is low in intellectual ambitions; (2) it completely excludes grand theory; (3) it will fragment the discipline into unrelated special theories; and (4) a positivist conception of theory will be the result. There is no evidence that these criticisms have been realized. Nursing's current middle range theory foundation: reflects scholarly work conceptualized at a lower level of abstraction that rises to intellectual challenge; builds on grand theory that continues to offer a foundation for development; and projects a historical context to begin the millennium with theories at the middle range in the perspective of the discipline.

Disciplinary Perspective of the Middle Range Theory Foundation

An association between the existing middle range theory foundation and the disciplinary perspective synthesized as a caring, healing process in which the human developmental potential for health and transformation emerge[2,3] is depicted in Table 48-3. Through the reflective process of dwelling with the essence of the disciplinary perspective and the middle range theories as named, two themes surfaced. These themes were caring—healing processes and transforming struggle-growth. These themes offer a view of the existing middle range theory foundation in the context of a disciplinary perspective as well as an integrated paradigm for spinning middle range theory in the new millennium.

The Future: Where Does Nursing Theory Go From Here?

In conclusion, a lot of thoughtful spinning of middle range theory has been done in the past decade; and although knots and tangles have been created along the way, one must remember that spinning theory is a creative human endeavor that can best be described as a work in progress. It is expected that the knots and tangles will be sorted out with the spinner's persistence and careful attention to

Table 48-3
Middle Range Theories by Disciplinary Themes

Caring—Healing Process	Transforming Struggle—Growth
Caring	Self-Transcendence
Facilitating Growth and Development	Resilience
Interpersonal Perceptual Awareness	Psychological Adaptation
Cultural Brokering	Uncertainty in Illness
Nurse-Expressed Empathy and Patient Distress	Unpleasant Symptoms
Nurse Midwifery Care	Chronic Sorrow
Acute Pain Management	Peaceful End of Life
Balance between Analgesia and Side Effects	Negotiating Partnerships
Individualized Music Intervention for Agitation	Hazardous Secrets and Reluctantly Taking Charge
Chronotherapeutic Intervention for Post-Surgical Pain	Affiliated Individuation as a Mediator of Stress
	Women's Anger
	Homelessness-Helplessness

creating and combining fibers. Based on the description and analysis of the current middle range theory foundation, several recommendations are presented for developing middle range theory in the future. The recommendations are that the creators of middle range theory:

1. Take care to clearly articulate the theory name and approaches used for generating the theory;
2. Strive to clarify the conceptual linkages of the theory in a diagrammed model;
3. Give deliberate attention to articulating the research-practice links of the theory;
4. Create an association between the proposed theory and a disciplinary perspective in nursing; and
5. Move middle range theory to the front lines of nursing practice and research for further analysis, critique, and development.

Twenty-first century theorists are offered the challenge of these recommendations. The challenge is to move nursing theory forward by spinning research and practice in the creation of middle range theories congruent with the current historical context. It is this forward movement that will give substance and direction to the discipline. Middle range theory will create the disciplinary fabric of the new millennium as nurse theorists spin and twist fibers from the past-present into the future.

REFERENCES

1. Anderson TA. Post modern person. *Noetic Sciences Review.* 1998;45:28–33.
2. Watson J. Postmodernism and knowledge development in nursing. *Nurs Sci Quarterly.* 1994;8:60–64.
3. Reed PG. A treatise on nursing knowledge development for the 21st century: beyond postmodernism. *ANS.* 1995;17:70–84.
4. Merton RK. On sociological theories of the middle range. In: *Social Theory and Social Structure.* New York: Free Press: 1968.
5. Smith MJ, Liehr P. Attentively embracing story: a middle range theory with practice and research implications. *Sch Ing Nurs Prac.* In press.
6. Suppe F. Middle range theory—Role in nursing theory and knowledge development. In: *Proceedings of the Sixth Rosemary Ellis Scholar's Retreat, Nursing Science Implications for the 21st century.* Cleveland. OH: Frances Payne Bolton School of Nursing, Case Western Reserve University: 1996.
7. Lenz ER, Suppe F, Gift AG, Pugh LC, Milligan RA. Collaborative development of middle-range nursing theories: toward a theory of unpleasant symptoms. *ANS.* 1995;17:1–13.
8. Reed P. Toward a nursing theory of self-transcendence: deductive reformulation using developmental theories. *ANS.* 1991; 12:64–74.
9. Fawcett J. *Analysis and Evaluation of Nursing Theories.* Philadelphia, PA: F. A. Davis: 1993.
10. Morris D. Middle range theory role in education. In: *Proceedings of the Sixth Rosemary Ellis Scholar's Retreat, Nursing Science Implications for the 21st century.* Cleveland, OH: Frances Payne Bolton School of Nursing, Case Western Reserve University; 1996.
11. Jacox A. Theory construction in nursing: an overview. *Nurs Res.* 1974;23:4–12.

12. Lenz E. Middle range theory—Role in research and practice. In: *Proceedings of the Sixth Rosemary Ellis Scholar's Retreat, Nursing Science Implications for the 21st century.* Cleveland, OH: Frances Payne Bolton School of Nursing, Case Western Reserve University; 1996.

13. Dluhy NM. Mapping knowledge in chronic illness. *J Adv Nurs.* 1995;21:1051–1058.

14. Jenny JJ, Logan J. Caring and comfort metaphors used by patients in critical care. *Image.* 1996;28:349–352.

15. Lenz ER, Pugh LC, Milligan RA. Gift AG, Suppe F. The middle range theory of unpleasant symptoms: an update. *ANS.* 1997;19:14–27.

16. Good M, Moore SM. Clinical practice guidelines as a new source of middle range theory: focus on acute pain. *Nurs Outlook.* 1996;44:74–79.

17. Good M. A middle range theory of acute pain management use in research. *Nurs Outlook.* 1998;46:120–124.

18. Powell-Cope GM. Family caregivers of people with AIDS: negotiating partnerships with professional health care providers. *Nurs Res.* 1994;43:324–330.

19. Swanson KM. Empirical development of a middle range theory of caring. *Nurs Res.* 1991;40:161–166.

20. Levesque L, Ricard N, Ducharme F, Duquette A, Bonin J. Empirical verification of a theoretical model derived from the Roy Adaptation Model: findings from five studies. *Nurs Sci Q.* 1998;11:31–39.

21. Nolan M. Grant G. Mid-range theory building and the nursing theory-practice gap: a respite care case study. *J Adv Nurs.* 1992; 17:217–223.

22. Chenitz WC. Entry into a nursing home as status passage: a theory to guide nursing practice. *Geriatric Nurs.* 1983; Mar/Apr: 92–97.

23. Beck CT, Reynolds MA, Rutowski P. Maternity blues and postpartum depression. *JOGNN.* 1992;21:287–293.

24. Beck CT. The lived experience of postpartum depression: a phenomenological study. *Nurs Res.* 1992;41:166–170.

25. Beck CT. Teetering on the edge: a substantive theory of postpartum depression. *Nurs Res.* 1993;42:42–48.

26. Beck CT. Postpartum depressed mothers' experiences interacting with their children. *Nurs Res.* 1996;45:98–104.

27. Chinn P. Why middle range theory? *ANS.* 1997;19:viii.

28. Auvil-Novak SE. A mid-range theory of chronotherapeutic intervention for postsurgical pain. *Nurs Res.* 1997;46:66–71.

29. Olson J, Hanchett E. Nurse-expressed empathy, patient outcomes, and development of a middle-range theory. *Image.* 1997;29:71–76.

30. Polk LV. Toward a middle range theory of resilience. *ANS.* 1997;19:1–13.

31. Eakes GG, Burke ML, Hainsworth MA. Middle-range theory of chronic sorrow. *Image.* 1998;30:179–184.

32. Kinney CK. Facilitating growth and development: a paradigm case for modeling and role-modeling. *Issues Ment Health Nurs.* 1990;11:375–395.

33. Acton GJ. Affiliated-individuation as a mediator of stress and burden in caregivers of adults with dementia. *J Holistic Nurs.* 1997;15:336–357.

34. Erickson HC, Tomlin EM, Swain MAP. *Modeling and Role-Modeling: A Theory and Paradigm for Nursing.* Englewood Cliffs, NJ: Prentice-Hall; 1983.

35. Chinn PL, Kramer MK. *Theory and Nursing: A Systematic Approach.* St. Louis, MO: Mosby; 1995.

36. Thompson JE, Oakley D, Burke M, Jay S, Conklin M. Theory building in nurse-midwifery: the care process. *J Nurs-Midwifery.* 1989;34:120–130.

37. Reed PG. Toward a nursing theory of self-transcendence: deductive reformulation using developmental theories. *ANS.* 1991;13: 64–77.

38. Mishel MH. Uncertainty in illness. *Image.* 1988;20:225–232.

39. Burke SO, Kauffmann E, Costello EA, Dillon MC. Hazardous secrets and reluctantly taking charge: parenting a child with repeated hospitalizations. *Image.* 1991;23:39–45.

40. Jezewski MA. Evolution of a grounded theory: conflict resolution through culture brokering. *ANS.* 1995;17:14–30.

41. Tollett JH, Thomas SP. A theory-based nursing intervention to instill hope in homeless veterans. *ANS.* 1995;18:76–90.

42. Gerdner L. An individualized music intervention for agitation. *J Am Psych Nurs Assoc.* 1997;3:177–184.

43. Brooks EM, Thomas S. The perception and judgment of senior baccalaureate student nurses in clinical decision making. *ANS.* 1997;19:50–69.

44. Thomas SP. Toward a new conceptualization of women's anger. *Issues Ment Health Nurs.* 1991;12:31–49.

45. Huth MM, Moore SM. Prescriptive theory of acute pain management in infants and children. *JSPN.* 1998;3:23–32.

46. Ruland CM, Moore SM. Theory construction based on standards of care: a proposed theory of the peaceful end of life. *Nurs Outlook.* 1998;46:169–175.

The Authors Comment

Middle Range Theory: Spinning Research and Practice to Create Knowledge for the New Millennium

We wrote the Spinning article because we were entrenched in making sense of middle-range theory. Our graduate students repeatedly told us that it was challenging to attempt to figure out what theory was middle range. When sent to the literature in search of meaningful middle-range theory, the students returned with questions and quagmire. We thought it was important to make some sense of the existing literature on middle-range theory if the discipline ever expected to use it as a base for practice and research. We believe that middle-range theory offers a promising direction for the next generation of nursing scholars. We have recently coedited a book, *Middle Range Theory for Nursing,* which extends the knowledge developed in the Spinning article and describes eight middle-range theories useful for nursing practice and research.

—Patricia Liehr
—Mary Jane Smith

Characteristics and Criteria of Nursing Theories

The chapters in this unit address the characteristics of scientific theory. The Hardy articles present theory evaluation criteria that are used widely across disciplines. Fawcett and Parse outline criteria that, in addition to criteria used to evaluate theories across disciplines, target evaluation of nursing theories in particular. Dickoff and James' classic article provides readers a historical perspective in the thinking about what makes a theory a nursing theory. Lasiuk and Ferguson provide an exemplary article on a contemporary view of nursing theory as related to nurses' theoretical thinking, research, and practice.

This unit and others (for example, Units One, Three, Six, and Seven) demonstrate that what is meant by *nursing theory* has advanced beyond the original set of conceptual models that once defined the realm of nursing theory. In general, the term *nursing theory* refers to a wide variety of theories developed in nursing, most of which are mid-range in scope and abstraction. However, as more nurses in practice take on roles in knowledge development, other types of nursing theories (for example, situation-producing theories, situation-specific theories, micro-theories) may be generated that differ from midrange theories in important ways.

Questions for Discussion

- What makes a theory a nursing theory?
- Are there certain characteristics that distinguish nursing theories from other theories?
- What is the role of theory in advancing nursing knowledge?
- What role does theory evaluation have in advancing practice?

CHAPTER 49

Theories: Components, Development, Evaluation

Margaret E. Hardy

The roles of concepts, statements of relationship, and models in theory development are examined. Criteria for evaluating theories are outlined, and the tentative nature of theories is discussed.

Although nurses in their everyday work are expected to evaluate health conditions of persons under their care, usually little thought is given to evaluating the soundness of the theory and knowledge which guides their action. If the theory is poorly suspended by evidence (i.e., the theory is not "true"), the health of the persons for which nurses are responsible may be severely jeopardized. As health professionals, nurses need to be able to make sound judgments about the rationale for various treatments, therapies, and care. It is often assumed that because an idea is in print (particularly if in a textbook or professional journal), it must be true. Many of the theories on which health professionals base their activities, however, are open to severe criticisms. With the speed with which new ideas are published, nurses now more than ever need to keep abreast of the development of relevant knowledge and be able to evaluate that knowledge in order to make informed judgments.

Unless nurses can assess the knowledge generated in such diverse areas as stress, systems, decision making, leadership, self-concept, body image, family, groups, body systems, they cannot use that knowledge wisely and constructively. Failure or inability to assess knowledge relevant to her area of work means the

About the Author

MARGARET E. HARDY was born in Edmonton, Alberta, Canada, in 1938. She received her BSN in 1960 from the University of British Columbia in Vancouver, Canada; her MA in 1965 from the University of Washington School of Nursing, with a major in community mental health; and her PhD in sociology in 1971 from the University of Washington. Her employment includes a faculty position at Boston University from 1971 to 1985, where she held a joint appointment in the School of Nursing and the Department of Sociology. From 1985 to her early retirement in 1993, she was Professor at the University of Rhode Island School of Nursing. Her major contribution to nursing evolved serendipitously as a result of her teaching assignment at Boston University; development of courses for the graduate program led to the publication of her award-winning books *Theoretical Foundations for Nursing* and *Role Theory*, as well as a book *Research Readings*. Through her publications and teaching hundreds of graduate students throughout New England during the 1970s and 1980s, Dr. Hardy provided foundational knowledge on metatheory and inspired many to initiate theory development for nursing. Dr. Hardy enjoys watercolor painting, reading, walking, hiking, traveling, and camping in the mountains with her husband and two dogs.

nurse must function as a technician, depending on others to interpret the knowledge-base which guides her actions. If nurses intend to direct their own actions in a responsible manner, they must become well informed on developing knowledge, they must be able to evaluate critically the knowledge developed, and they must make informed judgments based on this knowledge. They also must learn to function optimally as generalists. A competent practitioner really does not have the luxury of concentrating her efforts in a restricted area (psychiatry is currently under attack for the narrowness of its activities), but must take into account a wide variety of phenomena which have bearing on her clients.

Our comprehension of the world around us is based on the use of concepts, hypotheses, and theories. Nurses, as practitioners in the health field, apply and use knowledge generated from theories. In spite of the pervasiveness of theories in guiding and controlling our everyday life, the literature on theory development is diverse and confusing, and it generally is little related to the activities of practitioners. This article attempts to identify the structure of theory, to differentiate between different types of theoretical statements, and to identify criteria for evaluating theories.

Concepts

Concepts are labels, categories, or selected properties of objects to be studied; they are the bricks from which theories are constructed. Concepts are the dimensions, aspects, or attributes of reality which interest the scientist. Patients, illness, cardiovascular diseases, nurses, or physicians are examples of concepts used in health-related fields on which research may be based. The scientist constructs theories in his domain of interest by linking concepts of one class or attribute to concepts of other classes or attributes. When he has a set of interrelated statements or hypotheses concerning the relationships between concepts (i.e., when he has filled between the bricks with mortar), he has a theory. Concepts are the basic elements of theory. A major part of the evaluation of a theory is the identification and assessment of the concepts.

Components and Structure of Theory

A theory may be viewed from a variety of perspectives. For the purpose of exploring the structure of a theory, one may view theory as a language (Rudner, 1966). Like any language, theory consists of elements, formulations, and a set of definitions, i.e., it is comprised of syntax and semantics. When an investigator studies a scientific theory, he is interested in the logical structure or the relation between the elements (concepts) of the theory (the syntax) and the meaning given to the elements (the semantics). Syntax, then, is concerned with the occurrence of concepts in the axioms, postulates, or hypotheses of a theory and the relationship between the concepts and between the hypotheses of a theory, while semantics is concerned with the specific meaning attributed to the concepts. When a theory is made explicit or is formalized, one can examine the syntax and determine if the structure of the theory is consistent with the rules of logic.

The Semantics of Theory

Theories consist of two types of elements or terms. One set, the *derived* terms, are specifically introduced through definition whereas the other set, the *primitive* terms, remain undefined (Hempel, 1952). The primitive terms (or concepts) are the primary building blocks of theories from which new terms are derived. Both primitive and derived terms appear in a theory's axioms and postulates and give meaning to an otherwise uninterpreted or formalized system.

Concepts are defined and their meanings are understood only within the framework of the theory of which they are a part. Much conceptual confusion exists in theoretical areas upon which nurses draw. Concepts are often vaguely defined; the same concept may be defined and described many different ways (each writer providing his own definition). For example, within the area of role theory the concepts of role, status, and role behavior overlap and are often used interchangeably. Concepts develop as part of theory and are altered and refined as a body of knowledge grows. The concern for clarifying concepts involves a dilemma of trying to achieve consistency in meaning without premature closure of theories. Conceptual confusion and vagueness in theories appear to be a necessary and an important condition for creativity in science as elsewhere. Persons in the more applied professions often find this state of confusion difficult to cope with.

The refinement of concepts (improving the bricks) is a continuous process which involves not only sharpening of theoretical and operational definitions, but also modification of existing theory. Theories and concepts are reformulated by relating the theoretical world to the empirical, by organizing a great many concrete items into a small number of classes (regrouping the bricks), and by relating diverse concepts within a more general system of concepts.

General or Abstract

Concepts may be ordered on the basis of their level of abstractness. A specific occurrence, such as a patient's chest pain, is treated as a special case of a more general condition, such as heart disease. Heart disease, in turn, is a special condition of the more general area, the circulatory system.

Concepts are also appraised for their degree of generality; they are assessed according to the extent they change or vary. Concepts which refer to classes or categories of phenomena may be called *nonvariable* (Hage, 1972). Such concepts are found in typologies in which classes are clearly defined; an observation either fits or does not fit into a given category, depending upon the presence or absence of the property of interest, e.g., male, female. Concepts which are used to order phenomena according to some property or concepts which refer to dimensions of phenomena are called *variables* (Hage, 1972). When the results of observations fall on a continuum, the property being observed is a variable concept, e.g., 27 years, 82 years. It has been argued (Hage, 1972) that concepts that have a continuum should be utilized more frequently in conceptualizing and theory construction because such concepts facilitate theory development, are not restricted to time and place, and are more subtle for description and classification. The following illustrates the difference between nonvariable and variable concepts: Schizophrenia, manic depression, phobic reactions, and passive-aggressive traits are nonvariable concepts; they are bound by culture. The following general variable concepts are not so bound: anxiety, the degree of depression, intensity of affect, extent of contact with reality, frequency of phobic reactions. These general variable concepts may be utilized to describe the specific mental disorders listed above as well as other normal and abnormal mental states, whereas the nonvariable concepts (disease entities) are specifically either-or types of abnormal phenomena. By using both abstract and variable concepts, the scientist is able to develop laws and theories which have a wide range of applicability.

Theoretical or Operational

Concepts, whether nonvariable or variable, may have both a theoretical definition and an operational definition. The theoretical definition gives meaning to the terms in context of the theory and permits any reader to assess the validity of that definition. The operational definition tells how the concept is linked to concrete situations. An operational definition, which is used in the process of giving experiential meaning to the concept of a theory, describes a set of physical procedures which must be carried out in order to assign to every case a value for the concept. For example, the concept of level of aggression may be operationally defined as the number of times a child hits another child during an hour of play. How adequately the operational definition reflects the theoretical concept is another matter for consideration. That is, not only do concepts need operational definitions but the operational definition must be a valid reflection of the theoretical meaning of the concept. In this example, the operational definition certainly permits an observer to assign a level of "aggression" to each child observed. The level of aggression score for a child, however, may not reflect the theoretical meaning of the concept. The operational definition does not take into account the intent of the child, aggressive acts other than hitting, or the intensity of the act. The dilemma encountered in trying to link observable events to theoretical constructs is that the more concretely concepts are defined, the more restricted is the scope of the theory and the less useful is the theory. In spite of the difficulty in developing operational definitions, it is necessary to define theoretical terms in a way that the concepts can be measured. Only through developing

measurements of concepts can hypotheses and, in turn, theories be tested.

Operational definitions are a necessary part of theory construction. Operational definitions permit the validity of concepts to be assessed. They permit hypotheses to be tested and the empirical relevance of a theory to be assessed. They also permit other scientists to replicate the study. Operational definitions, which form the bridge between the theory and the empirical world, are modified over time as both theoretical and technological knowledge grow.

Theoretical concepts only make sense when considered within the framework of the theories of which they are a part. Such concepts may be examined on the basis of the degree of observability of their referent. Observable concepts (concepts that refer directly to observable objects) are likely to be found in derived theorems which are to be tested, whereas nonobservable concepts are found in axioms. Nonobservable concepts—intervening variables or hypothetical constructs—are derived on the basis of inferences from observable referents. Intervening variables are concepts that are based on inferences from observations. To illustrate this point, consider the following: A state of anxiety is often inferred on the basis of observations of increased heart rate, sweaty palms, and nausea. Anxiety per se is not observable.

Hypothetical concepts are more abstract than intervening variables. Belief in their existence is based primarily on theoretical support, and only indirectly on supporting empirical data. The id and the unconscious are examples of hypothetical constructs. The distinctions between intervening variables and hypothetical constructs are not at all clear. In one theory, a concept may be a hypothetical construct; in another theory, the same concept may be an intervening variable.

Attributes of Concepts Utilized for Evaluation

Concepts are abstractions from concrete events; concepts themselves can have a varying degree of abstraction. As one moves up the level of abstraction in order to develop systematic explanations of general phenomena, one is faced with the problem of relating back from the symbolic concepts to concrete phenomena. Part of the difficulty in doing this is dependent on the adequacy of the rules of correspondence (or the links one is able to make) between the theoretical concepts and their empirical referents. The generality (abstraction) of concepts and the relationship between the concepts and the empirical referent (testability) are criteria used to evaluate a theory. Examination of the semantics of a theory provides another means for evaluation. This may, in part, be examined by assessing the intersubjectivity of meaning. The intersubjectivity of the meaning of concepts refers to whether the concepts are given a meaning similar to the meaning used by other scientists in related areas (Reynolds, 1971).

Statements of Relationships Between Concepts

Syntax of Theory

If a theory is formalized or made explicit, the syntax, or relationship, between concepts can be examined and the logical adequacy of the theory can be assessed. In assessing a theory's logical structure, the meanings of the concepts themselves are not taken into consideration. That is, symbols may be used to represent the concepts. This facilitates the examination of the logical structure without confusing the issue by considering the explicit meaning of the concepts. For example, the statement that social stress "results in" heart disease can be expressed symbolically. If social stress is represented by X, heart disease by Y, and results in by $\rightarrow$ then the statement social stress results in heart disease can be expressed by $X \rightarrow Y$. A formalization of statements like this and other interrelated statements in a theory facilitate the examination of the structure of a theory.

Types of Relationships

To analyze the structure of a theory it is necessary to identify the relationships between concepts. Some types of relationships and their meanings are summarized in Figure 49-1. Relationships listed are not mutually exclu-

Nature of Relation[1]	Meaning
Symmetrical	If A, then B; if B, then A
Asymmetrical	If A, then B; but if no A, no conclusion about B
Causal	If A, always B
Probabilistic	If A, probably B
Time order	If A, later B
Concurrent	If A, also B
Sufficient	If A, then B, regardless of anything else
Conditional	If A, then B, but only if C
Necessary	If A and only if A, then B

[1]The relations are not all mutually exclusive

Figure 49-1 *Relationships between concepts.*

sive. Some of the relationships between concepts may be illustrated by using Selye's (1956) theory of stress. This stress formulation indicates that stressors result in a physiological syndrome identified as General Adaptive Syndrome (GAS). If in this formulation the relationship between stressors and GAS is determinate, then this implies that the concepts are *time-ordered* (stressors occur prior to the development of GAS), *sufficient* (if stressors occur, then GAS occurs regardless of anything else), and *necessary* (if stressors and only if stressors occur, then GAS occurs). The determinate relationship between stressors and GAS is asymmetrical (if stressors occur, then GAS occurs; if no stressors occur, then no conclusions may be reached about the occurrence of GAS) rather than symmetrical (if stressors occur, GAS occurs; if GAS occurs, then stressors occur). It is possible, however, that the relationship between stressors and GAS is not determinate but probabilistic (if stressors occur, there exists a 90 percent chance that GAS will occur) or conditional (if stressors occur, then GAS occurs, but only if specific physiological condition W exists). For clarity in theoretical formulations, it is necessary to specify the type of relationships between concepts. Although the identification of causal relationships in the health sciences is the reason for considerable success in disease prevention, relationships which are stochastic and relationships which are conditional are valuable in the prediction and control of disease-related events and hence should be identified rather than ignored.

Sign of the Relationship

An additional characteristic of the relationship between concepts is the sign $(+/-)$ of the relationship. Concepts may be either positively $(+/-)$ or inversely $(-)$ related. The sign of relationships, though being discussed here in the context of theory development, really relates to the concept of measures of association or correlation. Thus, in the postulates—the greater X, the greater Y, and the greater Y, the greater Z—a positive relationship is implied between concepts as measured by some measure of association. Knowing that Y increases with X and Z increases with Y, it can be logically deduced that Z increases with X. The sign of the relationship between X and Z depends upon the sign of the relationships between the concepts X and Y, and Y and Z in the postulates. The sign rule has been summarized from work by Zetterberg (1963); Costner and Leik (1964) stated that the sign of the deduced relationship is the algebraic product of the signs of the postulated relationships. If Y is positively correlated with X and Z is positively correlated with Y, then it can be concluded by deduction and the sign rule that Z is positively correlated with X. This process of deduction may be expressed as:

$$
\begin{array}{ll}
\text{If} & X \xrightarrow{+} Y \\
\text{and} & Y \xrightarrow{+} Z \\
\hline
\text{then} & X \xrightarrow{+} Z
\end{array}
$$

It is still an empirical question as to whether this logically deduced relationship actually exists. A relationship which is true according to logic is not necessarily true empirically.

Formalizing and Examining a Set of Statements

This discussion has emphasized that the evaluation of a theory's structure is facilitated if the concepts and the relationships between the concepts are formalized. The following stress formulation will be utilized to illustrate ways of assessing the syntax of theory: Social stress results in emotional tension whereas cognitive dissonance and social stress are inversely related; emotional tension results in somatic dysfunctioning. These statements may

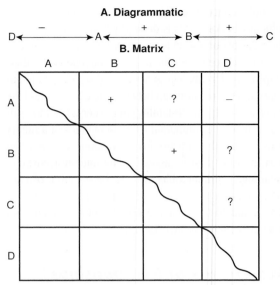

^{1}Concepts: Social stress, A; emotional tension, B; somatic dysfunctioning, C; cognitive dissonance, D. Sign of the relationship: Positive, +; inverse, −; unspecified,? Relationships between concepts: Symmetrical, ←→ ; asymmetrical, ⟶.

Figure 49-2 *Diagrammatic (A) and matrix (B) representation of stress formulation: concepts and their relationships.*[1]

be formalized and displayed diagrammatically or in a matrix (Figure 49-2). The matrix used here is an adaptation of a data correlation matrix. The visual representation of the formalized model makes it relatively simple to examine the theory's structure. The diagram shows the relationship between the concepts while the matrix readily displays the completeness and logical consistency of the formulation. Discontinuities in the stress formulation are evident in both the diagram (lack of connections between the concepts) and the matrix (empty cells). Deductions can be made from the postulates stated. Using the sign rule and the deduced relationship, we may conclude that A and C are positively associated. That is, an increase in social stress is associated with an increase in somatic dysfunctioning. From this deduction the formulation is made more complete; no logical inconsistencies exist. The formalization of a theory to facilitate an evaluation of it will be discussed later.

Types of Statements

Although "postulates," "proposition," "hypothesis," "axiom," "laws," "principles," and "empirical generalizations" refer to different types of statements, they have a common characteristic in that they link together two or more concepts. A theory is made up of a set of interrelated propositions, theorems, or hypotheses derived from axioms, initial hypotheses, or postulates. Hypotheses refer to facts that are as yet unexperienced; they are corrigible in view of fresh knowledge. Principles and empirical generalizations are statements about data and are generally believed to be true. The distinguishing characteristic between empirical generalizations and hypotheses is that a hypothesis may be formulated in the absence of data, while an empirical generalization summarizes empirical evidence. Statements differ in their degree of generality and degree of empirical support. Empirical generalizations, since they summarize data, are closer to reality than are hypotheses. However, hypotheses, because they are at a higher level of generalization, are invaluable in aiding our understanding of events which have not yet been systematically tested.

Scientific hypotheses are more or less *grounded* on previous knowledge, i.e., they are partially supported (or at least not refuted) by empirical evidence and by theory. Hypotheses are developed from a rationale; they are not wild, groundless guesses. They should show reasonable conjecture—not fly in the face of existing knowledge.

Laws are well grounded; they have strong empirical support. They state a constant relation among two or more variables, each representing (at least partly and indirectly) a property of concrete systems. An example of a law is $E = Mc^2$. In the psychosocial area few, if any, laws exist. Laws are propositions that assert universal connections between properties.

Statements on the highest level of generality are laws and axioms. Statements on a lower level of generality (propositions, theorems, hypotheses) can be deduced from laws. The purpose of deduction is to test the general statements. In a deductive system, high-level statements can be falsified by the falsification of lower-level (deduced) statements. In any hypotheticodeduc-tive theory, the less universal statements or lower-level statements are themselves still, strictly speaking, universal statements; they are empirical generalizations and must have the character of hypotheses. Postulates, axioms, and laws are primitive statements about an infinite universe, whereas hypotheses and empirical generalizations are statements about a finite universe.

The following examples may illustrate the difference between laws and hypotheses: A law in physiology is: Cardiac output = heart rate $\times$ stroke volume. This statement is true under all conditions (i.e., for all human hearts regardless of time or culture and also for nonhuman hearts). An hypothesis in physiology is: Resting potentials in nerve and muscle cells depend only on the difference in potassium ion concentration across the cell membrane. The statement has not reached the status of a law. Although there is reasonable evidence to support this statement, experimental evidence suggests that other ions may affect resting potentials. The generalization holds true for most muscle and nerve cells rather than for all cells. An hypothesis in social psychology is: In any task-oriented group, inequality in task activity among group members occurs and results in role differentiation. This generalization has mixed empirical support. Some experimental studies corroborate this hypothesis, while other experimental studies identify conditions under which role differentiation in task-oriented groups does not occur. The generalization may only apply under specific conditions and only in the American culture.

Models

Although a scientific theory is considered to be a deductive system, the relationship between variables may best be expressed in terms of a model. That is, an investigator may formalize a theory, identify its postulates, identify or derive the remaining propositions, and then decide that the problem of relationships is best represented by a model. A model is a simplified representation of a theory or of certain complex events, structures, or systems. Constructing a model forces the theorists to specify the precise relationship between components.

Models, like theories, are isomorphic systems; they are selective representations of the empirical world with which the scientist is concerned; crucial aspects of the phenomena are identified and aspects not considered important are ignored. Models are descriptive; they simplify the area of concern and can help the scientist grasp key elements and the relationships between these elements. The distinction between theories and models is not always clear. For example, what is considered a well-established theory in one academic area may be used as a model to represent phenomena in another area. Modeling is a technique used to describe and explain as well as to generate ideas and predictions.

Types

One type of model is an *analog* model, or an analogy. This model directs attention to resemblances between theoretical entities and familiar subject matter (Kaplan, 1964). For example, a nurse may use the analogy of a mechanical pump to explain to a patient the workings of his heart. In doing this, the nurse is using properties of the pump (an entity with which the patient is familiar) to explain characteristics about the heart (an entity with which the patient is unfamiliar). A problem which is difficult to understand may be made more comprehensible by the use of an analogy. The study of social organizations has been based on an organic model, e.g., Parsons' (1951) description of social systems, and social interactions have been described in terms of economic exchanges (Blau, 1964). Because the model is "true" in one area of science, however, does not mean that it will be true or hold up on another area. The model must be tested for its validity in each area of application. Although many characteristics of the organic model are inappropriate for describing social systems, the organic model has been a useful starting point for the study of social phenomena.

Iconic models are used if a direct representation of the subject is wanted (DiRenzo, 1966). The model may vary as to the number of properties represented and the level of abstraction. A kidney machine, for example, although it does not resemble the kidney in appearance, does represent relatively accurately some of the kidney processes. A model of the heart (built to scale), a scaled model of a DNA molecule, an organizational chart of a hospital, and a miniature social system depicting the hierarchical structure and communication processes in an organization are examples of iconic models. These models represent the original phenomena but in another form. Such models are useful to the extent that they increase our sense of understanding of the entity. This type of modeling has been utilized more perhaps in the physical sciences than in the social sciences. The usefulness of iconic models for understanding social phenomena may be directly related to our ability to identify key variables and to abstract these characteristics. For many persons it is easier to accept a plastic model of the heart as a useful model than it is to accept a three-person decision-making network as a useful model of a social organization. The value of models is dependent upon the extent to which they increase understanding, explain phenomena, or give us a sense of what is going on and why.

Another type of model is the *symbolic* model which represents phenomena figuratively (DiRenzo, 1966). A set of connected symbols, objects, or concepts may be used to represent a problem of interest. The relationship between concepts may be represented diagrammatically to facilitate conceptualization and understanding.

Use

Although models have proved to be extremely helpful in theory construction, they should be used carefully. Models have no truth value themselves. There is no guarantee that a model that has been successfully used in one area of study will be useful in another area. A major question to consider is the extent to which the model faithfully represents the phenomena of interest. There may be a tendency to overlook the differences between the phenomena of interest and the model since the scientist is more interested in the similarities. The differences, however, may completely negate the usefulness of the model. Models are tools for understanding reality which should be used judiciously and be replaced or modified when outmoded or inappropriate.

Criteria for Evaluating Theories

Theories are sets of interrelated hypotheses which are subject to reformulation and refinement. The development of adequate theories to describe, explain, predict, and control phenomena is a slow process and requires the cooperative effort of many persons. Knowledge is not acquired by one person in isolation but results from the cumulative efforts of many persons over a long period of time. Various writers, primarily philosophers, have suggested criteria to assist in the evaluation of theory. A theory may be evaluated in terms of its logical adequacy, abstractness, testability, empirical adequacy, and pragmatic adequacy (Schrag, 1967). These criteria are not meant to hinder the development of theories but to provide guidelines.

Theories are developed to help describe, explain, predict, and control phenomena in the world around us whether the theory is concerned with the area of astronomy, genetics, physics, chemistry, psychology, sociology, physiology, or biology. Implicit in the discussion of theories is the assumption that a theory can be evaluated according to certain universal standards. Regardless of the content of the theory, an investigator examines the underlying assumptions, the validity of the concepts and of the general perspective, the degree of generality of the theory, the soundness of the reasoning, the testability of the hypotheses, the empirical support for the hypotheses, the ability to control and manipulate the phenomena, and the degree of accuracy with which predictions can be made.

Meaning and Logical Adequacy

That few theories successfully meet all these criteria does not mean that theories should not be evaluated. A first step in evaluating theory is to identify basic assumptions (these may not be stated), the concepts, and the relationships between the concepts and to consider the validity of the assumptions, the validity of the meaning attributed to the concepts (are the concepts defined in a manner similar to that used by other scientists in the area?), and the logic of the theoretical system.

When an investigator has reached a conclusion about the validity of the concepts and proposed theory,

he can assess the logic of the argument. In doing this, the scientist is concerned with the reasonableness of the argument. The logical adequacy of a theory can be evaluated by formalizing the theory and examining it for discontinuities, discrepancies, and contradictions. In the example cited earlier (Figure 49-2a and b), discontinuities in the theory were evident. When the theory was formalized, it was apparent that nothing was said about the relationship between social stress and somatic dysfunctioning or about the relationship between cognitive dissonance and emotional tension and cognitive dissonance and somatic dysfunctioning. From the postulates and using the sign rule, it was deduced that A and C are positively associated. Since D is related (inversely) only to A, nothing can be said about its relationship to B or C. Because the relationships between A and B and B and C are asymmetrical (A B, B C), the conclusion that A is positively correlated with and results in C is logical. Had the relationship between the variables been symmetrical (A = B, B C), then the conclusion that A is related to C might not hold up. The relationship between A and B, for example, says that A and B vary together; the relationship is not necessarily causal. A and B may be related because of their common relationship to another variable, i.e., the relationship could be spurious.

Likewise, the symmetrical relationship between B and C might be spurious. If either or both of the relationships in these postulates are spurious, then the relationship between the concepts in the deduced proposition is open to question. No contradictions were evident in the stress formulation. Formalizing a theory increases the probability that discontinuities and contradictions will be identified.

Operational and Empirical Adequacy

Next, the theory can be assessed for its testability. To be testable, a theory must have operationally defined concepts. Since Bridgman's (1927) introduction of the phrase, "operational definition," scientists in all areas have been concerned with identifying adequate operational definitions for their concepts. When operational definitions for theoretical concepts have been established, the theory can be tested. Assessing the operational adequacy of a theory requires consideration of (a) whether the concepts can be measured and (b) how accurately the operational definitions reflect the theoretical concepts.

In testing a theory, it can be subjected to falsification (be found false) rather than to confirmation (Popper, 1959). If a sincere attempt is made to refute a theory and the theory stands up, the theory is considered supported or tentatively confirmed. Terms such as "confirmation," "verification," "support," "corroboration," "disconfirmation," "falsification," "failure to support," relate to the empirical base for a theory. Hypotheses may not be proved true, verified, or falsified by limited evidence, but evidence gathered over time from a variety of sources may tend to support, bear out, corroborate, or be in accord with an hypothesis, and thus be confirming evidence. If the evidence does not support the hypothesis, the evidence may be viewed as disconfirming rather than falsifying; the hypothesis is not "proved false." The use of the term "evidence" and the terms "disconfirming," "supporting," and "corroborating" suggests that one recognizes the status of the hypothesis as tentative— awaiting further testing. An hypothesis is not an absolute statement or a truth statement; it should be stated in a way that it can be tested and refuted. For data from any one study and for cumulative evidence from numerous studies, the question of the empirical adequacy of the theory is raised, i.e., how well does the evidence support the theory?

Over time, evidence that both supports and fails to support a theory accumulates. When the relative strengths of the evidence are evaluated, some conclusion about the empirical adequacy of a theory may be reached. Assessing the empirical adequacy of a theory requires the determination of the degree of congruence between the theoretical claims and the empirical evidence.

Generality

Another criterion used to evaluate a theory is the degree of generality or the degree of abstractness which characterizes it. The more general a theory, the more useful it is. A theory of the grieving process which can be applied to persons of all ages, to persons in any culture, and to losses of any object is more useful than a theory of grieving which can be applied only to middle-aged persons who lose a spouse.

Contribution to Understanding

A theory may be assessed as to how much it increases understanding. Does it describe the phenomena and give a sense of insight? Does it suggest new ideas and a new way of looking at the phenomena? The scientist constantly looks for theories that will increase his understanding of phenomena, which are relatively simple explanations, and which suggest new lines of reasoning and new avenues of exploration.

Predictability

Another criterion used to assess theory is the extent to which predictions can be made. A theory may describe a process, may increase the understanding of the process, but it may not assist in making any predictions about the outcomes of that process. A theory, for example may permit a description and explanation of a process after it has occurred; i.e., it is possible to look at a family which has suffered a "loss" and describe the family behavior in terms of adjustment to a crisis, but it may not be possible to predict accurately the behavior of family members in response to this crisis before the crisis occurs.

Pragmatic Adequacy

Since the purpose of a theory is to explain, predict, and control, the ability to control phenomena of interest is one means for assessing a theory. This criterion is pragmatic adequacy (Schrag, 1967). A theory may permit explanation and accurate prediction, but the theory may not permit the scientist to control the phenomena of interest.

The business of the applied professions (nursing, engineering, social work, medicine, architecture, political science) is to make *use* of existing theory to predict certain processes or outcomes and to control "events" in such a way that desired outcomes are achieved. The usefulness of a theory (pragmatic adequacy) for changing conditions is of major importance to the health professions. In the biological sciences many theories enable scientists or professionals to control outcomes; e.g., disease control, (prevention) of degenerative process in the body, and control or replacement of defective body parts. Although it is recognized that science has as its goal the production of knowledge for predicting and controlling phenomena, the ethics of using this knowledge is only now being examined in detail. Some of the decisions as to whether man should use the knowledge he had generated to control and alter the forces around him are being questioned more in some areas than in others, i.e., few question the use of vaccines to prevent disease, but the use of abortions to prevent overpopulation has been severely attacked by some segments of the population. Although there are relatively few theories (particularly in the area of social behavior) which permit the scientist to control phenomena, the development of such theories is likely to increase. The problems associated with the use of these theories by the applied professions will also increase.

Tentative Nature of Theories

Although rules and guidelines can be postulated to aid in the development and evaluations of theories, theories are tentative. With new knowledge, old facts are subject to different interpretations, and different data are brought to light. The development of theory is man's attempt to establish structure and meaning in his world. In assessing existing knowledge, one needs to take into account the culture of the scientific community as well as the values of society in general. The values of both communities come into play in many aspects of the process of establishing knowledge. The selection of problem areas and the development and use of concepts involve arbitrary choices. The theories that develop reflect the interests of the scientific community and of society and do not necessarily represent the areas that are in most need of examination.

REFERENCES

Blau, P. M. (1964). *Exchange and power in social life*. New York: John Wiley & Sons.

Bridgman, P. W. (1927). *The logic of modern physics*. New York: Macmillan.

Costner, H. L., & Leik, R. K. (1964). Deductions from axiomatic theory. *American Sociological Review, 29*, 819–835.

Di Renzo, G. J. (Ed.). (1966). *Concepts, theory and explanation in the behavioral sciences*. New York: Random House.

Hage, J. (1972). *Techniques and problems of theory construction in sociology*. New York: John Wiley & Sons.

Hempel, C. G. (1952). Fundamentals of concept formation in empirical science. In *International encyclopedia of unified sciences*. Chicago: The University of Chicago Press.

Kaplan, A. (1964). *The conduct of inquiry*. San Francisco: Chandler.

Parsons, T. (1951). *The social system*. Glencoe, IL: Free Press.

Popper, K. (1959). *The logic of scientific discovery*. New York: Basic Books.

Reynolds, P. D. (1971). *A primer in theory construction*. Indianapolis: Bobbs-Merrill.

Rudner, R. S. (1966). *Philosophy of social science*. Englewood Cliffs, N.J.: Prentice-Hall.

Schrag, C. (1967). Elements of theoretical analysis in sociology. In L. Gross (Ed.), *Sociological theory: Inquiries and paradigms* (pp. 220–253). New York: Harper & Row.

Selye, H. (1956). *The stress of life*. New York: McGraw-Hill.

Zetterberg, H. (1963). *On theory and verification in sociology (A much revised edition)*. Totowa, NJ: Bedmeister Press.

The Author Comments

Theories: Components, Development, Evaluation

The motivation for writing this article was the need for students to have an organizing framework for selecting one theory over another when faced with a clinical situation, regardless of clinical specialty or unit of study, from the physiologic to the organizational. Students also needed to link theoretic areas, which, at the time, often included the concepts of stress, crisis, and adaptation. To do this, students had to know the characteristics and components of a theory and the criteria for selecting and evaluating theory. This metatheoretic knowledge was and still remains a necessary prerequisite for comparing and selecting theories for nursing practice, as well as for evaluating one's own theories. At the time this article was written, there was no literature published on this topic. This article, along with the book publications, forged new and important territory in knowledge development for nursing.

—MARGARET E. HARDY

CHAPTER 50

From Practice to Midrange Theory and Back Again

Beck's Theory of Postpartum Depression

Gerri C. Lasiuk

Linda M. Ferguson

This article presents a brief overview of theory as background for a more detailed discussion of midrange theory—its origins, the critical role for midrange theory in the development of nursing practice knowledge, and the criteria for evaluating midrange theory. We then chronicle Cheryl Tatano Beck's program of research on postpartum depression (PPD) and advance the thesis that her theory of PPD, titled Teetering on the Edge, *is an exemplar of a substantive midrange nursing theory. We demonstrate Beck's progression from identification of a clinical problem to exploratory-descriptive research, to concept analysis and midrange theory development, and finally to the application and testing of the theory in the clinical setting. Through ongoing refinement and testing of her theory, Beck has increased its generalizability across various practice settings and continually identifies new issues for investigation. Beck's program of research on PPD exemplifies using nursing outcomes to build and test nursing practice knowledge.*

In today's world of *evidence-based nursing* and *knowledge utilization,* few question the centrality of theory to nursing knowledge development and the importance of that process to the ongoing evolution of the discipline.

Although even Florence Nightingale knew that the practice of nursing requires specialized, discipline-specific knowledge,[1] it would he several decades before the science of nursing had evolved sufficiently to systematically

From G. C. Lasiuk & L. M. Ferguson, From practice to midrange theory and back again: Beck's theory of postpartum depression. Advances in Nursing Science, *28(2), 137–151. Copyright © 2005. Reproduced with permission of Lippincott Williams & Wilkins.*

About the Authors

GERRI LASIUK was born and grew up in Saskatchewan, Canada, where the subtle beauty of the flat prairie landscape is juxtaposed against the glorious drama of wide-open skies. Her interest in women's health and health research stems from her clinical nursing practice with individuals across the life span and from a range of geographic, social, economic, and cultural backgrounds. Through first-hand experience, she came to appreciate the profound and far-reaching impact that women's health has on families and on society as a whole. In particular, she is interested in the health effects of interpersonal violence and other severe stressors. Her doctoral research in progress (she will graduate in November 2007) focuses on the experience of pregnancy and birthing of women with histories of childhood sexual abuse. Other scholarly contributions include participation in a multidisciplinary, multisite study on the sensitive health care of individuals with histories of childhood sexual abuse; a three-part examination of the sufficiency of the posttraumatic stress disorder construct to capture the range of human responses to trauma; and contributions to the first Canadian psychiatric nursing textbook.

LINDA FERGUSON was raised in Saskatchewan, Canada, and has worked as a nurse educator for most of her career. She teaches obstetrical nursing in a baccalaureate nursing program at a major medical-doctoral university, and has always been affected by those young women for whom birth and the care of a young family have been difficult. The emotional responses to the demands of childbirth and parenting are significant and need to be addressed within the biosocial events of birthing. Beck's work as a midrange theory is fundamental to how health care providers interact with these women. She also has a focus on nursing education research and is committed to the development of the science of nursing education. To this end, she is the director of the Center for the Advancement of the Study of Nursing Education and Interprofessional Education (CASNIE) at the University of Saskatchewan. Her funded research focuses on preceptorship and mentorship in nursing, and the epistemology of nursing as it relates to the development of practice knowledge and clinical judgment by new nurses entering practice.

develop that knowledge. In the early part of the last century, nursing practice knowledge took the form of "rules, principles, and traditions"[1(p34)] derived from experience and taught by rote. The competent practitioner needed only a caring disposition coupled with a handful of technical skills, which were taught in hospital-based apprenticeship-training programs. The little theoretical knowledge that did exist in nursing was co-opted from other disciplines.

This situation began to change when the public health movement took hold in the Western world. By 1913, the National League for Nursing Education in the United States recognized that the increasing scope and complexity of nursing practice required a broader knowledge base that must include "some knowledge of the scientific approach to disease, causes, and prevention . . . ."[2(p60)] The social

upheaval that accompanied two world wars and the intervening Depression years spawned major shifts in the social order; changes to the delivery of healthcare; and a growing demand for skilled nurses. In response, national governments invested new resources into the study of nurse education and work life. This was a critical juncture for the discipline because it presented both an opportunity and an imperative for nurses to articulate the nature of the discipline, to define its domain, and to set a course for future development. Consideration of these weighty issues precipitated a cascade of events that culminated in a consensus about the need for a body of distinctly nursing knowledge, developed and tested through research (for reviews, see references 1 and 3).

The importance of theory to nursing knowledge development received official sanction in 1965 when the

American Nurses Association (ANA) issued a position paper declaring theory development to be the primary goal of the profession.[3] Nursing scholars responded and the earliest nursing theories went to press in the late 1960s and through the 1970s. These highly abstract grand theories and conceptual models defined the boundaries of the discipline and established the theoretical foundations for nursing curricula.[1,3,4] While many practicing nurses saw them as having little direct relevance to their work, their articulation was a necessary precondition for subsequent phases in nursing knowledge development.[4] In their seminal article, Dickoff et al[5] reiterated the theory-practice gap and sketched out a course for the development of research-based knowledge to guide nursing practice. At the same time, the sociologist Merton[6] introduced the notion of middle-range theory as a means to guide empirical inquiry and to test that discipline's organizing theories. Jacox[7] would later endorse middle-range theory development as an important vehicle for the development of practice knowledge needed in nursing.

By the late 1980s, nursing was primed to respond to Meleis[8(p123)] impassioned plea for a "reVisioning" of the goals of nursing scholarship. For the discipline to go forward, she said, it must refocus its efforts on developing substantive nursing knowledge built on concepts grounded in practice. This marked the entry of nursing into the current era, one in which the main thrust is toward the generation and testing of midrange and situation-specific theory.

This article opens with a brief review of theory as a way to create a context for a more detailed discussion of midrange theory—its origins, the critical role for midrange theory in the development of nursing practice knowledge, and criteria for evaluating midrange theory. We then chronicle Cheryl Tatano Beck's program of research on post-partum depression (PPD) and advance the thesis that her theory of PPD, titled *Teetering on the Edge,* is an exemplar of a substantive midrange nursing theory. We demonstrate Beck's progression from identification of a clinical problem, to exploratory descriptive research,[9–12] to concept analysis[13] and midrange theory development,[14] and finally to the application and testing of her theory in the clinical setting.[15–18] Through ongoing refinement and testing of the theory, Beck has increased its utility and applicability across various practice settings and continually identifies new issues for investigation. This research program on PPD exemplifies of using nursing outcomes to develop practice knowledge through midrange theory development.

Theory: A Primer

Chinn and Kramer describe theory as the "creative and rigorous structuring of ideas that projects a tentative, purposeful, and systematic view of phenomena."[1(p91)] More specifically, it consists of concepts and the relationships among those concepts, for the purpose of describing and explaining the phenomenon, predicting outcomes, or prescribing nursing actions.[3,19,20] Theory serves to organize disciplinary knowledge and to advance the systematic development of that knowledge.[6] It may also identify the parameters of a discipline; provide a means for addressing disciplinary problems; furnish a language with which to frame ideas of interest to a discipline[3]; and provide unifying ideas about phenomena of interest to a discipline.[20]

By its nature, theory is abstract and does not exist in the material world per se; rather, it is a mental conception or an idea that represents things or events in that world. Because it is abstract, theory does not necessarily represent a particular thing or event, but may refer more generally to a class of similar things or events. In contrast, something that is concrete does exist in material form and "is embodied in matter, actual practice, or a particular example."[21] In elucidating the nature of a particular theory, we might construct an imaginary line or continuum (an abstraction in itself!) anchored on one end by things or events that are *concrete* and on the other by things or events that are *abstract.* Theories that are relatively more abstract are broader in scope and can be generalized to a greater number of things or events, whereas those that are more concrete are narrower in scope and applicable to a smaller range of phenomena.

A concept is "a complex mental formulation of experience."[1(p61)] It is the totality of a phenomenon, as it is perceived and—if it is empiric—can be verified by others. Like theories, concepts also exist at varying levels of concreteness and abstractness. A concept such as "biological sex" is more concrete (or empiric) because we can directly observe evidence of it. On the other hand, phenomena that can be measured only indirectly (such as depression) are somewhat more abstract and exist somewhere in the middle of our continuum. At the other end of the scale are highly abstract concepts like "self esteem" or "social support." Measurement of these concepts is also done indirectly, via agreed-upon indicators. The relationships between and among the concepts of a theory are stated as *propositions*.[1] These are "postulates, premises, suppositions, axioms, conclusions, theorems, and hypotheses,"[1(p266)] each of which reflects the proposition's purpose, type of logic used in its construction, and the context in which the propositions occurs.

Types of Theory

Having described key elements of theory, we can begin to label theories on the basis of their nature and purpose. Here we will consider metatheories, grand theories, midrange theories, and situation-specific theories.

Metatheory is global in nature and stipulates, in the broadest terms, the phenomena of interest to a discipline. Because of its high degree of abstraction, metatheory does not lend itself to empirical testing. This level of theory furnishes the concepts and propositions that are epistemological building blocks for disciplinary knowledge development. To a lesser degree than metatheory, *grand theory* is also very abstract. It offers conceptual frameworks, which define and organize disciplinary knowledge into distinct, though still broad, perspectives.[1]

The sociologist Merton[6] introduced the notion of *middle range theory* as a tool for empirical inquiry. He described it a "limited set of assumptions from which specific hypotheses are logically derived and confirmed by empirical investigation."[6(p68)] Midrange theories are less abstract and more limited in scope than grand theories. They involve fewer concepts, have clearly stated propositions, and readily lend themselves to the generation of testable hypotheses.[3]

Situation-specific or microtheories focus on specific phenomena in a particular setting. They are very limited in scope and are not intended to transcend time, place, or social-political structure.[3] Two such nursing theories are Gilliland and Bush's[22] theory of social support for family caregivers and Im and Meleis'[23] theory of Korean immigrant women's menopausal transition.

Midrange Theory

A major limitation of grand-theory is that its concepts are too broad and abstract for empirical testing. In contrast, situation-specific or single-domain theories[3] contribute little to building a cohesive and unified body of disciplinary knowledge because they are very concrete and too narrow in scope. Merton[6] argues that middle range theory circumvents both of these problems. To his way of thinking, efforts to explicate a unifying grand theory in sociology had just the opposite effect. That is, they resulted in the proliferation of a "multiplicity of philosophical systems in sociology and, further, led to the formation of schools, each with its cluster of masters and disciples."[6(p3)] Merton believes that sociology's advance as a discipline rests on the development of middle-range theory whereas continued focus on total sociological systems (ie, grand theories) impede that progress. In nursing, early efforts to define the parameters of nursing's domain and to identify its phenomena of interest led to the development of metatheory and grand-theory. While these did serve to differentiate nursing from other disciplines and explicated the discipline's ontological values, they provided little direction for nursing research to say nothing of the day-to-day practice of nursing.

According to Merton,[6] middle range theory can be developed from grand-theory (deductively) or from empirically grounded concepts (inductively). He emphasized, however, that the strength of middle-range theory is its capacity to describe, explain, and make predictions about concrete phenomena of interest to a discipline. The range of theoretical problems and testable hypotheses generated by middle range theory potentates its utility and productivity. While Merton believes that the larger conceptual schemes of the discipline should evolve from the conceptual consolidation of tested middle-range theories, he does not advocate exclusive focus on them.

Early nursing advocates of midrange theory[24] envisioned that a particular midrange theory might support a single or multiple grand-theories, thus cohering nursing knowledge. As well, Cody[25] suggests that midrange theory testing provides a way to analyze the adaptability of nonnursing theories to nursing practice. On a cautionary note, however, he adds that researchers and clinicians must first determine whether this *borrowed* theory is consistent with the ontological values of nursing. If it is not, he warns, it will not advance nursing science.

Evaluating Midrange Theory

In a 1993 address to the ANA's Council of Nurse Researchers Symposium, Suppe proposed that midrange theory is identifiable by its scope, level of abstraction of the concepts, and testability.[26] The scope or generalizability of a theory refers to the range of phenomena to which the theory applies[1] or to the number of situations addressed by a particular theory.[3] Because midrange theory is more concrete than grand theory—but less so than situation-specific theory—it applies across several client populations and practice settings, but not to all.[1,18,26] The concepts of a midrange must be clearly delineated and sufficiently concrete as to be testable.[19,20,26-28] Testability requires that these concepts can be coded objectively, as operational definitions, empirical measures, or hypothesized relationships, and that researchers can test the relationships between and among these concepts under different conditions.[19,26,27]

In the following section, we examine Cheryl Tatano Beck's theory of PPD. Our method for doing this is adapted from an approach to theory analysis described by Meleis[3] and on the more specific criteria for analysis and evaluation of midrange theory proffered by Whall.[29] Meleis' approach encourages attention to the theorist's

background and important life influences; the paradigmatic origins of the theory; as well as analysis of the theory's rationale, scope, goal, and system of relations among other factors. This provides a context for the theory, locates the theorist in the larger scientific community, and fosters an understanding of where their work resides within the disciplinary knowledge structure. On the other hand, Whall's approach to theory evaluation is more directly oriented to an analysis of whether or not a theory bears the characteristics of a midrange theory. The latter considers (1) the assumptions underlying the theory; (2) the relationship of the theory to philosophy of science; (3) any loss of information due to concepts not being interrelated via propositions; (4) presence/absence of internal consistency and congruence among all components of the theory; (5) empirical adequacy of the theory; and (6) evidence as to whether it has been tested in practice and/or through research and has held up to that scrutiny.

Teetering on The Edge: Is It a Midrange Nursing Theory?

Beck's Background and Life Influences

According to her curriculum vitae.[30] Beck received a bachelor's degree in nursing in 1970 from Western Connecticut State University. Two years later, she earned a master's degree in both maternal-newborn nursing and nurse-midwifery from Yale University. She specifically chose the Yale program because of this blend of research training and clinical specialization (written communication, November 25, 2002). A decade later, in 1982, Beck completed a doctorate in nursing science from Boston University. During that time, we see foreshadowing of Beck's later interest in PPD. The first of these is an article[31] examining the contributions of role conflict and learned helplessness to women's depression The second comes during her doctoral research (involving time perception during labor and delivery) when she is intrigued to discover a link between depression and alterations in time sensibility (written communication, November 25, 2002). Ten years later, in an analysis of maternal-newborn nursing literature published between 1977 and

1986.[9] Beck concluded that nurse researchers need to aim for methodological congruence in their choice of research designs; that the reliability and validity of instruments employed in maternal-child research must be evaluated; and that maternal-child nurse researchers need to identify areas of potential research.

Paradigmatic Origins of the Theory

Beck's initial study in the area of PPD explored early discharge programs in the United States through a literature review and critique, in which she identified a significant gap in maternal care. She wrote:

> What has not been given equal priority in post-partum follow-up care, however, is the mother's psychological status, more specifically, the phenomenon of maternity blues. Early discharge mothers are at home when the blues usually occur during the first week after delivery. Specific assessments for maternity blues should routinely be part of the nurse's assessment of these mothers during home visits.[10(p137)]

The next year, she reviewed the existing literature on maternity blues[11] and began clarifying the differences among the concepts of *postpartum psychosis, postpartum depression,* and *maternity blues.* She also identified the need to improve the instruments employed in this area and called for "both qualitative and quantitative research designs . . . to completely investigate the phenomenon of the blues."[11(p298)]

Beck[32] takes exception to the notion that qualitative research belongs exclusively to the early stage of a research program. She contends that at the outset of a research program it is impossible to predict its trajectory. Rather, she says, the "path of a nurse scientist's research program is truly determined by the state of knowledge that is known at each juncture when the research questions for the next study are being determined."[32(p266)] In response to Morse's[33] caution against investigators moving back and forth between inductive and deductive research approaches at the expense of methodological rigor, Beck counters that researchers can acquire the knowledge and skills about a variety of research methods through continuing education and/or via collaboration with others who have the methodological expertise needed for a particular study. In her rejection of the incommensurability of different inquiry perspectives, she provides the basis for her program of research: the need to address the question that arises with the most appropriate research method.

Philosophical Foundations

Beck reflects characteristics of a postmodern philosophy of science. Many postmodernists are also constructivists who believe that each of us constructs an understanding of the material world on the basis of our perceptions of it. Because observation and perception are fallible, these understandings are invariably incomplete. Our best hope for approximating a full understanding of phenomena of interest, is through systematic research employing multiple methods. According to Beck, "Each successive research project should be guided by the previous research study. The objective of this systematic, continuous inquiry is the cumulative production of new knowledge in a substantive area of nursing."[32(p265)]

Scope of the Theory

In 1992, Beck[13] published a phenomenological study of the lived experience of PPD. Data for the study were the text of transcribed interviews with women attending a PPD support group, which Beck cofacilitated for a number of years. From those, Beck identified 45 significant statements about the women's experience of PPD and clustered them into the following 11 themes, which explicate the "fundamental structure of postpartum depression"[13(p170)]:

1. Unbearable loneliness
2. Contemplation of death provides a glimmer of hope
3. Obsessive thoughts about being a bad mother
4. Haunting fear that "normalcy" is irretrievable
5. Life is empty of all previous interests and goals
6. Suffocating guilt over thoughts of harming their infants
7. Mental fogginess
8. Envisioning self as a robot, just going through the motions

9. Feeling on the edge of insanity due to uncontrollable anxiety
10. Loss of control of emotions
11. Overwhelming feelings of insecurity and the need to be mothered

The next year Beck[13] extended those findings into a grounded theory of PPD, titled *Teetering on the Edge*. She chose a qualitative approach to the topic because she believed that the Beck Depression Inventory (BDI),[34] a widely used instrument to detect depression, failed to accurately capture the 'horrifying experiences" (written communication, November 25, 2002) of PPD that she saw in her clinical practice. Research evidence corroborated Beck's observations,[35,36] calling into question the content validity of the BDI for PPD and identified a need for further investigation.

Beck's grounded theory inquiry involved a purposive sample of women attending her PPD support group.

Data were collected over a period of 18 months and included field notes from the support group meetings and transcriptions of in-depth interviews with 12 of the group's participants. Through constant comparative analysis. Beck identified the core variable or basic psychological problem in PPD as being *loss of control,* which the women experienced as teetering on the edge of insanity. Participants' attempt to cope with PPD through 4 stages—*encountering terror, dying of self, struggling to survive,* and *regaining control* (Fig 50-1).

In the first stage of PPD, *encountering terror,* the women live with horrifying anxiety, relentless obsessive thinking, and enveloping fogginess. During the stage of *dying of self,* they experienced alarming unrealness, isolation, and thoughts/attempts at self-harm. The third stage of PPD, *struggling to survive,* reflects the women's attempts to survive by praying for relief, battling the system, and seeking solace in support groups. In the final stage, *regaining control,* participants experience

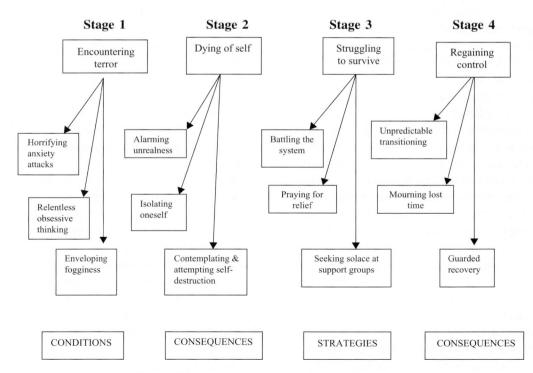

Figure 50-1 *The 4-stage process* of Teetering on the Edge.

unpredictable transitioning, mourning of lost time, and guarded recovery. These 4 stages of PPD subsume the 11 themes generated in Beck's earlier phenomenological study,[13] which, according to Beck,[14] extends and enhances the trustworthiness of her conceptualization of PPD.

Internal Consistency

The major concepts in Beck's theory of PPD (*loss of control, encountering terror, dying of self, struggling to survive,* and *regaining control*) are moderately abstract and relatively narrow in scope. All of the important concepts in Beck's theory are clearly identified, as are the propositions that explicate the relationships among them. The author explains each of the concepts and supports them with direct quotes from participants. With respect to the concept of *dying to self,* Beck furnishes[14(p44)] a partial audit trail illustrating how she derived the concept from the data. The fact that the 11 themes from her phenomenological study[13] readily subsume into the codes in her grounded theory study[14] indicates a high degree of transferability, dependability, and congruence of results between the studies. Not only is information not lost, but the findings from a prior phenomenological study[13] are integrated into Beck's[14] ground theory research project. This suggests a high degree of internal consistency and congruency among elements of the theory.

An assumption underlying Beck's theory is that PPD is a significant women's health problem that not only affects individual women but also has deleterious effects on their children's health and development.[37–40] Despite the fact that PPD had received considerable research attention by 1993, little of it was qualitative in nature. That being the case, Beck believed that some aspects of the experience of PPD remained underexplored. As well, because previous studies had never demonstrated an unequivocal link between PPD and the physiological changes associated with pregnancy and childbirth, there were undoubtedly other factors at play (eg, psychosocial, environmental, etc).

Other assumptions supporting Beck's theory of PPD are those embedded in the qualitative inquiry paradigm, which is consistent with nursing's values. Participants in qualitative research are viewed as competent *knowers* of their own experience and, as such, are collaborators in the inquiry process. In this tradition, there is emphasis on understanding phenomena by attending closely to participants' lived experience. Furthermore, because qualitative research is discursive in nature and emergent in design, the researcher examines data for patterns of meaning with the aim of objectifying those patterns for scientific inquiry, while at the same time endeavoring to remain true to the participants' construction of their experience. Qualitative research arises from traditions of human science inquiry in which the intent is to construct a holistic and ecological understanding of the phenomenon in question.

Empirical Adequacy and Testing

The empirical adequacy of Beck's theory of PPD becomes apparent in her subsequent work. She went on to develop the Postpartum Depression Predictors Inventory[16] (PDPI), a tool to identify women at risk for developing PPD. The PDPI is a checklist of 8 risk factors, determined through 2 meta-analyses[39,41] to relate to PPD. These factors include prenatal depression, prenatal anxiety, history of previous depression, social support, marital satisfaction, life stress, childcare stress, and maternity blues. The PDPI is used in clinical settings across North America and in Iceland.[42] In 2002, Beck published a revised version of the PDPI—the PDPI-R, which incorporates the results of another, more recent meta-analysis.[16]

Beck has also collaborated with Gable[15,17,18] to develop the Postpartum Screening Scale (PDSS) for detection of PPD. The PDSS is a 35-item, Likert-type, self-report instrument whose psychometric properties are supported in the literature and by content experts.[15] Confirmatory factor analysis of the scale supports the existence of its 7 hypothesized dimensions. Analyses of the 5-point response categories supported meaningful score interpretations and the internal reliability ranged from 0.83 to 0.94. Recently Beck[43] published a Spanish version of the PDSS.

Beck's research program clearly adopts a holistic approach to understanding the experience of PPD, consistent with the perspective and values of nursing. She explores views about women as whole beings operating in the context of a person-health-environment-nursing complex. In all of her writing. Beck discusses the implications of the work for nursing care. At the same time, her work resonates with those in other clinicians and researchers who work in the area of PPD. We find evidence of this in the congruence between Beck's theory with the work of Sichel and Driscoll (cited in reference 18) "earthquake model" of PPD. The latter explains that a woman's vulnerability to PPD reflects her unique genetic, hormonal, and reproductive makeup in the context of her life stressors. Depression, like an earthquake, can erupt when pressures increase at already highly stressed points of the system.

Conclusion

This article reviewed the basic elements of theory and chronicled the development of *Teetering on the Edge.* Cheryl Tatano Beck's theory of PPD.[14] We argue that Beck's theory is an exemplar of substantive midrange nursing theory. Through ongoing refinement and testing of her theory of PPD, Beck has increased its generalizability across various practice settings and continually identifies new issues for investigation. Beck's program of research on PPD represents a significant contribution to nursing practice knowledge through midrange theory development, which, in turn, advances the discipline of nursing.

Midrange theory has the potential to address the theory-practice gap that continues to plague nursing and to develop the substantive practice knowledge needed to advance nursing as a discipline.

REFERENCES

1. Chinn PL. Kramer MK. *Integrated Knowledge Development in Nursing.* 6th ed. St Louis. Mo Mosby 2004.
2. Gortner SR. Knowledge development in nursing our historical roots and future opportunities *Nurs Outlook.* 2002:48:60–67
3. Meleis Al *Theoretical Nursing: Derelopment and Progress.* 3rd ed. Philadelphia: Lippincott Williams & Wilkins: 1997.
4. Blegen MA. Tripp-Reimer T. Implications of nursing taxonomies for middle-range theory development. *Adv Nurs Sci.* 1797: 19:37–49.
5. Dickoff J. James P. Wiedenbach E. Theory in a practice discipline. Pt I: practice oriented theory. *Nurs Res.* 1968: 17:415–435.
6. Merton RK. *Social Theory and Social Structure* New York: The Free Press: 1968.
7. Jacox A. Theory construction in nursing an overview *Nurs Res.* 1974:23:4–13.
8. Meleis Al. ReVisions in nursing knowledge development: a passion for substance. In Nicoll LH. ed. *Perspectives on Nursing Theory* 3rd ed. Philadelphia Pa: Lippincott Williams & Wilkins 1997:123–132.
9. Beck CT. Maternal-newborn nursing research published from 1977 to 1986. *West J Nurs Res.* 1989:11:621–626.
10. Beck CT. Early postpartum discharge: literature review and critique. *Women and Health.* 1991:17:125–138.
11. Beck CT. Maternity blues research: a critical review. *Issues Mental Health Nurs.* 1991:12:291–300.
12. Beck CT. Postpartum depression a meta-synthesis. *Qual Health Res.* 2002:12:453–472.
13. Beck CT. The lived experience of postpartum depression: a phenomenological study. *Nurs Res.* 1992:41:166–170.
14. Beck CT. Teetering on the edge: a substantive theory of postpartum depression. *Nurs Res.* 1993:42:42–48.
15. Beck CT, Gable RK. Postpartum Depression Screening Scale: development and psychometric testing. *Nurs Res.* 2000:49: 272–282.
16. Beck CT. Predictors of postpartum depression an update. *Nurs Res.* 2001:50:275–285.
17. Beck CT, Gable RK. Further validation of the Postpartum Depression Screening Scale. *Nurs Res.* 2001:50:155–164.
18. Beck CT, Gable RK. Comparative analysis of the performance of the Postpartum Depression Screening Scale with two other depression instruments. *Nurs Res.* 2001:50:242–250.
19. Fawcett J. *Analysis and Evaluation of Contemporary Nursing Knowledge: Nursing Models and Theories.* Philadelphia FA Davis: 2000.
20. Walker LO, Avant KC. *Strategies for Theory Construction in Nursing.* 3rd ed. Norwalk Conn: Appleton & Lange; 1995.
21. Oxford University Press. *Oxford University Dictionary.* Available at http://dictionary. oed.com/. Accessed April 16, 2005.
22. Gilliland MP, Bush HA. Social support for family care-givers: toward a situation-specific theory. *J Theory Constr Testing.* 2001:5: 53–62.
23. Im E, Meleis AI. Situation-specific theories: philosophical roots, properties, and approach. *ANS.* 1999:22:11–24.
24. Suppe F, Jacox AK. Philosophy of science and the development of nursing theory. *Ann Rev Nurs Res.* 1985:3:241–267.
25. Cody WK. Middle-range theories: do they foster the development of nursing science? *Nurs Sci Q.* 1999:12:9–14.
26. Higgins PA, Moore SM. Levels of theoretical thinking in nursing. *Nurs Outlook.* 2000:48:179–183.
27. Lenz ER, Suppe F, Gift AG, Pugh LC, Milligan RA. Collaborative development of middle-range nursing theories: toward a theory of unpleasant symptoms. *ANS.* 1995:17:1–13.
28. Lenz ER, Pugh LC, Milligan RA, Gift A, Suppe F. The middle-range theory of unpleasant symptoms: an update. *ANS.* 1997:19: 14–27.

29. Whall AL. The structure of nursing knowledge analysis and evaluation of practice, middle-range, and grand theory. In: Fitzpatrick JJ, Whall AL, eds. *Conceptual Models of Nursing: Analysis and Application.* Stamford, Conn: Appleton & Lange: 1996:13–25.

30. Cheryl Tatano Beck's Web Page. Available at: http://www.nursing. uconn.edu/FACULTY/CherylT.html. Accessed April 6, 2005.

31. Beck CT. The occurrence of depression in women and the effect of the women's movement. *J Psych Nurs Mental Health Serv.* 1979:17:14–16.

32. Beck CT. Developing a research program using qualitative and quantitative approaches. *Nurs Outlook* 1997:45:265–269.

33. Morse J. Qualitative nursing research: a free for all? In: Morse J. ed. *Qualitative Nursing Research: A Contemporary Dialogue.* Newbury Park Calif: Sage; 1991:14–22.

34. Beck AT, Ward CH, Mendelson M, Mock J, Erbaugh J. An inventory for measuring depression. *Arch Gen Psychiatry.* 1961:4:561–571.

35. O'Hara MW, Neunaber DJ, Zekoski EM. Prospective study of postpartum depression prevalence course and predictive factors. *J Abnorm Psychol.* 1984:93:158–171.

36. Whiffen VE. Screening for postpartum depression a methodological note *J Clin Psychol.* 1988:44:367–371.

37. Beck CT. The effects of postpartum depression on maternal-infant interaction: a meta-analysis. *Nurs Res.* 1995:44: 298–304.

38. Beck CT. Postpartum depressed mothers experiences interacting with their children. *Nurs Res.* 1996:45:98–104.

39. Beck CT. A meta-analysis of the relationship between postpartum depression and infant temperament. *Nurs Res.* 1996:45:225–230.

40. Beck CT. Maternal depression and child behavior problems: a meta-analysis. *JAN* 1999:29:623–629.

41. Beck CT. A meta-analysis of predictors of postpartum depression. *Nurs Res.* 1996:45:297–303.

42. Stefansdouir H. Eiriksdouir IK. Karlsdouir S. Ingolfsdouir E. *How Do Icelandic Women Express Their Feelings During the Last Trimester of Pregnancy?* [Unpublished BS dissertation]. University of Iceland: 2000.

43. Beck CT. Postpartum Depression Screening Scale (Spanish version). *Nurs Res.* 2003:52:296–306.

The Authors Comment

From Practice to Midrange Theory and Back Again: Beck's Theory of Postpartum Depression

This article evolved from an assignment in a graduate-level nursing theory course that challenged us to examine the scholarship of a nursing theorist and decide whether it meets the criteria for midrange theory. We both chose to explore the work of Cheryl Tatano Beck, and through independent analysis we concluded that her theory of postpartum depression (*Teetering on the Edge*) exemplifies a substantive midrange nursing theory. Beck's theory reflects a holistic approach to understanding women's experience of postpartum depression that is consistent with the values of nursing and demonstrates nursing praxis in action. Beck's and other midrange theories diminish the theory–practice gap and advance nursing into the twenty-first century through development of empirically grounded practice knowledge.

—GERRI LASIUK
—LINDA FERGUSON

CHAPTER 51

A Theory of Theories: A Position Paper

James Dickoff
Patricia James

This paper takes a position on two important issues: first, on the issue of what a theory is; then, on the issue of what a nursing theory should be. Even more fundamentally, the position is taken that the difficulty in identifying and developing nursing theory stems in important part, on the one hand, from a conceptual muddle as to what theory is in any of its manifestations and, on the other hand, from the tendency in nursing, or in any discipline or individual, to grasp any structural security—even one that vitiates the basic purpose of individual or discipline—rather than to rest without security or even to brave fumbling toward a more significant security.

The Position in Four Theses

The position taken can be seen in outline through four theses:

1. Theory is a conceptual system or framework invented to some purpose; and as the purpose varies so too must vary the structure and complexity of the system.
2. Professional purpose requires a commitment beyond mere understanding or describing.
3. Significant nursing theory must be theory at the highest level—namely, so-called situation-producing theory.
4. A profession or practice discipline has built-in advantages that facilitate theory development for that discipline.

These four theses will be elaborated and then the third thesis—that significant nursing theory must be theory at the highest level, must be *situation-producing* theory—will be presented as the thesis most central to the position taken.

From J. Dickoff and P. James, A theory of theories: A position paper. Nursing Research, *1968, 17(3), 197–203. Copyright © 1968.*
Reprinted with permission of Lippincott Williams & Wilkins.

About the Authors

At the time this article was reprinted in the 3rd edition (1997) of *Perspectives on Nursing Theory*, JAMES DICKOFF and PATRICIA JAMES were professors of philosophy at Kent State University in Kent, Ohio. DR. DICKOFF had been teaching at Kent State since 1970 and was Chair of the Department of Philosophy. He studied philosophy at Washington University, where he received a BA in 1954. He continued his study of philosophy at Yale, where he received an MA in 1958 and a PhD in 1962. He worked with nurses and wrote about nursing for many years.

DR. JAMES graduated from the University of Detroit in Michigan with a BS in mathematics in 1955. She was a Fulbright Scholar in Belgium and then studied at Yale, where she obtained an MA in 1958 and a PhD in 1962. She was a visiting professor at the Oregon Health Sciences University School of Nursing. She collaborated with Dr. DICKOFF in writing many articles on nursing, education, and health care ethics.

What Is Theory?

In some nebulous way we all know what theory is. But if we want to deal with theory at close quarters—if we want to develop, criticize, or use theory—then a more explicit awareness or agreement is needed as to what is meant by theory, at least within the context of any given discussion. Our claim is that a real advance in clarity and potential usefulness is made if we view theory in this perspective: A theory is a conceptual system or framework invented to some purpose.

To emphasize theory as a *conceptual* device is to urge careful discrimination of theories and theoretical entities from things or reality, on the one hand, and from the inarticulate and incommunicable mental awareness, on the other hand. Theory is essentially verbalizable and hence communicable; but theory is a structuring proposed as a guide, control, or shaper of reality, and is not itself reality. Things, situations, matters of fact, histories—all these are to be distinguished from conceptual entities that are or go to make up theories. Entities on the conceptual or theoretic level are *concepts, propositions, laws, set of propositions* (and sometimes the linguistic expression of these conceptual entities are considered as theoretic entities). The question of the relation to reality of theoretical entities either in isolation or as systematically interrelated is the question of valida-

tion for theories. But, as we will urge later, no such simple-minded notion as isomorphism or mirroring exhausts or even helps much with the question of this relation—particularly in the higher reaches of theory.

Ontologically, then, theory is an entity at the conceptual level. But what is the structure of this "conceptual entity?" Practically speaking, no concept in isolation and rarely any proposition or law in isolation is deemed a theory, though strictly speaking even such single-element systems might be proposed as theories. Speaking most generally, a theory is a *conceptual system or framework*. That is, a theory is a set of elements in interrelation. All elements of a theory are at the conceptual level, but theories vary according to the number of elements, the characteristic kind and complexity of the elements, and the kind of relation holding between or among the theory's elements or ingredients. The factor (or concept) is the simplest element; a proposition or law is a certain relation among concepts. Theory at one level might be a coordinate set of factors or a coordinate set of propositions. But theory at its highest level has elements that are not merely coordinate, elements that differ from one another in level of complexity and even some elements that contain whole theories as elements.

A theory, then, is a conceptual system—but a conceptual system invented to some purpose. To emphasize that theory is invented rather than found in, or discovered in, or abstracted from, reality calls attention not only to the conceptual status of theory but also to the necessity for imagination and risk-taking in the proposing of a theory. Reality is not prefactored; and even more obviously, no relation among factors comes automatically noted or automatically labeled.

Though theory is no mere picture of reality, neither is theory an invention that is a mere fancy. Rather theory is a conceptual system invented to some purpose. And a good theory—or in perhaps more familiar terms a true or valid theory—is a theory that in fact fulfills the purpose for which the theory was proposed or invented. As the purpose of the theory varies, the structure or level of the theory varies—and so also will vary the mode of validating and even of proposing the theory. Theory whose purpose is prediction is the most familiar kind of theory, and the most developed methodology is that for testing the "goodness" of such a theory (or at least of the component elements of such a theory). But the position is taken here that important types of theory are presupposed by predictive theory and that moreover a more sophisticated kind of theory exists within which predictive theory functions as an element of an element of the theory. Nursing theory is of this elaborate kind.

What Is a Professional Purpose?

To consider what kind of theory is needed for a professional discipline requires articulating professional purpose. A true professional as opposed to a mere academic is action-oriented rather than being a professional spectator or commentator. But a professional as opposed to a mere technician is a doer who shapes reality rather than merely a doer who merely tends the cogs of reality according to prescribed patterns. A true professional—as opposed to a mere visionary—shapes reality according to an articulate purpose and in the light of means conceptualized in relation not only to purpose but also in relation to existent reality. In short, a professional cannot just watch, cannot just do, and cannot just hope or dream. The position taken here is that a theory for a profession or practice discipline must provide for more than mere understanding or "describing" or even predicting reality and must provide conceptualization specially intended to guide the shaping of reality to that profession's professional purpose.

What Would Constitute a Nursing Theory?

If nursing is a profession, then, the position taken here is that nursing must have an action orientation that aims to shape reality, not hit or miss, but by a conception of ends as well as means. This conception of ends and means is based somehow on conceptual awareness deemed adequate to take into account reality in its structure, course, and potential. A proper nursing theory, then, would be a conceptual system invented to serve the requisite purpose. Given the purpose, quite clearly the conceptual apparatus wanted is necessarily more elaborate than any merely predictive theory. The position taken here is that nursing theory must be theory at the fourth or highest level—namely, situation-producing theory. Situation-producing theory is called fourth-level theory because it presupposes the existence of three prior levels of theory, where predictive theory is a kind of third-level theory.

Situation-producing theory is called highest level theory because each of the other levels of theory exists in part at least to allow or provide basis for the next level of theory. But situation-producing theory is not as such developed for the sake of producing a theory of more elaborate structural level but rather for the production of or shaping of reality according to the situation-producing theory's conception. In plainer terms, situation-producing theory is produced to guide action to the production of reality. The major contention here is that all theory exists finally for the sake of practice (since in a sense every lower level of theory exists for the next higher level and the highest level exists for practice) and that nursing theory must be theory at the highest level since either the nursing aim is practice or else nursing is no longer a profession as distinct from some mere academic discipline.

How Could Nursing as a Profession or Practice Discipline Hope to Produce so Sophisticated a Theory?

On the surface it seems unreasonable to expect that a discipline newly dedicated to producing its own theory should have the capacity to produce a theory whose structural sophistication is necessarily greater than the sophistication of, say, physics, psychology, or biochemistry. But the position taken here is that nursing—like any practice discipline—has certain built-in advantages that could, if properly exploited, facilitate theory development within the discipline. As one level of theory presupposes another, so theorizing itself presupposes prior nontheoretical awareness (and prior activity other than theorizing). The privileged and habitual intercourse with empirical reality carried on in a practice discipline—often within the bounds of rote-like or carefully specified procedures—is a rich source of such preconceptual awareness. In the terms of "the father of empiricism" Francis Bacon, nursing or any profession is richly endowed with so-called "polychrest instances"—i.e., without artifice a "night watch" can be taken on highly complex phenomena and patterns of behavior and other changes.[1]

Not only is there a privileged and nonartificial field of observation at any present instance but also—thanks to the unity and history of the profession—there is a fund of practical wisdom passed on now often by word of mouth or apprenticeship. This wisdom could, if properly viewed, be precipitated and surveyed with keener scrutiny not just as a guide to the immediate practice of the scrutinizing individuals but for the sake of being put into more communicable, more stable, more generalized, and hence more amendable form. Not only is nursing rich in nonthetic awareness since its "professionals" engage habitually in practice and so encounter reality at least nonconceptually; nursing possesses also certain regularized patterns of behavior which are inherited and persistent over time—a built-in body of accepted practice, if not a body of knowledge in some other sense. That is, nursing has at the very least some awareness of the basis from which a constructive criticism should start. Moreover, not all this "basic wisdom" remains at the preconceptual level. Within nursing practice and tradition there is a certain abundance of written sources—among these the lowly or mighty procedure books—which could constitute a veritable gold mine of "incipient theory," recoverable and refineable given appropriate tools, energies, and aims.

In the pursuit of a scientific body of knowledge, nursing or any profession must be on guard against the two-fold temptation: 1) on the one hand, of a too quick contempt for anything already possessed or developed before the newest phase within the profession, or developed without or independently of skills newly acquired and hard won by current leaders in the profession; and 2) on the other hand, the temptation of embracing seemingly safe procedures from any other discipline, without very critical scrutiny of what those procedures have done for that discipline, let alone what they might do for nursing.

What must be admitted is the complexity and difficulty of producing a nursing theory in accordance with the position taken here. The temptation will be to do something easier, even though perhaps useless to nursing; to do something less novel and more in keeping with rigid stereotypes of researchers and theorists in natural and social sciences; to do what will make an acceptable doctoral thesis, whether or not useful to nursing; to do what is fundable, whether or not useful to nursing. These are temptations to which succumbing is easy, resistance difficult. But recognizing that to succumb is to sell your birthright as a nurse may give the impetus, and energy needed: 1) to entertain the proposed notion of theory with the burden of its detail; 2) to persist in nursing inquiry despite the allurements of smoother sailing and quicker payoff in status and funds to be found in repetition or imitation of inquiry in a more academic discipline; and 3) to exploit the advantages, history, and special peculiarities of nursing toward an appropriate bias within nursing inquiry.

Nursing Theory as Situation-Producing Theory

The four theses explored, let's sketch out what we take to be the levels of theory and some of the distinctive features of theory at each level. We but sketch these levels and features here for two reasons. First of all, too much

---

[1] Bacon, Francis. New Organon Book II, especially Aphorisms 50 and 41.

detail here on these matters moves the focus away from the four-thesis position taken by this paper. The more detailed consideration of these matters is offered in a paper "Theory in a Practice Discipline"—a paper basic in a sense to the present discussion, written by us with Ernestine Wiedenbach, and to be published in a forthcoming issue of *Nursing Research*.[2] Secondly, the task of the present paper is in part to create the need for that more detailed consideration. Unless there is some awareness of the practical import of seeing the relation of professional purpose to the mode of theorizing, exploring in depth levels and structure of theory could constitute just one more academic distraction for nursing. The point here is to emphasize the structure of fourth-level or situation-producing theory, so as to render somewhat more concrete the kind of structure we deem any viable nursing theory should have. Without initial awareness, awareness of the needed structure of theory, it is hard to see how any progress can be made in assessing any purported theory as to its adequacy or in deciding: 1) where work is already done; 2) where work must be done; and 3) how to guide in economical and feasible ways the time, energies, and talents at nursing's disposal so that the inquiry made will neither founder in despair nor constitute a mere status search or distraction.

The Kinds or Levels of Theory

A severe limitation in many current notions of theory stems from the oversimple view that takes as theory only sets of causal laws, so that the only conceptual systems regarded as theories are those that allow prediction on their bases. We have suggested that we can profitably see as theory conceptual frameworks which allow something less than prediction (for example, theories of classification or more simply systems or even conventions for naming or marking off significant elements) as well as conceptual frameworks that go beyond mere prediction.

It seems to us that careful attention to the structure of predictive theory suggests three things: 1) predictive theory presupposes the prior existence of more elementary types of theory; 2) predictive theory is not the only kind of theory dealing essentially with relations conceived as between states of affairs; and 3) there is a type of theory which presupposes and builds on theories at the level of relations between states of affairs.

The point of emphasis here is that in addition to factor-isolating and depicting theories (presupposed by predictive theories) and to predictive or causal theories (including what we elsewhere call promoting or inhibiting theories), there does or could exist another kind of theory which presupposes and builds on these other levels of theory. This fourth-level of theory can be called prescriptive theory, goal-incorporating theory, or perhaps most graphically, situation-producing theory. Situation-producing theories are not satisfied to conceptualize factors, factor-relations, or situation relations, but go on to attempt conceptualization of desired situations as well as conceptualizing the prescription under which an agent or practitioner must act in order to bring about situations of the kind conceived as desirable in the conception of the goal.

In "Theory in a Practice Discipline," (section on "The Four Levels of Theory"), the lands of theories are charted thus:

I. Factor-isolating theories
II. Factor-relating theories (situation depicting theories)
III. Situation-relating theories
    A. Predictive theories
    B. Promoting or inhibiting theories
IV. Situation-producing theories (prescriptive theories)

Situation-Producing Theory

A theory is here viewed as a conceptual framework invented to some purpose, and since the purpose of a situation-producing theory is to allow for the production of situations of a desired kind, the three essential ingredients of a situation-producing theory are: 1) goal-content specified as aim for activity; 2) prescriptions for activity to realize the goal-content; and 3) a survey list to serve as a supplement to present prescription and as preparation for future prescription for activity toward the goal-content. The goal-content specifies features of situations to be produced; the prescriptions give directives for activity productive of such situations; the survey list calls attention to those aspects of activity and to those theories at whatever level deemed by the theorist relevant to the production of desired situations but not (or not yet) explicitly or fully incorporated into goal-content or prescriptions.

We suggest that six aspects of activity fruitful to highlight as well as to use to organize a theory's survey list are these:

1. Agency
2. Patiency
3. Framework
4. Terminus
5. Procedure
6. Dynamics

In "Theory in a Practice Discipline" these ingredients and organization of situation-producing theory are charted as follows:

Ingredients of a Situation-Producing Theory

Goal content
Prescriptions
Survey list (organized, e.g., as follows)
1. Agency (explored, e.g., with respect to)
   a. Dimensions of the aspect (here agency) deemed especially relevant
      (1) External resources of agents
      (2) Internal resources of agents
      (3) Factors of agency proposed as significant in the statement of the theory or for acting under the theory
   b. Theories from other disciplines (at whatever level) deemed relevant
2. Patiency
   a. Relevant dimensions or realities
   b. Relevant theories
3. Framework
   a. Relevant dimensions or realities
   b. Relevant theories
4. Terminus
   a. Relevant dimensions or realities
   b. Relevant theories
5. Procedure
   a. Relevant dimensions or realities
   b. Relevant theories
6. Dynamics
   a. Relevant dimensions or realities
   b. Relevant theories

The Structure of Nursing Theory

Our contention is that any practice-minded nursing theory must be a theory at the situation-producing level. Looking at the ingredients typical of a situation-producing theory and at a survey list organized along the suggested dimensions is a first step toward rendering the contention plausible. Once initial plausibility is granted, the further investment of energy in the articulation of such theory becomes less academic and moves us one step closer to seeing whether practice bears out the contention.

What is the point of calling attention to goal, prescription, and survey list as essential ingredients of any nursing theory in a context where we are emphasizing the explicit conceptual nature of theory and the practical orientation of theory for any professional discipline? Emphasizing goal as a theoretical entity has three advantages: we dare or deign to become articulate about the explicit features of what we desire to produce; secondly, we see goals as giving explicit practical direction rather than merely emotional tone; and thirdly, we see the essential and respectable function of professional bias in the formulation of a practice theory. That is, goals become speakable—and hence communicable and alterable, functional, and finally viewable as professional rather than personal prejudices.

Calling attention to prescription as an essential ingredient of nursing theory, first of all, stresses the extra-academic features of a professional and of his situation-producing theory. Demand for prescriptions toward the realization of stated goals furnishes not only a stimulation to practical thought but also an antidote to the "beautiful soul" syndrome of the self-righteous reformer who won't sully ideals in any interplay with demands of practice. More specifically, a call for prescriptions constitutes a demand for bringing into the practical realm—in terms of real personnel and circumstances—the ideally desirable.

Presence of the survey list is a healthy reminder that the basis of professional judgment is incredibly complex and probably at no time fully articulate rather than something mysterious, ineffable, or inborn. The suggested six-fold organization pattern for the survey list gives at least one mode of rendering more manageable the admittedly wide and rich and deep scope of nursing activity. Any suggested patterning would provide an initial basis of exploration or command of this scope. The six-fold analysis suggested—along the dimensions of Agency, Patiency, Framework, Terminus, Procedure, Dynamics—brings the mind to bear on certain features of nursing which though perhaps noted dumbly in practice are often unnoted in theory or actively repressed from theory.

Considering Agency—or the question, Who or what performs the activity?—could be useful in at least bringing up for theoretical consideration the practical value of considering as agents of nursing activity not just registered nurses but also other professionals and non-professionals who might be directed or exploited to contribute to realization of nursing goal. Shouldn't a nursing theory take theoretical account of the proper function of at least, say, licensed practical nurses and aides? And is the sick person ever an agent? With similar generality, considering the aspect of Patiency (Who or what is the recipient of the activity?) makes us realize that even if we consider only the registered nurse as agent her activity is received or "suffered" by many others in addition to the sick "patient." And realizing that sometimes inanimate things such as charts or machines "receive" a registered nurse's activity might broaden the conception of both agent and patient not just beyond the registered nurse and the sick but also to include things other than persons. But what's the purpose of so irreverent an extension of agent and patient? Perhaps this: seeing their analogy to inanimate things may increase the theoretical sensitivity to the limits of elasticity and of repertoire and to the need for upkeep and fuel-input not only for immediate service but for any long-range expectation of serviceability.

Attending to Framework makes less plausible the insistence on registered-nurse-sick-patient dyad functioning in isolation as the sole focal point of a viable nursing theory. Part of professional purpose may in fact be to support or maintain not only the "patient" but also the profession and its supporting institutions. Practice would never deny this; why does theory not note it?

Emphasis on the aspect of Terminus (What is the end point of the activity?) calls for not recipes for service but apt characterizations of practical units of work. Conceiving these practical units might stimulate articulation of alternative modes of realization. But perhaps more importantly, considering Terminus calls attention to the function of the mode of conceptualizing activity as a possible contributor to the ease of doing or receiving the activity in question.

Giving explicit status to the Procedure aspect of activity requires attending to the safety, economy, and controlled performance that constitutes some of the virtues of rote, ritual, and policy: and seeing procedures as distinct from terminus demands an attempt at integrating appropriate detail with appropriately sensed direction.

Focusing on Dynamics (What is the energy source for the activity?) brings up for specific consideration, for example, psychological input, and makes discussable in theoretical terms the question of the appropriate place of, say, motivation other than service motivation in the rendering of professional services. Moreover, the very multiplicity of the noted dimensions makes evident the need to consider in theory as well as in practice the mutual interaction of these dimensions and their relation to prescription and to goal.

Given this general notion of nursing theory as a situation-producing theory with the three characteristic ingredients and with the survey list ingredient organized along the lines of the six distinguished aspects of activity, now it might be proper to ask where particular theories of biology, psychology, and sociology, to name a few, would fit within a nursing theory? Any one of these theories—or some specific part of any one of them—might (considering only structural demands) be a cited theory under any heading of the nursing theory survey list.

More generally, a nursing theory is a situation-producing theory which presupposes the existence of many lower level theories. Natural and social science theories are likely to be important contributors for these lower level theories of prediction, correlation, and terminology. But to say that nursing science or theory is merely applied biology, or applied psychology, or applied anything is misleading if it makes us overlook that conceptualization at a very sophisticated level constitutes the integration of the so-called pure sciences into nursing theory. These theories are building blocks, so to speak, in the mansion of nursing theory. This remark is not meant to demean the importance of these supporting theories, but to call attention to the mighty labor needed to exploit these basic sciences intelligently toward the nursing function.

This Theory of Theories—Its Novelty and Its Viability: An Immodest Proposal

Novelty alone is no reason to accept a theory or anything else. To the timid or conservative the tinge of novelty may in fact be reason sufficient to reject any proposal. Nonetheless, for two special reasons we point out what are the novel aspects of the position offered here. First of all, to label as inappropriate—before it appears—a rejection of the position offered on the mere grounds that the position differs from certain currently accepted theories of theory. This reason for rejection, though inappropriate, is the more likely to appear the more recently acquired is the awareness of other theories of theory and the more pain spent in acquiring that awareness. Secondly, to emphasize that no apology is made for the novelty—quite the contrary.

The first point of novelty to be urged is the contention that nursing or any so-called applied theory is more, rather than less, conceptually sophisticated than are so-called "pure" theories. To exclude the possibility of specific conceptual guidance in the attempts to put to use descriptive theories of reality is to confuse the present state of theory production with the theoretic possibilities for theory production. This remark leads to the

main point of novelty claimed. We suggest that proposing a theory of theories that sees theory as a conceptual system invented to some purpose—when seen in its full consequences—has revolutionary possibilities. The proposal allows at last for theory to be viewed as a proper tool to man even in his role of providing himself with purpose. But how is the novel related to the old? As Einstein's theory of relativity is to the Newtonian physician, so is our theory of theories to the, shall we say, classical theories of theory. The theories of Hempel, Carnap, Toulmin, Nagel, and so on, are special cases of the broader theory proposed here; these earlier views are not wrong so much as they are overly restrictive, concentrating only on one kind of theory without backing up to inquire as to theoretic activity itself and without seeing that one kind of theory—predictive—in relation to other possible kinds.[3]

The theory of theories offered here may be novel; but is it correct? To answer this question requires answering whether or not the proposed position constitutes a fruitful view of theory. It is important to realize that—whether the domain be nursing or theory—the theory of that domain must be invented rather than "discovered" from a hidden store of truth or "abstracted" somehow from the real. But consulting empirical reality is an important way of assessing fruitfulness. Reality may be so consulted by carefully controlled experiments with all action on the basis of the questioned theory postponed until research results are in and interpreted. But sometimes action cannot and should not wait on such niceties: the face validity, so to speak, of a theory or hypothesis may be sufficient to lead us to the acceptance of a conceptual framework as a tentative guide to action,

---

[3] For example : HEMPEL, C. G. Fundamentals of concept formation in empirical science. IN *International Encyclopedia of Unified Science*, ed. by Otto Neurath and others. Chicago, Ill., University of Chicago Press, 1952, Vol. 2, No. 7; Hempel, C. G. *Philosophy of Natural Science*. New York, Prentice-Hall, 1966; CARNAP, R. Methodological character of theoretical concepts. IN *Foundations of Science and the Concepts of Psychology and Psychoanalysis*, ed. by H. Feigl and M. Scriven. (Minnesota Studies in Philosophy of Science, Vol. 1) Minneapolis, University of Minnesota Press, 1956; TOULMIN, S. E. *Philosophy of Science*. London, Hutchinson & Co., Ltd., 1953; NAGEL, ERNEST. *Structure of Science*. New York, Harcourt, Brace, 1961.

with the resolution to note the results of following the guide so as to be prepared for needed amendments or to be sure of knowing how to repeat the happily followed path. For—as will be clear in our remarks on research—sometimes time, money, or energy demands make research narrowly defined too costly a mode of reassurance. And more importantly, there are some things about which we seek reassurance but for which research narrowly conceived can never be justly expected to constitute a reliable guide.

A major part of this paper was also presented by Doctors Dickoff and James at the Fourth Inter-University Faculty Work Conference of the New England Council on Higher Education for Nursing, held in Chatham, Massachusetts on June 18–23, 1967, and is also published in their report, *Physical-Biological Bases for Nursing Care: Implications for Newer Dimensions in Generic Nursing Education,* under the title, "Putting the Biological Sciences in Their Place(s)."

The Authors Comment (taken from Perspectives on Nursing Theory, *3rd edition, 1997)*

A Theory of Theories: A Position Paper

"Our conception of theory for nursing evolved from our interaction with nurses. It was fashioned in response to two things: (1) our philosophically educated awareness and enthusiasm for possibilities of concepts as guides for action and (2) our intensive work with nurses involved in enhancing nursing research, nursing practice, and nursing education by developing the conceptual dimension of nursing" (p. 112).

"As philosophers, our interest centered on 'concepts as they mattered for action.' Within philosophy we had concentrated on normative philosophy, including ethics but especially logic; even in the more speculative parts of philosophy we gravitated to problems of action-oriented thought ..." (p. 115).

"Our conception of theory was a purposive and innovative move—a reconception of theory itself" (p. 113).

—James Dickoff
—Patricia James

discipline, (2) serves as a way of organizing perceptions, (3) defines what entities are of interest, (4) tells the scientists where to find these entities, (5) tells them what to expect and (6) tells how to study them (i.e., the research methods available).

What do paradigms have to do with nursing theory? Kuhn's (1970) discussion of paradigms suggests that the metaparadigm and the exemplar paradigm are endorsed by a discipline and its subgroups because of their scientific-empirical support. The existence of a prevailing paradigm facilitates the normal work of science. Research is purposeful, orderly and raises few unanswerable questions.

When a dominant paradigm does not exist, a discipline may be in a crisis situation characterized by competing paradigms or it may be in a *preparadigm* stage with different, ill-defined perspectives that are heatedly argued and defended. In the preparadigm stage of a discipline, there is little agreement among its scientists as to what entities are of particular concern, where to locate these entities or how to study them. Such is the status of nursing today, with energy going into attempts to justify one of several embryonic paradigms rather than into purposeful, orderly research. Confusion prevails as to what exactly nursing should be studying; the research that is conducted is often poorly focused and unsystematic.

Kuhn's theory of paradigms and scientific revolution suggests that the development and evaluation of knowledge in nursing may proceed at a very slow pace, not because nurse-scientists lack the necessary ability to develop empirically-based scientific knowledge but because so much time is being devoted to justifying the various preparadigms. Until there is a prevailing paradigm and exemplar paradigms to give focus to the thinking and work of nurse-scientists, knowledge in nursing will develop slowly and somewhat haphazardly. This leaves the practicing nurse in a difficult position of deciding what knowledge is usable and how it should be evaluated for use.

Nursing as a Preparadigm Science

If Kuhn's conception of science is correct and if nursing is indeed in the preparadigm stage, then the time spent in defending one of the existing nursing conceptualizations (Riehl & Roy, 1974), the present concern with conceptual frameworks, models, theory construction and research methods are all part of an evolutionary process that other disciplines have either experienced already or have yet to face. Although this period of theory development in a discipline is characterized by ambiguity and uncertainty, nurse-scientists can help build the knowledge base that will help formulate an acceptable paradigm. They can do this by being well informed in a substantive area and participating actively in both theory construction and research. Nursing cannot decree that a specific paradigm will be adopted; the adoption of a paradigm will be based on its scientific credence and its potential for advancing scientific knowledge in nursing.

The preparadigm stage of science is one of confusion and frustration, with much dispute over theory, research and frequent factional power struggles. Nurse-scientists who realize this may be able to raise themselves above the battleground and focus their efforts and skills on developing sound nursing knowledge. Their work to solve very specific nursing-care problems may contribute significantly to developing exemplar paradigms and a predominant paradigm in nursing. The predominant nursing paradigm, when developed, will make it possible for other nurses to define more clearly their own "turf" or subject matter. While working on knowledge for practice, nurse-scientists must at present tolerate loosely constructed theoretical notions. This preparadigm stage of nursing science is difficult not only for those developing theory and research but also for those attempting to evaluate and use nursing knowledge.

The Development of Theory

The Nature of Theory

Before addressing the question of theory evaluation, the term theory must be defined. In common usage, the meaning of theory ranges from a hunch or a speculative explanation to a body of established knowledge. Kaplan (1964), in *The Conduct of Inquiry,* elaborates on the process of theorizing, suggesting that theory formation may well be the most important and distinctive attribute of human being. He does not perceive theorizing as a process removed from experience as opposed to brute fact.

In science, the term *theory* refers to a set of verified, interrelated concepts and statements that are testable. In his discussion of the human ability to develop scientific theory, Kaplan says:

> In the reconstructed logic, . . . theory will appear as the device for interpreting, criticizing, and unifying established laws, modifying them to fit data unanticipated in their formulation, and guiding the enterprise of discovering new and more powerful generalizations. To engage in theorizing means not just to learn by experience but to take thought about what is there to be learned. (Kaplan, 1964, p. 295)

Nurses will do well to remember the vital part that experience plays in theorizing.

Since a theory is a validated body of knowledge about some aspect of reality, it is appropriate that in developing theory nurses should concern themselves with identifying aspects of reality they wish to focus on, developing relevant theory and evaluating the soundness of the knowledge they develop. The scientist, in developing theory, looks for lawful relationships, patterns or regularities in the empirical world. Such relationships between concepts, sets facts or variables are carefully studied in order to identify conditions that modify or alter the original relationship.

Few "theories" in nursing or related disciplines are sufficiently well developed to permit specification of both lawful relationships and the condition under which these relationships vary. One possibility is behavior modification theory, which expresses a lawful relationship between specified behavior and reinforcement. Furthermore, this relationship may alter according to the type of reinforcement schedule employed.

Relationship Between Theory and Practice

Kaplan stresses the interrelatedness of theory and experience. In nursing, scientists and practicing nurses are frequently out of touch with one another. The nurse-scientist is a thinker unconcerned with the practice setting, while the practitioner is a provider of nursing care and is sometimes referred to as a technician. But it is from the practice setting that the nurse-scientist should derive ideas, and it is for the nurse in the clinical setting that ideas are developed. If the nurse-scientist is to be the major developer of theoretical knowledge, the practitioner must be in a position to provide the nurse-scientists with research-worthy problems and, at the same time, must be able to evaluate the knowledge generated for its soundness and applicability. A similar symbiosis has been highly successful in other fields. For instance, the theoretical physicist develops ideas and the engineer applies those ideas for the practical benefit of human beings.

Nursing has a mandate from society to use its specialized body of knowledge and skills for the betterment of humans. The mandate implies that knowledge and skills must grow in such a way as to keep up with the changing health goals of society. Furthermore, nursing must regulate its own practice, control the qualifications of its practitioners and implement *newly developed knowledge*.

The majority of nurses are clearly "doers" or practitioners. However, the discipline must also include scientists dedicated to generating knowledge. These scientists must be committed to finding things out, to obtaining an understanding and explanation of phenomena in their world and to identifying means for controlling significant phenomena. Nursing practice and nursing science, as pointed out earlier, are not antithetical; each depends on the other. It is important that theory be useful and encompass significant concepts and conditions that can be applied and favorably altered in the clinical setting.

Drawing on Work in Other Disciplines

Nursing draws on theories and knowledge from the disciplines of psychology, sociology and physiology. This is entirely legitimate; there is no reason for nurse-scientists to spend years of hard work duplicating knowledge that already exists but is housed in other disciplines. However, theory from another discipline must first be empirically validated to determine if its generalizations are applicable to nursing and its particular problems and needs. For example, generalizations from cognitive dissonance theory should be assessed to see if they can be used by nurses in practice settings; it is conceivable and, in fact likely, that modifications will first be necessary.

A large number of hours has been expended by social scientists in developing empirically based theoretical frameworks on role and social exchange. If nurses and nurse-scientists wish to employ these two sets of knowledge, they will need to determine how, when and where the concepts and empirical generalizations are applicable. In making this evaluation, they are likely to identify conditions unique to nursing practice which alter the social scientists' generalizations; they may also find they need to expand the original theory.

Types of Theory: Grand Versus Circumscribed

If the discipline of nursing is indeed in the preparadigm stage, consideration must be made for the level of theory development. Given a set of criteria for evaluating theory, the evaluator must make a decision as to what can be considered to be theory. A body of knowledge which is in the preparadigm stage cannot be evaluated as rigorously as a theory, nor can formulations which are "grand theories" or philosophies about nursing. They provide neither solid nor practical foundations for nursing practice; they are difficult to evaluate for their scientific value.

A theory in the early stage of development is characterized by discursive presentation and descriptive accounts of anecdotal reports to illustrate and support its claims. The theoretical terms are usually vague and ill defined, and their meaning may be close to everyday language. A paradigm at this embryonic stage is very readable and provides a perspective rather than a set of interrelated theoretical statements. This type of formulation *lacks empirical support;* the empirical illustrations accompanying it are not tests of the theoretical perspective.

This type of formulation, the "grand theory" or "general orientation," is aimed at explaining the totality of behavior (Merton, 1957). Grand theories tend to use vague terminology, leave the relationships between terms unclear and provide formulations that cannot be tested. Examples of grand theory might be Parsons's

theory of Social Systems, Rogers's (1970) formulations of nursing theory, crisis theory, and some of the stress formulations. All present unique ways of looking at reality, but their ill-defined terms and questionable linkages between concepts make them impossible to put into operation and test empirically—and testability of a theory is one of the most important conditions a formulation must meet (Gibbs, 1972).

In addressing the problem of grand theories, Merton (1957) makes a plea for scientists to move into the study of partial theories. Since this plea, social scientists seem to have been successful in developing and testing partial or circumscribed theories. These circumscribed formulations may become exemplar paradigms; the move from grand formulations to circumscribed theory may take a discipline from a preparadigm stage to a paradigm stage with exemplar paradigms.

Circumscribed theories focus on selective aspects of behavior such as communication, social exchange, role behavior and self-consistency. In time, these formulations may lead to explication of theoretical terms and hypotheses which can be tested by carefully designed studies. The cumulative research and resulting theory is sound. Of the paradigms developed, one may eventually predominate, several may combine into a new paradigm which will address a larger part of reality, and several may coexist as exemplar paradigms.

The circumscribed theories on which scientists focus may seem irrelevant and unimportant when compared to the complex day-to-day problems confronted by nurses. Yet nurses must recognize that such complex problems cannot be solved quickly—as is evident in the enormous number of hours this country has spent trying to determine what cancer is and how it develops. Complicated scientific problems usually must be broken down into smaller, more manageable parts and tackled one by one. The scientific process for developing knowledge is slow, but it is the only sure one we have.

The norms that guide scientific activities seem to be universal; they are not specific to a discipline or country (Hardy, 1978). These norms include the need for public discourse on knowledge; the need for establishing the validity of scientific work; the need for critical assessment of both theory and research; and the need for empirical, objective work which can be replicated by others. It is in a milieu influenced by these norms that knowledge is generated and theory is developed; thus the outcome of the scientific process, the scientist's major goal, is achieved. If theory application is to contribute to the advancement of knowledge and to the professional code of ethics, nurse-scientists must adhere to these norms when developing knowledge.

Evaluation of Theory

Scientists have a variety of criteria for assessing knowledge. They examine their theories for explanatory and predictive power, for parsimony, generality, scope and abstractness (Hage, 1972; Hardy, 1978). For nurse-scientists, there is also a subset of criteria relating to the application of a particular theory in clinical practice. The following questions might be asked for such a theory: Is it internally consistent or *logically adequate?* How sound is its *empirical support?* Does the theory present concepts and conditions which the nurse can actually *modify?* Can the theory be used in bringing about *major, favorable changes?*

Logical Adequacy (Diagramming)

Since a theory is a set of interrelated concepts and theoretical statements, its structure can be analyzed for internal consistency or logic (Hardy, 1978; Rudner, 1966). This involves examining the syntax of the theory rather than its content. If the structure is inconsistent or illogical, then empirical testing may not provide a test of the theory itself but only of unrelated or loosely related hypotheses.

One method for examining a theory's internal consistency involves identifying all the major theoretical terms. These may include constructs, concepts, operational definitions or referents. Once identified, each term can be represented by a symbol. Use of symbols serves to decrease the evaluator's bias and thus lessens the likelihood that substantive meaning will be attributed to the theory when it is not present.

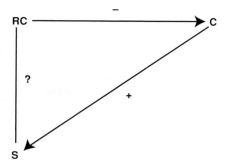

RC = role conflict
C = communication
S = satisfaction
+ = positive linkage
− = negative linkage
? = unspecified linkage

Figure 52-2 *Typical linkage diagram.*

The next step is to identify the relationships or linkages between terms. The linkages are usually expressed as follows: direction, type of relationship (positive or negative) and form of relationship (Hage, 1972). Symbols are used to signify the linkages; if the theory does not specify a linkage, this will become obvious as the structure of the theory is diagrammed.

To illustrate this process, consider the statement "high role conflict experienced by a person results in less communication with coworkers" and the statement "frequent communication with coworkers is associated with job satisfaction." The structure of these two statements would then be as shown in Figure 52-2. Diagramming these statements shows clearly that there are no contradictions in the specified linkages, and that there is no link specified between role conflict and satisfaction. This type of diagramming makes it possible to identify gaps, contradictions and overlaps. Linkages between constructs, concepts and operational definitions can also be diagrammed. (See Figure 52-3.) Diagramming a theoretical formulation will clearly show whether the hypothesis to be tested flows logically from the more abstract theoretical statements.

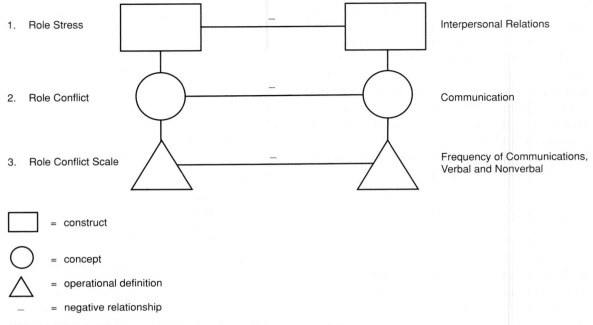

1. Role Stress

2. Role Conflict

3. Role Conflict Scale

Interpersonal Relations

Communication

Frequency of Communications, Verbal and Nonverbal

 = construct

 = concept

 = operational definition

 = negative relationship

Figure 52-3 *Linkage diagram showing relationships between terms.*

Empirical Adequacy

Empirical validity is perhaps the single most important criterion for evaluating a theory which is to be applied in a practice setting. However, a theory cannot be empirically valid if it is logically inadequate. Many theories are proposed but only a few are testable. Unfortunately, it is all too easy to select a theory which seems plausible or fits our own belief system and then use it in teaching students and working with patients. Among others, popular theories which have such questionable empirical support are psychoanalytic theory, crisis intervention theory and Erikson's theory of developmental crisis.

Assessment of Empirical Support

Assessing the empirical support for a theory is a rigorous but exciting puzzle-solving activity which involves several independent but closely related steps. Suppose an individual is planning to go to a major theoretical work and attempt to identify the key theoretical terms and the linkages between them. This process is identical to the processes used in determining the internal consistency

of the theory, and a linkage diagram is used. When the individual has diagrammed the theory and identified predictions and hypotheses, it is necessary to examine the empirical support which actually exists. This requires going to the literature and identifying related studies.

After the pertinent studies have been reviewed, they may be classified according to the strength of their research methodology and the empirical support given to the hypotheses tested. Care must be taken in judging which studies represent valid empirical tests of the theory. Case studies, anecdotal reports or descriptions of processes presented in discursive accounts of the theory do not constitute empirical tests. Such accounts are generally presented to give the reader the feeling that the theory is plausible and congruent with life events. This type of material may, however, be used to assess the theory's potential scope and generality.

It should not be forgotten that researchers usually have vested interests in their studies and may have introduced biases that alter the interpretation of the findings. During the critical reading, a study's hypotheses and their empirical referents may be diagrammed, as may the empirical relationship found between the concepts. The congruence between theoretical predictions and empirical outcomes can then be readily assessed in a relatively objective manner.

Factors to Consider

In evaluating research, possible changes in meaning of terms and concepts should be kept in mind. For example, in the literature of the 1950s on therapeutic communication theory, the concept of negative feedback may have been defined as derogatory (negative) communication, while in the 1970s, negative feedback has been redefined to mean any communication that alters (increases or decreases) the communication of the other person.

In analyzing a theory and its empirical support, it is necessary to determine that the hypotheses tested are clearly deduced from the theory. If they are not, the research is not testing that theory. In examining theoretical terms and their corresponding operational definitions, one's immediate concern is with the validity of the operational definitions. A theory may be logically sound—the hypotheses may follow clearly from it and be stated in a form that can be confirmed or rejected—but if the operational definitions do not reflect the meaning of the theoretical concepts, the research is not really addressing the theory and results will have limited or no bearing on it.

To complete the assessment, the entire body of relevant studies must be evaluated in terms of the extent to which it supports the theory, or some part of the theory. This assessment should result in a decision as to whether empirical support is sufficient to warrant the theory's application. The absolute necessity for determining the empirical adequacy of a theory cannot be overemphasized. If nurses are taught "theories" that have little or no empirical support, the nursing care interventions based on such "theories" may have deleterious effects on clients who believe in the nurse's skill, expertise and competence. And indeed there has been a tendency to base nursing actions on tradition, intuition and conceptual frameworks which seem sound but have

not been empirically tested. Though they may be creative and may give nurses a sense of security in what they do, these sources of knowledge remain in the realm of myth and nonscientific knowledge.

For example, even if a conceptual framework for crisis intervention makes intuitive sense to a nurse, using it as a basis of action when it does not have sound empirical support is a serious error in judgment and one that has considerable ethical implications. There is a need to develop and use empirically sound scientific knowledge if nursing is to retain its reputation as a profession. And the process of evaluating a theory empirically should be shared with students since they, as practicing nurses, should carry out this same process for the remainder of their nursing careers.

Usefulness and Significance

Since nursing is an applied profession, it follows that relevant theories are those which nurses may use in the clinical setting. After a theory has been identified as having internal consistency and strong empirical support, can it actually be put to use by a nurse? The theory is *useful* to the degree that the practitioner is able to control, alter or manipulate the major variables and conditions specified by the theory to realize some desired outcome. Knowing multiple sclerosis is caused by a virus that lies dormant in a person for 30 years does not provide nurses with a basis for immediate intervention. On the other hand, the awareness of the empirical association between smoking and both lung cancer and heart disease allows the nurse to manipulate variables that can decrease the occurrence and severity of these diseases. Here theoretical knowledge is useful. Inhaling carcinogens from cigarettes is an activity over which the nurse can exert some influence, either through persuading individual patients not to smoke or by assisting in more general public education efforts.

Related to the usefulness of a theory is its *significance*. Given two theories which are internally consistent, have strong empirical support and encompass variables that the nurse is able to modify, what else should influence the choice of which theory to use? Assuming that both are focused on the same nursing problem,

The Author Comments

Perspectives on Nursing Theory

This article reflects my thinking regarding the knowledge needed by doctoral students to evaluate theories that are germane to nursing. The ideas in this article were first presented at a nursing conference at Case Western Reserve in response to an invitation from Dr. Rosemary Ellis to speak to doctoral students. The notions of metaparadigm and theory development were important metatheoretical ideas for students to understand to effect the status and progress of knowledge in nursing. The ideas in this article, including the often-used diagrammatic model of the structure of a theory, were borrowed from sociology. This diffusion of knowledge from sociology helped launch the explosion of theory development activity that occurred in nursing during the decade this article was written and continues to this day.

—MARGARET E. HARDY

CHAPTER 53

Criteria for Evaluation of Theory

Jacqueline Fawcett

This column presents criteria for evaluation of nursing theories specified by Jacqueline Fawcett and Rosemarie Rizzo Parse. Fawcett's criteria are significance, internal consistency, parsimony, testability, empirical adequacy, and pragmatic adequacy. Some of those criteria are differentiated for grand theories and middle-range theories but are not differentiated by type of data—qualitative or quantitative—used to develop the theory. Parse's criteria are structure and process. Structure encompasses historical evolution, foundational elements, and relational statements. Process encompasses correspondence, coherence, and pragmatics. Parse's criteria are appropriate for the critical appraisal of all frameworks and theories, regardless of level of abstraction. Parse also presents a comparison of her own and Fawcett's criteria.

Several different sets of criteria for evaluation of theories have been published (Barnum, 1988; Duffy & Muhlenkamp, 1974; George, 2002; Marriner-Tomey & Alligood, 2002; Meleis, 1997; Parse, 1987). Just one set of criteria, however, differentiates between grand theories and middle-range theories (Fawcett, 2000, 2005).

Although none of the authors of those publications have indicated that the source of the data for a theory influences the selection of evaluation criteria, a recent conversation with a colleague raised the question of whether theories grounded in qualitative data should be evaluated using criteria that differ from those used to

From J. Fawcett, Nursing Science Quarterly, *2005;18(2):131–135. Copyright © 2005 SAGE Publications. Reprinted with permission by SAGE Publications, Inc.*

About the Author

JACQUELINE FAWCETT received her Bachelor of Science degree from Boston University in 1964, her Master's in Parent–Child nursing from New York University in 1970, and her PhD in Nursing, also from New York University, in 1976. Dr. Fawcett currently is Professor, College of Nursing and Health Sciences, University of Massachusetts, Boston. She is Professor Emerita at the University of Pennsylvania. Starting with her dissertation, Dr. Fawcett conducted a program of research dealing with wives' and husbands' pregnancy-related experiences that was derived from Martha Rogers' conceptual system. Subsequently, she undertook a program of research dealing with responses to Cesarean birth derived from the Roy Adaptation Model of Nursing. A third program of research, also derived from the Roy Adaptation Model, focuses on function during normal life transitions and serious illness. Dr. Fawcett is perhaps best known for her meta-theoretical work, including many journal articles and several books. Since 1996, Dr. Fawcett has lived in the mid-coast region of Maine with her husband John and a now-tame feral cat, Lydia Dasher. She and her husband own Fawcett's Art, Antiques, and Toy Museum. She swims laps and walks on a treadmill at a fitness center for exercise and relaxation and sails on a windjammer off the Maine coast during the summer.

evaluate theories grounded in quantitative data. That conversation resulted in an invitation to Rosemarie Rizzo Parse to engage in a dialogue about what criteria are appropriate for evaluating grand theories and middle-range theories and whether those criteria can be applied to theories regardless of the type of data (qualitative or quantitative) in which a theory is grounded.

Consensus exists that theories are made up of ideas called concepts and statements about the concepts, called propositions (King & Fawcett, 1997). Consensus also exists that components of nursing knowledge, including theories, vary in levels of abstraction (King & Fawcett). I regard grand theories as more abstract than middle-range theories but less abstract than conceptual models (Fawcett, 2005). Accordingly, my framework includes some differences in the evaluative criteria for grand theories and middle-range theories. I do not, however, differentiate criteria for evaluation of either grand or middle-range theories based on the type of data (qualitative or quantitative) used to develop the theory.

I developed a framework for both the analysis and evaluation of nursing theories several years ago and refined the framework twice (Fawcett, 1993, 2000, 2005). Analysis involves objective and nonjudgmental descriptions of theories, whereas evaluation involves judgments about the extent to which nursing theories

meet certain criteria. For the purposes of this dialogue, my comments are limited to the criteria for evaluation of grand theories and middle-range theories. Those criteria are significance, internal consistency, parsimony, testability, empirical adequacy, and pragmatic adequacy.

The criterion of *significance* focuses on the context of the theory. That criterion requires justification of the importance of the theory to the discipline of nursing and is met when the metaparadigmatic, philosophical, and conceptual origins of the theory are explicit, when antecedent nursing and adjunctive knowledge is cited (Levine, 1988), and when the special contributions made by the theory are identified. The four questions to be asked when evaluating the significance of a theory, which are applicable to both grand and middle-range theories, are listed in Table 1.

The criterion of *internal consistency* focuses on both the context and the content of the theory. That criterion requires all elements of the theorist's work, including the philosophical claims, conceptual model, and theory concepts and propositions, to be congruent. The internal consistency criterion also requires the concepts of the theory to reflect semantic clarity and semantic consistency. The semantic clarity requirement is more likely to be met when a theoretical definition is given for each concept than when no explicit definitions are given. The semantic consistency requirement is met when the same term and the same definition are used for each concept in all of the author's discussions about the theory. Semantic inconsistency occurs when different terms are used for a concept or different meanings are attached to the same concept. In addition, the internal consistency criterion requires that propositions reflect structural consistency, which means that the linkages between concepts are specified and that no contradictions in relational propositions are evident. The three questions to be asked when evaluating the internal consistency of a theory, which is applicable to both grand and middle-range theories, are listed in Table 53-1.

The criterion of *parsimony* focuses on the content of the theory. Parsimony requires a theory to be stated in the most economical way possible without oversimplifying the phenomena of interest. This means that the fewer the concepts and propositions needed to fully explicate the phenomena of interest, the better. The parsimony criterion is met when the most parsimonious statements clarify rather than obscure the phenomena of interest. The question to be asked when evaluating the parsimony of a theory, which are applicable to both grand and middle-range theories, is given in Table 53-1.

The criterion of *testability* also focuses on the content of the theory. That criterion frequently is regarded as the major characteristic of a scientifically useful theory. Marx (1976) declared, "If there is no way of testing a theory it is scientifically worthless, no matter how plausible, imaginative, or innovative it may be" (p. 249). Testability typically is regarded as an empirically based criterion. Yet the relatively abstract and general nature of grand theories means that their concepts lack operational definitions stating how the concepts are measured, and their propositions are not amenable to direct empirical testing. Therefore, I identified different criteria for the evaluation of the testability grand theories and middle-range theories.

Description of personal experiences may be used to evaluate the testability of grand theories (Silva & Sorrell, 1992). That approach requires specification of an inductive, qualitative research methodology that is in keeping with the philosophical claims and content of the grand theory and that has the capacity to generate middle-range theories. The product of the descriptions of personal experiences approach is "generalities that constitute the substance of [middle-range] nursing theories" (Silva & Sorrell, 1992, p. 19). In essence, then, evaluation of the testability of a grand theory involves determining the middle-range theory-generating capacity of a grand theory. The criterion of testability is met when the grand theory has led to the generation of one or more middle-range theories. Three questions, which were adapted from requirements proposed by Silva and Sorrell (1992), are asked when evaluating the testability of a grand theory (Table 53-1).

The relatively concrete and specific nature of middle-range theories means that their concepts can have operational definitions and their propositions are amenable to direct empirical testing. Consequently, an approach called traditional empiricism is used to evaluate the testability of middle-range theories. That approach requires the concepts of a middle-range theory to be observable and the propositions to be measurable. Concepts are empirically observable when operational definitions identify the empirical indicators that are used to measure the concepts. Propositions are measurable when empirical indicators can be substituted for concept names in each proposition and when statistical procedures can provide evidence regarding the assertions made. The criterion of testability for middle-range theories, then, is met when specific instruments or experimental protocols have been developed to observe the theory concepts and statistical techniques are available to measure the assertions made by the propositions. Three questions, which were adapted from requirements identified by Silva (1986) and Fawcett (1999), are asked when evaluating the testability of a middle-range theory (Table 53-1).

The criterion of *empirical adequacy* requires the assertions made by the theory to be congruent with empirical evidence. The extent to which a theory meets that criterion is determined by means of a systematic review of the findings of all studies that have been guided by the theory. The logic of scientific inference dictates that if the empirical data conform

Table 53-1
Fawcett's Criteria for Evaluation of Nursing Theories and Pertinent Questions

Criteria	Pertinent Questions
Significance	Are the metaparadigm concepts and propositions addressed by the theory explicit? Are the philosophical claims on which the theory is based explicit? Is the conceptual model from which the theory was derived explicit? Are the authors of antecedent knowledge from nursing and adjunctive disciplines acknowledged and are bibliographical citations given?
Internal Consistency	Are the context (philosophical claims and conceptual model) and the content (concepts and propositions) of the theory congruent? Do the concepts reflect semantic clarity and semantic consistency? Do the propositions reflect structural consistency?
Parsimony	Is the theory content stated clearly and concisely?
Testability: Grand Theories	Is the research methodology qualitative and inductive? Is the research methodology congruent with the philosophical claims and content of the grand theory? Will the data obtained from use of the research methodology represent sufficiently in-depth descriptions of one or more personal experience(s) to capture the essence of the grand theory?
Testability: Middle-Range Theories	Does the research methodology reflect the middle-range theory? Are the middle-range theory concepts observable through instruments that are appropriate empirical indicators of those concepts? Do the data analysis techniques permit measurement of the middle-range theory propositions?
Empirical Adequacy: Grand Theories	Are the findings from studies of descriptions of personal experiences congruent with the concepts and propositions of the grand theory?
Empirical Adequacy: Middle-Range Theories	Are theoretical assertions congruent with empirical evidence?
Pragmatic Adequacy	Are education and special skill training required before application of the theory in nursing practice? Has the theory been applied in the real world of nursing practice? Is it generally feasible to implement practice derived from the theory? Does the practitioner have the legal ability to implement and measure the effectiveness of theory-based nursing actions? Are the theory-based nursing actions compatible with expectations for nursing practice? Do the theory-based nursing actions lead to favorable outcomes? Is the application of theory-based nursing actions designed so that comparisons can be made between outcomes of use of the theory and outcomes in the same situation when the theory was not used? Are outcomes measured in terms of the problem-solving effectiveness of the theory?

NOTE: From Fawcett (2005 p. 447–448. Copyright 2005) by F. A. Davis. Adapted with permission.

to the theoretical assertions, it may be appropriate to tentatively accept the assertions as reasonable or adequate. Conversely, if the empirical data do not conform to the assertions, it is appropriate to conclude that the assertions are false. Evaluation of the empirical adequacy of a theory should take into consideration the potential for circular reasoning. More specifically, if data always are interpreted in light of a particular theory, it may be difficult to *see* results that are not in keeping with that theory. Indeed, if researchers constantly uncover, describe, and interpret data through the lens of a particular theory, the outcome may be limited to expansion of that theory and that theory alone (Ray, 1990). Therefore, unless alternative theories are considered when interpreting data or the data are critically examined for both their fit and nonfit with the theory, circular reasoning will occur and the theory will be uncritically perpetuated. Circular reasoning can be avoided if the data are carefully examined to determine the extent of their congruence with the concepts and propositions of the theory, as well as from the perspective of alternative theories (Platt, 1964). In other words, evaluation of a theory always should take alternative theories into account when interpreting data collected within the context of the theory in question.

It is unlikely that any one test of a theory will provide the definitive evidence needed to establish its empirical adequacy. Thus decisions about empirical adequacy should take the findings of all related studies into account. Meta-analysis and other formal procedures can be used to integrate the results of related studies. It is important to point out that a theory should not be regarded as the truth or an ideology that cannot be modified. Indeed, no theory should be considered final or absolute, because it is always possible that subsequent studies will yield different findings or that other theories will provide a better fit with the data. Thus the aim of evaluation of empirical adequacy is to determine the degree of confidence warranted by the best empirical evidence, rather than to determine the absolute truth of the theory. The outcome of evaluation of empirical adequacy is a judgment regarding the need to modify,

refine, or discard one or more concepts or propositions of the theory.

The extent to which a grand theory meets the criterion of empirical adequacy is determined by a continuation of the description of personal experiences approach discussed earlier in the section on testability of grand theories. The data used to determine the empirical adequacy of a grand theory may come from multiple personal experiences of an individual or similar personal experiences of several individuals. The extent to which a middle-range theory meets the criterion of empirical adequacy is determined by a continuation of the traditional empirical approach discussed earlier in the section on testability of middle-range theories. The questions to be asked when evaluating the empirical adequacy of grand and middle-range theories are listed in Table 53-1.

The criterion *of pragmatic adequacy* focuses on the utility of the theory for nursing practice. The extent to which a grand theory or a middle-range theory meets this criterion is determined by reviewing all descriptions of the use of the theory in practice. The pragmatic adequacy criterion requires that nurses have a full understanding of the content of the theory, as well as the interpersonal and psychomotor skills necessary to apply it (Magee, 1994). Although that may seem obvious, it is important to acknowledge the need for education and special skill training before theory application.

The pragmatic adequacy criterion also requires that the theory actually is used in the real world of nursing practice (Chinn & Kramer, 1995). In addition, the pragmatic adequacy criterion requires that the application of the theory-based nursing actions is generally feasible (Magee, 1994). Feasibility is determined by an evaluation of the availability of the human and material resources needed to establish the theory-based nursing actions as customary practice, including the time needed to learn and implement the protocols for nursing actions; the number, type, and expertise of personnel required for their implementation; and the cost of in-service education, salaries, equipment, and protocol-testing procedures. Moreover, the willingness of those who control financial resources to pay for the theory-based nursing actions, such as healthcare system administrators and third-party payers, must be determined. In sum, the nurse must be in a setting that is conducive to application of the theory and have the time and training necessary to apply it.

Furthermore, the pragmatic adequacy criterion requires the nurse to have the legal ability to control the application and to measure the effectiveness of the theory-based nursing actions. Such control may be problematic in that nurses are not always able to carry out legally sanctioned responsibilities because of resistance from others. Sources of resistance against implementation of theory-based nursing actions include attempts by physicians and healthcare system administrators to control nursing practice, financial barriers imposed by healthcare institutions and third-party payers, and skepticism by other health professionals about the ability of nurses to carry out the proposed actions (Funk, Tornquist, & Champagne, 1995). The cooperation and collaboration of others may, therefore, have to be secured.

Moreover, the pragmatic adequacy criterion requires that theory-based nursing actions be compatible with expectations for practice (Magee, 1994). Compatibility should be evaluated in relation to expectations held by the public and the healthcare system. If the actions do not meet existing expectations, they should be abandoned or people should be helped to develop new expectations. Johnson (1974) commented, "Current [nursing] practice is not entirely what it might become and [thus people] might come to expect a different form of practice, given the opportunity to experience it" (p. 376).

The pragmatic adequacy criterion also requires the theory-based nursing actions to be socially meaningful by leading to favorable outcomes for those who participate in the actions. Examples of favorable outcomes include a reduction in complications, improvement in health conditions, and increased satisfaction with the theory-based actions on the part of all who participate.

The outcomes of theory-based nursing actions are further judged by use of what Silva and Sorrell (1992) called the problem-solving approach. That approach emphasizes the problem-solving effectiveness of a theory and seeks to determine "whether what is purported or experienced accomplishes its purpose" (Silva & Sorrell, 1992, p. 19). The problem-solving approach is based on the position that theories are developed "to solve human and technical problems and to improve practice" (Kerlinger, 1979, p. 280). It requires deliberative application of a theory. Chinn and Kramer (1995) explained that the application "involves using research methods to demonstrate how a theory affects nursing practice and places the theory within the context of practice to ensure that it serves the goals of the profession . . . [and] provides evidence of the theory's usefulness in ensuring quality of care" (p. 164). The problem-solving approach can be used with all types of theories but is most effective when applied to middle-range predictive theories. In that case, the application seeks to determine the effects of interventions specified in middle-range predictive theories on the health conditions of the human beings who participate in the interventions (Hegyvary, 1992). The eight questions to be asked when evaluating pragmatic adequacy are given in Table 53-1. Two last two questions, which were adapted from requirements identified by Silva and Sorrell (1992), are asked when evaluating the problem-solving effectiveness of nursing theories.

REFERENCES

Barnum, B.J.S.(1998). *Nursing theory: Analysis, application, evaluation* (5th ed.). Philadelphia: Lippincott.

Chinn, P. L., & Kramer, M. K. (1995). *Theory and nursing. A systematic approach* (4th ed.). St. Louis, MO: Mosby.

Duffy, M., & Muhlenkamp, A. F. (1974). A framework for theory analysis. *Nursing Outlook, 22,* 570–574.

Fawcett, J. (1993). *Analysis and evaluation of nursing theories.* Philadelphia: F. A. Davis.

Fawcett, J. (1999). *The relationship of theory and research* (3rd ed). Philadelphia: F. A. Davis.

Fawcett, J. (2000). *Analysis and evaluation of contemporary nursing knowledge: Nursing models and theories.* Philadelphia: F. A. Davis.

Fawcett, J. (2005). *Contemporary nursing knowledge: Analysis and evaluation of nursing models and theories* (2nd ed.). Philadelphia: F. A. Davis.

Funk, S. G., Tornquist, E. M., & Champagne, M. T. (1995). Barriers and facilitators of research utilization. *Nursing Clinics of North America, 30,* 395–407.

George, J. B. (Ed.). (2002). *Nursing theories: The base for professional nursing practice* (5th ed.). Upper Saddle River, NJ: Prentice Hall.

Hegyvary, S. T. (1992). From truth to relativism: Paradigms for doctoral education. In *Proceedings of the 1992 forum on doctoral education in nursing* (pp. 1–15). Baltimore: University of Maryland School of Nursing.

Johnson, D. E. (1974). Development of theory: A requisite for nursing as a primary health profession. *Nursing Research, 23,* 372–377.

Kerlinger, F. N. (1979). *Behavioral research: A conceptual approach.* New York: Holt, Rinehart, & Winston.

King, I. M., & Fawcett, J. (Eds.). (1997). *The language of nursing theory and metatheory.* Indianapolis, IN: Sigma Theta Tau International Center Nursing Press.

Levine, M. E. (1988). Antecedents from adjunctive disciplines: Creation of nursing theory. *Nursing Science Quarterly, 1,* 16–21.

Magee, M. (1994). Eclecticism in nursing philosophy: Problem or solution? In J. F. Kikuchi & H. Simmons (Eds.), *Developing a philosophy of nursing* (pp. 61–66). Thousand Oaks, CA: Sage.

Marriner-Tomey, A., & Alligood, M. R. (2002). *Nursing theorists and their work* (5th ed.). St. Louis, MO: Mosby.

Marx, M. H. (1976). Formal theory. In M. H. Marx & F. E. Goodson (Eds.), *Theories in contemporary psychology(2nd* ed., pp. 234–260). New York: Macmillan.

Meleis, A. I. (1997). *Theoretical nursing: Development and progress* (3rd ed.). Philadelphia: Lippincott.

Parse, R. R. (1987). *Nursing science: Major paradigms, theories, and critiques.* Philadelphia: Saunders.

Platt, J. R. (1964). Strong inference. *Science, 146,* 347–353.

Ray, M. A. (1990). Critical reflective analysis of Parse's and Newman's research methodologies. *Nursing Science Quarterly, 3,* 44–46.

Silva, M. C. (1986). Research testing nursing theory: State of the art. *Advances in Nursing Science, 9*(1), 1–11.

Silva, M. C., & Sorrell, J. M. (1992). Testing of nursing theory: Critique and philosophical expansion. *Advances in Nursing Science, 14*(4), 12–23.

The Author Comments

Criteria for Evaluation of Theory

I developed a framework for analysis evaluation of nursing grand theories and middle-range theories that is a companion to my framework for analysis and evaluation of conceptual models of nursing. Both frameworks are published in my book, *Contemporary Nursing Knowledge: Analysis and Evaluation of Nursing Models and Theories (2nd ed.),* Philadelphia: F. A. Davis, 2005. I developed the theories framework in an attempt to distinguish theories from the more abstract conceptual models and to convey my belief that grand theories are not the same as conceptual models. The article reprinted here is part of a dialogue with Rosemarie Parse that we undertook in an attempt to clarify whether the same evaluation criteria could be used for theories based on qualitative data and those based on quantitative data. Although the evaluation criteria that I identified were intended for all theories, regardless of the type of data used, the dialogue led me to begin to think about the need for different criteria for theories based on different types of data; I have not yet reached any conclusions.

—Jacqueline Fawcett

Parse's Criteria for Evaluation of Theory With a Comparison of Fawcett's and Parse's Approaches

Rosemarie Rizzo Parse

I am pleased to share with Dr. Fawcett my criteria for evaluation of theory and a comparison of our work. First, I should clarify my position on middle-range theory, since it is in direct contrast to Dr. Fawcett's. The term middle-range theory is ubiquitous in the nursing literature without any substantive definition. Cody (1999) said that there is "a lack of clarity as to what constitutes middle-range" (p. 10). He raised this question: Are those "working in the middle range on myriad topics . . . really developing nursing science or merely elaborating the vast patchwork quilt of applied-science nursing" (Cody, 1999, p. 11)? Dr. Fawcett and I generally agree that nursing is a basic science with its own unique body of knowledge and that theory is defined as a set of concepts combined uniquely and written at an abstract level to describe, explain, or predict phenomena (Parse, 1997). My view is that propositional statements written at lower levels of abstraction, often called middle-range theories, are really hypotheses that can be tested only through quantitative research methods using appropriate instrumentation (Parse, 2000). Thus, my comments here do not address middle-range theories and are relevant only to theory as described above.

I set forth criteria for the evaluation of nursing theory in my 1987 book, *Nursing Science: Major Paradigms, Theories, and Critiques*. At that time, I developed a design for critical appraisal appropriate for all frameworks and theories, no matter how they are constructed. I have modified these ideas considerably to be consistent with my current thinking, but I still believe

From R. R. Parse, Nursing Science Quarterly *2005;18(2):135–137. Copyright © 2005 SAGE Publications.*
Reprinted with permission by SAGE Publications, Inc.

About the Author

ROSEMARIE RIZZO PARSE was born in Pittsburgh, PA. She is a graduate of Duquesne University in Pittsburgh, and received her master's and doctorate from the University of Pittsburgh. Dr. Parse is Distinguished Professor Emeritus, Loyola University Chicago, and Visiting Scholar and Consultant, New York University. She is founder and editor of *Nursing Science Quarterly,* and president of Discovery International, which sponsors international nursing theory conferences. Dr. Parse is also founder of the *Institute of Human Becoming,* where she teaches the ontological, epistemological, and methodological aspects of the human becoming school of thought, including classes on topics such as birthing-dying, suffering, and hope. She has authored many books on her theory and science including *Illuminations: The Human Becoming Theory in Practice and Research; The Human Becoming School of Thought: A Perspective for Nurses and other Health Professionals;* and *Qualitative Inquiry: The Path of Sciencing.* Additional information about Dr. Parse and human becoming can be found at: www.discoveryinternationalonline.com.

in the basic premise that criteria for evaluation of theory should be broad enough to accommodate all perspectives in the discipline. The two major areas of critical appraisal in my design are structure and process (Parse, 1987). Questions applicable to both areas are listed in Table 54-1.

Structure criteria refer to the physiognomy of the theory, that is, the historical evolution, foundational elements, and relational statements. *Historical evolution* refers to the details of the development of the theory including the philosophical and theoretical antecedents and the changes in the theory over time. *Foundational elements* refer to the philosophical assumptions underpinning the theory and the major concepts of the theory. These are written at an abstract level and are the theorist's beliefs about the phenomenon of concern to the discipline, the human-universe-health process. *Relational statements* refer to the principles that are created from the unique weaving of the concepts into descriptions of the human-universe-health process, and they also are written at an abstract level.

The process criteria encompass correspondence, coherence, and pragmatics (Parse, 1987). *Correspondence* refers to semantic integrity and simplicity. *Semantic integrity* is recognized by the consistency of meanings among the terms used to explain the human-universe-health process in the philosophical assumptions and in the definitions of the concepts and principles. Two

aspects of semantic integrity are substance and clarity (Parse, 1987). Substance refers to the durability of the meaning assigned to terms, the breadth of the descriptions, and the consistency in levels of discourse within and among the assumptions, concepts, and principles. Clarity refers to the distinctness and mutually exclusive nature of the definitions. *Simplicity* is recognized by the uncluttered abstract descriptions and economy of words used to explain the theory.

Coherence refers to syntax and aesthetics. *Syntax* is recognized by the precision with which ideas are presented, that is, the logical flow in organization and movement of the central ideas from philosophical assumptions to major concepts to principles. *Aesthetics* is recognized in the beauty of the presentation of the theory, that is, the symmetry and harmony present in the descriptions of the major concepts, principles, basic concepts, and the connection of these to the philosophical assumptions.

Pragmatics refers to effectiveness and heuristic potential. *Effectiveness* is recognized by the way the theory is used as a guide to research and practice. This is shown through publications and presentations of research findings and reports of projects related to practice. *Heuristic potential* refers to the possibilities for further inquiry arising from the contributions made through the use of the theory in research and practice. The potential is shown in the ways that the research

Table 54-1
Parse's Criteria for Evaluation of Theories and Pertinent Questions

Criteria	Pertinent Questions
Structure Criteria	
Historical evolution	How was the theory developed?
	What are the philosophical and theoretical antecedents to the theory?
	What changes have been made since the first publication of the theory?
Foundational elements	Are the philosophical assumptions explicitly stated?
	Are the major concepts explicitly stated?
	Do the philosophical assumptions and major concepts refer to the human-universe-health process?
	How is the human-universe-health process defined?
Relational statements	How are the philosophical assumptions reflected in the principles?
	How do the principles reflect the unique weaving of the basic concepts?
Process Criteria	
Correspondence	
Semantic integrity	Are the meanings of the terms that appear in the assumptions, the concepts, and the principles consistent?
	Does clarity prevail in the descriptions of the assumptions, concepts, and principles?
	Are consistent levels of discourse evident within and among the assumptions, concepts, and principles?
	Are the meanings of words consistent throughout the description of the theory?
	Do the principles interrelate concepts at the same abstract level of discourse to describe, explain, or predict about the human-universe-health process?
	With what paradigmatic perspective does the theory correspond?
Simplicity	Are the descriptions of the assumptions, concepts, and principles clearly written at an abstract level?
	Is the word usage economical?
Coherence	
Syntax	Is there a logical flow from the philosophical assumptions to major concepts to principles?
	Are the foundational elements presented precisely at the same level of discourse?
	Are the relational statements presented precisely at the same level of discourse?
Aesthetics	How is the beauty of the theory expressed?
	Is the theory structured symmetrically?
Pragmatics	
Effectiveness	How is the theory used as a guide for research?
	How is the theory used as a guide for practice?
	What publications and presentations have emanated from the research studies and practice projects?
Heuristic potential	What possibilities for further inquiry arise from the research findings of studies guided by the theory?
	How have the research findings from studies guided by the theory advanced nursing knowledge?
	What new knowledge surfaced from the research studies?
	What possibilities for different practice projects arise from the reports of projects guided by the theory?

findings advance knowledge and further develop the theory.

In comparing Fawcett's criteria for evaluation of theories with the criteria I set forth, it is clear that there are similarities and differences. Fawcett's criteria for significance, internal consistency, and parsimony are similar to my criteria for historical evolution, semantic integrity, simplicity, and syntax. The differences arise with Fawcett's criteria for testability, empirical adequacy, and pragmatic adequacy. The language used to describe these criteria is slanted toward validation of theory through quantitative research methods and evidence-based practice. Thus, theories grounded in philosophical assumptions that preclude use of quantitative research methods and predetermined outcomes as evidence for effective practice cannot be fairly evaluated with Fawcett criteria's (see Table 54-1 in Fawcett, 2005). These would include theories that describe the human-universe-health process as indivisible, unpredictable, and ever-changing. Parse's criteria (Table 54-1) are specified to include all perspectives of the human-universe-health process in the discipline of nursing.

I am grateful to have this opportunity to share my views on the evaluation of nursing theory in this column. A diversity of perspectives is essential for the advancement of knowledge of a discipline. This scholarly dialogue sparked by Dr. Fawcett's interest in clarification is one of many dialogues that contribute significantly to the advancement of nursing knowledge.

REFERENCES

Cody, W. K. (1999). Middle-range theories: Do they foster the development of nursing science? *Nursing Science Quarterly, 12*, 9–14.

Fawcett, J. (2005). Criteria for evaluation of theory. *Nursing Science Quarterly, 18*, 131–135.

Parse, R. R. (1987). *Nursing science: Major paradigms, theories, and critiques.* Philadelphia: Saunders.

Parse, R. R. (1997). The language of nursing knowledge: Saying what we mean. In I. M. King & J. Fawcett (Eds.), *The language of nursing theory and metatheory* (pp. 73–77). Indianapolis, IN: Sigma Theta Tau International Center Nursing Press.

Parse, R. R. (2000). Obfuscation: The persistent practice of misnaming. *Nursing Science Quarterly, 13*, 91–92.

The Author Comments

Parse's Criteria for Evaluation of Theory With a Comparison of Fawcett's and Parse's Approaches

The article was written to offer an alternative to the linear perspective apparent in the language used in the extant published works on the evaluation of nursing theory. The extant works exclude the theories grounded in philosophical perspectives that honor the human–universe process as indivisible, unpredictable, and ever-changing. The criteria set forth in the Parse article allow for the evaluation of theories from all perspectives of the human–universe process in the discipline of nursing.

—ROSEMARIE RIZZO PARSE

Ethics Inquiry

Ethics, like epistemology, metaphysics and logic, is a branch of philosophy. Ethical theory has existed since antiquity. Ethics is also a significant albeit underdeveloped area of theorizing in nursing and other professions. These chapters present various philosophical perspectives on ethics, particularly in reference to theorizing and nursing inquiry.

Ethics can become a potent area of inquiry for nursing. Following is a sample of some of the provocative questions raised in this unit.

Questions for Discussion

- Is there a 'nursing' ethics as distinct from ethics or bioethics?
- Is a particular perspective, unified or pluralistic, of ethics more useful in nursing knowledge development?
- How has postmodern thinking influenced views about nursing ethics?
- Should ethical theory be considered as important as empirically-based theory in developing nursing knowledge?

Ethics Inquiry

Questions for Discussion

CHAPTER 55

Integration of Nursing Theory and Nursing Ethics*

Michael Yeo

Nursing theory and nursing ethics are two main areas of inquiry in nursing scholarship today. Each addresses common themes and each, in its own way, speaks not only about but for nursing. In spite of this commonality there is remarkably little dialogue between them. Both theory and ethics shall benefit from increased integration.

Nursing today is a profession in flux and a profession profoundly self-critical and self-examining. This self-examination is primarily taking place in two proliferating areas of scholarship, nursing theory and nursing ethics. A rich dialogue exists within each of these areas but remarkably little communication occurs between them.

One important shared factor behind the rapid growth of scholarship both in nursing theory and nursing ethics is the ascending importance of professionalism in nursing. Although the rhetoric of professionalism has been around for some time—as early as 1900

Nightingale[1] was proclaiming that nursing had become a profession—developments in the 1950s marked a decisive turning point.[2,3] This is evidenced by increased emphasis on fundamental questions having to do with the education, role, and responsibility unique and proper to nursing. A more radical questioning has occurred about the nurse's role and responsibility in relation to patients, other health care professionals, and society in general. Both nursing theory and nursing

*This article was supported by a grant from Associated Medical Services and the Richard and Jean Ivey Fund.

From M. Yeo, Integration of nursing theory and nursing ethics. Advances in Nursing Science, 11(3), 33–42. Copyright © 1989. Reproduced with permission of Lippincott Williams & Wilkins.

about patient autonomy. Given the considerable advocacy movement in nursing, this is quite remarkable. It is, however, understandable, given Roy's scientific orientation. When the person is defined as an adaptive system (a definition mainly fleshed out in physiologic terms) there is not much room for autonomy (or for the person to be humanistically understood). Roy may be an extreme example, but it is generally true that questions having to do with autonomy and paternalism, questions that reach to the core of the nursing profession, are seldom tackled directly by nursing theorists.

Nursing theory is rife with value dimensions—only a few have been touched here—but too often these are not brought to the fore and made the theme of analysis. There is a tendency for nursing theory to obscure its own operative norms. Typically, theorists present their work as if it were merely descriptive (science is not supposed to be normative), as if they were merely stating what nursing is. In fact, all of them, directly or indirectly, are also taking a stand on what nursing should be, and offering recommendations for the future direction of the profession—recommendations that cannot be evaluated on scientific grounds alone.

Thus, it is conceptually muddled and highly misleading to divide nursing theories into those that are valuational (normative) and those that are descriptive (scientific) as does Walker,[13] positing different standards of evaluation for each. All nursing theories, however scientific, are in some considerable measure normative or valuational, although some more self-consciously than others. They are structurally cemented with values throughout. The key definitions of nursing theory—human beings, nurse, health, environment (society)—are thickly laden with value. Disputes about them, for the most part, are not of a sort that science alone can be expected to resolve. As Gadow writes, "the very definition of nursing is an ethical problem—moreover the most fundamental and pressing ethical problem facing nursing today."[14(p93)]

One should not have to decipher the ethical face of a nursing theory behind the mask of science. The values dimension of nursing theories should be brought more out into the open and tackled more directly.

Ethical issues should be identified as such and confronted head on. Here nursing theorists would stand to benefit from increased dialogue with those working in nursing ethics, who have taken as their focus the values dimension of nursing. This dimension has been somewhat obscured in nursing theory owing to the value it places on science, or perhaps even on a narrow view of science, it being an open question whether other views of science might not be more congruent with ethical interests.

Evaluation of Nursing Theories

The potential for overenthusiasm about science to eclipse ethical considerations in nursing theory is even more evident at the level of theory evaluation. To pick a somewhat early example, King,[15] placing a great deal of value on the scientificity of nursing theories, lists ten criteria for theory evaluation, none of which explicitly addresses the ethical dimension of nursing theories. Theory evaluation has become much more sophisticated since then, but the scientific paradigm (and frequently a very narrow interpretation of it) continues to dominate at the expense of sensitivity to ethical dimensions of nursing theory.

Parse,[16] a theorist who is more explicit about values than most, nevertheless sacrifices ethical concerns at the altar of science when it comes to speaking about theory evaluation. Following Kaplan,[17] she distinguishes between structure and process criteria for evaluation. Value considerations are implicit in the detailed analysis she gives of these criteria, but nowhere are they explicitly stated. This omission is telling, but all the more so given that she deems esthetic criteria significant enough to warrant special reference.[16] Surely if esthetics is worthy of honorable mention, ethics is all the more so, especially given nursing's traditional sensitivity to ethical matters.

Even Chinn and Jacobs,[18] who are otherwise refreshingly open-eyed about the limitations of the scientific ideal, do not escape its allure when it comes to theory evaluation. They are certainly to be lauded for acknowledging that there are other patterns of knowing besides the scientific one, and for assigning a legitimate place to moral knowledge or ethics in nursing as distinct from empirics. They call for the "integration of all patterns."[18(p17)] of knowing, and this *holistic* ideal approximates what this article advocates. Furthermore, they point out that "the assumptions and purposes of scientific theory form the template against which nursing theories have been judged, although many traits of theories in general and nursing theories in particular both draw on and reflect other patterns of knowing besides empirics."[18(p7)] Nevertheless, when it comes to presenting their criteria for evaluation, the guidelines they offer, although broader than many, remain dominated by the scientific ideal and concentrated on empirics. They list clarity, simplicity, generality, empirical applicability, and consequences (more or less a rehash of the familiar scientific standards), and neglect to include an evaluative category addressing the values dimension of theory in a direct manner.[18] Presumably, the value assumptions of nursing theory with respect to such matters as patient autonomy, nursing autonomy, advocacy, and so on, do not count. If, as the authors state, the integration of the various patterns of knowledge is desirable, what better place to start than in the evaluation of nursing theory?

Nursing theorists and those writing about nursing theory evaluation need to become more reflective about the fact that evaluation is valuation. More scrutiny needs to be given to the various elements that are valued and why this is so. Why are ethical (value) considerations typically overlooked or even excluded in theory evaluation? Why should simplicity be valued or evaluated while something like the moral basis of the theory is not valued at all? Could it be that, dazzled by the allure of science and obsessed with being scientific, evaluators have been somewhat blinded to questions of ethics and values?

Relevance of Nursing Theory to Nursing Ethics

If nursing theory stands to benefit from the kind of questioning that takes place in nursing ethics, so too nursing ethics stands to benefit from the not inconsiderable achievements of nursing theory. Just as nursing theorists have sought to carve an identity for nursing distinct from the medical model, there is also growing concern to develop nursing ethics as a unique field of enquiry, and something "more than a footnote to medical ethics,"[19(p72)] as Yarling and McElmurry have put it:

> Nursing theorists and those writing about nursing theory evaluation need to become more reflective about the fact that evaluation is valuation.

Nursing ethics today is reaching to find its own voice, an endeavor in which nursing theory, even if overly concerned about sounding scientific, is qualified to furnish some guidance. Gadow comments that in framing ethical problems, "nursing regrettably has retained medicine as its referent in an area of concern where nurses most need to engage in independent, critically reflective self-examination."[14(p92)] Gadow's remark should be qualified, since it would not apply to everyone working in nursing ethics, but overall her characterization of the state of affairs is insightful. The general tendency has been to adopt a ready-made ethics and bring it to bear on the nursing profession.

Scholarship in nursing ethics can be divided roughly into two streams, each borrowing its conceptual paradigm from a different source. On the one side, the ethical theory approach borrows heavily from moral philosophy. On the other the moral development approach borrows heavily from developmental psychology.

The Ethical Theory Approach

What James and Dickoff[20] have claimed about Beckstrand[21] could be applied to the ethical theory approach. They charge that "Beckstrand takes some selected version of what is ethics,"[20(p58)] as being authoritative, seemingly unaware that ethics is itself a contentious discipline, embracing a broad diversity of often conflicting opinions. To be sure, nursing ethicists do acknowledge some diversity. Almost everyone makes the standard distinction between deontologic and teleologic theories. However, the scope of this diversity is narrowly circumscribed.

Nursing ethics primarily borrows its framework for ordering ethical theories from medical ethics. By itself, this would not be so significant were it not that medical ethics has been very selective in circumscribing the discipline of ethics. The focus is placed almost exclusively on Kant and Mill, while other legitimate contenders are buried in the background. A list of neglected or even excluded voices would include names like Aristotle, Plato, Spinoza, Kierkegaard, and Nietzsche, all of whom wrote substantial works in ethics. Why has nursing ethics uncritically subscribed to the same canon as medical ethics? How different might the ethical landscape of nursing appear if existentialism, for example, enjoyed the same privilege accorded to utilitarianism in the nursing ethics literature?

Nursing ethics has borrowed from medical ethics not only its list of canonical authors, but also certain ways of relating to ethical issues. What White[22] calls formula ethics is a case in point. Formula ethics "involves applying ethical theories to specific situations and suggesting, for instance, what the contractarian versus the utilitarian position might be."[22(p42)] Carroll and Humphrey's[23] *Moral Problems in Nursing* is typical: "I feel I used Kant's theory when I refused to call the police and have Ms B committed for I was respecting her autonomy."[23(p82)] It is a mistake to think that Kant's theory can be used like a cookie cutter to shape the moral situation of nursing into tidy resolutions. Moreover, if one has to derive one's respect for autonomy from an ethical theory, one is in deep trouble. Nurses have practiced respect for autonomy long before Kant was brought into the hospital setting.

Formula ethics is misguided for several reasons, and not least of all because it simplifies ethical positions almost to the point of caricature. More importantly, however, it reduces ethical practice to correct technique, and promotes an overly mechanical (and therefore insensitive) comportment to ethical problems. The moral situation of nursing is squeezed into imported categories that are applied in a top-down fashion. The danger is that the experience of nursing will be distorted or otherwise denied.

While it would be folly to ignore the rich untapped resources of ethical theory, it is important to be critical in bringing them to bear on the moral situation of nurs-ing. Those working in nursing ethics are becoming increasingly critical of the ethical theory approach. There is a growing desire for an ethic that issues from nursing itself, rather than one borrowed from elsewhere and applied from the top down. Bishop and Scudder exemplify this in urging that nursing ethics should begin "with the moral sense of nursing rather than with ethical theory."[24(p42)] This sentiment is echoed by Packard and Ferrara, who maintain that "the moral foundation of nursing will have to derive from bold excursions into the meaning of nursing."[25(p63)] What does it mean to speak of the "meaning of nursing," however? Where would one look to find such a thing?

Nursing theory would be a good place to start. If nursing ethics must borrow, why not borrow from the rich tradition of nursing theory, which at least has the advantage over ethical theory of being derived from nursing experience? Nursing theory could play an important role in a bottom-up approach to nursing ethics. It offers an alternative made-in-nursing framework (or rather several) in which to think about humans, health, environment, society, and the meaning of nursing. Nursing theory tackles these fundamentals at the very outset, whereas nursing ethics has tended to be somewhat more narrow in its focus. The tendency has been to focus on cases, which are analyzed along the traditional lines of autonomy, paternalism, and beneficence. Nursing theory can teach nursing ethics to think more profoundly about the meaning of nursing and help to broaden the frame of reference in which ethical questions are being examined. It may be illuminating in ways hardly imaginable to rethink the stock ethical terms—autonomy, justice, beneficence—in light of nursing theory.

The Moral Development Approach

The moral development approach in nursing ethics differs from the ethical theory approach by being more empirical. It looks at the moral situation of nursing with an eye to how nurses actually respond to ethical issues, and analyzes the moral behavior of nurses in light of models of moral development. At one level, one could contrast the ethical theory approach to the moral development approach as the normative to the descriptive, but this would be misleading. Models of moral development are not value neutral, and norms come into play in describing moral behavior in the framework of a given model.

> The moral development approach in nursing ethics shares with the ethical theory approach the habit of borrowing uncritically.

The moral development approach in nursing ethics shares with the ethical theory approach the habit of borrowing uncritically. In particular, the work of Kohlberg[26] has exerted a profound influence on research on the moral development of nurses. Ketefian[27–31] has been a major catalyst in this area. Without negating the value of her work, it is fair to say that she has not been very critical in her acceptance of the paradigm for moral development laid out by Kohlberg. For the most part, she has accepted it as being authoritative without interrogating its fundamental norms. This is ironic, since the model's overarching norm is autonomy, which calls for such interrogation. Kohlberg has always had his detractors, but recent work by Gilligan[32] has cast his model in a critical light that is particularly illuminating for nursing. Gilligan found that, as a group, women score differently than men on Kohlberg's moral development scale. If one accepted Kohlberg's value premises, one would have to say that women score lower than men. Gilligan's innovation was to interpret this difference in a positive way. Rather than accepting the norms supporting Kohlberg's scale and interpreting this difference as deficiency, she made a virtue of it, and used it to call into question the fundamental values of Kohlberg's theory. Women do indeed define moral issues differently, but this difference is not a minus. Gilligan calls this difference the ethic of care, which is different from, but not subordinate to, the ethic of justice presupposed as norm in Kohlberg's theory. She celebrates the ethic of care as being the different voice of women.[32] Interestingly, Gilligan's work converges with that of James and Dickoff,[20] who, inspired by the French feminist Helene Cixous,[33] advanced a new ethic for nursing based on reciprocal nurturance.

The moral lesson to be drawn from Gilligan's critique of Kohlberg is a profound one: rather than trying to speak the language that happens to be authoritative, one should learn to speak unashamedly in one's own voice and to celebrate one's difference rather than apologize for it. This lesson has special relevance for nursing. Applying Gilligan's work to nursing, Huggins and Scalzi write, "If an ethical base for nursing practice is built on the ethics of justice, and the nurse's orientation is the ethic of care of another model, there will continue to be a denial of the nurse's own voice."[34(p46)] Uncritical borrowing can lead to the denial of the unique experience of nursing and to the disvaluation of the ethic of care to which Gilligan,[32] turning Kohlberg upside down, assigns a positive evaluation.

Directing their concerns specifically to Ketefian,[27–31] Huggins and Scalzi caution, "A theory of ethical practice, as is sought by Ketefian, is essential to the maturation of the nursing profession, but it must be carefully built to speak to the true voice and experience of nursing."[34(p44)] This is a very important point, but it raises a difficult question: What is the true voice and experience of nursing? Perhaps there is no one true voice, but there are several voices, the voices of nursing theorists speaking about the experience of nursing. Anyone undertaking to develop an ethic for nursing based on the experience of nursing would do well to begin by listening carefully to those voices.

Nursing theory and nursing ethics speak about and for nursing, an onerous challenge and responsibility for a profession so self-conscious and self-examining. Each, in its own way, is searching to find its own voice. To this end, would it not be desirable for each to broaden the parameters of its conversation and listen to the voice of the other? Only by joining together can the voices of nursing theory and nursing ethics hope to lay legitimate claim to be the voice of nursing.

REFERENCES

1. Nightingale, F., cited in Palmer IS.: From whence we came, in Chaska NL. (ed): The *Nursing Profession: A Time to Speak.* New York, McGraw-Hill, 1983.
2. Crowley, D. M.: Perspectives of pure science. Nurs Res 1968;17:497–499.

3. Aydelotte M. K.: Issues of professional nursing: The need for clinical excellence. *Nurs Forum* 1968;7(1):73675.

4. Conway, M. E.: Prescription for professionalization, in Chaska NL (ed): *The Nursing Profession: A Time to Speak.* New York, McGraw-Hill, 1983.

5. Greenwood, E.: Attributes of a profession, in Baumrin B., Freedman B. (eds): *Moral Responsibility and the Professions.* New York, Haven, 1983.

6. Roy, C.: Introduction to Nursing: An Adaptation Model, ed. 2. Englewood Cliffs, NJ, Prentice-Hall, 1984.

7. Muyskens, J. L. *Moral Problems in Nursing: A Philosophical Investigation.* Totowa, NJ, Rowman and Littlefield, 1982.

8. Meleis, A. I.: *Theoretical Nursing: Development and Progress.* New York, Lippincott, 1985.

9. Watson, J.: Nursing's scientific quest. *Nurs Outlook* 1981;29: 413–416.

10. Johnson, D. E.: The nature of a science of nursing. *Nurs Outlook* 1959;7:291–294.

11. Tucker, R. W.: The value decisions we know as science. *Adv Nurs Sci* 1979;1(2):1–12.

12. Roy, C., Roberts, S. L.: *Theory Construction in Nursing: An Adaptation Model.* Englewood Cliffs, NJ, Prentice-Hall, 1981.

13. Walker, L. O.: Theory and research in the development of nursing as a discipline: Retrospect and prospect, in Chaska, N. L. (ed): *The Nursing Profession: A Time to Speak.* New York, McGraw-Hill, 1983.

14. Gadow, S.: ANS open forum. *Adv Nurs Sci* 1979;1(3):92–95.

15. King, I.: *Toward a Theory for Nursing: General Concepts of Human Behaviour.* New York, Wiley, 1971.

16. Parse, R. R.: Paradigms and theories, in Parse, R. R. (ed): *Nursing Science: Major Paradigms, Theories and Critiques.* Philadelphia, Saunders, 1987.

17. Kaplan, A.: *The Conduct of Scientific Inquiry.* Scranton, Penn, Chandlisher, 1964.

18. Chinn, P. L., Jacobs, M. K.: *Theory and Nursing: A systematic Approach,* St. Louis, Mosby, 1983.

19. Yarling, R. R., McElmurry, B. J.: The moral foundation of nursing. *Adv Nurs Sci* 1986;8(2):63–73.

20. James, P., Dickoff, J.: Toward a cultivated but decisive pluralism for nursing, in McGee (ed): *Theoretical Pluralism in Nursing.* Ottawa, University of Ottawa Press, 1982.

21. Beckstrand, J.: The notion of practise theory and the relationship of scientific and ethical knowledge to practise. *Res Nurs Health* 1978;1(3):131–136.

22. White, G. B.: Philosophical ethics and nursing—a word of caution, in Chinn, P. L. (ed): *Advances in Nursing Theory and Development.* Rockville, Md, Aspen, 1983.

23. Carroll, M. A., Humphrey, R. A.: *Moral Problems in Nursing: Case Studies.* Washington, University Press of America, 1979.

24. Bishop, A. H., Scudder, J. R.: Nursing ethics in an age of controversy. *Adv Nurs Sci* 1987;9(3):34–43.

25. Packard, J. S., Ferrara, M. S. N.: In search of the moral foundation of nursing. *Adv Nurs Sci* 1988;10(4):60–71.

26. Kohlberg, L.: The cognitive developmental approach to moral education, in Scharf, P. (ed): *Readings on Moral Education.* Minneapolis, Minn: Winston Press, 1978.

27. Ketefian, S.: Critical thinking, educational preparation, and development of moral judgment among selected groups of practising nurses. *Nurs Res* 1981;30:98–103.

28. Ketefian, S.: Moral reasoning and moral behavior among selected groups of practising nurses. *Nurs Res* 1981;30: 171–176.

29. Ketefian, S.: Tool development in nursing: Construction of a scale to measure moral behavior. *J NY State Nurs Assoc* 1982;13: 13–18.

30. Ketefian, S.: Professional and bureaucratic role conceptions and moral behavior in nursing. *Nurs Res* 1985;34:248–253.

31. Ketefian, S.: A case study of theory development: Moral behavior in nursing. *Adv Nurs Sci* 1987;9(2):10–19.

32. Gilligan, C.: *In a Different Voice: Psychological Theory and Women's Development.* Cambridge, Harvard University Press, 1982.

33. Marks, E., de Courtivron, I. (eds): *New French Feminisms, an Anthology.* New York, Schocken Press, 1981.

34. Huggins, E. A., Scalzi, C. C.: Limitations and alternatives: Ethical practice theory in nursing. *Adv Nurs Sci* 1988;10(4):43–47.

The Author Comments

Integration of Nursing Theory and Nursing Ethics

Professor Marguerite Warner, who was then on the Faculty of Nursing at the University of Western Ontario, first introduced me to nursing theory. Her passion for the subject was infectious, and I learned much from her (and miss our conversations). As I worked through the nursing theory literature, I was struck by what I believed to be an uncritical and unwise deference to science and lack of attention to ethics, which was surprising to me, given nursing's rich tradition of ethical reflection. I believe that nursing theory should be grounded primarily not in science but in ethics. The articulation of this viewpoint in this article is my modest contribution to dialogue in and about nursing theory.

—MICHAEL YEO

CHAPTER 56

Nursing Theorizing as an Ethical Endeavor

Pamela G. Reed

This article addresses the ethical dimensions of nursing theorizing. Nursing theorizing, whether it occurs primarily at the outset or emerges during the process of inquiry, is inescapably linked to the theorist's value choices and beliefs about human beings, the environment, and health. These choices are reflected in the conceptual frame of one's research. The normative commitment of the conceptual frame is explored using examples from nursing and nonnursing research. Elements of critical ethical reflection are outlined. It is suggested that the discipline's understanding of what constitutes health and how best to promote health, as well as solutions to ethical dilemmas posed by research, may be enhanced by purposeful ethical inquiry that occurs as an integral component of theorizing activities.

Nurses and other scientists who are embracing the post-positivist tradition in science recognize the historical evolution of knowledge: that knowledge is not absolute but changes in interaction with the culture as a whole and with the scientists, theologians, practitioners, philosophers, and others who contribute to perceptions of truth. There is no one truth about the pathway to health that allows theorists, once it is discovered and described, to sit back, content in knowing that they had laid out the facts and cannot be held accountable for the consequences of their theories. No one dominant paradigm exists as a guide for nursing inquiry in the selection of the right worldview, the right perspective on human health and nursing, the right questions and goals, the right method, or the right answers. Instead, development of nursing knowledge seems to be flourishing in what

About the Author

PAMELA G. REED is Professor at the University of Arizona College of Nursing in Tucson, Arizona, where she also served as Associate Dean for Academic Affairs for 7 years. She is a three-time graduate of Wayne State University in Detroit, receiving a BSN in 1974, an MSN in 1976 (with a double major in child–adolescent psychiatric mental health nursing and teaching), and her PhD, with a major in nursing, (focused on life-span development and aging) in 1982. Dr. Reed pioneered research into spirituality and well-being with her doctoral research with terminally ill patients. She also developed a theory of self-transcendence and two widely used research instruments, the *Spiritual Perspective Scale* and the *Self-Transcendence Scale*. Her publications and funded research reflect a dual scholarly focus: spirituality and other facilitators of well-being and decisions in end-of-life transitions, and nursing metatheory and knowledge development. Dr. Reed also enjoys time with her family, reading, classical music, swimming, and hiking in the mountains and canyons of Arizona.

Laudan (1984) described as a "dissensus" rather than consensus among nursing paradigms. Philosophical aims of nursing are changing toward a focus on "continuing a conversation rather than discovering truth" (Rorty, 1979, p. 373).

The nature of the discipline of nursing is such that the ethical implications of nursing science in general and the ethical implications of the selected conceptual perspective of the individual's research in particular are enormous. This is so not only because the consequences of nursing conceptualizations are intimately linked to promotion of a good of society—health—but also because of the shifting axiology of the discipline. Criteria for what characterizes essential knowledge and for making value choices and judgments in conceptualizing the phenomena of nursing vary across extant nursing paradigms. The indeterminate nature of nursing phenomena is such that these criteria may never, and perhaps should never, be definitively described. Nevertheless, the "assumptions, value choices, and judgments" (Chinn & Jacobs, 1987, p. 80) on which theory is based are ultimately translated into nursing knowledge for actions that directly affect human health. According to Bellah, "what [our theories] say human beings [and health] fundamentally are has inevitable implications about what they ought to be" (Bellah, 1981, p. 15).

Nursing theorizing, then, is an ethical endeavor. Theorizing refers here to the reasoning processes involved in constructing what Kaplan (1964) has termed the "conceptual frame," or the framework or theory in scientific inquiry. Choices made in theory have ethical consequences in practice. In addition, the act of theorizing alone constitutes a "moral situation" (Dewey, 1948) in that it entails reflective choice and deliberate consideration of what may be better or worse. Thus, both the purpose of nursing inquiry and the nature of the phenomena studied render nursing theorizing its ethical dimension.

Nursing theorizing, whether it occurs at the outset or emerges during the process of inquiry, is inescapably linked to the theorist's value choices and beliefs about human beings, the environment, and health. The message in Nietzsche's "dogma of immaculate perception" (Nietzsche, 1966) extends to qualitative and quantitative methodologies alike. No observation is free from conceptual contamination; observation is already cognition, valuing, and believing (Kaplan, 1965). More precisely, there is no such thing as immaculate conceptualization in theorizing. Regardless of the methodology by which theories are advanced, theorizing likely entails value choices made by the nursing theorist or researcher that ultimately influence the good of society. Kaplan's thesis "that not all value concerns are unscientific, that indeed some of them are called for by the scientific enterprise itself" (Kaplan, 1965, p. 373) is an understatement for nursing science where value-laden terms such as health are the prime focus of inquiry.

The Normative Commitment of the Conceptual Frame

All phases of scientific inquiry in nursing are embedded in "normative commitments" (Bellah, 1981). Deontological judgments of moral value and obligation occur in nursing theorizing, evidenced for example in the theorist's speculations about what may be good for health or well-being, why it may be good, and what ought to be done to promote that good. The distinction between cognitive and normative knowledge is hazy at best and, because of this, ethical inquiry must accompany inquiry into human processes (Bellah, 1981).

Critical ethical reflection is important not only in the testing and application of knowledge, but also in the conceptualization of knowledge. Ethical knowing has been put forth as an essential component of nursing knowledge (Carper, 1978) and fundamental to the development of theory (Chinn & Jacobs, 1987). However, the ethical dimension of selecting or developing a conceptual frame for research has been addressed in the literature by only a few, such as Archbold (1987) or mentioned only in passing (White, 1983).

Ethical issues continues to be addressed in nursing research most characteristically in reference to methodology (Connors, 1988; Moccia, 1988; Munhall, 1988), but also in reference to health care policy (Hinshaw, 1988) and allocation of resources for research (Fowler, 1987). Conspicuous references to the ethical aspects of research methodology and overall purpose of research are found in the American Nurses' Association's *Code of Ethics* (ANA, 1985) and *Human Rights Guidelines* (ANA, 1984). However, selection of a research strategy, generally recognized as a value-laden decision, is often so because the conceptual frame out of which this decision flows is value laden. Careful attention to the values and assumptions operant in the conceptual perspective of a study could facilitate solutions to ethical dilemmas encountered at other points in the research process. Ethical inquiry into the components of an individual's conceptual frame, as prerequisite to the ethical inquiry into the methodology suggested by Munhall (1988) and others, could further

enhance the likelihood that the means and ends of research will be morally justified.

The ethical responsibilities associated with scientific knowledge cannot be relegated entirely to the implementors of the research design nor to those who translate the findings in clinical practice. Normative commitments are made in the earliest efforts in theorizing. Dewey (1928) rejected the positivist, continental European image of the scientist as one whose dedication to reason and truth sets him or her apart from the ethical concerns related to the products of science. Dewey denied any dualism between scientific and moral thinking and proclaimed that scientific activity is inherently moralistic in its concern with understanding natural processes and their relationship to the welfare of humankind.

Laudan's (1977, 1981) historicist view on scientific progress reinforces the normative commitment of the conceptual frame in research. Scientific progress is evaluated, according to Laudan, in terms of the problem-solving effectiveness of the discipline's theories. A major problem of interest in nursing is the facilitation of health as a good of society. The nature of nursing is such that, if nurses are to contribute to the scientific progress of their discipline, their theorizing must incorporate a moral dimension that includes logical reasoning and creative reflection on what may be considered good or best vis-à-vis the health of individuals and groups. If nursing theories are to have problem-solving effectiveness, clarification of an individual's ontology, values, and goals must occur not only in reference to implementing the research design as pointed out by Moccia (1988), but also in reference to the act of conceptualizing.

Value-based choices about the sorts of conceptualizations or theories invoked in research influence decisions regarding the problems deemed worthy of study, the perceived societal benefits, definition and measurement of concepts, the types of participant risks worth taking, acceptable threats to internal and external validity, the interpretation and significance of the findings, and most importantly the knowledge offered for use in effecting health in human beings. It is not inconceivable that the conceptual nets (Popper, 1968) cast out by scientists could be used for catching fish only for their liking and not necessarily for the good of society.

So powerful is the conceptual frame of a study that Kaplan (1964) noted one could more easily dispense with the physical operations of a study than with the framework that gives meaning to all of the research activities. The same methodology can constitute a different study and result in different outcomes if the conceptual framework changes. Secondary analysis is an example of this. Moreover, Laudan (1981) explained that changes in scientific knowledge occur more often due to conceptual issues rather than questions of empirical support.

Ethical Implications of Selected Conceptual Frameworks

The ethical implications of theorizing can be illustrated in examples from nursing and nonnursing literature. In the nonnursing literature, examples of the ethical significance of conceptual frameworks can be found in classic studies of human development. Human development, like health, is a value-laden concept and not easily defined. Personal biases have entered into conceptualizations of development with moral consequences.

Developmental Psychology Literature

The late 17th-century conceptualization of the tabula rasa view of people held moral implications related to the potential for human development and well-being. Neither the environment nor the person was perceived as having an active role in development. The infant, in particular, was viewed as insignificant in terms of his or her value in effecting change in the environment; infants were perceived as ineffectual, empty vessels waiting to be filled with information. Research hypotheses derived from this conceptual stance were directed toward the study of maturity in terms of the acquisition of a quantity of information using the adult white male as the standard. This framework limited the scope of study about sources of human potential and ways in which development could be enhanced from early life onward. Primary intervention for the emotional development of infants, for example, was unheard of, since the infant was not conceptualized as a unique and dynamic being.

The nature vs. nurture controversy was brought to public scrutiny with Jensen's (1973) well-known conclusions about genetically based racial differences in intelligence. Jensen was proclaimed as having hoodwinked large segments of government and society into believing that IQ was genetically based, and as having an oppressive effect on disadvantaged, primarily black individuals (Jensen, 1973; Kamin, 1974). The ethical implications of Jensen's work relate to provision of educational opportunities, hiring practices, and to the self-concept and self-expectations of certain ethnic groups. The debate about the heritability of intelligence continues to be fueled by contrasting views about the development of intelligence, particularly by conceptual frameworks such as Jensen's, which dichotomize the contributions of heredity and environment in development and do not account for the possibility of interaction between the two factors.

The decrement model of human aging provides an example of the influences that a conceptual frame may have on human welfare. This model was most popular 15 years ago, although its influences can still be felt today. The decrement model emphasized quantitative biological changes that occur with age, such as cardiovascular and perceptual losses (Botwinick, 1973; Horn, 1976). These losses were generalized to the overall process of aging; regression of capabilities was regarded as a normal process. Young adulthood marked the time of maximal level of development, after which linear and irreversible decrement occurred.

Aging was conceptualized as a first in, last out process, whereby the most recent and complex abilities are lost first and the earliest and simplest are retained (Labouvie-Vief & Schell, 1983). The older adult was conceived of as becoming more childlike with development. In addition, the environmental context was not valued as significant in the process of aging. Research based on this model focused solely on ontogenetic rather than contextual factors in development (Labouvie-Vief, 1977). Thus, for example, plasticity, the ability to learn from the environment (now recognized as a characteristic ability of the elderly), was not identified as an issue of aging worthy of study.

The decrement model, in which developmental changes were conceptualized primarily as losses rather than as adaptive or progressive, did little to facilitate means to improve health care, educational programs, and career opportunities of the elderly, not to mention promotion of self-esteem among older adults and a basic societal value for the elderly persons. Research efforts guided by this conceptual frame and directed toward its support could be regarded as unethical, particularly in view of the theorizing and scientific evidence to the contrary that were emerging at the time (Baltes & Baltes, 1977; Labouvie-Vief, 1980; Schaie, 1973).

Nursing Literature

Examples of ethical issues in theorizing exist in current nursing literature, although perhaps they are not yet viewed as being as dramatic as the historical accounts from the developmental psychology literature. A research report on social support by Ellison (1985) increases awareness of the potential dangers in conceptualizing social support as a purely positive phenomenon. Her findings suggest that social support is most health promotive only during certain phases of the lifespan and that social support in other developmental phases may be detrimental to individuals. Personal biases about the desirability of social support that enter the research framework unchecked can have costly effects on well-being when applied in clinical practice.

Boyd's (1985) analysis of the concept of "identification" demonstrates the different meanings the term acquires within various theoretical frameworks. A key point presented was that identification in the parent-child relationship typically has been conceptualized as a one-way, time-limited process in which the child is influenced by the parent. This view contrasts sharply with the mutually interactive and dynamic view of interpersonal relationships depicted in some nursing conceptual frameworks. Research and intervention approaches stemming from a one-sided framework have neglected the potential influence of the child on the parent, including influences on fulfillment of the parental role and the parent's well-being as parent and as a human being.

Narayan and Joslin's (1980) critique of the medical conceptual model of human crisis and their proposal of a nursing model of crisis illustrate the striking difference that a conceptual perspective could make in terms of clinical intervention. In one model, pathogenic risks of crisis are emphasized and a return to the precrisis level of functioning is the treatment goal; in the other model, opportunities for growth enhancement are emphasized and treatment goals acknowledge the human potential for change and further development. Because the definitions of health and goals for intervention differ markedly between the medical and nursing models, it is likely that different outcomes in the client's health and well-being would occur as well. Explicating a conceptual framework of crisis is an ethical endeavor, requiring reflection on one's beliefs about human potential, the level of functioning of which the client is perceived capable, and the ideals the clinician may envision for the client.

There are many nursing phenomena that, when conceptualized for research, stimulate if not demand ethical reflection by the theorist. Personal biases and assumptions about emotional illness, adolescent development, and female sexuality, for example, which typically elicit presumptive notions about the value of time, independence, and other assumed goods, can have moral influences on the types of conceptualizations constructed in the study of these phenomena as they relate to health.

Ethical Reflection— Response to a Calling

In the spirit of Nightingale's ideas, Kaplan stated that science is a "calling" and "cannot flourish if it is always an occupation only" (Kaplan, 1964, p. 379). He explains further that, while one chooses an occupation, a calling chooses the individual and commits him or her to the professional ethic of science—values that guide the conduct of inquiry. The professional ethic of scientific inquiry extends beyond basic moral principles such as beneficence, nonmaleficence, and justice. This ethic is also evident in theorizing about nursing phenomena in a manner unwavered by "habit, by tradition, by the Academy, or by the powers that be" (Kaplan, 1964, p. 380). Normative commitments made in theorizing must not be limited by traditions that exist, either in practice or theory, in hospitals or schools of nursing. The potential for human health is not static, but is ever expanding. Ideas put forth in the conceptual frame must not compromise or constrain this human potential.

Theorists are morally obligated to deliberately examine their motives and values as reflected in their conceptualizations about health and health-related issues. Propositions implicit and explicit to the conceptual frame should be judged not only in reference to what they state but also in reference to what they make more likely (Kaplan, 1964).

Ethical inquiry into one's conceptual frame requires examination of both intrapersonal factors (e.g., worldview, personal and professional experiences) and extrapersonal factors (e.g., historical context, influential others) (DeGroot, 1988) as they influence the motives and purposes underlying one's conceptual frame. Ethical reflection also entails:

- Assessment of the moral ideals underlying the concepts of health, human being, environment, and nursing practice that may be represented in the framework;
- Creative imagining of the consequences of one's framework;
- Depth of personal knowledge;
- Moral vision, described by McInerny (1987) as awareness of the deepest beliefs about such things as the value of life and death, and the nature and worth of the environment; and
- An openness to undergo a "transformation of values" (Chinn, 1985) when it is determined that concepts need redefining or theories need reformulating.

An ethical framework in nursing reflects not only a basic concern for human welfare, but also a moral commitment to the discipline. The theorizer must refrain from being lured into conceptualizations "framed in the unique perspective of other disciplines" (Smoth, 1988, p. 3) that offer more certainty or specificity for the theorists but make little contribution to the aims of nursing. Smith (1988) admonishes nurses to stay tough during the process of theorizing. Moral timidity creates trivial theory. Bellah was highly critical of those who lacked moral vision in their inquiry, who misrepresented human processes with reductionistic and deterministic conceptualizations, and who hid behind the excuse that "our science is still young" (Bellah, 1981, p. 17).

Toward Boldness in Nursing Theorizing

There is movement underfoot to become more deliberate in exploring the philosophical bases of nursing theorizing. Evidence for this can be found not only in the nursing literature over the past decade, but also among graduate students' requests for more courses and course content on the history and philosophy of science, in lunch-hour seminars in which various philosophical views are debated, and in conference proceedings that address philosophical issues as integral to theory development. Doctoral students are embracing a new philosophy of their science, a philosophy that thrives on the indeterminate nature of nursing phenomena, entertains radically new hypotheses, welcomes diversity among paradigms, and values independent thought. At the same time, it is a philosophy that challenges scientists to examine the ethical questions associated with their value choices, judgments, and patterns of reasoning. As nursing turns toward a greater focus on substance rather than structure in the science (Downs, 1988; Fitzpatrick, 1987), increased attention may be given to the ethical dimensions of conceptual processes in research as has been given to the ethical dimensions of the methodological processes in research.

The discipline's understanding of what constitutes health and how best to promote optimal well-being, quality of life, and other values may be clarified by purposeful ethical reflection as a routine occurrence in theorizing. Carper, in explaining the importance of the ethical pattern of knowing, stated that differences in normative judgments may have more to do with disagreements over conceptualizations of health than with a lack of empirical evidence (Carper, 1978). Ethical knowledge about the underpinnings of the conceptual frame may also facilitate solutions to ethical dilemmas encountered in other stages of the research process and in the eventual clinical applications of knowledge.

Nursing scientists today are being challenged to make choices in their theorizing—choices that touch their own identity as well as affect the good of society. Tensions between theory and practice, the conceptual and the operational, help bring into focus the variety of philosophical views and values inherent among nursing paradigms, and the choices one makes in explicating a framework. Is human health best measured and promoted from a reductionistic or holistic perspective or is there yet another perspective? Is the environment best conceptualized as integral or external to human functioning? Is the human cell or human field, or some other human dimension, the fundamental unit of study in nursing?

In nursing's present phase of development as a science, scientists need to explicate the value choices underlying their frameworks in a bold, self-informed manner. Knowledge can be used as sociopolitical power to enforce a theorized good and to affect human health in unforeseeable ways. Ethical inquiry into one's conceptual frame can provide needed constraints on the human tendency to blur the distinction between a researcher's beliefs and societal needs and can also provide the moral vision needed to effectively and humanely solve nursing problems.

REFERENCES

American Nurses' Association (1985). *Code of ethics.* Kansas City: Author.

American Nurses' Association (1984). *Human rights guidelines.* Kansas City: Author.

Archbold, P. G. (1981). Ethical issues in the selection of a theoretical framework for gerontological nursing research. *Journal of Gerontologic Nursing, 7,* 408–411.

Baltes, M. M., & Baltes, P. B. (1977). The ecopsychological realtivity and plasticity of psychological aging: Convergent perspectives of cohort effects and operant psychology. *Psychology, 24,* 179–197.

Bellah, R. N. (1981). The ethical aims of social inquiry. *Teachers College Record, 83*(1), 1–18.

Botwinick, J. (1973). *Aging and behavior.* New York: Springer.

Boyd, C. (1985). Toward an understanding of mother-daughter identification using concept analysis. *Advances in Nursing Science, 7*(3), 78–86.

Carper, B. A. (1978). Fundamental patterns of knowing in nursing. *Advances in Nursing Science, 1*(1), 13–24.

Chinn, P. L. (1985). Quality of life: A values transformation. *Advances in Nursing Science, 8*(1), vii-ix.

Chinn, P. L., & Jacobs, M. K. (1987). *Theory and nursing* (2nd ed.). St. Louis: C. V. Mosby.

Connors, D. D. (1988). A continuum of research-participant relationships: An analysis and critique. *Advances in Nursing Science, 10*(4), 32–42.

DeGroot, H. A. (1988). Scientific inquiry in nursing: A model for a new age. *Advances in Nursing Science, 10*(3), 1–21.

Dewey, J. (1928). In J. Rather (Ed.). *The philosophy of John Dewey.* New York: Holt, Rinehart & Winston.

Dewey, J. (1948). *Reconstruction in philosophy.* Boston: Beacon Press.

Downs, F. (1988). Doctoral education: Our claim to the future. *Nursing Outlook, 36*(1), 18–20.

Ellison, E. S. (1985). Social support and the constructive-developmental model. *Western Journal of Nursing Research, 9,* 19–28.

Fitzpatrick, J. J. (1987). Philosophical approach: Empiricism. In C. Bridges & N. Wells (Eds.). *Proceedings of the Fourth Nursing Science Colloquium: Strategies for Nursing Theory Development.* Boston: Boston University School of Nursing.

Fowler, M. D. (1987). Ethical issues in nursing research. *Western Journal of Nursing Research, 9,* 269–271.

Hinshaw, A. S. (1988). Using research to shape health policy. *Nursing Outlook, 36*(1), 21–24.

Hirsch, J. (1975). Jensenism: The bankruptcy of "science" without scholarship. *Educational Theory, 25,* 3–28.

Horn, J. L. (1976). Human abilities: A review of research and theory in the early 1970s. *Annual Review of Psychology, 27,* 437–485.

Jensen, A. R. (1973). Race, intelligence, and genetics: The differences are real. *Psychology Today, 12,* 80–86.

Kamin, L. J. (1974). *The science and politics of IQ.* New York: Halstead.

Kaplan, A. (1964). *The logic of scientific discovery.* New York: Thomas Y. Crowell.

Labouvie-Vief, G. (1977). Adult cognitive development: In search of alternative interpretations. *Merrill-Palmer Quarterly of Behavior and Development, 23*(4), 227–263.

Labouvie-Vief, G. (1980). Adaptive dimensions of adult cognition. In N. Datan & N. Lohmann (Eds.). Transitions in aging. New York: Academic Press.

Labouvie-Vief, G., & Schell, D. A. (1983). Learning and memory in later life: A developmental view. In B. Wolman & G. Striker (Eds.). *Handbook of developmental psychology.* Englewood Cliffs, NJ: Prentice-Hall.

Laudan, L. (1977). *Progress and its problems: Toward a theory of scientific growth.* Berkeley, CA: University of California Press.

Laudan, L. (1981). A problem-solving approach to scientific progress. In I. Hacking (Ed.). *Scientific revolutions.* New York: Oxford University Press.

Laudan, L. (1984). *Science and values.* Berkeley, CA: University of California Press.

McInerny, W. F. (1987). Understanding moral issues in health care: Seven essential ideas. *Journal of Professional Nursing, 3,* 268–277.

Moccia, P. (1988). A critique of compromise: Beyond the methods debate. *Advances in Nursing Science, 10*(4), 1–9.

Munhall, P. L. (1988). Ethical considerations in qualitative research. *Western Journal of Nursing Research, 10,* 150–162.

Narayan, S. M., & Joslin, D. J. (1980). Crisis theory and intervention: A critique of the medical model and proposal of a holistic nursing model. *Advances in Nursing Science, 2*(4), 27–40.

Nietzche, F. (1966). *Beyond good and evil* (W. Kaufmann, trans). New York: Vintage.

Popper, K. R. (1968). *The logic of scientific discovery.* New York: Harper & Row.

Rorty, R. (1979). *Philosophy and the mirror of nature.* Princeton, NJ: Princeton University Press.

Schaie, K. W. (1973). Methodological problems in research on adulthood and aging. In J. R. Nesselroade & H. W. Reese (Eds.). *Life-span developmental psychology: Methodological issues.* New York: Academic Press.

Smith, M. J. (1988). Wallowing while waiting, *Nursing Science Quarterly, 1*(1), 3.

White, G. B. (1983). Philosophical ethics and nursing—a word of caution. In P. L. Chinn (Ed.). *Advances in nursing theory development.* Rockville, MD: Aspen.

The Author Comments

Nursing Theorizing as an Ethical Endeavor

This article was written to address a gap in the ethics literature and course content that I noticed early in my teaching career. Ethics was depicted as an important component of practice and research but not theory. This was so despite the links professed to exist between theory, research, and practice. Theorizing is a powerful tool in knowledge building, affecting the focus and outcomes of research. It calls for ethical reflection on the variables we choose to study, how we define them, and how they fit into a theoretic framework to influence the nursing that is practiced. I anticipate that ethics will move into the center of nursing theory development as the 21st century progresses.

—Pamela G. Reed

CHAPTER 57

Relational Narrative:
The Postmodern Turn in Nursing Ethics

Sally Gadow

A philosophy of nursing requires an ethical cornerstone. I describe three dialectical layers of an ethical cornerstone: subjective immersion, objective detachment, and relational narrative. Dialectically, the move from immersion to detachment is the turn from communitarian to rational ethics, replacing traditions with universal principles. The move from universalism to engagement is the turn from rational to relational ethics, replacing detached reason with engagement between particular selves. Conceptually, the three layers correspond to premodern, modern, and postmodern ethics. I propose that the layers be viewed not as stages, but as elements that coexist in an ethically vital profession, and I conclude with an illustration of their coexistence in a clinical situation.

A philosophy of nursing requires an ethical cornerstone, because a profession is informed by moral ends. Discussions of ethics in nursing usually are framed in the categories of philosophical ethics, such as deontology, virtue, and consequentialism. While useful for locating nursing ethics within the disciplinary context of philosophy, the categories are not helpful because they manifest no internal relationship to each other, no connection within an encompassing framework. Without a coherent framework, ethics cannot provide the cornerstone for a philosophy of nursing.

In the hope that establishing philosophical connections among different ethical approaches will lead to the construction of an ethical cornerstone, I offer a method

From Scholarly Inquiry for Nursing Practice: An International Journal, 13(1), Gadow, S., Relational narrative: The postmodern turn in nursing ethics, pp. 57–70. Copyright © 1999, Springer Publishing Company. Used with permission.

About the Author

SALLY GADOW was born in Boston. She received a baccalaureate degree in nursing from the University of Texas at Galveston; a master's degree in nursing from the University of California, San Francisco; and a PhD in philosophy from the University of Texas at Austin. Her academic career has included faculty positions at Johns Hopkins University, the University of Maryland, Georgetown University, the University of Florida, the University of Texas, and the University of Colorado. Her scholarship focuses on the philosophy of nursing, with emphasis on ethics and phenomenology. Her key contribution to the discipline is her philosophic examination of the nurse-patient relationship within a broad humanities framework. Her principal hobby is long-distance sailing.

for understanding different ethical views within a dialectical framework. The framework I describe is a triad of ethical layers: subjective immersion (ethical immediacy), objective detachment (ethical universalism), and intersubjective engagement (relational narrative)—corresponding, respectively, to premodern, modern, and postmodern ethics (see Figure 57-1). After a brief discussion of dialectic, I describe each of the three layers and conclude with an illustration of their coexistence in a clinical situation.

Dialectic

The method of developing a philosophical dialectic is adapted here from the work of Hegel (1807/1977). A brief elaboration of method is important to the thesis of this discussion, namely, that premodern, modern, and postmodern ethics represent a dialectical relationship among different ethical approaches in which none of the three can stand alone and only their coexistence constitutes a sound basis for practice.

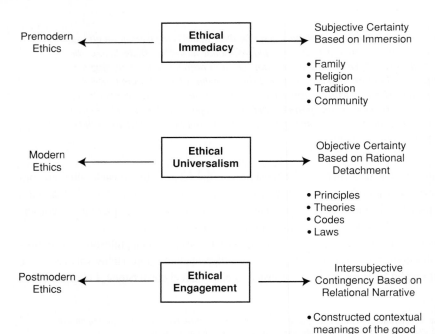

Figure 57-1 *Triad of ethical layers.*

Premodern Ethics ← **Ethical Immediacy** → Subjective Certainty Based on Immersion
- Family
- Religion
- Tradition
- Community

Modern Ethics ← **Ethical Universalism** → Objective Certainty Based on Rational Detachment
- Principles
- Theories
- Codes
- Laws

Postmodern Ethics ← **Ethical Engagement** → Intersubjective Contingency Based on Relational Narrative
- Constructed contextual meanings of the good

The nature of dialectic can be expressed as mediation. Mediation is the negation of simplicity, resulting in increasing complexity as each new level of differentiation is in turn negated, producing further distinctions. At the same time, the opposition among distinctions is itself mediated. Negativity, in other words, becomes increasingly positive as the original opposition is qualified by a new relationship in which once antithetical elements are no longer mutually exclusive but become mutually enhancing.

A clinical example of dialectic is the experience of injury and rehabilitation (Bloom, 1992; Gadow, 1982). (1) Before injury, the body is experienced as a taken-for-granted immediacy that accomplishes the aims of a person, such as climbing stairs, without reflection or even awareness. (2) An injury negates that immediacy in two ways: the body opposes the aims of the self by its inability to climb, and the inability is itself the antithesis of the lost immediacy. (3) Rehabilitation negotiates a new relationship between body and self. While the body remains an other for the self (an otherness the injury produced), harmony between them is cultivated through attentiveness to the injured part. That cultivated unity based on care entails the possibility for climbing stairs as a cooperative, rather than an unconscious, activity of body and self.

A characteristic rhythm is associated with dialectic because of the three phases of simplicity, opposition, and reconciliation. The formulaic description of dialectic as thesis-antithesis-synthesis, however, can be deceptive; it masks the principle of ongoing *self*-negation at the heart of dialectic. No phase is exclusively thesis, antithesis, or synthesis. Each phase serves as antithesis of the one before, and each synthesis becomes a new thesis as its own unity is further differentiated. The rehabilitated body, for example, can train for a marathon, involving further cycles of immediacy, opposition, and reconciliation.

If an inherent telos is assumed, a dialectic will move inexorably toward culmination. Hegel insisted on a telos, but I do not. Without a telos, the movement of mediation can proceed indefinitely. Without closure, a dialectic of ethical levels such as I propose can give rise to further cycles of differentiation. Ethics, in other words, need not culminate in the postmodern. Indeed, the most interesting question evoked by a dialectic of premodern-modern-postmodern ethics may be, "What now?" Given the nihilism sometimes associated (mistakenly, I believe) with postmodern ethics, treating it as the thesis for a new set of negations might be a fruitful sequel to the discussion that follows.

Premodern Immersion: Ethical Immediacy

In a dialectical framework the first level is immediacy. In ethical terms, immediacy is an unreflective and uncritical certainty about the good. A certainty powerful enough to resist reflection originates outside an individual in order to avoid being undermined by particularity. Certainty about the good, if it is to be more than personal conviction, must derive from a source that transcends the individual, such as religion, family, customs, or the ethos of a profession.

Ethical immediacy is an experience of certainty that needs and allows no explication; it is nondiscursive. That, in fact, is its power. A discursive description of a morally good nurse can be argued and revised, requires consideration, and has to be consciously accepted in order to have power. In contrast, a nondiscursive portrayal—an image rendered in film, a virtue modeled by a mentor—bypasses deliberation to gain acceptance. With a cultural, professional, or religious basis for certainty, a nurse intuits the good directly, without recourse to reflection. That immediacy is the phenomenon I call immersion: a nurse is immersed in a tradition that provides an ethical appraisal of the situation, as well as immersed in the situation itself. Depending on the tradition, that appraisal may dictate, for example, that nurse-assisted suicide is wrong (or that it is right). Whatever the tradition, immersion offers a degree of certainty unavailable to the other ethical layers because it is nonreflective. It needs no defense.

The strength of immersion as an ethical approach is the solidarity it achieves. Nurses and patients sharing an unquestioned view of the good are united in their attempt to realize that good. Differences in interpretation may

either of their individual narratives as they seek a new form of the good.

A Dialectical Framework in Practice

I have proposed that the philosophical cornerstone of nursing is dialectically layered rather than unitary. The question now emerges: What would the dialectic among different ethical layers look like in practice?

A dialectic can be reduced to ideology by theorizing a telos that draws the movement toward a final level. To avoid that reduction and its coerciveness, I suggest that the three ethical approaches be regarded not as successive stages in the profession's advance, but as possibilities coexisting in an ethically vital practice. Dialectic offers a way of envisioning contradictory approaches as intrinsically related. None of the three is fully intelligible without its connection to the others. Each complements the limitations of the other two.

Dialectic as a philosophical framework is more than a heuristic device for conceptualizing nursing. It is a also a framework for the continuing development of the discipline. If otherwise opposing approaches can be appreciated as inseparable, they may then be acknowledged in practice as being mutually enhancing instead of oppositional. Nursing becomes more than a moral high ground from which difference is excluded. It becomes, instead, a region of existence large enough to accommodate, even encourage, diversity among those who live there.

Just as a geographic region cannot be conveyed in its totality by a map, an existential region cannot be captured in a theory, but something of its vitality can be rendered by images. In a beginning attempt to answer the question of how a dialectical framework might look in practice, I offer instead of theory a metaphor and a clinical example that may serve as an impetus to further exploration.

The flourishing of premodern, modern, and postmodern ethics in nursing can be imagined metaphorically as the biodiversity of a coral reef where different life forms integrate and where organisms even after their death provide a structure that supports life. At the level of immediacy, we are immersed in ethical currents that carry us safely through situations where reflection would be impossible. When crosscurrents require us to reflect and to hold a position, an edifice of ethical principles offers a structure for steadying ourselves. Finally, there are situations where no edifice can alleviate our vulnerability, and in those cases we can only turn to each other and together compose a fragile new form of the good.

To illustrate, I consider the reef-like situation described by Schroeder (1998) in which Carole (mother) and Morgan (daughter) found themselves while Morgan spent the first 3 months of life undergoing surgical heart repairs, inept and relentless technical procedures, and near-fatal nursing and medical errors. Schroeder's description does not indict professionals for being unethical, but displays instead the inevitable collisions when a mother's immersion in her daughter's danger meets the detachment of ethical objectivity.

> "How can she be in congestive heart failure if I'm rooming-in?" He looked impatiently at me. "You're a nurse. Call the intensive care nursery if her respirations go over 60" (p. 14).

Instead of calling, Carole brought her baby into bed with her, pulled the blanket over them, and unplugged the phone, mutely sinking into the quicksand of isolation that immersion becomes when no hand is offered.

Hands eventually were offered from each of the three ethical layers. All of them were essential to the survival of both mother and child.

1. From the urgency of another mother's immersion in her own child's situation:

> "Get her out of here no matter what," she whispered, . . . "Get her out of here if she is getting better at all" (p. 13).

And from the same mother, the offer of community in an informal group where mothers' stories to each other kept them from drowning in the immediacy of their children's pain.

2. From the honesty of a nurse who countered institutional hierarchy with her own ethical autonomy:

> One day, Lea told me that the physicians at this hospital were unable to do anything further for Morgan . . . Although she merely confirmed what I had already been thinking, I was unable to summon the strength to act upon my thoughts without her support. I now know that Morgan would have died in that hospital cubicle if Lea had not risked angering the physicians and telling me the truth (p. 19).

3. From a nurse whose overtures opened the door to a different story, to engagement instead of isolation:

> Carolyn would ignore my hostile looks and sit with me at Morgan's bedside on work breaks . . . Her words and presence began to fill some of the emptiness inside me. Although I would never admit it to her, I began to look forward to her visits, and eventually we began to communicate on a level very foreign to our previous working relationship (p. 19).

And from a nurse who transcended moral duties:

> Cathy came out of the ICU and said that they were trying to get her off the heart-lung machine now; "I'll be right back to let you know," she said, and walked back into the ICU. I stared at the door, awestruck at her bravery. She'll have to let me know, I marveled, now she can't just stay behind those doors and let someone else tell me the news. I felt ready to handle anything, almost exhilarated that someone would risk so much when it wasn't even required (p. 21).

The coral reef that I believe Schroeder describes is ethically layered. Modern, premodern, and postmodern elements alternately prevailed. The situation would have been ethically diminished by an absence of any of the elements. Philosophically, the dialectical nature of nursing entails the presence of all of them. Without a telos to drive the dialectic, there is no basis on which to insist that nursing limit itself to one. The postmodern turn only makes explicit an element that has been implicit; it does not establish a superior ground from which to dismiss the others. In the case of Carole and Morgan, no single element was decisive in determining the ethical course to pursue. They did escape, as the first mother urged, but not before a nurse had urged moving to a better hospital where surgery was successful, and not until other nurses had offered engagement as alternative to immersion.

A dialectical ethical narrative such as Schroeder provides is the equivalent of a relational narrative that a nurse and patient together create. Both narratives are layered with voices from immediacy and objectivity in a continuing tension that cannot be resolved in favor of either without destruction of the narrative's relational nature, its contingency and vitality. The postmodern turn is not an advance that dismisses immersion and detachment as ethical approaches. It is instead a turn toward the absurd, as Camus (1955) would call it, the cultivation of a life "without appeal" (p. 39) in which the longing for certainty and the impossibility of certainty are both embraced passionately. From a modern or premodern perspective, that contradiction is absurd in the sense of being hopeless. From the postmodern perspective, an absurd life is filled with "a wild kind of hope" (Schroeder, 1998, p. 20).

The practice of an absurd life, an absurd ethics, is dialectical because it grants at once the validity of subjective and objective ethics. In nursing the story of that practice can only be intersubjective, a relational narrative. The narrative is layered with voices of immersion and detachment like a medieval motet in which several voices simultaneously sing parts of the text that counter and complement one another (Gadow, 1999). Perhaps the fact that a philosophical cornerstone can be compared metaphorically to a phenomenon as ephemeral as a song is one more indication of the postmodern turn in nursing ethics.

REFERENCES

Akhmatova, A. (1983). *Poems.* New York: Norton.

Bauman, Z. (1993). *Postmodern ethics.* Oxford, England: Blackwell Publishers.

Bauman, Z. (1995). *Life in fragments: Essays in postmodern morality.* Oxford, England: Blackwell Publishers.

Beauchamp, T., & Childress, J. (1994). *Principles of biomedical ethics* (4th ed.). Oxford, England: Oxford University Press.

Benhabib, S. (1992). *Situating the self: Gender, community and postmodernism in contemporary ethics.* London: Routledge.

Benjamin, M., & Curtis, J. (1992). *Ethics in nursing* (3rd ed.). Oxford, England: Oxford University Press.

Bloom, L. R. (1992). How can we know the dancer from the dance?: Discourses of the self-body. *Human Studies, 15,* 313–334.

Bordo, S. (1993). *Unbearable weight: Feminism, western culture, and the body.* Los Angeles: University of California Press.

Camus, A. (1955). *The myth of Sisyphus and other essays.* New York: Vintage Books.

Carr, D. (1986). *Time, narrative, and history.* Bloomington, IN: Indiana University Press.

Cixous, H. (1993). We who are free, are we free? In B. Johnson (Ed.), *Freedom and interpretation: The Oxford Amnesty Lectures, 1992* (pp. 14–44). New York: HarperCollins.

Connelly, F., & Clandinin, D. (1990). Stories of experience and narrative inquiry. *Educational Researcher, 19*(5), 2–14.

Dillon, R. (1992). Respect and care: Toward moral integration. *Canadian Journal of Philosophy, 22,* 105–131.

Foucault, M. (1979). *Discipline and punish: The birth of the prison* (A. Sheridan, Trans.). New York: Vintage Books. (Original work published 1975)

Friedman, M. (1993). *What are friends for? Feminist perspectives on personal relationships and moral theory.* Ithaca, NY: Cornell University Press.

Gadow, S. (1982). Body and self: A dialectic. In V. Kestenbaum (Ed.), *The humanity of the ill: Phenomenological perspectives* (pp. 86–100). Knoxville, TN: University of Tennessee Press.

Gadow, S. (1994). Whose body? Whose story? The question about narrative in women's health care. *Soundings, 77,* 295–307.

Gadow, S. (1995). Clinical epistemology: A dialectic of nursing assessment. *Canadian Journal of Nursing Research, 27,* 25–34.

Gadow, S. (1999). *I felt an island rising: Interpretive inquiry as motet.* Manuscript submitted for publication.

Gouldner, A. (1978). *The dialectic of ideology and technology: The origins, grammar, and future of ideology.* Oxford, England: Oxford University Press.

Hegel, G. W. F. (1977). *The phenomenology of spirit* (A. V. Miller, Trans.). Oxford, England: Clarendon. (Original work published in 1807)

LeGuin, U. (1989). Some thoughts on narrative. In U. LeGuin (Ed.), *Dancing at the edge of the world: Thoughts on words, women, places* (pp. 37–45). New York: Harper & Row.

MacIntyre, A. (1981). *After virtue.* Notre Dame, IN: University of Notre Dame Press.

Poole, R. (1991). *Morality and modernity.* London: Routledge.

Rorty, R. (1989). *Contingency, irony, and solidarity.* Cambridge, England: Cambridge University Press.

Sandelowski, M. (1994). We are the stories we tell: Narrative knowing in nursing practice. *Journal of Holistic Nursing, 12,* 23–33.

Scarry, E. (1985). *The body in pain: The making and unmaking of the world.* Oxford, England: Oxford University Press.

Schroeder, C. (1998). So this is what it's like: Struggling to survive in pediatric intensive care. *Advances in Nursing Science, 20,* 13–22.

Tester, K. (1993). *The life and times of post-modernity.* London: Routledge.

Young, I. (1990). *Justice and the politics of difference.* Princeton, NJ: Princeton University Press.

The Author Comments

Relational Narrative: The Postmodern Turn in Nursing Ethics

All my work reflects an appreciation for philosophic dialectic as described by Hegel. This article was my attempt to use a dialectic perspective to understand ethics as a whole and to integrate opposing ethical approaches that were, to me, incompatible. I wanted to demonstrate how relational ethics could evolve naturally in nursing as a response to the limitations of traditional and rational ethics. I hope the article contributes to an emerging view of not only ethical theory but also nursing theory as postmodern.

—SALLY GADOW

CHAPTER 58

A Pluralist View of Nursing Ethics

Joan McCarthy

This paper makes the case for a pluralist, contextualist view of nursing ethics. In defending this view, I briefly outline two current perspectives of nursing ethics—the Traditional View and the Theory View. I argue that the Traditional View, which casts nursing ethics as a subcategory of healthcare ethics, is problematic because it (1) fails to sufficiently acknowledge the unique nature of nursing practice; and (2) applies standard ethical frameworks such as principlism to moral problems which tend to alienate or undermine nursing ethical concerns. Alternatively, the Theory View, which aims to build an independent and comprehensive theory of nursing ethics, is also found wanting because it (1) fails to sufficiently acknowledge the heterogeneous nature of nursing practices; (2) overemphasizes the differences and undervalues the similarities between nurses and other health professionals; and (3) assumes that one ethical framework can be meaningfully applied across diverse moral problems and contexts.

My alternative, is to argue that nursing ethics inquiry should take a pluralist and critical stance towards available ethical frameworks and the negotiation of the ethical realm. On this view, the search for moral consensus or a unique ethical framework for nursing is replaced by the task of working strategically with multiple frameworks in order to expand the moral agency of nurses and empower them to positively engage with moral uncertainty as an inevitable feature of living a moral life. I conclude by indicating some of the implications that this has for the teaching of nursing ethics.

About the Author

JOAN MCCARTHY is the youngest of five children born to working-class parents in 1959, in Killarney, Co. Kerry, Ireland. She has worked as a typesetter, administrator, and fundraiser, and has had part-time teaching jobs in women's studies, development studies, and community education. When she was 35, she started her PhD in philosophy, her thesis on the narrative self will be published this year by Humanity Books, New York. She has also co-authored *The Ethics of New Reproductive Technologies* (with Dooley et al., 2003, Oxford: Berghahn Books) and *Nursing Ethics, Irish Cases and Concerns* (with Dooley 2005, Dublin: Gill and Macmillan). Her scholarly interests include feminist and narrative ethics, and she is currently working on a research project on end-of-life decision making. She has been employed as a full-time lecturer in nursing and health care ethics in the School of Nursing and Midwifery, University College Cork, since 2002. When not working, she enjoys music, friendships, and walking around the beautiful city and country where she lives. She also loves detective novels and films, and debating about the state of the world over food that she has cooked and wine that someone else has chosen.

Introduction

Two perspectives on nursing ethics are currently debated in the literature: the first, the Traditional View, casts nursing ethics as a subcategory of healthcare ethics; the second, the Theory View, aims to build an independent and comprehensive theory of nursing ethics. In this paper, I raise a number of objections to these views; while I agree that traditional ethical frameworks are limited, I also suggest that the search for a more comprehensive theory of nursing ethics ought to be abandoned. I propose a third alternative, that nursing ethics is best understood as a pluralist and contextualist form of moral inquiry. On the Pluralist View of nursing ethics, the search for moral consensus or a unique ethical framework for nursing is replaced by the task of working strategically with multiple frameworks in order to expand the moral agency of nurses and adequately address the diversity among nursing practices, nurses, patients, and families.

What Is Nursing Ethics?

'Nursing ethics' does not describe a single academic discipline or subject area. Rather, it is best understood as an umbrella term for a number of different but related areas of inquiry. Firstly, it examines nursing practices and critically reflects on the ethical issues that arise therein. I see this domain as standing on the fault-line between the discipline of ethics and the profession of nursing. Secondly, it attempts to account for the values and standards of the nursing profession that are articulated in national and international nursing codes. This field of inquiry takes a critical look at the role nursing codes play in guiding the profession in relation to ethical issues. Thirdly, nursing ethics includes ethics research, a developing field of inquiry that combines theoretical reflection with empirical research. It involves the identification and description, based on empirical methodologies, of the ethical decisions nurses actually make or are involved in. Finally, nursing ethics is a subject or part of a subject that is taught on undergraduate and postgraduate nursing programmes (Fry, 1995; Yeo & Moorhouse, 1996, pp. 2–23).

My interest is largely in the first of these areas of nursing ethics, that domain of inquiry which involves the application of ethical theories and concepts to nursing practice and, in turn, the consideration of ethical theories and concepts in the light of insights drawn from nursing practice. The development of this field of inquiry has taken, roughly, two different directions in recent years. What I am calling the Traditional View, understands nursing ethical inquiry as significantly *similar* to other evolving disciplines in the broader field of healthcare ethics such as medical ethics and dentistry ethics. In light of this, it deploys similar ethical concepts and frameworks in considering nursing practice. What I am calling The Theory View, sees nursing ethical inquiry as significantly *different* from other disciplines, so much that it requires a distinct nursing ethical framework or theory to undergird the ethical decision making of nursing. I will explain and consider each, in turn.

Traditional View

The Traditional View of nursing ethics casts it as a subcategory of healthcare ethics. One proponent of this view, Søren Holm, for example, argues that similar moral issues arise in healthcare settings for doctors, nurses, and other care professionals. These include concerns arising out of the professional-patient relationships such as autonomy, consent, veracity, and confidentiality. In addition, Holm argues that general concerns arise among and between professional groups and between professionals and organizations such as whistle-blowing, advocacy, and scarce resources (Holm, 1997, pp. 150–151).

Furthermore, while acknowledging that the nursing ethics literature usually draws sharp distinctions between nursing ethics and medical ethics, Holm, nevertheless, argues on the basis of his research with different professional groups in Denmark, that there is little difference between the ways in which doctors and nurses identify and assess ethical problems there (Holm, 1997, pp. 197–203).

It follows, on the Traditional View, that the task of identifying, analysing, and assessing nurses' ethical issues and decisions is similar to the task of identifying and analysing the decisions of other healthcare professionals. Proponents of the Traditional View argue that nurses, like other health professionals, must draw insight from ethical frameworks such as deontology, utilitarianism or principlism in order to negotiate the ethical challenges they meet with in the course of their work. Steven Edwards, for example, while he differs from Holm in his analysis of nurse-patient relationships and doctor-patient relationships, nevertheless suggests that nursing ethics should adapt and adopt the principlist ethical framework developed by Beauchamp and Childress for medical ethics. He defends principlism and its four foundational principles of autonomy, non-maleficence, beneficence, and justice, on several grounds including the following: that it provides a clear and coherent framework for ethical decision making, that it is easily applicable to very many problems that nurses face, that it requires that nurses consider moral problems in the light of a different perspectives and that it is consistent with the norms of international nursing codes (Edwards, 1996, p. 1, 48–49).

Criticism of the Traditional View

Opposition to the Traditional View of nursing ethics has gained momentum in the last 20 years. Firstly, objections have been levelled at its basic premise; that different health professional groups share the same moral concerns. Nursing ethics, it is argued, can be distinguished from other fields in healthcare ethics because it is connected with the history of nursing, with nursing goals and nursing practices. Especial attention is focused on the nurse-patient relationship which Sara Fry argues ought to be a central concern of nursing ethics:

> Any theory of nursing ethics should consider the nature of the nurse-patient relationship within health care contexts and should adopt a moral point of view that focuses directly on this relationship. (Fry, 1989, p. 20)

Fifteen years on, in 2004, Janet Storch similarly places emphasis on the holistic role of the nurse in the care of patients:

> Nursing is a profession with a moral mandate that differs from the medical mandate in that nurses address the full diversity of need, with less emphasis on treatment and cure. (Storch, 2004, p. 2)

In the same vein, Helen Brown *et al.*, (2004) argue that principlism is too 'medicocentric' because '[t]he exotic issues of medical science are relevant to nursing but do not constitute the bulk of nurses' moral concerns of everyday practice of caring for patients and families (Brown *et al.,* 2004, p. 127).

However, even if proponents of the Traditional View were to pay increased attention to, specifically, nursing ethical issues (as Edwards, 1996 does) they must still, according to critics, defend their particular choice of theory. Principlism, for example, while it is widely deployed across many different healthcare settings, has been challenged by ethicists in the broader field for being overly scientific, abstract, and impersonal (Clouser & Gert, 1990; DuBose *et al.,* 1994; Davis, 1995). Its specific application to nursing practice has also been criticized by theorists, such as Patricia Benner. She places emphasis on more traditional virtues and acknowledges that while theories such as principlism may permit reflection and reveal some issues, 'it is in disembodied and conceptual distance that [it] fails to grasp essential embodied human distinctions of worth, such as honor, courage, and dignity' (Benner, 1991, p. 4). More recently, Elizabeth Peter and Joan Liaschenko make the even stronger claim that in the course of their careers of writing, research and teaching, they have found 'bioethical theory to be essentially irrelevant' (Peter & Liaschenko, 2003, p. 259).

> [S]tandard bioethical theory fails to reflect nurses' moral concerns; [. . .] we believe that it is part of the process through which nurses' moral concerns actually 'get disappeared'. (Peter & Liaschenko, 2003, p. 259)

Peter and Liaschenko argue that having knowledge of ethical theories does not entail that nurses can participate fully in the process of ethical decision making. In their view, the very naming of what is or is not morally relevant is not neutral—different theories foreground different concerns and ignore or 'disappear' others. Moreover, even after a particular feature of a moral situation is highlighted, the processes of reflection and analysis that are invoked, play a role in the eventual outcome of the deliberations. Their particular concern is that adherence to traditional moral frameworks leads nurses to doubt their own moral reading of situations and they fear that they will become 'morally paralysed in

their attempt to embrace theoretical ideas far removed from their world' (Peter & Liaschenko, 2003, p. 261).

Theory View

In light of the concerns that some theorists have with the Traditional View, the idea of an independent and comprehensive theory of nursing ethics—the Theory View—has been promoted in recent years. Such a theory is usually grounded in a particular nursing philosophical approach, or, it appeals to an ethical framework, such as virtue ethics, care ethics or feminist ethics, which is seen as particularly compatible with nursing interests. A comprehensive theory of ethics, developed along these lines, is advanced as an antidote to the supposed abstraction, irrelevance, and empty generalizations of traditional bioethics and as holding out the promise of capturing and articulating a, specifically, nursing ethical focus.

Fry & Johnstone (2002), for example, propose a view of nursing ethics that draws from both the history of the nursing profession and virtue ethics theory. They posit a number of ethical concepts such as advocacy, accountability, cooperation, and caring, which they see as historically associated with nursing, as a starting point for nursing ethics inquiry in the 21st century (Fry & Johnstone, 2002, pp. 37–47). They argue that a theory of nursing should set aside the primacy of principles and rules in bioethics in favour of an emphasis on care as a central nursing value. They propose the idea of the nurse as a virtuous character, motivated to promote human well-being (Fry & Johnstone, 2002, pp. 30–31). Drawing on nursing practices, research, and professional codes, Fry argues that

> The 'good' nurse of the 21st century will be a composite ideal shaped by empirical evidence about the ethical reality of nurses' practices and by the ethical standards for nursing practice set forth by organizations such as ICN. (Fry, 2002, p. 2)

To act ethically on this view is to act in accordance with best nursing practice and professional standards.

Similarly, theorists such as Nel Noddings (1984), Jean Watson (1988), and Sally Gadow emphasize caring and relationship as central features of nursing ethics. For instance, Gadow's account of existential advocacy (Gadow, 1980), and, later, her account of relational narrative (Gadow, 1994), appeal to existentialist and narrative ethics to characterize good ethical practice as grounded in relationships:

In 1980,

> [The] essence of nursing is the nurse's participation with the patient in determining the unique meaning which the experience of health, illness, suffering, or dying is to have for that individual. (Gadow, 1980, p. 81)

In 1994, Gadow describes a relational narrative as an ethical stance which starts from the idea that relationship is the foundation of moral valuing. Within the relationship, an ethically acceptable narrative is composed between nurse and patient that is:

> An interpretation of their situation together and an imagining of alternatives to which they could both be committed. Together they address the questions, What is the story that makes sense of this situation? What are other stories (situations) in which we could live instead of this one and toward which we want to move? (Gadow, 1994, p. 306)

Finally, feminist theories of ethics have also been recruited to serve the ends of nursing ethics theory. In general, feminist ethics is the application of feminist theory to understanding the ethical realm: it critiques traditional ethical frameworks from a feminist perspective and considers the impact of gender roles and gendered understandings on the moral lives of individual human beings. Specifically, it draws attention to the power and power differentials inherent in moral relationships at individual, societal, and organizational levels (Dooley & McCarthy, 2005, pp. 255–258). Peter and Liaschenko, mentioned above, see feminist perspectives as a rich resource for the development of nursing ethics theory. They describe the work of feminist philosopher, Margaret Urban Walker, as a 'superior approach' for all healthcare ethics and the 'best understanding of morality available for nursing' (Peter & Liaschenko, 2003, p. 262).

Briefly, Walker (1997, 1998) rejects the possibility of there being any objective or near objective moral system of decision making and tries, instead, to offer an account of morality that is contextual but not relativist. Walker critiques moral frameworks such as principlism, which, on her view, represent morality as a compact code of impersonal propositions guiding the actions of moral agents. She replaces it, with a moral framework that represents morality as a process, rather than a set of prescriptions or outcomes. For Walker, morality and politics cannot be pulled apart. Individuals are not the bounded integrated decision makers that traditional moral approaches seem to presuppose. Rather, who we are and how we decide upon a course of action at any given time must be understood contextually. Morality, for Walker, is a socially embedded process which determines what is morally significant, who is assigned responsibility for decision making and who is permitted and enabled to participate (Walker, 1998, pp. 7–9; Peter & Liaschenko, 2004).

Peter and Liaschenko, pointing to the contested role of nurses in decision making in healthcare situations argue that Walker's work can be usefully deployed to help nurses to navigate their way in the moral and social spaces where they work, and to support them to identify, articulate and defend their moral concerns (Peter & Liaschenko, 2003, p. 262; 2004).

Criticism of the Theory View

All of the above mentioned theories of nursing ethics and their related philosophical paradigms—virtue ethics, care ethics, narrative ethics, feminist ethics—have garnered both praise and criticism in the course of their development and refinement and it is beyond the scope of this paper to consider these on an individual basis. Instead, I will suggest three objections that can be levelled at the Theory View—at the very possibility of a comprehensive theory of nursing ethics.

First of all, any one ethical framework, no matter how comprehensive, cannot possibly address all of the ethical issues that arise in healthcare settings. Nursing practice, involving care, cure, prevention, and promotion gender and hierarchy enable and limit the moral agency of individuals are particularly relevant to nursing in many countries. These take seriously key problems that have long exercised generations of nurses ethically, personally, and professionally. However, the political acuity of these perspectives does not imply that nursing ethics should align itself exclusively with these approaches.

Can I tell you in advance and independently of context which ethical framework should trump in any given situation? The short answer is no, because, while nursing ethics is concerned about what nurses ought to do, its focus is on the quality of the decision making process rather than any specific conclusions that nurses might draw in any given situation. The quality of that process is dependent on a number of different features some of which have a lot to do with moral reasoning skills and others that do not. The features of good decision making include: awareness of the socio-political context, sensitivity to the moral dimensions of the situation, conceptual clarity, imaginative and rigorous argumentation, critical evaluation of theoretical presuppositions. Applying standards such as comprehensiveness, coherence, and clarity may help to distinguish between good and bad theories. So also may the search for features such as inclusiveness and practicality. Even so, these standards and features can only be truly tested in real time and in relation to decisions about a particular ethical policy, case or relationship. And even then, the end of the decision-making process is not the solace of certainty. In the end, the Pluralist View acknowledges that making ethical decisions is often a messy and heart wrenching business and that our finest ethical decisions are not those about which we are certain; they are those with which we can live and which prompt us to do better next time.

A nursing ethics syllabus based on this pluralist perspective of nursing ethics has the advantage of being able to draw on the pedagogical resources of many theories. For example, like the feminist perspective of Peter and Liaschenko, it attaches significance to where nursing students are starting out from. Account is taken of national health policies and health organizations, of perceptions of the role of nurses in health provision, of gender and class relations, of institutional practices and standards of patient care. Attention is also given to the needs that nurses themselves say they have in relation to the moral problems that they encounter. Specific moral concepts, theories and forms of engagement may have particular resonance for groups of nurses and individual nurses at specific historical junctures and locations. The educator must ask, which questions, concepts, frameworks, teaching, and learning strategies will encourage critical reflection, stimulate moral imagination, deepen moral understanding, extend moral agency? Tools of analysis may include traditional paradigms such as principlism, as well as more politically intelligent frameworks such as feminism.

Whatever the tools used, what drives the agenda of nursing ethics education based on the Pluralist View, is a view of ethical work as a critically engaged process whose object is to negotiate, rather than eliminate, ethical uncertainty. The task is to foster a range of ethical skills and sensitivities, and in particular, to deepen students' understanding of the context of ethical decision making so that they can wisely draw on the most appropriate of these. In sum, nurses, not theorists of nursing ethics, decide to accept, reject or modify the applications of available ethical frameworks.

REFERENCES

Almond B. (1995) *Introducing Applied Ethics.* Blackwell, Oxford.

Benner P. (1991) The role of experience, narrative and community in skilled ethical comportment. *Advances in Nursing Science,* 14(2), 1–21.

Brown H., Rodney P., Pauly B., Varcoe C. & Smye V. (2004) Working within the landscape: nursing ethics. In: *Toward a Moral Horizon* (eds J.L. Storch et al.), pp. 126–153. Pearson Education Canada, Toronto.

Clouser K.D. & Gert B. (1990) A critique of principlism. *Journal of Medicine and Philosophy,* 15, 219–236.

Davis R.B. (1995) The principlism debate: a critical overview. *Journal of Medicine and Philosophy,* 17, 511–539.

Doane G., Pauly B., Brown H. & McPherson G. (2004) Exploring the heart of ethical nursing practice: implications for ethics education. *Nursing Ethics,* 11(3), 240–253.

Dooley D. & McCarthy J. (2005) *Nursing Ethics, Irish Cases and Concerns.* Gill and Macmillan, Dublin.

DuBose E.R. *et al.,* (1994) *A Matter of Principles? Ferment in US Bioethics.* Trinity Press International, Valley Forge, PA.

Edwards S.D. (1996) *Nursing Ethics, a Principle-Based Approach.* Macmillan, Basingstoke.

Edwards S.D. (2001) *Philosophy of Nursing,* Palgrave, Basingstoke.

Fry S.T. (1989) Toward a theory of nursing ethics. *Advances in Nursing Science,* 11(4), 9–22.

Fry S.T. (1995) Nursing ethics. In: *Encyclopedia of Bioethics* (ed. W.T. Reich), revised edn., pp. 1822–1823. Simon and Schuster Macmillan, New York.

Fry S.T. (2002) Denning nurses' ethical practices in the 21st century. International Council of Nurses. *International Nursing Review,* 49,1–3.

Fry S.T. & Johnstone M. (2002) *Ethics in Nursing Practice,* 2nd edn. Blackwell, Oxford.

Gadow S. (1980) Existential advocacy: philosophical foundation of nursing. In: *Images and Ideals: Opening Dialogue with the Humanities* (eds S.F. Spicker & S. Gadow), pp. 79–101. Springer, New York.

Gadow S. (1994) Whose body? Whose story? The question about narrative in women's health care. *Soundings,* 77(3–4), 295–307.

Holm S. (1997) *Ethical Problems in Clinical Practice.* Manchester University Press, Manchester.

Noddings N. (1984) *Caring: A Feminine Approach to Ethics and Moral Education.* University of California Press, Berkeley.

Peter E. & Liaschenko J. (2003) Whose morality is it anyway? Thoughts on the work of margaret urban walker. *Nursing Philosophy,* 4(3), 259–262.

Peter E. & Liaschenko J. (2004) Feminist ethics is not a subject matter. *8th International Philosophy of Nursing Conference,* 7–9 September, University of Swansea.

Storch J.L. (2004) Nursing ethics: a developing moral terrain. In: *Toward a Moral Horizon* (eds J.L. Storch, P. Rodney & R. Starzomski), pp. 1–16. Pearson Education Canada, Toronto.

Walker M. (1997) Picking up pieces, lives, stories, and integrity. In: *Feminists Rethink the Self* (ed. D.T. Meyers), pp. 62–84. Westview Press, Boulder, CO.

Walker M. (1998) *Moral Understandings.* Routledge, London.

Watson J. (1988) *Nursing: Human science and Human Care: A Theory of Nursing.* National League for Nursing, New York.

Yeo M. & Moorhouse A. (1996) *Concepts and Cases in Nursing Ethics.* Broadview Press, Ontario.

The Author Comments

A Pluralist View of Nursing Ethics

I have no nursing or medical qualifications whatsoever. My work in nursing and health care ethics is based on my philosophical education of course, but it also comes from my experience of life, illness, and death as a human being, a daughter, a lover. I have also spent many years listening to and working with nursing students and colleagues whose testimonies inspire me to work harder as a teacher and a writer. This chapter is based on an article that I delivered at the International Philosophy of Nursing Conference in Swansea in 2004, and it has benefited greatly from the feedback that I received from the workshop participants. I wrote the article because I truly believe that intellectual spaces must be forged to engage with what happens at the edges of life; what exceeds the dominant explanatory frameworks that are assumed to make sense of the world. When it comes to nursing theory, my article makes a very simple point: What is interesting about any account of what humans do, is what that account misses, excludes, or silences; that's why nursing perspectives need to be diverse, tentative, and situated.

—JOAN MCCARTHY

reasoning processes used in ethics. For the purpose of this column, the body of knowledge known as ethics will include theories, standards, and inquiry into what should comprise ethical behavior as well as study of how people actually behave and reason about ethical situations.

There is no agreement in the nursing literature as to the meaning of the term, *nursing ethics.* Unfortunately, many authors use the term without any explanation of definition or intended meaning. And of those who do articulate a conceptualization of what constitutes an ethic of nursing, no clear consensus emerges. For example, Bishop and Scudder (2001) state that "nursing ethics primarily concerns articulating the moral sense of nursing and appraising how it is fulfilled rather than applying ethical theories to nursing practice" (p. v). Whereas, Thomasma (1994) asserts "nursing ethics is about the primary healing relationship. It is essential for healing, and so are the ethical issues that arise from the task" (p. 91). Other descriptions of nursing ethics include moral decision-making and behaviors, ethical and values conflicts, beliefs about right and wrong behavior, and analysis of ethical issues that arise within nurses' practice. Yet, it is not clear whether such conceptualizations represent a phenomenon unique to nursing's professional domain. Presumably, a distinct nursing ethic should address unique theories, standards, and inquiry into what comprises nurses' ethical behavior and study of how nurses actually behave and reason about ethical issues. A review of the nursing ethics literature reveals four core themes that speak to the possibility of a distinct nursing ethic. These include the moral foundation of the nurse-patient relationship, the ethic of care, organizational and interdisciplinary relationships, and theories of nursing ethics.

The Moral Foundation of Nursing

Yarling and McElmurry (1986) argued that a unique nursing ethic must be embedded in the moral foundation of nursing. They concluded that, although nurses have numerous relationships and obligations to a variety of parties, the moral foundation of a nursing ethic must be that of an autonomous nurse-patient relationship. The primacy of this relationship is the fundamental basis of the nursing process and the "human quality of the patient's experience" (p. 65). They asserted, however, that nurses are constrained from advocating for patient interests (for example, behaving in an ethically responsible manner) due to overwhelming situational and sociopolitical constraints. They called for development of a distinct nursing ethic which is a social ethic aimed at social reform.

Yarling and McElmurry (1986) set a rather adversarial tone for interactions between nurses and their employers. Their argument perpetuates the helpless victim stance that some nurses use to excuse their reluctance to practice in compliance with state practice acts and professional standards, both of which clearly outline a focus on patient advocacy. True, most nurses practice within difficult institutional bureaucracies. But Yarling and McElmurry failed to recognize that institutional constraints are not unique to nurses. Physicians, social workers, and even housekeepers all answer to employers of sorts, whether they are hospitals, third party payers, managed care gatekeepers, and so on. Although the primacy the nurse-patient relationship *should* be at the core of nursing practice, it does not follow logically that engaging in social reform is at the heart of a unique nursing ethic.

Yarling and McElmurry's (1986) work became the target of a number of response articles in subsequent publications. Bishop and Scudder (1987) took a more conciliatory tone by shifting the moral focus away from the moral autonomy or independence of the nurse to the moral responsibility for patients via excellence in practice. They observed that all healthcare team members have the same moral commitment to patients, and that moral decisions in healthcare must be cooperative among all parties. Bishop and Scudder did not advocate for a distinct nursing ethic, but rather concluded that the moral foundation of nursing was excellence in patient care. Similarly, Packard and Ferrara (1988) also criticized Yarling and McElmurry for their emphasis on the political ideology of achieving autonomy as nursing's moral foundation. Instead, they suggested that nursing actions, nursing knowledge, and the desire to *serve the good* constitute moral foundation. Yet they also conceded that this foundation is still developing and evolving.

Others have questioned the relevance of traditional biomedical ethical frameworks that are based on the time-honored, core principles of justice, beneficence, non-maleficence, and respect for autonomy. Instead, the concept of a distinct nursing ethic based on the unique, moral foundation of the nurse-patient relationship is promoted. Moral concepts central to the nurse-patient relationship include advocacy (Gadow, 1980), integrity (ANA, 2001), and fidelity (Milton, 2002). Certainly these constitute important qualities that provide a moral substrate for implementing nursing actions. Yet, these concepts are important qualities for all healthcare providers and do not constitute a unique aspect of nursing practice.

The Ethic of Care

A second core theme in the nursing ethics literature is that of the ethic of care. Given the focus on the nurse-patient relationship as an essential feature of a nursing ethic, many nurses characterize the nature of this relationship as that of caring. The concept of an ethic of care in nursing is derived from the work of feminist philosopher, Carol Gilligan. In her classic work, *In a Different Voice,* Gilligan (1982) examined the process of moral development and reasoning, and influence of gender. She questioned prevailing thought that men and women resolve moral dilemmas by applying a detached, hierarchical set of rules and principles about what constitutes ethical behavior. Instead, she postulated that women use concern for relationship with others, contextual factors, and responsibilities toward others in addition to consideration of competing rules, rights, and principles. Gilligan observed that, when tested, women consistently did not score as highly as men in moral development studies due to concern about interpersonal and situational relationships. Given Gilligan's emphasis on gender differences and focus on caring and relational aspects of moral reasoning, her ideas have been embraced by many nurses.

Although Gilligan's (1982) work frequently is associated with the ethic of care, nurses have also looked to others as philosophical support for a caring paradigm of nursing. In an ethic of care, moral reasoning and behavior involves empathy, compassion, and connectedness; consideration of abstract ethical principles is secondary concern. Contextual factors and interpersonal relationships are key elements to understanding and resolving ethical dilemmas that occur in practice.

The literature is replete with assertions and assumptions that nursing is the practice of caring. As such, an ethic of care is a reasonable partner to guide nursing practice. Benner, Tanner, and Chesla (1996) asserted that ethical and clinical knowledge are inseparable; the dominant ethic in everyday practice is that of care. Thomasma (1994) suggested that nursing adopt an ethic of care, noting that nursing ethics should be "seen as a separate discipline [from medical ethics] with its own patterns of development" (p. 85). He proposed a new model of ethical decision-making that rejects the application of the traditional bioethical principles of beneficence, autonomy, nonmaleficence, and justice. Instead, he described a process of interpreting the patient's body, the spirit, the relation of body and spirit, and the patient's relationships with others. Similarly, Bishop and Scudder (2001) and many others have rejected the primacy of bioethical principles in ethical nursing practice and called for the adoption of an ethic of care.

The concept of a separate, distinct ethic of care is intuitively attractive to many nurses because it appeals to enduring, core values which underpin our practice. Principled ethical thinking is portrayed as cold, detached, and associated with the medical model of practice. Yet, promotion of a single model of ethical practice based on the caring paradigm may be misguided and even harmful to nurses. Pinch (1996) cautioned against the indiscriminate use of the ethic of care, citing that it could become a moral trap for nurses. She suggested that such traps could include continued oppression of nurses by encouraging self-sacrifice, self-denial, obedience, and burnout. Further, the concept of an ethic of care may be too vague to provide theoretical and practical guidance for clinical decision-making. For example, two very caring nurses could hold different opinions as to whether a patient is benefiting from artificial life support. Consideration of context and relationships may lead one nurse to argue that discontinuing support is a caring action based on an understanding that the patient is in irreversible, multi-system failure and physically suffering from the effects of burdensome medical interventions to sustain life. On the other hand, a second nurse might argue that the more caring action would be to continue life support because of family values about the sanctity of life. An ethic of care does not provide guidance as to how to solve this ethical conflict.

The debate about existence of a separate nursing ethic of care is further clouded by empirical work done to date. Studies of ethical practice in nursing tend to support whichever theoretical paradigm the researcher selects to guide the work. For example, Corley and Selig (1994) used a justice-oriented developmental framework to examine moral reasoning processes of critical care nurses. The framework consisted of a detached, hierarchical set of rules and principles to guide ethical decisions. They found that their subjects all used varying components of the framework to solve ethical problems. Conversely, Gaul (1995) used Gilligan's model to guide the study of ethical dilemmas in critical care and emergency nursing; she found that caring constituted a major component of her subjects' ethical reasoning process. Not surprisingly, studies that do not impose one or the other framework find that subjects reflected a mixture of justice and care moral orientations.

Does the ethic of care framework constitute a distinct ethic of nursing? That conclusion is not substantiated in the research literature as yet. Although caring represents a central feature of nursing practice, the profession must be cautious about claiming care as its unique domain. Patients would do well to have all healthcare providers who care, regardless of professional identity.

Organizational and Interdisciplinary Relationships

Organizational and interdisciplinary relationships have an impact on the ethical practice of nursing. A practice setting influences both the type of ethical issues a nurse encounters, and the way in which the nurse responds.

Because nurses are often employees within healthcare organizations, they confront ethical challenges associated with manipulating an unwieldy, bureaucratic system in order to obtain necessary services for patients. In an analysis of five studies of nurses' ethical issues and concerns, Redman and Fry (2000) observed that many study participants experienced ethical problems related to institutional or health policy constraints. Issues included deceptive documentation and billing practices as a response to nonreimbursable services, institutional reluctance to treat the uninsured, and incentives to increase revenue and keep costs down. But, as mentioned earlier, the hegemony of the healthcare system does not exclusively target nurses. All who provide healthcare struggle with the constraints imposed by organizational systems and structures.

Ethical issues do arise within the context of interdisciplinary relationships. Nurse-physician conflicts regarding patient care decisions are a significant source of ethical tension (Redman & Fry, 2000). Nursing has been characterized as an *in-between* role; that is, nurses function in between patients and physicians, and other healthcare providers (Bishop & Scudder, 2001). Unfortunately, conflict often arises due to nurse-physician conflict over the age-old care versus cure debate. Although nurses experience ethical conflict with physicians, this reality reflects differing professional goals and values, unilateral decision-making, gender inequity, and poor communication, as opposed to substantiating the existence of a separate ethic. To be sure, the quality of nurse-physician relationships remains a core concern for nurse recruitment and retention in healthcare facilities. However, such concern is better resolved by equipping nurses with skills in conflict management and communication.

Nursing Theory

Nurse ethicists have called for the development of a theory of nursing ethics that reflects nurses' unique moral experiences and guides the study of nurses' moral development. According to Fry (1989), such a theory should include consideration of the nature of the nurse-patient relationship, the healthcare context, the value of caring, and a moral view of persons (as opposed to moral behavior or action). Nurses have attempted to formulate ethical nursing theories and models. Most of these frameworks are ethical reasoning or decision-making models.

Ethical decision-making models for nurses are designed to guide behavior in the context of ethical dilemmas. Three models are reviewed as examples of the wide range frameworks suggested for nursing practice. Gadow (1980) proposed a framework for ethical decision-making based on the advocacy role of nurses to ensure patient autonomy. Gadow's prescriptive model morally aligns the nurse with the patient (as opposed to the family, physician, or healthcare institution) and outlines a process in which the nurse mediates between the patient's right to self-determination and other competing (and conflicting) interests. Fry (1994) outlined a four-step process for decision-making that includes examination of (a) the story and context of the ethical problem, (b) the significance of the values pertinent to problem, (c) the meaning of the conflict to involved individuals, and (d) potential solutions to the problem. Cameron's (2000) model of ethical decision-making is based on virtue ethics, characterized by the behaviors and attributes of a morally good person. The model consists of answering three questions: (a) What should I believe about my purpose in life, (b) who should I be in order to be a person of integrity, and (3) what should I do [about the ethical dilemma at hand]?

These models of ethical decision-making all include aspects of ethical reasoning processes experienced by nurses. Yet no model seems to represent or capture core constructs unique to an ethical nursing practice. A more useful model would include consideration of a range of ethical dilemmas, values of the nurse and the patient, the uniqueness of a specific nurse-patient relationship, the context in which the dilemma occurs, and a full spectrum of potential outcomes, including cognitive, affective, and behavioral possibilities.

Discussion

As previously stated, a unique nursing ethic would be expected to encompass unique theories, standards,

inquiry into what comprises nurses' ethical behavior, and study of how nurses actually behave and reason about ethical issues. Although much work has been completed in all of these areas, a unique nursing ethic has yet to emerge. The moral basis of the nurse-patient relationship is grounded in qualities desirable in all healthcare professionals. The ethic of care has not been substantiated as the nursing profession's exclusive domain. Similarly, healthcare professionals experience organizational and interdisciplinary ethical conflicts that arise from practicing in environments fraught with shrinking resources and conflicting values. Proposed theories of nursing ethics focus on components of ethical decision-making but do not move beyond that realm to address other aspects of the nursing profession.

To be sure, nurses must practice in an ethical manner. Although nurses bring their own values to the nurse-patient relationship and function in a wide variety of roles, society must be able to expect a certain standard of ethical behavior from all nurses. This standard is articulated in the ANA (2001) *Code of Ethics for Nurses* and other ANA position statements on ethical issues. Although use of the *Code* and position statements cannot solve all ethical nursing problems, they do provide direction for thoughtful consideration of *right behavior* in nursing practice. For example, the Code directs a nurse to support a patient's right to self-determination. This is a clear mandate to protect a patient's right to make informed decisions about treatment even if such decisions may be contrary to the nurse's sense of what may be best for a patient. Although the Code sets the standard for ethical behavior, it does not provide the theoretical basis for understanding the nature of ethical practice in nursing.

Although nurse scholars have yet to establish a unique nursing ethic, much work remains to further understanding of ethical practice in nursing. Ketefian (2001) recently completed a meta-analysis of 12 quantitative nursing ethics studies in order to examine relationships between education and moral reasoning to ethical practice. Although she found a positive relationship between education and ethical practice, Ketefian noted numerous challenges and questions that warrant further investigation. The meta-analysis included studies that focused on nurses' responses to hypothetical ethical dilemmas. Future work must include actual, *real life* behavior, consideration of other variables that may influence ethical behavior, and analysis of the many qualitative studies of ethical issues in nursing. Indeed, use of qualitative methods to collect and analyze stories of nurses' lived experience with ethical issues may be better suited to understanding the nature of ethical practice.

Noureddine (2001) and others have proposed an interesting alternative to development of a unique nursing ethic; that is, nurses' ethical issues and decision-making should be understood and supported via integration of ethics within nursing theories. Based on a review of nursing ethics and theory literature, Noureddine offered nine criteria for evaluating the ethical dimension of nursing theories. These criteria address articulation of values, duties, biases, rights, responsibilities, relevant ethical principles and codes, guidance for ethical practice, and the like. In essence, the criteria ask whether these factors are articulated and question whether there is congruence among the factors. Surely all nursing theories have an ethical basis. Yet, in order to evaluate such theories for utility in addressing nursing' ethical issues, a nurse first must have a strong working knowledge of ethical theory and concepts.

Unarguably, nursing is a moral act. The provision of nursing care is an inherently good service to society. But in the quest to identify the knowledge, theory, and practice that constitute nursing, some nurses may have confused the picture by claiming a unique knowledge, theory and practice that constitute nursing ethics. Instead of focusing on a search for a separate ethical turf, researchers should focus on expanding understanding of ethical issues in that occur in nursing. In the meantime, all nurses would better serve patients by fostering collaborative interdisciplinary relationships among all healthcare providers, teaching and role modeling the relational, caring behaviors which temper the technology of medicine, and developing expertise in a variety of ethical frameworks in order to respond to ethical issues in a thoughtful, reasoned fashion.

REFERENCES

American Nurses Association. (2001). *Code of ethics for nurses with interpretive statements.* Washington, DC: Author.

Beauchamp, T. L., & Childress, J. F. (2001). *Principles of biomedical ethics* (5th ed.). New York: Oxford University Press.

Benner, P., Tanner, C., & Chesla, C. (1996). *Expertise in nursing practice: Caring, clinical judgment, and ethics.* New York: Springer.

Bishop, A., & Scudder, J. (1987). Nursing ethics in an age of controversy. *Advances in Nursing Science, 9*(3), 34–43.

Bishop, A., & Scudder, J. (2001). *Nursing ethics: Therapeutic caring presence* (2nd ed.). Boston: Jones and Bartlett Publishers.

Cameron, M. (2000). An ethical perspective: Value, be, do: Guidelines for resolving ethical conflict. *Journal of Nursing Law, 6*(4), 15–24.

Corley, M., & Selig, P. (1994). Prevalence of principled thinking by critical care nurses. *Dimensions of Critical Care Nursing, 3,* 96–103.

Fry, S. T. (1989). Toward a theory of nursing ethics. *Advances in Nursing Science, 11*(4), 9–22.

Fry, S. T. (1994). *Ethics in nursing practice: A guide to ethical decision making.* Geneva: International Council of Nurses.

Gadow, S. (1980). A model for ethical decision making. *Oncology Nursing Forum, 7*(4), 44–47.

Gaul, A. (1995). Casuistry, care, compassion, and ethics data analysis. *Advances in Nursing Science, 17*(3), 47–57.

Gilligan, C. (1982). *In a different voice: Psychological theory and women's development.* Cambridge, MA: Harvard University Press.

Ketefian, S. (2001). The relationship of education and moral reasoning to ethical practice: A meta-analysis of quantitative studies. *Scholarly Inquiry for Nursing Practice, 15*(1), 3–23.

Milton, C. L. (2002). Ethical implications for acting faithfully in the nurse-patientrelationship. *Nursing Science Quarterly, 15,* 21–24.

Noureddine, S. (2001). Development of the ethical dimension in nursing theory. *International Journal of Nursing Practice, 7,* 2–7.

Packard, J. S., & Ferrara, M. (1988). In search of the moral foundation of nursing. *Advances in Nursing Science, 10*(4), 60–71.

Pinch, W. J. (1996). Is caring a moral trap? *Nursing Outlook, 44,* 84–88.

Redman, B., & Fry, S. (2000). Nurses' ethical conflicts: What is really known about them? *Nursing Ethics, 7*(4), 360–366.

Thomasma, D. C. (1994). Toward a new medical ethics: Implications for ethics in nursing. In P. Benner (Ed.), *Interpretive phenomenology: Embodiment, caring, and ethics in health and illness* (pp. 85–98). Thousand Oaks, CA: Sage.

Yarling, R., & McElmurry, B. J. (1986). The moral foundation of nursing. *Advances in Nursing Science, 8*(2), 63–73.

The Author Comments

Is There a Unique Nursing Ethic?

This article was written as a component of my doctoral qualifying exam at The University of Texas at Austin. As an oncology clinician with many years of experience in working with interdisciplinary health care teams, I questioned the relevance of creating a unique nursing ethic that sets our discipline apart. I believe that this article contributes to the evolution of nursing theory in the twenty-first century by pointing out the pitfalls of creating a separate framework or "turf" for nursing action in the context of complex ethical patient care issues. Such challenges require shared planning and close collaboration among interdisciplinary caregivers who share a common ethic that respects patient and family choice.

—DEBORAH LOWE VOLKER

Philosophic Views on Nursing and Its Practice

This unit focuses on the **ontology** of nursing, that is, the content, focus, or substance of theory development. This is in contrast to the *epistemology of nursing*, which focuses on the process, methods, or syntax of theory development. The authors of these articles put forth metaparadigmatic statements about nursing—how it is defined and what its unique focus is as a discipline. Others address the meaning of nursing in relation to practice, clients, praxis, art, and science.

May readers be inspired to develop and defend their own metaparadigmatic statements about nursing and then reflect on how these statements could influence their focus and methods in research and practice.

Questions for Discussion

- What is the substantive focus of theory development in nursing?

- How is this focus distinct from that in other disciplines? How is it similar?

- What, if any, are the differences in the knowledge that exists in nursing science, nursing practice, and nursing education?

- What is your own metaparadigmatic statement about nursing?

- How would your metaparadigmatic statement about nursing influence your focus and methods in research and practice?

CHAPTER 60

The Focus of the Discipline of Nursing

Margaret A. Newman
A. Marilyn Sime
Sheila A. Corcoran-Perry

The focus of nursing as a discipline has not been clearly defined but is emergent in the centrality of the concepts of caring and health. The authors propose a focus for nursing as a professional discipline in the form of a statement that identifies a domain of inquiry that reflects the social relevance and nature of its service. Several perspectives from which the focus can be studied are described. The authors assert that a unitary-transformative perspective is essential for the full explication of nursing knowledge.

A discipline is distinguished by a domain of inquiry that represents a shared belief among its members regarding its reason for being. A discipline can be identified by a focus statement in the form of a simple sentence that specifies the area of study. For example, physiology is the study of the function of living systems; sociology is the study of principles and processes governing human society.

A professional discipline, in addition, is defined by social relevance and value orientations.[1,2] The focus is derived from a belief and value system about the profession's social commitment, nature of its service, and area of responsibility for knowledge development. These requisites need expression in the focus statement. For example, medicine is the study of the diagnosis and treatment

Discussions in the School of Nursing Curriculum Coordinating Committee stimulated ideas for this article. The authors acknowledge the contributions of other members of the committee: Monica Bossenmaier, Dorothy Fairbanks, Carol Reese, Mariah Snyder, and Patricia Tomlinson. The authors also thank Ellen Egan and Kathleen Sodergren for manuscript critiques.

the discipline, and to examine the philosophic and scientific questions provoked by the focus statement.

Differing Paradigmatic Perspectives

What may appear to be confusing and inconsistent meanings of concepts in the proposed focus may actually be a reflection of the use of different paradigms for knowledge explication.[20,23] Nursing research has been conducted from an orientation consistent with at least two, and possibly three, paradigms. Each paradigm specifies a point of view from which the field of study is conceptualized, the assumptions that are inherent in that view, and the basis upon which knowledge claims are accepted. These differing paradigms reflect the shift in focus from physical to social to human science. The three perspectives extant in nursing literature could be described as: particulate-deterministic, interactiveintegrative, and unitary-transformative. To explain the effect of a paradigm on the development of nursing knowledge, each perspective will be addressed briefly.

From the particulate-deterministic perspective, phenomena can be viewed as isolatable, reducible entities having definable properties that can be measured. These entities have orderly and predictable connectedness to each other. Change is assumed to be a consequence of antecedent conditions—conditions that, if sufficiently identified and understood, could be used to predict and control change in the phenomena. Relationships within and among entities are viewed as linear and causal. Kinds of knowledge sought include facts and universal laws. Knowledge claims that cannot be refuted are admitted to the body of knowledge. From the perspective of this paradigm, caring in the human health experience could be studied by examining the concepts that comprise the focus. For example, caring could be isolated for study as a human trait having definable and measurable characteristics. Similarly, health could be reduced and dichotomized in terms of characteristics considered healthy versus those considered unhealthy. Caring also could be studied as a therapeutic intervention affecting patients' health in terms of measurable responses.[23]

From the interactive-integrative perspective (an extension of the particulate-deterministic perspective that takes into account context and experience and legitimized subjective data), phenomena are viewed as having multiple, interrelated parts in relation to a specific context. To explain a phenomenon, the interrelationships of parts and the influence of the context are taken into consideration. Thus, reality is assumed to be multidimensional and contextual. Change in a phenomenon is a function of multiple antecedent factors and probabilistic relationships. Relationships among phenomena may be reciprocal. Knowledge claims may be context dependent and relative. From this perspective, caring in the human health experience would be studied as interactive-integrative phenomena within specific contexts, but still with probabilistic predictability.

The unitary-transformative perspective represents a significant paradigm shift. From this perspective, a phenomenon is viewed as a unitary, self-organizing field embedded in a larger self-organizing field. It is identified by pattern and by interaction with the larger whole. There is interpenetration of fields within fields and diversity within a unified field. Change is unidirectional and unpredictable as systems move through stages of organization and disorganization to more complex organization. Knowledge is personal, involves pattern recognition, and is a function of both viewer and the phenomenon viewed. The subject matter includes thoughts, values, feelings, choices and purpose.[24] Inner reality depicts the reality of the whole. From this perspective, caring in the human health experience would be studied as a unitary-transformative process of mutuality and creative unfolding.

Relationship of Focus to Paradigmatic Perspective

The explication of knowledge relevant to caring in the human health experience is affected by the paradigmatic perspective. As described earlier, concepts in the focus statement could be isolated for study within the first two perspectives, while the unitary-transformative perspective requires the focus to be studied as an indivisible whole. For example, knowledge generated from the particulate-deterministic perspective includes behaviors that characterize caring, physiologic and psychologic aspects of human health, and acontextual rules that relate observable caring behaviors with measurable health outcomes. Examples of knowledge generated from the interactive-integrative perspective include the reciprocal nature of nurse-client interactions, culture-specific caring responses to life process events that are disruptive to health, and rules regarding the influence of specific caring behaviors on the health-related behaviors of particular groups of clients. Knowledge from a unitary-transformative perspective is more difficult to characterize. An example generated from this perspective might be an understanding of the synchrony and mutuality of nurse–client encounters that transcend the time and space limitations of a present situation.

Although multiple perspectives are appropriate for knowledge development in nursing, we are convinced that a unitary-transformative perspective is essential for full explication of the discipline. This position is consistent with a changing world view of the conduct of inquiry into human experience[25–27] and with other nurse scholars who recognize the value of a unitary perspective to nursing inquiry.[22,28–30] Insights from our research and practice reveal a rich and fertile glimpse into caring in the human health experience.

The focus of a professional discipline is an area of study defined by the profession's shared social and service commitment. We conclude that the focus of nursing is the study of caring in the human health experience. The explication of nursing knowledge based on this focus takes different forms depending on the perspective of the scientist. We conclude that a unitary perspective is essential for full elaboration of caring in the human health experience. A unified focus derived from the coalescing of theory on caring and health has the potential for claiming the shared vision of nursing.

REFERENCES

1. Johnson DE. Development of theory: A requisite for nursing as a primary health profession. *Nurs Res.* 1974;23(5):372–377.
2. Donaldson SK, Crowley DM. The discipline of nursing. *Nurs Outlook.* 1978;26(2):113–120.
3. Torres G, Yura H. *Today's Conceptual Framework: Its Relationship to the Curriculum Development Process.* New York, NY: National League for Nursing, 1974.
4. Fawcett J. The metaparadigm of nursing: Present status and future refinements. *Image.* 1984;16(3):84–87.
5. Newman MA. *Health as Expanding Consciousness.* St. Louis, Mo: Mosby, 1986.
6. Meleis AI. Being and becoming healthy: The core of nursing knowledge. *Nurs Sci Q.* 1990;3(3):107–114.
7. Pender NJ. *Health Promotion in Nursing Practice.* Norwalk, Conn: Appleton & Lange, 1987.
8. Newman MA. Health conceptualizations and related research. *Ann Rev Nurs Res.* 1991;9.
9. Leininger M, ed. *Care: The Essence of Nursing and Health.* Thorofare, NJ: Slack, 1984.
10. Watson J. *Nursing: The Philosophy and Science of Caring.* Boulder, Col: Colorado Associated University Press, 1985.
11. Benner P, Wrubel J. *The Primacy of Caring.* Menlo Park, Calif: Addison-Wesley, 1989.
12. Stevenson JS, Tripp-Reimer T, eds. *Knowledge About Care and Caring.* Proceedings of a Wingspread Conference, February 1–3, 1989. Kansas City, Mo: American Academy of Nursing, 1990.
13. Duffy ME, Pender NJ, eds. *Conceptual Issues in Health Promotion.* Proceedings of a Wingspread Conference, April 13–15, 1987. Indianapolis, In: Sigma Theta Tau, 1987.
14. *ANS.* 1981:3(2); 1984:6(3); 1988:11(1); 1990:12(2); 1990:13(1).
15. *Nurs Sci Q.* 1990:3(3).
16. Leininger M. Historic and epistemologic dimensions of care and caring with future directions. In: Stevenson JS, Tripp-Reimer T, eds. *Knowledge About Care and Caring.* Proceedings of a Wingspread Conference, February 1–3, 1989. Kansas City, Mo: American Academy of Nursing, 1990.
17. Watson MJ. New dimensions of human caring theory. *Nurs Sci Q.* 1988;1(4):175–181.
18. Benner P. *Nursing as a caring profession.* Presented at meeting of the American Academy of Nursing: October 16, 1988; Kansas City, MO.
19. Pender NJ. Expressing health through lifestyle patterns. *Nurs Sci Q.* 1990;3(3):115–122.
20. Newman MA. Nursing paradigms and realities. In: Chaska NL, ed. *The Nursing Profession: Turning Points.* St. Louis, Mo: Mosby, 1990.
21. Phillips JR. The different views of health. *Nurs Sci Q.* 1990;3(3):103–104.
22. Parse RR. *Man-Living-Health: A Theory of Nursing.* New York, NY: Wiley, 1981.
23. Morse JM, Solberg SM, Neander WL, Bottorff JL, Johnson JL. Concepts of caring and caring as a concept. *ANS.* 1990;13(1):1–14.
24. Manen MV. *Researching Lived Experience: Human Science for an Action Sensitive Pedagogy.* Albany, NY: State University of New York Press, 1990.
25. Bohm D. *Wholeness and the Implicate Order.* London, England: Routledge & Kegan Paul, 1980.
26. Prigogine I. Order through fluctuation: Self-organization and social system. In: Jantsch E, Waddington CH, eds.

Evolution and Consciousness. Reading, Mass: Addison-Wesley, 1976.

27. Briggs J, Peat FD. *Turbulent Mirror*. New York, NY: Harper & Row, 1989.

28. Rogers ME. *An Introduction to the Theoretical Basis of Nursing*. Philadelphia, Pa: FA Davis, 1970.

29. Munhall PL. Nursing philosophy and nursing research: In apposition or opposition? *Nurs Res*. 1982;31(3):176–177, 181.

30. Sarter B. Philosophical sources of nursing theory. *Nurs Sci Q*. 1988;1(2):52–59.

The Authors Comment

The Focus of the Discipline of Nursing

This article came about as I listened to the ongoing harangue of nursing scientists regarding the validity of different modes of research. The answer, I believed, was "all a matter of paradigm." Concurrently, colleagues at the University of Minnesota (Marilyn Sime and Sheila Corcoran-Perry) and I were involved in curriculum development and recognized that the focus and methods of the research of our faculty colleagues varied considerably. How could all these viewpoints be reconciled in nursing? Hence, this article emphasizes the different paradigms that prevailed in nursing and suggests an overarching focus to define the discipline.

—MARGARET A. NEWMAN
—A. MARILYN SIME
—SHEILA A. CORCORAN-PERRY

CHAPTER 61

An Ontological View of Advanced Practice Nursing

Cynthia Arslanian-Engoren
Frank D. Hicks
Ann L. Whall
Donna L. Algase

Identifying, developing, and incorporating nursing's unique ontological and epistemological perspective into advanced practice nursing practice places priority on delivering care based on research-derived knowledge. Without a clear distinction of our metatheoretical space, we risk blindly adopting the practice values of other disciplines, which may not necessarily reflect those of nursing. A lack of focus may lead current advanced practice nursing curricula and emerging doctorate of nursing practice programs to mirror the logical positivist paradigm and perspective of medicine. This article presents an ontological perspective for advanced practice nursing education, practice, and research.

The profession and discipline of nursing has struggled for decades to define and refine its disciplinary focus and unique contributions to health care. Although multiple theoretical perspectives exist to assist in guiding practitioners and scientists in their respective work, we continue to be hindered in fostering a unifying framework that is helpful to all of nursing's varied practition-ers. Across the globe, nurses are pursuing advanced education to keep up with the demands of an ever-expanding knowledge base and the omnipresent need for effective health care services. Graduate nursing education has been prevalent in the United States for more than 50 years. Yet, trends in nursing education in the US may not necessarily be headed toward an advancement

From Research and Theory for Nursing Practice, *19(4), Arslanian-Engoren C., Hicks F. D., Whall A. L., & Algase D. L. An ontological view of advanced practice nursing, pp. 3, 5–322. Copyright © 2005, Springer Publishing Company. Used with permission.*

About the Authors

CYNTHIA ARSLANIAN-ENGOREN was born and raised in Detroit, MI. She earned her BSN from Wayne State University in Detroit, MI; her MSN in adult health nursing as a clinical nurse secialist from the Medical College of Ohio, Toledo, OH; and her PhD in nursing from the University of Michigan. Currently, she is an Assistant Professor at the University of Michigan School of Nursing. Dr. Arslanian-Engoren's scholarship focuses on nurses cardiac triage decisions and the treatment-seeking decisions of women with symptoms suggestive of acute coronary syndromes.

FRANK D. HICKS was born and raised in Hammond, IN. He has a BSN from Indiana University and an MS and PhD in nursing science from the University of Illinois at Chicago, and he completed a 2-year postdoctoral fellowship at the University of Michigan School of Nursing. Currently, Dr. Hicks is Associate Professor of Adult Health and Director of Generalist (prelicensure) Education at Rush University College of Nursing. His scholarly foci are decision-making, self-management behaviors, and theory development. He enjoys cooking, reading, coffee, and his dog, Alex.

ANN L. WHALL is a native Michiganian and three-time graduate of Wayne State University in Detroit. She is an Advanced Nurse Practitioner in Michigan and was a Fulbright Distinguished Scholar in the United Kingdom, examining expert nurses' use of implicit memory in dementia care. The focus of her scholarship is gero-mental health, especially improving and/or maintaining the function of persons with dementia. Throughout her career, Dr. Whall has been "driven by the desire to explicate the depth and exquisite nature of nursing knowledge which has historically been unrecognized exterior to nursing." As a diploma graduate, she was denied admittance to graduate programs exterior to nursing on the basis of a belief that nursing was "manual art, not a science." Among her most significant accomplishments is recipient of the John A. Hartford Doris Schwartz Award in 2003 for "visionary and exemplary contributions advancing the field of gerontologic nursing research" and (ANA) Book of the Year awards for her theory development textbooks. Dr. Whall has published widely, held several visiting professorships, and completed multiple research studies and related publications, often with an identifiable emphasis upon the metatheoretical nature of nursing knowledge. Dr. Whall enjoys classical music, golfing, interacting with her three children, and developing international connections within nursing.

DONNA L. ALGASE is Professor in the School of Nursing, Director of the Center on Frail and Vulnerable Elders, and Faculty Associate in the Institute of Gerontology at the University of Michigan in Ann Arbor. She received a diploma from St. Vincent Hospital School of Nursing in Toledo, OH; her BSN from the University of Toledo; an MSN from the Medical College of Ohio at Toledo; and her PhD from Case Western Reserve University in Cleveland, OH. She is the editor of the outstanding journal, *Research and Theory for Nursing Practice.* Her scholarly work and research focus on behavioral issues in dementia and Alzheimer's disease, particularly wandering behavior, and therapeutic use of the environment. She also writes on complex measurement issues, observational methods, and theory development and testing. Dr. Algase has developed and published an instrument, the *Wayfinding Effectiveness Scale,* and on its use in the understanding and effective management of wandering behavior.

of nursing knowledge or nursing practice if these programs are based on a medical model that has as its main goal the transmission of medical knowledge. With the multiplicity of educational entrees to nursing at the graduate level, it is more crucial than ever to define the unique perspective of nursing and its relation to health care. The purpose of this article, therefore, is to explicate an ontological view of nursing that may be helpful to advanced practice nurses (APNs) and nurse scientists. Advances in developing nursing knowledge are synthesized into a coherent framework, and suggestions presented for nurses to incorporate into clinical practice.

The Case for a Disciplinary Focus

Identifying, developing, and incorporating nursing's unique ontological and epistemological perspective into APN practice places priority on delivering care based on knowledge derived from the disciplinary perspective of nursing. Moreover, practicing from a strong nursing perspective that is theoretically grounded and steeped in specialized knowledge assists our efforts to gain recognition and respect as a profession and an academic discipline. Without such grounding, the very future of the profession and discipline is at stake. It is imperative that APNs be able to delineate their unique contribution and perspective to health care delivery. For without a clear distinction of our meta-theoretical space, we risk blindly adopting the practices, views, and values of other disciplines (Whall, 2005), which may not necessarily reflect those of nursing. A lack of disciplinary focus may lead current APN curricula and emerging doctor of nursing practice (DNP) programs in the US to mirror the logical positivist, reductionistic paradigm and perspective of medicine.

Equally disturbing are national certifications that may embrace a medical focus, thus neglecting the nursing focus that should be inherent in APN programs. The question that must then be asked is: Does the current system of educating APNs mirror the focus of medicine (i.e., laboratory data interpretation, medication management, and medical diagnoses) or nursing? A review of such educational content should include an emphasis on nursing diagnoses, questions that address the meta-paradigm of nursing, and inquiries that address holistic,

patient-centered care. If national examinations for advanced practice nursing are limited in scope to medical phenomena of interest, these examinations will not reflect the essence or values of nursing. Failing to differentiate the practice of APNs compared to physicians and physician assistant colleagues further blurs the essential nursing core of disciplinary knowledge that should be inherent in any advanced nursing degree program. While diagnostic reasoning processes are essential to all health care professions, the questions, data, and clinical labels applied in these processes are specific to each profession and reflect knowledge generated through related research in the discipline.

Advanced Practice Nurses and Knowledge Development

By virtue of their education and experience, and the emphasis on holistic care and health promotion, APNs are in a prime position to provide affordable, expert, and efficient health care to diverse populations. Moreover, as clinical experts, APNs have a unique and significant part to play in advancing the development of nursing knowledge. Often believed to be the sole responsibility of academicians, clinical practice in essence is *the field* for knowledge development, for it is in the practice arena that nursing's phenomena of interest are encountered. Indeed, there is a largely untapped source of nursing knowledge embedded within nurses' daily practice (Benner, 1984; Benner, Tanner, & Chesla, 1996). By virtue of their exposure and participation in clinical nursing, APNs are in a prime position to add to and shape the body of nursing knowledge from a nursing perspective.

Knowledge development from a unique nursing perspective defines the boundaries of nursing and delineates the nature and application of nursing knowledge that explicates nurses' unique contribution to the health care team. Without this, nurses merely interpret what other disciplines have come to know. Without a unique and clearly articulated body of knowledge, nursing will never truly achieve the independence and stature of a profession. Thus, nursing practice will depend upon others to legitimate and guide it.

understood by society. The social contract between nursing and the public will be jeopardized and it will be difficult to ascertain the role of nurses as compared to other health care providers. Nursing has a service to offer that has been historically understood by society. Not recognizing this unique nursing perspective and philosophic view will jeopardize nursing existence. This perspective should underpin APN education, practice, and research.

APN Education

As specialty curricula are developed and implemented for the education of APNs and nurses with DNP degrees, ontological and epistemological perspectives necessary to actualize these roles must be carefully considered. While not negating the importance of natural, biological, organizational, and social science knowledge (e.g., pathophysiology, statistics, and psychology), commonly found within APN curricula, these alone do not provide the student with the advanced skills and knowledge necessary to deliver high-quality, advanced practice nursing. Indeed, many theoretical foundations shared with the medical discipline are used to prepare expert clinical practitioners. However, what distinguishes APNs from medical health care providers is the unique contribution of nursing's ways of knowing and holistic approach to the delivery of patient care. The clinical care provided by APNs focuses on the whole of a person's health and illness experiences (American Association of Colleges of Nursing, 1996). APN education, therefore, must focus on educating nurses to understand the essential nursing processes inherent in the human conditions, and teach students to analyze the relationship of complexity, integration, and well-being. The mission of advanced practice nursing, "to provide expert, quality, and comprehensive nursing care to clients" (American Nurses Association, 1996, p. 1) must be grounded in the ontological and epistemological perspectives of the nursing discipline and reflected in professional competencies unique to nursing's pattern of knowing (Vinson, 2000).

APN Practice

The clinical practice of APNs must actualize the values and beliefs inherent within the discipline of nursing.

Therefore, it is imperative that APNs who address the health care needs of patients do so from an advanced nursing perspective. APNs must not limit the focus of their care to just the differential medical diagnoses and prescribed pharmacological therapy. Instead, APNs must be mindful to include the integration of the family, the environment, and the human response to health and illness in the provision of health care, for this is what sets APNs apart from other health care professionals.

APNs must begin to reconceptualize their practice and endeavor to examine the multiplicity of patterns that evolve from the intersection of complexity, integration, and well-being. As such, the discernment of human health patterns may be able to capitalize on the existing nursing diagnosis taxonomy. Delineating and incorporating relevant nursing diagnoses into the plan of care illuminates the nursing component of APN practice. Firmly rooted in the epistemological and ontological values of the discipline, nursing diagnoses represent the essence of nursing; its focus, function, and future at an advanced practice level.

APN Research

Another available means to accentuate the nursing perspective within APN practice is through the utilization and generation of nursing research. Conceptual and philosophic consistency is obtained when scientists work under an overarching ontologic worldview. If nurse scientists and APNs both operated from this ontologic worldview, incorporating empirical knowledge with diverse ways of knowing, it would facilitate a richer and more holistic approach to patient care. Moreover, the application of nursing research to APN clinical practice anchors the delivery of care within a nursing perspective and communicates the value and importance of nursing investigations to clients, families, communities, and other health care professionals. The generation of nursing knowledge through scientific research advances the science of nursing from which APNs practice.

Conclusion

As the discipline of nursing continues to develop, the direction will be set by the philosophy and theories selected and the values espoused. To truly practice professional nursing at an advanced practice level requires a vast repertoire of skills coupled with a mastery of conceptual, empirical and clinical knowledge of nursing. Embracing a paradigmatic perspective that unifies the values of the discipline of nursing will advance the profession, direct clinical practice, and enhance our understanding. Ignoring the complexity of nursing phenomena will lead to an incomplete nursing science (Whall & Hicks, 2002) that fails to serve its members or the public's health care needs.

REFERENCES

American Association of Colleges of Nursing. (1996). *The essentials of master's education for advanced practice nursing.* Washington, DC: Author.

American Nurses Association. (1996). *Scope and standards of advanced practice registered nursing.* Washington, DC: Author.

Benner, P. A. (1984). *From novice to expert: Excellence and power in clinical nursing practice.* Menlo Park, CA: Addison-Wesley.

Benner, P. A., Tanner, C. A., & Chesla, C. A. (1996). *Expertise in nursing practice: Caring, clinical judgment and ethics.* New York: Springer Publishing Company.

King, I. M. (1971). *Toward a theory for nursing.* New York: Wiley.

King, I. M. (1995). The theory of goal attainment. In M. A. Frey & C. L. Seiloff (Eds.), *Advancing King's systems framework and theory of nursing* (pp. 23–33). Thousand Oaks, CA: Sage.

Neuman, B. (2002). *The Neuman systems model* (4th ed.). Upper Saddle River, NJ: Prentice Hall.

Nightingale, F. (1969). *Notes on nursing: What it is and what it is not.* New York: Dover Publications. (Original work published 1860)

Orem, D. E. (1991). *Nursing: Concepts of practice* (4th ed.). St. Louis: Mosby Year Book.

Parse, R. R. (1981). *Man-living-health: A theory of nursing.* New York: Wiley.

Parse, R. R. (1998). *The human becoming school of thought: A perspective for nurses and other health professionals.* Thousand Oaks, CA: Sage Publications.

Reed, P. G. (1997). Nursing: The ontology of the discipline. *Nursing Science Quarterly, 10*(2), 76–79.

Rogers, M. E. (1970). *An introduction to the theoretical basis of nursing.* Philadelphia: F. A. Davis. Rogers, M. E. (1990). Nursing: Science of unitary, irreducible human beings. Update 1990. In E. A. M. Barrett (Ed.), *Visions of Rogers' science-based nursing* (pp. 5–11). New York: National League for Nursing.

Roy, C. L. (1995). Developing nursing knowledge: Practice issues raised from four philosophical perspectives. *Nursing Science Quarterly, 8*(2), 79–85.

Vinson, J. A. (2000). Nursing's epistemology revisited in relation to professional educational competencies. *Journal of Professional Nursing, 16*(1), 39–46.

Watson, J. (1985). *Nursing: Human science and human care.* Norwalk, CT: Appleton-Century-Crofts.

Watson, J. (1995). Postmodernism and knowledge development in nursing. *Nursing Science Quarterly, 8*(2), 60–64.

Whall, A. L. (2005). "Lest we forget": An issue concerning the doctorate in nursing practice (DNP). *Nursing Outlook, 53,*1.

Whall, A., & Hicks, F. D. (2002). The unrecognized paradigm shift within nursing: Implications, problems, and possibilities. *Nursing Outlook, 50,* 72–76.

The Authors Comment

An Ontological View of Advanced Practice Nursing

The genesis of this article was a conversation between Drs. Arslanian-Engoren and Hicks about the lack of a nursing theoretical base in many Advanced Practice Nursing (APN) programs. From our years of studying and teaching nursing theory, we believed that there was a wealth of information to be gleaned from nursing theory. Our purpose in writing this article was to begin to explicate that belief and show that nursing theory has a place in APN. We were thrilled when Drs. Whall and Algase, mentors and supporters of nursing theory, agreed to assist us in writing this article. We hope that this article will serve as a resource and an inspiration for others who wish to emphasize nursing in APN.

—CYNTHIA ARSLANIAN-ENGOREN

—FRANK D. HICKS

—ANN L. WHALL

—DONNA L. ALGASE

CHAPTER 62

Nursing: The Ontology of the Discipline

Pamela G. Reed

The purpose of this article is to contribute to clarifying the ontology of the discipline by extending existing meanings of the term nursing to propose a substantive definition. In this definition, nursing is viewed as an inherent human process of well-being, manifested by complexity and integration in human systems. The nature of this process and theoretical implications of the new nursing are presented. Nurses are invited to continue the dialogue about the meaning of the term and explore the implications of nursing, substantively defined, for their practice and science.

Distinguishing the term *nursing* as a noun from its use as a verb was put forth most profoundly by Rogers (1970), whose vision extended the scholarship of earlier nursing theorists to thrust nursing forward to be recognized as both a scientific discipline as well as a professional practice. It is time, however, to push back the frontier once again, beyond these two important understandings of nursing, by proposing a new meaning of nursing. With this new meaning, the term itself represents the nature and substance of the discipline. In other words, *nursing* is the ontology of the discipline.

The ideas put forth here are done so in the spirit of accepting Watson's (1995) "postmodern challenge" to exploit the climate of deconstruction of nursing (see

About the Author

PAMELA G. REED is Professor at the University of Arizona College of Nursing in Tucson, where she also served as Associate Dean for Academic Affairs for 7 years. She is a three-time graduate of Wayne State University in Detroit, receiving a BSN in 1974, an MSN in 1976 (with a double major in child–adolescent psychiatric mental health nursing and teaching), and her PhD with a major in nursing, (focused on life-span development and aging) in 1982. Dr. Reed pioneered research into spirituality and well-being with her doctoral research with terminally ill patients. She also developed a theory of self-transcendence and two widely used research instruments, the *Spiritual Perspective Scale* and the *Self-Transcendence Scale*. Her publications and funded research reflect a dual scholarly focus: spirituality and other facilitators of well-being and decisions in end-of-life transitions, and nursing metatheory and knowledge development. Dr. Reed also enjoys time with her family, reading, classical music, swimming, and hiking in the mountains and canyons of Arizona.

Rampragus, 1995; Reed, 1995) to extend and, by some degree, reconstruct current understandings of nursing. Smith's (1988a) article outlined the ongoing dialogue about two meanings of nursing, as a verb and a noun. This dialogue is revisited here for the purpose of further clarifying what is the ontology of the discipline, long considered a crucial question by seminal thinkers in nursing (Ellis, 1982; Rogers, 1970; Roy, 1995).

Continuing the Dialogue: Nursing as a Process of Well-Being

It is proposed here that there exists a third and perhaps most basic definition of nursing in which nursing represents the *substantive* focus of the discipline. Disciplines are characterized by their substantive focus: archaeology is the study of the archaeo, or what is ancient and primitive; astronomy is the study of the astro, astronomical phenomena such as the motion and constitution of celestial bodies; biology is a branch of knowledge about biol, or living matter; chemistry deals with the processes and properties of chemical substances; physics is the study of physical properties and processes; psychology is the study of the psyche, referring to mental processes and activities associated with human behavior; and nursing, the discipline, is proposed here to be the study

of nursing processes of well-being, inherent among human systems.

This meaning of nursing, as an inherent process of well-being, derives in part from the root word, nurse, defined as a process of nourishing, of promoting the development or progress of something. The meaning also derives from synonyms of nurse meaning to heal, to foster, to sustain (Laird, 1971; *Webster's New Collegiate Dictionary,* 1979). These descriptions signify that nursing involves a process that is developmental, progressive, and sustaining, and by which well-being occurs.

The Inherent Nursing Process

The theme of human beings' inherent nursing processes as the substantive focus of the discipline is supported in nursing theorists' works from Nightingale in 1859, to the mid-20th century writings of Henderson, to the contemporary turn-of-the-century ideas of Schlotfeldt. Nightingale (1859/1969) wrote about the person's "innate power" and the inner "reparative process." Henderson (1964) eloquently symbolized the power of the nurse within, describing nursing as "the consciousness of the unconscious, the love of life of the suicidal, . . . the eyes of the newly blind, a means of locomotion for the infant, . . . the voice for those too weak or withdrawn to speak" (p. 63). Watson (1985) referred to "self-healing processes," and Schlotfeldt (1994) stressed human beings' "inherent ability and propensity to seek and attain health." In addition, this nursing process is not necessarily based upon a reversal of a disease process, but more upon a moving forward, to gain a sense of well-being in the absence or presence of disease.

The discipline's understanding of how a nursing process is manifested is shifting away from the mid-20th century mechanistic conception of nursing as a process external to patients and conducted by the nurse, that is, the old nursing process. The process of nursing is viewed now more from a relational perspective, congruent with contextual and transformative conceptions of the world (see Newman, 1992; Pepper, 1942). Nursing is a participatory process that transcends the boundary between patient and nurse and derives from a valuing of what Rogers (1980, 1992) described as human systems' inherent propensity for "innovation and creative change."

"Human systems" refers to an individual or a group of human beings (Rogers, 1992, p. 30). As such, human systems, whether in the form of individuals, dyads, groups, or communities, emanate and participate in nursing processes. Nursing processes may be manifested, for example, in the grieving that an individual experiences, in the caring that occurs among people and their families and nurses, in the healing practices shared by a culture, or in many other as yet undiscovered patterns of nursing. Today, these patterns may be described as intentional or unconscious, automatic or contemplative, relational or chemical, or simply unknown. Nevertheless, with continued nursing research, education, and practice, nursing processes can be learned and knowingly deployed to facilitate well-being. Murphy's (1992) visionary book, for example, addresses some of these possibilities. He proposes a future wherein people are more aware of their innate healing potential and employ it to more purposefully enhance health.

Nightingale did not invent nursing, described here in terms of an inherent propensity for well-being. Just as earthquakes existed before geologists and photosynthesis before botanists, nursing processes existed in human beings, ultimately described by Nightingale (1859/1969) as that which nurses were to facilitate by placing the patient in the best situation possible. It follows, then, that nursing does not belong exclusively to certain groups of people, such as "well" persons or professional nurses; it belongs to human nature.

Defining the substance of the discipline of nursing in terms of a well-being process inherent among human beings does not negate the importance of knowledge of factors that interface with nursing to influence well-being and healing. Examples of these factors, often the focus of study in ancillary professions and disciplines, include the environmental, financial, cultural, surgical, and pharmacological. However, any sense of well-being involves, most basically, a nursing process. The quest for nursing is to understand the nature of and to facilitate nursing processes in diverse contexts of health experiences.

The Nature of Nursing Processes

What is the nature of nursing processes that distinguishes them from other human processes? It is proposed that the intersection of at least three characteristics—complexity, integration, well-being—distinguishes human processes as nursing; specifically, nursing processes are manifested by changes in complexity and integration that generate well-being. Importantly, other distinguishing characteristics of nursing processes may be identified as the dialogue continues beyond this article.

This new understanding of the nature of nursing processes derived from various theorists' work, such as von Bertalanffy's (1981) systems view of human beings; Rogers' (1970, 1992) science of unitary human beings; Lerner's (1986) developmental contextualism; and complexity theory (see Kauffman, 1995; Waldrop, 1992). While the translation of these theorists' ideas may not be entirely congruent with those presented here, their ideas nonetheless can help inform development of a new nursing ontology.

Human beings are viewed as open, living systems and not as passive but intrinsically active and innovative. As an open system, human systems are capable of self-organizing, where *self* refers to the system as a whole. Self-organization is an inherent capacity for generating qualitative change out of ongoing events in the life of a system and its environment.

In his seminal work on development, Werner (1957) explained this process of qualitative change as his "orthogenetic principle," which posits that living organisms change over time from lower to higher levels of differentiation and integration. Werner (1957) called this change "development," in contrast to mechanistic processes of change, which are not developmental.

Similarly, Rogers' (1980) principles of homeodynamics describe the inherent innovative patterning of change that occurs in open systems, both environmental and human. Her three principles of helicy, resonancy, and integrality together depict the nature of qualitative change in human beings in terms of ongoing movement from lower to higher levels of diversity.

Complexity theorists (for example, Kauffman, 1995; Waldrop, 1992), and developmentalists (for example, Lerner, 1986; Werner, 1957) in particular have clarified a distinction between quantitative and qualitative change, both of which are necessary for development; contrasting terms such as complexity and order, and differentiation and organization, depict this distinction. Similarly, two distinct forms of change can be identified in Rogers' (1980, 1992) works, namely diversity and innovation (Reed, 1997).

Because of the articulation between quantitative and qualitative change, human systems are not simply complex systems (SCS) but rather are complex innovative systems (CIS) (see Stites, 1994). In the context of nursing, then, nursing processes entail at least two forms of change, complexity and integration.

Complexity. Complexity refers to the number of different types of variables that can be identified in a given situation. A variable is simply something that varies (*Webster's,* 1979). Complexity occurs when human systems experience or express variables (for example, life events, physiologic events) as parts, separated from the whole, rather than as patterns of the whole. So, for example, complexity is evident when loss of a loved one or chronic illness introduces many new and seemingly disconnected variables into an individual's life, on various levels of awareness. Increasing complexity means change

in quantity (size or number) not change in quality of the whole; this would become chaotic were it not accompanied by corresponding changes in integration.

Integration. Integration refers to a synthesizing and organizing of variables such that there is a change in form, not just change in size or number of events. A certain level of complexity is needed for integration to occur. Integration is evident, for example, when people construct meaning or identify a pattern in the variables or events experienced. Integration may also occur on levels of awareness that are not yet so readily apparent. Integration is trans*form*ative, involving qualitative change in form.

Well-Being

While changes in complexity and integration may be used to explain many facets of human development and systems' changes, this process may also be used to understand health, healing, and well-being. The rhythm between complexity and integration is proposed here to be a means by which innovative change occurs, as a manifestation of the underlying process called nursing. Thus, well-being may be explained in part by changes in complexity that are tempered by changes in integration. Complexity provides life with diversity, specialization, and depth in experiences, whereas integration provides organization, coherence, and breadth.

Examples of nursing processes are abundant. For example, groups incorporate new attachments or children into an organization called family. Persons with spinal cord injuries develop different pathways that link together shattered parts of life and bodily functions. Premature infants' behaviors become more innovative as they organize the complexity of their environment. Adults reminisce to integrate past life events and inevitable death. Healing after the loss of a loved one or the occurrence of chronic illness requires an integration of what seem like disjointed events and experiences, including memories of the past, future dreams, altered rhythms and routines, physical pain and other bodily symptoms, sadness, anguish, and self-doubt. Further, Sachs (1995) depicted what can be called nursing processes, through his stories about people with various maladies, such as a colorblind painter and a surgeon with Tourette's syndrome. These people were able to create a new organization that fit with their altered needs and world. These health events, in all their initial complexity and heartbreak, gave way to metamorphoses and innovation. Regardless of whether there is a "cure" that can reverse a particular ailment, well-being occurs when the particulars of a life experience are brought together and synthesized in a coherent way. Any less, and people risk feeling dis-integrated, dis-associated, dis-organized.

While the centrality of well-being as a focus in nursing has been established, other disciplines also may be concerned with well-being and its correlates. However, promoting well-being based upon a perspective of the inherent process of complexity and integration is distinctly nursing.

Challenging the Status Quo: Nursing Reconstructed

The definition of nursing proposed here is that of an inherent process of well-being, characterized by manifestations of complexity and integration in human systems. The substantive focus of the discipline, then, is not how *nurses* per se facilitate well-being but, rather, how *nursing processes* function in human systems to facilitate well-being. The focus is, in a very basic sense, how nurses can facilitate nursing.

Refocusing the Lens

This new construction of nursing provides another lens of focus for nursing researchers and practitioners. Smith (1988b) wrote metaphorically about three different camera lenses used to view human wholeness. One in particular, the motion lens, focuses on process and rhythmic flow, and requires a "creative leap" to identify this process. Nurses typically encounter people in motion, in dynamic flow with their environment, whether in life-threatening experiences or perceived memory loss, chronic illness or acute pain.

The creative leap necessary for formulating the motion lens of nursing inquiry may be to address the rhythmic processes of complexity and integration that enhance well-being across these health experiences. From premature infants to dying adults and their families and communities, it is proposed that human systems have nursing processes, that is, inherent resources for well-being based on a capacity to integrate their complexities.

Debates on holism and on what represents the critical focus of nursing may be enlivened by including a new ontology of nursing—an ontology that transcends debates about part versus whole, person versus environment. Nursing processes are not necessarily bound by dimensions such as biologic, environmental, or social. Instead, the lens is focused on any human process that manifests complexity and integration related to well-being. Looking through this new lens, researchers and practitioners may identify a myriad of human manifestations of wholeness, whether they be labeled physiologic, phylogenic, or philosophic, that are integral to well-being.

Nursing as a Metaparadigm Concept

Given this reconstructed view of nursing, as a substantive focus of the discipline, the term *nursing* should be a central concept in the nursing metaparadigm. In the past, for good reason, some have suggested the elimination of the term nursing from the metaparadigm (Conway, 1985). However, rather than remove the term nursing from the metaparadigm, this fin-de-siècle may be the time in nursing history to consider renaming the discipline to something other than a verb, to better distinguish the disciplinary label from the substantive focus of the science and practice.

To help clarify this distinction, a term such as Paterson and Zderad's (1976) "nursology," or another disciplinary label with the "nurs" prefix could be developed, while reserving the term nursing as the *process* word and verb that it is, for the metaparadigm. By identifying nursing as a substantive, metaparadigm concept, nurses can better claim their unique focus and clarify the ontology of their discipline.

Approaching the Frontier

Rogers (1992) explained that one could not push back the frontier of knowledge until one approached it. This article has not been about maintaining the status quo, but about approaching a frontier so that others might join in a dialogue that pushes back the frontier a bit more. In this era of healthcare reform, the discipline must define nursing as nurses truly envision it and not necessarily as others would have it be defined. Nurses may decide against renaming the discipline as was suggested here. Nevertheless, within a broadened and partially reconstructed view of the discipline that embraces nursing at its most fundamental meaning, new understandings that blend with the old can emerge to present a fuller picture of the discipline.

Nursing (as practice and praxis) is a way of doing that creates good actions that facilitate well-being. Nursing (as syntax and science) is a way of knowing that creates goods in the form of knowledge. And nursing (the substance and ontology) is a way of being that creates patterns of changing complexity and integration experienced as well-being in human systems.

Nurses are invited to try on the substantive definition of nursing to see how it fits within the context of their practice and science. Ongoing philosophic dialogue about the ontology of the discipline will help ensure that nurse theorists are theorists of nursing in its fullest sense, and likewise, that nurse researchers are researchers of nursing, and nurse practitioners are practitioners of nursing.

REFERENCES

Conway, M. E. (1985). Toward greater specificity in defining nursing's metaparadigm. *Advances in Nursing Science, 7*(4), 73–81.

Ellis, R. (1982). Conceptual issues in nursing. *Nursing Outlook, 30*(7), 406–410.

Henderson, V. (1964). The nature of nursing. *American Journal of Nursing, 64*(8), 62–68.

Kauffman, S. (1995). *At home in the universe: The search for laws of self-organization and complexity*. New York: Oxford University Press.

Laird, C. (1971). *Webster's new world thesaurus* (rev. ed.). New York: Simon and Schuster.

Lerner, R. M. (1986). *Concepts and theories of human development* (2nd ed.). New York: Random House.

Murphy, M. (1992). *The future of the body: Explorations into the further evolution of human nature*. New York: J. P. Tarcher.

Newman, M. (1992). Prevailing paradigms in nursing. *Nursing Outlook, 40*, 10–13.

Nightingale, F. (1969). *Notes on nursing: What it is and what it is not*. New York: Dover (Original work published 1859)

Paterson, J. G., & Zderad, L. T. (1976). *Humanistic nursing*. New York: Wiley.

Pepper, S. P. (1942). *World hypotheses: A study in evidence*. Berkeley: University of California Press.

Rampragus, V. (1995). *The deconstruction of nursing*. Brookfield, VT: Ashgate.

Reed, P. G. (1995). A treatise on nursing knowledge development for the 21st century: Beyond postmodernism. *Advances in Nursing Science, 17*(3), 70–84.

Reed, P. G. (1997). The place of transcendence in nursing's science of unitary human beings. In M. Madrid (Ed.), *Patterns of Rogerian knowing* (pp. 187–196). New York: National League for Nursing Press.

Rogers, M. E. (1970). *Introduction to the theoretical basis of nursing*. Philadelphia: F. A. Davis.

Rogers, M. E. (1980). A science of unitary man. In J. P. Riehl & C. Roy (Eds.), *Conceptual models for nursing practice* (2nd ed., pp. 329–337). New York: Appleton-Century-Crofts.

Rogers, M. E. (1992). Nursing science and the space age. *Nursing Science Quarterly, 5*, 27–34.

Roy, C. L. (1995). Developing nursing knowledge: Practice issues raised from four philosophical perspectives. *Nursing Science Quarterly, 8*, 79–85.

Sachs, O. (1995). *An anthropologist on Mars: Seven paradoxical tales*. New York: A. Knopf.

Schlotfeldt, R. (1994). Resolving opposing viewpoints: Is it desirable? Is it practicable? In J. F. Kikuchi & H. Simmons (Eds.), *Developing a philosophy of nursing* (pp. 67–74). Thousand Oaks: Sage.

Smith, M. J. (1988a). Nursing: What's in a name? *Nursing Science Quarterly, 1*, 142–143.

Smith, M. J. (1988b). Perspectives of wholeness: The lens makes a difference. *Nursing Science Quarterly, 1*, 94–95.

Stites, J. (1994). Complexity research on complex systems and complex adaptive systems. *Omni, 16*(8), 42–50.

von Bertalanffy, L. (1981). *A systems view of man* (P. A. LaViolette, Ed.). Boulder: Westview Press.

Waldrop, M. M. (1992). *Complexity: The emerging science at the edge of order and chaos*. New York: Simon and Schuster.

Watson, J. (1985). *Nursing: Human science and human care*. Norwalk, CT: Appleton-Century-Crofts.

Watson, J. (1995). Postmodernism and knowledge development in nursing. *Nursing Science Quarterly, 8*, 60–64.

Webster's new collegiate dictionary. (1979). Springfield, MA: G. & C. Merriam Co.

Werner, H. (1957). The concept of development from a comparative and organismic point of view. In D. B. Harris (Ed.), *The concept of development* (pp. 125–148). Minneapolis: University of Minnesota Press.

The Author Comments

Nursing: The Ontology of the Discipline

The focus of this article is based on an epiphany I had when preparing a presentation for the 1993 National Forum on Doctoral Education. It struck me that nursing is so much more than we typically assume it to be—more than the practice we observe by people called "nurses" and more than a disciplinary body of knowledge. I proposed that nursing is a basic human process of healing that has evolved within and among human beings. This substantive focus (ie, ontology) of the discipline extends beyond the cell or the human field. Like any natural processes (eg, biologic or geologic) that define a disciplinary focus, understanding nursing processes requires the attention of educated practitioners and researchers who can study, appreciate, and facilitate nursing for human betterment.

—PAMELA G. REED

CHAPTER 63

Nursing as Normative Praxis

Colin Holmes

Philip Warelow

The purpose of this paper is twofold. First, it introduces a variety of concepts of 'praxis,' and argues in support of those which reflect the normative dimension of the critical social perspective. This begins with the Aristotelian concept, and moves through a variety of sources, including Hannah Arendt and Paulo Freire, but focuses primarily, and uniquely in the nursing literature, upon the work of the Yugoslavian 'praxis Marxists'. Second, specific ways of conceiving nursing as praxis are outlined, including political, aesthetic and ethical forms which have immediate import for nurses. The paper concludes with brief suggestions as to how these ways of conceiving praxis may be used by nurses to develop a more intimate and productive understanding of their own practices.

A number of authors have suggested that nursing can usefully be conceived as constituting a form of praxis (Holmes, 1992; Bent, 1993; Holmes, 1993; Rolfe, 1993; Lutz, et al. 1997; Thorne and Hayes, 1997; Warelow, 1997; Penney and Warelow, 1999). In this paper we explore the value of conceiving nursing as a form of praxis, undertaking some groundwork about what this may entail, and in particular trying to elucidate the part played by praxis in relation to nursing ethics. Many types of ethical viewpoint are 'normative'; that is, they are predicated on a particular view as to how a person should lead their life. In the case of praxis, the normative

About the Authors

COLIN ADRIAN HOLMES was born in Southampton, England, trained as a psychiatric nurse in 1972, and subsequently specialized in working in secure environments. He moved to Australia in 1989, and, in 1997, Dr. Holmes was appointed Foundation Clinical Professor of Nursing (Mental Health) at the University of Western Sydney. He is currently Professor of Nursing at James Cook University, Townsville, Queensland, and an Honorary Visiting Professor at the University of Central Lancashire, England. In addition to nursing and teaching qualifications, he holds an honors degree in psychology and philosophy, a research master's degree in history, and a PhD in nursing ethics. His research interests center on the care of mentally ill offenders, the history of psychiatry, and ethical and philosophic issues in health care. Dr. Holmes is married, with two adult children, and his hobbies include philately, the music of the 1920s and 1930s, and collecting materials relevant to the history of psychiatry.

PHILIP JOHN WARELOW was born in Kingston upon Hull, Yorkshire, England, but has lived for many years in Geelong, Victoria, Australia, where he works as a Lecturer in nursing, teaching undergraduate and postgraduate courses at Deakin University. He holds qualifications in psychiatric and general nursing and is currently undertaking a PhD through James Cook University, Townsville. His main area of scholarly interest is caring and how it may be conceptualized as nursing comes to grips with emerging intellectual, sociopolitical, and cultural challenges. Dr. Warelow cherishes lighthearted times with his family and friends, enjoys sports and fishing, and generally promoting the Australian value of giving people "a fair go."

element is the claim that human beings should become 'beings of praxis'. For this perspective, praxis can be seen as a standard of excellence, an ideal ethical goal for which to strive; it is also what Marxists would describe as an attempt to make an irrational world more rational, or a way of making useable sense of one's practice world.

Normative ethics is founded upon questions concerning how a person ought to live, what a person may or may not do, and especially how to define what constitutes a 'good life'. During the twentieth century, as a concomitant to the development of linguistic methods of philosophical analysis, this question gave way to a concern for the meaning and nature of ethical statements. Since the mid-1970s, however, normative ethics has gradually re-emerged as an important topic of political and ethical debate, focusing on problems arising from new technology and increasing public awareness of social injustices. More particularly, recent popular critiques of a whole range of social policies and practices by peace campaigners, advertising watchdogs, civil rights movements, governmental inquiries and so on has meant that the meta-ethics of philosophical analysis has become largely an irrelevance for all but the professional philosopher. The question 'what ought we to do?' has once again become one of the central questions of political and moral philosophy. It is not, however, simply a restatement of the classical debate: unlike previous generations, we are today faced with options that have the power to transform the world in all its aspects; and, at personal, social and global levels, the question of the good life is resurrected in a new and awesome way. Not surprisingly, the normative basis of personal and political decision-making is therefore under intensive scrutiny.

The guidance afforded to policy-makers by the broad objectives of traditional political ideologies has been outstripped by the variety of choices with which they are faced, and we discern a widespread acknowledgement that neither conservatism, liberalism, nor utopianism constitute an amalgam of politico-ethical principles adequate to the demands of modern political decision-making. Decisions as to the extent and nature of social, technological, political, and ecological change generate an increasing need for a normative social philosophy, which goes beyond traditional political ideologies. The need for a normative basis to political action has thus intensified considerably since Marx made the first attempts to construct a truly theoretico-practical political philosophy in the mid-nineteenth century, his political stance being based on a desire to eschew abstract theorisation in favour of applied philosophy, in accord with his famous observation that philosophers had hitherto only tried to describe the world, whereas the point was to change it.

There are three strands to the response of Marxists to these developments: critique of the present, a vision of the future, and a means by which theory and practice may unite in the realisation of that vision. First, it insists that before we consider the future, we must ask what exactly we find unsatisfactory about present conditions. This has led to Marxist critiques of just about every aspect of modern life, aiming to expose the pervasiveness of oppressive social processes, and to relate these to the material conditions of life. Second, Marxism offers a vision of a better form of society, in which inequalities and injustices are transcended by an egalitarian socialism within which each individual may find personal fulfilment. Third, it avoids the charge of utopianism or philosophical abstraction by making political practice inherent in its theory, and this is the notion of 'praxis.'

How might this notion of 'praxis' be useful as a means of conceiving the work of nurses? We may reasonably say that praxis is theory and practice in an intimate relationship, and this sounds promising as a way of describing nursing. The exact nature of that relationship is surprisingly elusive, however, and a number of interpretations are offered in the nursing literature (Warelow, 1997; Penney and Warelow, 1999). Nursing has not generally been sensitive to the distinctions on which these alternatives are based, however; nor to the social-political theories from which they have emerged (Holmes, 1992). Working through these shades of meaning will, we believe, lead us to a notion that may be

of the utmost importance to our understanding of our practice as nurses. Carr and Kemmis (1986) promoted a concept of praxis as informed action, which, by reflection on its character and consequences, reflexively changes the knowledge base that informs it. We suggest here that the more humanistic elements that many nurses advocate in their daily practice such as those of 'caring,' 'doing good,' and being guided by unwritten moral rules, are all nursing dispositions that contribute to praxis. They all encourage nurses to act truly and justly, incorporate the ideal of doing the right thing by others, notably patients, and are an essential element of being a theoretico-practical person or a 'being of praxis.' In this paper, praxis entails thought and action, or theory and practice, operating in a dialectical and complementary relationship.

On the Relationship Between Theory and Practice

Aristotelian Praxis

Views as to the relationship between theory and practice have a long history, centring on the unifying concept of praxis. In vernacular Greek, praxis was the action of free men in contrast to that of slaves. Indeed, Aristotle conceived praxis as constituting the moral and political life of the free man, made possible through a kind of disciplined knowing (practical knowledge or prudential judgment) called phronesis. It excluded the manual activities of slaves, and the domestic activities of women, which were considered basic activities of daily living. Aristotle also distinguished it from poesis, the production of artefacts, using techne or craftsman's skills. For Aristotle, praxis was citizenship itself, and the outcome was irrelevant: the good is in the exercise of praxis itself. Good actions (eupraxia) are those performed in accordance with phronesis, or good judgment, and praxis comes a strong second to theoria as the ultimate good. Theoria (theoretical knowing) is the supreme good because it transcends humanity through the pursuit of those things, which are unchanging and divine, whereas praxis is concerned with the moral and political organisation of the state/polis. We could say, then, that the contrast is between abstract knowledge (knowing) and concrete applications (doing).

Hannah Arendt

This Aristotelian notion of praxis was revived and developed by Hannah Arendt (1958) in *The human condition*, where she distinguishes between the contemplative life and the active life, and describes three varieties of the latter: labour, work and action (i.e., praxis). Labour produces the necessities of life; work produces artefacts, which transcend bodily requirements; and praxis seeks to solve the problem of meaninglessness generated by the instrumentality of labour and work by engaging in activities that are good in themselves. Praxis for Arendt is thus a means of confirming the humanity and uniqueness of the actor in relation to others. According to Crocker (1983), one of our distinctively modern dilemmas is that the pre-eminence of action in the Greek polis has been replaced by the superiority of labouring in a society of jobholders and consumers, and the opportunity to engage in true praxis has suffered accordingly.

Marx's Notion of Praxis

In *The German ideology* Marx refers to material praxis and social praxis, and some theorists have identified these with his notion of the labour process described in *Das Kapital*. Such labour is both biological, because it is the means to physical sustenance, and instrumental, in that it results in a product. It may be either unalienated, or (as at present) alienated. Although the Frankfurtian critical theorists, such as Marcuse and Habermas, make an advance on this notion of praxis as productive labour and as practical activity, they posit a relatively value-neutral concept, which refers to a 'normal' human mode of being. From their perspective, praxis is not the interaction with, or fashioning, an ordinary object but the generation of 'object domains'. This operates on the basis of two quasi-transcendental, 'knowledge-constitutive' cognitive interests: the technical and the practical, which result in two different types of science, the empirical-analytic and the hermeneutic, respectively. Technical interests are associated with pur-

posive-rational action of which there are two forms—instrumental action and strategic action. Instrumental action occurs when a person employs rules in order to achieve some desired, predicted state of affairs or goals. Strategic action involves a rational choice on the basis of information and values. The aim is not to control reality but to make a rational decision. Practical interests require a different form of praxis; this time aimed at securing personal identity and shared understandings. This is what Habermas (1972) calls 'communicative action,' and in a modern technocratic society it has tended to disappear under the weight of technical interests evidenced in the pervasive influence of positivism in the humanities and social sciences.

Praxis as Transformative Reflective Action: Freire

Freire's (1972, 1973) conception of praxis draws from the work of Lukács on the task of explaining to the people their own action, from Mao Tse Tung on antidialogical action, and from the humanistic Marxism of the Yugoslavian philosopher, Petrovic. For Freire, praxis is characterised by certain fundamental types of relation between persons, their actions, and the world, and Grundy (1987) describes it as the act of reflectively constructing or reconstructing the social world. Authentic praxis must involve both action and reflection, and a dialectical relationship between subjectivity and objectivity which is achieved through what Freire calls 'conscientisation,' or learning to perceive social, political, and economic contradictions, and the taking of action against the oppressive elements of reality as outlined by Ramos (Freire, 1972, p. 15), thereby changing the status quo.

Praxis is generally described by Freire as neither action nor reflection, but rather their synergistic combination in the human mind and body. Indeed, Freire (1973, p. 111) has gone so far as to say that men (sic) 'are praxis.' He is not entirely consistent concerning the epistemological status of his notion of praxis, however, and also says, for example, that 'men's activity consists of both action and reflection: it is praxis' (Freire, 1972, 96). Nevertheless, he is clear that praxis is a combination of reflection and action and that this combination may take the form of dialogue. Dialogue in which action is sacrificed is simply empty verbalism, he suggests, and dialogue in which reflection is sacrificed is blind activism; true dialogue only occurs when action and reflection are in combination. For Freire, therefore, to utter a true word is to engage in both action and reflection, i.e., praxis, and therefore to transform the world. Freire insists that there can be no dialogue without humility, love of life, or faith in one's fellow human beings. Dialogue is the motor force of social change, i.e., of revolutionary action, and such revolutionary praxis must stand opposed to the praxis of the dominant elites, for they are by nature antithetical.

Yugoslavian 'Praxis Marxism'

The humanistic Marxists in the former Yugoslavia, the 'Praxis Marxists,' most notably Markovic (1974a, 1974b) and Stojanovic (1981), tried to establish a normative concept of praxis in which their theory of the good life is combined with the epistemological and transformative concept described by Freire. They insist that the good life is achievable through human beings becoming 'beings of *praxis.*' The norm of praxis represents on one hand a standard for individual excellence, and on the other an axiological principle for social critique of present formations and possible futures. The principle that the optimal society is a praxis society, reflects this dual focus on the individual and the community, arguing that a praxis society promotes lived praxis rather than alienation, and creates structures and institutions which maximally exemplify communitarian principles, such as freedom, equality and justice.

The Marxist doctrine of the unity of theory and practice, which is basic to the concept of praxis, is understood by these writers in three ways, each embodying the notion that theory is the passive reflection of economic practice. First, for good or ill, theory directly influences human action. Second, social theory seeks to influence social behaviour: thus, Habermas, for example, has the practical intention that his theory play an emancipatory role enabling the surpassing of existing social formations, while for Markovic and Stojanovic,

the whole point of theory is to make an irrational world more rational. Third, the theorist's task is a dialectical one, not only deriving philosophical principles from life, but also raising life to the level of philosophical principles. In order to be what Crocker (1983, p. 29) calls a 'theoretico-practical being,' the theorist must practice his/her theory, and this is what we take to exemplify the meaning of the term 'praxis.'

For Markovic and Stojanovic, praxis is an ideal human activity because it realises in action one's best latent and actual dispositions, among which Markovic counts intentionality, self-determination, creativity, sociality, and rationality. It involves the realisation of some human potentials at the expense of others, and thus requires a valuing of some human qualities above others. It is 'ideal human activity . . . in which [wo]man realises the optimal potentialities of his[her] being, and which is therefore an end in itself' (Markovic, 1974a, p. 64). Markovic suggests that this ideal may be realised in a whole range of activities which Aristotle or Arendt would have excluded, such as domestic, intellectual and artistic activity, and therefore the concept does not elevate one particular aspect of life over others. It does exclude 'alienating activity' and value-neutral work, which are depicted as antipraxis. Markovic and Stojanovic both regard 'alienation' as occurring when others have control over one's work and creations, and as characteristically involving activities that are aimless, routine, and irrational, that lead to estrangement from others, and detract from the realisation of one's own optimal potentialities (Crocker, 1983, pp. 57–58). Value-neutral activity is equivalent to Marx's concept of labour as the means of survival: whilst it need not be alienating, it can never be praxis because it is purely instrumental. When one's work is also enjoyed for its intrinsic qualities, then it is regarded as praxis, but then it ceases to be defined by its qualities as work and is defined by its qualities as leisure or some other type of praxis. In other words, work can include praxis, but is never itself praxis. Markovic himself seems to regard work as morally neutral, in contrast to praxis, which is a moral ideal. It should be noted that, although it is normative and aspires to certain 'ideals,' praxis Marxism purports not to be

order to meet the normative standards of praxis, nurses must first critically reflect upon their practice in order to elaborate the implicit and often complex theories and attitudes, by which it is established, developed and sustained. It takes a considerable amount of effort, integrity, self-discipline and courage to work out anything which comes close to a comprehensive picture since, quite apart from the psychological difficulties involved, clearly, nursing's technical, aesthetic, ethical, communicative and other caring elements are linguistically differentiated, diverse and difficult to pin down. Second, nurses would need to critically reflect upon their feelings and beliefs about these linguistically differentiated elements, revising them in the light of the associated discourses, and bring this reflection to bear upon their nursing practices. Were they not to refer to the associated discourses, their reflections would be purely solipsistic, without regard for the experience and wisdom of others, thereby depriving nurses individually and collectively of a means for the realisation of their potential and subsequent improvements in nursing practice.

As we noted previously, praxis may take the form of dialogue, and by uttering true words and engaging in genuinely theoretico-practical actions—that is, by becoming beings of praxis—we transform the world of nursing, for ourselves, other nurses and patients, now and in the future, because we inevitably challenge dominant elites and demonstrate effective liberating alternatives. To paraphrase Freire, from a normative perspective, 'nurses are praxis,' actualising the full wealth of their best potential capacities, encompassing their distinctive talents and skills and engaging an emancipatory position in which they challenge received ways of thinking, feeling and practising. An approach to nursing based on the notion of praxis could thus take its cue from Freire's work.

One way in which nursing can be seen as constituting a form of praxis has been intimated by Holmes (1992), who introduces the notion of nursing as 'aesthetic praxis,' in which the performance of the task of nursing is viewed as an art form, combining practice skills, knowledge and values. The focus is on nursing as a skilled 'performance' along the lines described in Goffman's (1961) theory of 'dramaturgy,' but embodying the principles of a critical theory concept of praxis, as described above. Holmes refers to this performance as 'aesthetic praxis' and suggests that it represents 'a powerful form of self-expression, which has the potential to become liberating for the nurse and the patient' (Holmes, 1992, p. 941). A rather different approach, arguing that aesthetics and praxis offer alternative ways of conceiving practice, has been the subject of some interesting exchanges (De Raeve, 1998; Edwards, 1998; Van Hooft et al., 1998).

Another way of conceiving nursing as praxis is in terms of its normative or ethical dimension, which we have emphasised in our preceding outline, and praxis has indeed been linked by some scholars to concepts of nursing as caring (Owen-Mills, 1995; Thorne and Hayes, 1997; Bent, 1999). We wish merely to emphasise here how nursing can simultaneously embody both clinical expertise and ethical beliefs in ways that are liberating and authenticating, and constitute a form of 'ethical praxis.' A nurse who exercises his/her clinical skills without them being linked to a set of ethical principles would be like a sophisticated machine, practising without caring, making judgments without concern for their ethical assumptions or consequences. In reality, nurses always practice from a set of more or less consciously structured ethical principles, usually involving such notions as duty, rights, goodness, and caring. In ethical praxis, clinical expertise embodies these principles and become a vehicle for their expression and fulfillment. Clinical nursing practice sets the nurse ethicist apart from the nurse practitioner, the latter being both a practitioner and an ethicist, engaged in the reflexive dialectic that is ethical praxis. Taking this argument one step further, Warelow (1997) argues that using reflection and developing self-determination allows nurses who have previously functioned as objects in their practice worlds, to transform themselves into pro-active participatory subjects who then challenge the status quo. Street (1991) depicts this as a journey, suggesting that praxis and/or reflection should include the past and the future in the present, and contain a journey inward and outwards. The 'inner journey' uncovers our values, feelings, language (or 'discourse'), embodiment and ontology, whilst the 'outward' trip involves challenging our findings with an alternative perspective and consequently revising the situation as an emancipatory opportunity.

Conclusion

On its own, this paper sits inert and useless; it will take the imagination and responsiveness of particular readers to incorporate it into a transformatory process. To do this is to take the first steps along that path by which to realise the main objective of the nurse-scholar (to become a theoretico-practical being), and of the nurse practitioner (to become a practico-theoretical being). As we are referring to normative ideals, it is a matter of making progress toward these states, and we all can be located somewhere along the path. Our aim in this paper has been to alert readers to particular windows of opportunity offered under the normative nature and structure of praxis.

REFERENCES

Arendt H. 1958. *The human condition.* University of Chicago Press: Chicago.

Bent KN. 1993. Perspectives on critical and feminist theory in developing nursing praxis. *Journal of Professional Nursing 9*: 296–303.

Bent KN. 1999. The ecologies of community caring. *Advances in Nursing Science 21*: 29–36.

Carr W and S Kemmis. *Becoming critical: Knowing through action research,* 2nd edn. Geelong, Victoria: Deakin University Press.

Crocker D. 1983. *Praxis and democratic socialism: The critical social theory of markovic and stojanovic.* Atlantic Highlands, New Jersey: Humanities Press.

De Raeve L. 1998. The art of nursing: Aesthetics or praxis? *Nursing Ethics 5*: 401–11.

Edwards SD. 1998. The art of nursing. *Nursing Ethics 5*: 393–400.

Freire P. 1972. *Pedagogy of the oppressed.* Harmondsworth: Penguin.

Freire P. 1973. *Education for critical consciousness.* New York: Continuum.

Goffman E. 1961. *Encounters.* Indianapolis: Bobbs-Merrill.

Grundy S. 1987. *Curriculum: Product or praxis?* London: Falmer Press.

Habermas J. 1972. *Knowledge and human interests.* Boston: Beacon Press.

Holmes CA. 1992. The drama of nursing. *Journal of Advanced Nursing 17*: 941–50.

Holmes CA. 1993. Praxis: a case study in the depoliticization of a concept in nursing research. *Scholarly Inquiry for Nursing Practice 7*: 3–12.

Lutz KF, KD Jones and J Kendall. 1997. Expanding the praxis debate: contributions to clinical inquiry. *Advances in Nursing Research 20*: 23–31.

Markovic M. 1974a. *From affluence to praxis: Philosophy and social criticism.* Ann Arbour: University of Michigan Press.

Markovic M. 1974b. *The contemporary Marx: Essays on humanist communism.* European Socialist Thought series no. 3. Nottingham: Spokesman Books.

Owen-Mills V. 1995. A synthesis of caring praxis and critical social theory in an emancipatory curriculum. *Journal of Advanced Nursing 21*: 1191–5.

Penney W and P Warelow. 1999. Understanding the prattle of praxis. *Nursing Inquiry 6*: 259–68.

Rolfe G. 1993. Closing the theory-practice gap: A model of nursing praxis. *Journal of Clinical Nursing 2*: 173–7.

Stojanovic S. 1981. *In search of democracy in socialism: History and party consciousness.* Buffalo, NY: Prometheus Press.

Street A. 1991. *From image to action: Reflection in nursing practice.* Geelong, Victoria: Deakin University Press.

Thorne SE and VE Hayes, eds. 1997. *Nursing praxis: Knowledge and action.* Thousand Oaks, CA: Sage.

Van Hooft S, L De Raeve and P Nortvedt. 1998. The art of nursing: aesthetics or praxis? A response to Steven Edwards. *Nursing Ethics 5*: 545–52.

Warelow P. 1997. A nursing journey through discursive praxis. *Journal of Advanced Nursing 26*: 1020–7.

The Authors Comment

Nursing as Normative Praxis

In this article, we tried to encapsulate our long-held beliefs about the nature of nursing and the need to conceive it within a broad sociopolitical framework that can successfully depict a constructive relationship between theory, practice, and values. Although its idealism will find little sympathy among postmodernists, we believe that praxis is a realistic ideal that challenges orthodox accounts of nursing's value orientation and offers a useful way to bring that to bear on issues of theory and practice. We especially like the praxis approach because it suggests ways in which personal and communitarian ethics can be reconciled within a general account of action. We hope that others will take up the challenge and explore praxis as a framework within which to theorize aspects of the discipline of nursing.

—Colin Adrian Holmes
—Philip John Warelow

An Integrative Framework for Conceptualizing Clients: A Proposal for a Nursing Perspective in the New Century

Hesook Suzie Kim

It is exciting to view the year 2000 as the beginning for a new century and a new millennium that can be based on a new resolve and a refreshing insight. In thinking and reflecting about what aspects of nursing and nursing knowledge development that should be the focus for formulating such a new resolve or a refreshing insight, pluralism comes to mind as one of the critical issues that is both important and troublesome. Nursing has pursued multiple paths to develop knowledge with different commitments to philosophies and epistemological orientations during the past three decades. The resulting pluralism is evident not only in philosophical orientations regarding human nature and nursing, but also in theories, scientific explanations, and methods of inquiry adopted in nursing science.

During the past three decades we have put a great deal of our scientific effort into developing nursing knowledge in terms of (a) conceptualizing the key and essential phenomena of concern, (b) identifying the nature of nursing problems and different ways of solving such problems, (c) understanding fundamental human processes associated with health and illness through development of multiple theories, (d) identifying the impact of environment on human functioning and health, and (e) advancing technical supports that enhance human health. These efforts have resulted in truly pluralistic knowledge development in nursing in terms of theories, empirical findings, and practical approaches, along with differences in philosophical and

From H. S. Kim, Nursing Science Quarterly, *13(1): 37–44. Copyright © 2000 SAGE Publications.*
Reprinted with permission by SAGE Publications, Inc.

About the Author

HESOOK SUZIE KIM was born in Korea and came to the United States as an undergraduate student at Indiana University. She received a BS in nursing and an MS in nursing education from Indiana University and an MA and a PhD in sociology from Brown University. She has been in Rhode Island since 1964 and was a faculty member at the University of Rhode Island College of Nursing since 1973, and is now Professor Emerita there. Her scholarly work has focused on metatheoretical questions in nursing, and she considers her two books, *The Nature of Theoretical Thinking in Nursing* (2nd edition published in 2000) and *Nursing Theories: Conceptual and Philosophical Foundations* (edited with Ingrid Kollak, published in 1999), to be her major contributions to the discipline. Her empirical research has been on nursing practice issues from the cross-national perspective, including research on collaboration, pain assessment, clinical decision making, and the nature of nursing practice carried out in Finland, Japan, Korea, Norway, the United States, and Sweden. She reads (Günter Grass is her favorite author), listens to jazz, plays golf, and skis for sheer enjoyment and relaxation.

value orientations. A rich array of scientific results has provided the foundation to move nursing practice to be grounded in scientific knowledge. On the other hand, multiple theories, conflicting findings, and competing approaches to patient care have created confusion as well as a heightened sense of separation and schism between science and practice in nursing.

One of the most critical aspects of such pluralism is in regard to theories and conceptualizations about phenomena in the client domain. Client domain, identified as one of the four domains of nursing's subject matter (Kim, 1987), refers to the key area of nursing's concern for knowledge development. There has been a longstanding presumption that through the understanding and explanation about client phenomena, nursing could develop its approaches, that is, therapeutics and strategies of care regarding clients' problems. The conceptual works of early nurse scholars helped to shift nursing's orientation from medicine and pathologies to human needs. In the ensuing decades, the relevance of these frameworks as a basis for the practice of nursing became apparent, and a series of grand theories concerned with the knowledge domain of the client were proposed and studied.

Rogers's (1970, 1992) science of unitary human beings, Roy's (Roy & Andrews, 1997) adaptation model, Orem's (1995) self-care model, Neuman's (1995) systems model, and Parse's (1998) theory of human becoming are the major grand frameworks in nursing that try to formulaté and explain client domain phenomena from generalized conceptualizations of humanity and health. These and related nursing models can be categorized into six major types according to their views on humanity and health: (a) holistic processes as the modes through which humans coexist within their environment, (b) balance as the essential human characteristic that expresses human condition, (c) configuration of structural and functional aspects as an integrative basis for human functioning, (d) aggregation of parts as revealing states of the human condition, (e) experiencing as the basic form of human existence, and (f) meaning-making as the essential feature of human life.

This categorization suggests that in nursing there is diversity in the way clients and client phenomena are conceptualized and that there is no generally endorsed unified perspective regarding humans. It would be quite premature to state that nursing has firmly established specific paradigms or schools of thought based on these differing conceptualizations of humans and grand theories. However, these grand theories persist as the bases for empirical work and research, middle-range theory development, nursing curricula, and nursing practice models. In addition, knowledge development in nursing regarding client phenomena, particularly during the past decade, has also been rich and active not only in association with nursing's grand theories but in relation to general theoretical orientations such as biobehavioral, cognitive, psychosocial, and phenomenological frameworks. Multiple paradigmatic orientations are certainly in place in nursing and are viewed to be viable and necessary aspects of nursing knowledge development and practice (Gortner, 1993; Nagle & Mitchell, 1991).

Nevertheless, there are differing philosophical positions regarding this apparent pluralism in nursing. Many scholars seem to adhere to the notion that it is both acceptable and to some degree necessary to have multiple conceptualizations of persons and different grand theories in nursing. Others argue that for multiple paradigms and grand theories to be viable as the basis for scientific knowledge development, it is necessary to have a unifying perspective that provides the focus of the nursing discipline. It is from this second position that I propose a revisioning for the knowledge domain of client as necessary to establish firmly the unique focus of nursing in the larger context of healthcare. The conceptualization of the client domain as human living is presented as both a unifying perspective and a unique focus for nursing in the new century.

Human Living as a Metaparadigm Concept

From the 1960s and throughout the ensuing decades, nursing's focus has been to meet patients' needs related to maintaining health or to assist individuals in their responses to health and illness. As stated in the American Nurses' Association's (1980) first social policy statements, nursing is defined as "the diagnosis and treatment of human responses to actual or potential health problems" (p. 9). This view places an emphasis on clients' problems that are specified as *reactions* and *concerns* attendant with health problems. These widely accepted orientations have firmly grounded nursing to focus on states of clients, rather than on clients as humans. These client states are not only specified in the languages of the grand theories but also in the works of nursing diagnoses classifications and other concept

developments such as deficiencies, deficits, adaptation/maladaptation, balance/imbalance, homeostasis, or disturbances. Such seemingly unwitting focus on states of clients also has led nursing to view time as a discrete entity tied to states of responses and occurrences, rather than as a continuum in terms of history and trajectories, and in so doing has imposed an artificial interruption in connected human experience.

Furthermore, I believe this orientation and its subsequent developments have resulted in overemphasis on technical treatment of patients' problems, thereby shadowing the essential nursing philosophy of client care. Consequently, either by design or under pressure, professional nursing began handing over the care of certain states of clients traditionally associated with nursing to other healthcare workers and assistive healthcare personnel, while taking on tasks and responsibilities of other client states that were formerly within the professional domain of physicians. Often this reshaping of nursing's realm of responsibilities, which is usually considered unsatisfactory to us, has been attributed to political and economic pressures within the dynamics of the healthcare system. However, as Kitson (1997) states, it may also have resulted from nursing's "ineptitude and lack of appreciating what matters to us" (p. 114).

Hence, the heart of the matter is in articulating clearly what the essential and central focus of nursing is, so that it becomes the guiding post not only for knowledge development but also for nursing practice. It is not satisfactory just to say that nursing contributes to patient outcomes differently from medicine and other healthcare professionals, or to say that nursing is oriented to the promotion of health and to the care of people in illness. It is this ambiguity that needs to be addressed to avoid continued diffusion of nursing's unique contribution to healthcare. Therefore, I propose human living as the revisioning orientation of the knowledge domain of client for nursing in the new century. By orienting its mission to clients' living rather than limiting its focus to clients' states, nursing can clarify its distinctive role within the community of healthcare providers, formulate client-centered outcomes that are uniquely related to its knowledge-based practice, and ensure public recognition of its distinctive professional contribution in healthcare.

Dimensions of the Human Living Concept

Although I believe that as a profession nursing has been always concerned with clients' living, I do not believe that it has been articulated clearly as the central focus of the discipline. The following discussion is aimed at achieving this necessary articulation. Human beings are biological and symbolic entities entrusted with bodies, selves, and histories, intertwined to carry on living by continuing, responding to happenings, appropriating and accommodating, and controlling. The concept of human living is based on ontological assumptions that accept humanness in terms of its biology, personhood, and sociality. And living as it is embedded in situations cannot be clearly viewed or fully understood out of context. Given these assumptions of biology, personhood, sociality, and context, human living constitutes three dimensions—living of oneself, living with others, and living in situations—which are coalesced through integration and intersection. These three dimensions are not partitioned sectors of living or even different aspects of living, but are integrative orientations that make human living what it is.

The essential features of humanness that frame human living are body and personhood as aspects of human selves. A human body entrusted with its appearance, makeup, concreteness, and boundedness is, to begin with, biological. But this human entity is also existential, because it exists only through what is experienced in time and space. Furthermore, a human body can be considered as a vehicle through which humans are social beings, capable of symbolizing and interacting. Thus, a human body or entity is both biological/materialistic and symbolic/cultural. On the other hand, personhood is a specification of symbolic self constructed through reflexivity, consciousness, and meaning-making, which are uniquely human qualities. Hence, human living of oneself refers to body and personhood intricately connected and mediated to project

the nature of living that is uniquely human. For example, eating as one particular form of human living is not simply an act of getting food but is an act having specific personal meanings and modes of operation established through personal, social, and cultural habits and desires. Living of oneself, then, is oriented to aspects of one's life related to rhythms, intactness and appearance, capacities and limitations, body feelings and sensations, history and genealogy, desires and wants, dreams and hopes, ideas and opinions, choices, habits, and knowing. For a nursing perspective, living of oneself has a specific meaning in terms of how clients' living needs to be supported and/or guided when it is constrained by various sorts of health-related threats to the integrity of body and personhood or to the modes of living itself.

The second dimension, human living with others, is based on the sociality of humans and refers to communality of human existence. Living with others (i.e., with family, friends, colleagues, neighbors, countrymen, and citizens of the world—both intimates and strangers) involves coexisting, communicating, coordinating, exchanging, and interacting as human selves, sometimes by choice and design and other times through accidents or force, both natural and instrumental. Living with others pertains to relating one's instrumental, symbolic, and affective needs with those of others, and to making connections with others for sharing humanness. Living with others is intrinsically tied to living of oneself, in that for one to live of oneself, it is necessary instrumentally to live with others in specific ways. From the nursing perspective, living with others may be viewed to have potential for being constrained or needing to be arranged differently because of clients' health status or healthcare experiences.

Living in situations refers to the idea that living takes place in contexts and that modes of living are adjusted and modified to address contextual requirements of human existence. Situations of living may vary from ordinary life situations such as family, work, and community settings to more specialized situations such as hospitals or prisons. Situations also can be considered to be stable and continuous over time, or to be transient and changing. Living in situations involves responding to, accommodating and adapting to, managing of, engaging in, and choosing and creating contexts of one's existence. From the nursing perspective, living in situations raises questions regarding clients' relationships with their environment and accommodations or variations necessary in clients' living that are necessary, inescapable, or desirable because of situational contingencies accompanying health problems or healthcare.

Relevance for Theory and Practice

Focusing on human living as nursing's orientation gives a possibility to articulate nursing's unique contribution in healthcare. I believe nursing's orientation to human responses and conditions arising from actual or potential health problems, and resulting formulations in many of nursing's grand theories that emphasize clients' states, have limited the scope of that contribution. Revisioning nursing's focus emerges from shifting an attention on states to an attention on living, especially in response to the outcomes-based culture of healthcare practice. Nursing's concern with client outcomes, then, can focus on, for example, how well the client is living in this situation of healthcare, how the client is progressing with his or her living throughout this episode of care, how well the client is managing his or her living in the context of given health-related threats or problems, or with what sorts of continuity or alignment the client is carrying on his or her living. Nursing is primarily concerned with helping people to live as well as they can, whether they are experiencing acute episodes of illness or trauma, chronic disease trajectories, transient or persisting disabilities, or terminal illness. Nursing is also concerned with helping people to live as well as they can as they engage in anticipated developmental human living experiences such as giving birth, aging, and dying. Diagnosing and treating conditions, difficulties, and disturbances must not be an end in themselves but must be oriented to supporting and helping clients to find ways of living through these experiences—ways of living more creatively, more wisely, more meaningfully, and with more personal control.

The human living concept, elaborated in this way as a unifying focus for the discipline, is metaparadigmatic and hence is not tied to any specific theoretical formulation. Extant nursing theories and conceptualizations regarding clients and client phenomena, therefore, need to be reframed in relation to human living as an essential metaparadigm concept and knowledge domain in nursing. For many decades, nurse scholars have considered health, person, environment, and nursing as the essential metaparadigm concepts for nursing (Fawcett, 1984; Yura & Torres, 1975). However, as concepts these are so nonspecific that they have not been used to identify a distinctive nursing focus as a discipline and an area of study. Human living as an explication of the metaparadigm concept concerned with client and client phenomena can stipulate nursing to be concerned primarily not with health problems such as diseases, illness, or disability but with living in the context of health problems and healthcare. As shown in Figure 64-1, human living as a metaparadigm concept can embrace many theoretical concepts and phenomena of clients, which can be elaborated in terms of specific theoretical orientations.

Explanations and understanding about human responses, behaviors, processes, functioning, and subjectivity can thus be formulated, developed, and empirically examined from various theoretical orientations, such as from different grand theories of nursing as well as other theoretical frameworks. When such theoretical frameworks are interpreted within nursing practice, it would be necessary to frame nursing therapeutics in terms of the three dimensions of human living, considering it as an essential metaparadigm concept of nursing. For example, the phenomenon of being diagnosed with a chronic disease such as diabetes can be examined from various theoretical perspectives (adaptation, cognitive, or phenomenological). Ultimately, any theoretical explanation about this phenomenon must address possible ways of helping individuals who are diagnosed with chronic disease. At this point, the question of what nursing can do and needs to do for such clients must be framed in regard to human living in terms of living of oneself, living with others, and living in situations. This orientation means that nursing will focus on client outcomes

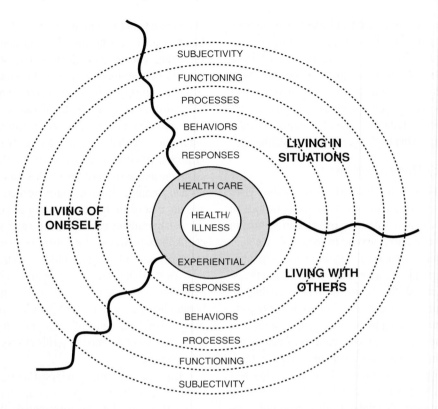

Figure 64-1   *Three dimensions of human living as a metaparadigm concept in nursing.*

of its practice in terms of promoting quality in human living that is understood as it is experienced—continuous, transitional, and trajectorial.

Conclusions

In this exposition, I have suggested that it is necessary to reposition nursing's focus within healthcare and uphold human living as its primary orientation. I have argued from the perspective of a pluralistic approach that allows for multiple paradigms and theories in nursing that is grounded in a unifying focus in the metaparadigm domain of client. Human living has been explained as a three-dimensional integrative dynamic of biology, personhood, and sociality. This unifying focus on human living provides a new, fresh image of nursing that can redefine and direct our role within healthcare in the emerging century. The

vision it gives us is a vitalized sense of mission for nursing, through which nursing can uniquely contribute to the lives of its clients. During the past decades, nursing has established a firm alliance with the culture of science and technology, which is primarily oriented to controlling health problems. Without diminishing our involvement in the scientific problem-solving traditions, we can renew our commitment to a human-practice perspective through a unifying disciplinary focus that orients our practice to helping clients in their living within the context of health and healthcare in the new century.

REFERENCES

American Nurses Association. (1980). *Nursing: A social policy statement.* Kansas City, MO: Author.

Fawcett, J. (1984). The metaparadigm of nursing: Present status and future refinements. *Image: Journal of Nursing Scholarship,* *16,* 84–87.

Gortner, S. R. (1993). Nursing's syntax revisited: A critique of philosophies said to influence nursing theories. *International Journal of Nursing Studies, 30,* 477–488.

Kim, H. S. (1987). Structuring the nursing knowledge system: A typology of four domains. *Scholarly Inquiry for Nursing Practice: An International Journal, 1,* 111–114.

Kitson, A. L. (1997). Johns Hopkins Address: Does nursing have a future? *Image: Journal of Nursing Scholarship, 29,* 111–115.

Nagle, L. M., & Mitchell, G. J. (1991). Theoretic diversity: Evolving paradigmatic issues in research and practice. *Advances in Nursing Science, 14,* 17–25.

Neuman, B. (1995). *The Neuman systems model* (3rd ed.). Norwalk, CT: Appleton & Lange.

Orem, D. (1995). *Nursing: Concepts of practice* (5th ed.). St. Louis, MO: Mosby.

Parse, R. R. (1998). *The human becoming school of thought: A perspective for nurses and other health professionals.* Thousand Oaks, CA: Sage.

Rogers, M. E. (1970). *An introduction to the theoretical basis of nursing.* Philadelphia: F. A. Davis.

Rogers, M. E. (1992). Nursing and the space age. *Nursing Science Quarterly, 5,* 27–33.

Roy, C., & Andrews, H. A. (1997). *The Roy adaptation model: The definitive statement.* Norwalk, CT: Appleton & Lange.

Yura, H., & Torres, G. (1975). *Today's conceptual frameworks with the baccalaureate nursing programs* (NLN Pub. No. 15-1558, pp. 17–75). New York: National League for Nursing.

The Author Comments

An Integrative Framework for Conceptualizing Clients: A Proposal for a Nursing Perspective in the New Century

Throughout the years, I have become increasingly concerned with the apparent difficulty nursing continues to have in articulating its independence of and separation from medicine in terms of the aspects of clients with which nursing is concerned. I believe this results from nursing's continuous emphasis on clients' conditions, states, responses, and behaviors, which are the ways client phenomena are conceptualized within many of the major nursing theories. I believe nursing must shift its major mission to focus on people's living and helping people to live well in the context of health and illness rather than dealing with and solving problems associated with clients' conditions, responses, and behaviors. Such a shift will certainly require rethinking regarding clients' problems that nursing should be concerned with, as well as the nature of nursing diagnoses. Hopefully, this shift in thinking will lead to new ways of conceptualizing and theorizing about clients and client phenomena in this new century and firmly establish the nursing perspective.

—Hesook Suzie Kim

technology as a designation for the complex practice called nursing has led nursing scholars to seek a definition of science more appropriate to nursing than the traditional rationalist approach.

One author who contends that traditional science does not adequately describe nursing science is Donaldson.[2] She believes that nursing science must include empirical and pragmatic science as well as traditional science. Rather than contending that nursing practice itself is a science, Donaldson maintains that nursing uses various scientific interpretations in carrying out nursing practice. Both Sandra Weiss,[3] who is wedded to an empiricist approach to science, and Christine Kasper,[4] who takes a pragmatic approach, agree with Donaldson. Weise stated this position well when she said that in nursing science, "Scientific inquiry must produce tangible concrete knowledge that promotes health, prevents illness, or increases the potential for recovery from illness."[3] All of these authors are concerned with the role of science in the study of nursing and believe that the purpose of that scientific study is to improve practice. Sara Fry states clearly why the practice of nursing itself cannot be a science: She contends that nursing "is a practical discipline" that has the moral end of fostering the well-being of the client.[5]

Nursing as an Artful Practice

If nursing practice cannot be a science because it is a practical discipline with a moral end, can it appropriately be called an art? The traditional purpose of art in the West has been to create beauty, whereas the purpose of nursing is to foster healing and wellness. Nurses do foster healing and wellness in ways that can legitimately be called artistic. However, regardless of how "aesthetically" a nurse cares for a patient, he/she would not be said to be engaged in the art of nursing if that care caused unneeded pain, inhibited healing, or enhanced the possibility of death. Because the purpose of the art of nursing is to foster health and healing, nursing at best could be called an artful practice.

The inadequacy of seeking the identity of nursing by labeling it as an art is evident in an article by Johnson[6] on the art of nursing. Johnson divides scholars who attempt to identify nursing as art into two groups: those who interpret the art of nursing as rational and those who oppose this definition of the art of nursing. She contends that those who define art as rational believe that "the artful nurse solves problems by selecting the intervention best suited to the intended end: Instrumental problem solving is said to be a thorough consideration of the facts of the situation, and is made rigorous by the application of scientific theory."[6] It is unclear from the article whether the many nursing scholars that she cites call this definition a definition of art or whether she has classified their work in this way. However, this definition describes well the position of Donaldson,[2] Weiss,[3] Kasper,[4] and Fry,[5] whose works appear not in a book on art but in a book entitled *In Search of Nursing Science.*

When the rationalistic interpretation of nursing, described by Johnson, is accurately labeled as science rather than art, the opponents of that interpretation would seem to favor nursing as an art, especially since they stress sensitivity and creativity. Johnson acknowledges that they do not call nursing an art, but she fails to recognize why. One leading opponent, Benner,[7] does not identify nursing as art because she believes that nursing is a practice that is appropriately studied as a human science. Johnson's treatment of the conflict between those who study nursing as an applied science and those who study nursing as a human science is confused by her attempt to treat this conflict as one concerning the art of nursing rather than the study of nursing. The conflict Johnson attempts to place in the art of nursing is identical to the one that is central to the book, *In Search of Nursing Science.* This struggle concerning the definition of nursing itself is being contested between those who believe that the meaning and direction of nursing should come from applied science and those who believe that nursing is a caring practice that can be best articulated and developed with enlightenment from the human sciences. Johnson discusses this struggle ably, but her attempt to treat it as an art suggests the inadequacy of trying to force nursing into the mold of an art or a science rather than interpreting nursing as a practice.

Nursing as a Practice

Nursing, as well as medicine, has traditionally called itself a practice. One physician, when asked to define practice, said, "It is the care that I give to my patients." His wife, who is a nurse, could make the same claim. Note that their ways of caring are necessarily different, not just because they are different persons but because they are engaged in different practices. The philosopher Hans Georg Gadamer[8] defines practice in a way that could include not only medicine and nursing but many other practices; he defines a practice as communally developed ways of being that promote human good. A practice is concerned not only with how to bring about the good, but what good or value is worth pursuing. In a practice the goods or values of a people become concretely instantiated in the world in which they live. The ways of being, doing, and the ends sought are integrally related to each other, unlike in an applied science, which is value neutral and detachable from the end sought. (For a more extensive treatment of nursing as a practice and the study of nursing as a human science, see Bishop and Scudder.[9,10])

One indication that nursing is a practice is that it has an essential moral sense. Neither an art nor a science has an essential moral sense in the way that nursing does. A study of fulfillment in nursing indicated that nurses recognize this moral sense.[9] We asked 40 practicing nurses at a community hospital and at a university medical center to describe their most fulfilling experience of nursing. On the basis of nursing literature, we expected that a large number of the fulfilling events would be ones in which nurses demonstrated great professional or technical proficiency. In actuality, all but one of the participants described experiences in which the moral sense of nursing was fulfilled. Even the nurse whose greatest fulfillment came from technical competence said that without the moral sense, she would not be a nurse.

The dominance of the moral sense in nursing as reported by nurses should not have surprised us; after all, nursing is caring for the well-being of others by fostering healing and wellness. Even when the description of fulfillment contained much technical and professional language, the moral sense was evident in this language. For example, a nurse who described a patient who had undergone an aneurysm clipping as "a GCS5T, E4, M1, VT [who] opened his eyes but [had] no movement and was trached," concluded her description by saying, "I can't describe the sensation I felt; but to see him follow a command for the first time—moving his thumb made me feel wonderful inside. All of our diligent nursing care, positioning, ROM, stimulation, etc., was working, and it felt good." Interestingly, in a follow-up interview with this nurse, she stated that although this work was very technical, she would not remain in nursing if it were not for personal and moral fulfillment.[9]

This example shows how the moral sense of practice is fulfilled when the technical is integrally incorporated into practice. Labeling a patient as a "GCS5T, E4, M1, VT" is beyond our (i.e., the authors') technical competence, and understanding the meaning of ROM requires an involvement in nursing practice that one of us (Scudder) lacks. Noting that ROM means range of motion is hardly adequate for understanding what the term means. Grasping the meaning of ROM involves understanding that the purpose of ROM is to assure the continued flexibility of the joint and to maintain muscle strength. This requires applying scientific understanding in nursing practice. However, the way that a nurse performs ROM for a patient requires experience in feeling muscles as they move in response to various movements by the nurse—an example of how nursing practice is artful. Nurses learn the meaning of ROM initially by appropriating it from other nurses, which is an example of why novice nurses rely on clinical experience rather than theory. The knowledge of the muscle movement cannot be acquired from a scientific treatment of muscles in a book; it has to be felt and recognized in the body. Sensitivity to the tension, relaxation, and strengthening of the muscle cannot be gained by reading a multiple-step procedure in a textbook. Obtaining such sensitivity requires first working with an experienced practitioner and gradually appropriating the communally developed ways of nursing practice.

When a nurse appropriates the practice of nursing, she/he becomes a competent nurse. The practice of nursing includes many practical skills and understandings that cannot be called an art or an applied science. Skillfully bathing a patient would not generally be considered an art. It could, however, be called artful practice, as the following example will illustrate.

> "It was after breakfast. I did not eat as much as I wanted to. I felt surprised, because I couldn't mobilize my will. I leaned back, as if I had used my body for hours. Suddenly she was there again, a nurse who had spent a lot of time with me the day before. She was smiling, full of energy. She went straight to the point, leaned onto the table and offered to help me have a shower in the bathroom. It seemed like climbing a mountain, but she was so convincing that I agreed. She explained the whole procedure, how she would cover the wound with plastic, etc. It began sounding like heaven. I had confidence in her; she seemed to have been doing this for a hundred years. And it was heaven. Never had I thought that I would appreciate water running slowly down my body as I did that morning. I was sitting on a chair, and the nurse was next to me. I relaxed. She had a special way of offering her help in concrete ways like washing my back and my feet, which I literally could not reach that morning. 'I suggest that you . . . ,' and 'what you could do is turn your body . . . '. Yes, she was assisting me, never taking over. I was in command, I felt. I mattered. Even though the only thing I could manage was steering the shower handle."[11]

Nursing is often called an art in recognition of the integral relationship of practical know-how with artistry that fulfills the moral sense of nursing by promoting healing and well-being.

Another reason that nurses call nursing an art is that they move from competency to excellence through creative action and interaction, as Benner[7] has shown. For Benner, nursing is a practice in which the highest level of practice is highly creative. A nurse becomes an excellent practitioner when she/he can draw on the resources of the practice in creative ways that foster healing and well-being.

Mary Cucci, a critical care unit nurse, described her experience of helping a patient learn to live his body once again after the removal of a misfiring defibrillator. The pain from the defibrillator misfiring plus the uncertainty in his life from his previous heart attacks had led this former well-ordered, self-directed businessman to retreat in fear from engagement with the world. He had become a prisoner in an alien body. Cucci creatively helped him learn to trust and live in his body again. "I teased him, cajoled him, and danced with him as he transferred to the chair. I challenged him more each day and ignored his fake whine when he half-heartedly pleaded abuse. It became a joke. He learned to monitor his pulse to guide his activity progression. This was a long, slow process of building belief in himself."[12] Cucci's artful practice is directed at fostering the healing and well-being of her patient. She uses the practice in ways that creatively express her way of being and that are sensitive and appropriate to her patient's way of being in his current circumstances.

A practice is a communally developed human way of being that fosters human good. A practice exists only in practitioners who appropriate these ways of being in ways that are appropriate to their own being and those of the persons for whom they care. Practices are continually being developed both by creative individual care and communal care. To account for this creative aspect of nursing practice, nurses have defined nursing as art. We believe it is more appropriately called an artful practice.

Conclusion

Although nursing cannot strictly be called a science or an art, the tendency of nursing to use these terms stems from recognition that nurses apply science in their care and that excellent care involves creativity and sensitivity. However, the involvement of science and art in nursing care does not mean that nursing itself is constituted as either an art or a science. The attempt to constitute nursing as an art or a science leads nursing scholars away from the issues of the day, such as applied science versus human science, and from seeking the identity of nursing in the practice itself. Nursing cannot be an art or a science because, rather than creating beauty or pursuing truth, nursing seeks to foster healing, health, and well-being. Having a dominant moral sense is the primary characteristic of a practice. Nursing is a practice in that it seeks to foster healing and wellness through communally developed ways of being with patients that sometimes involve applying science and other times artistic, creative care. At all times, artful practice and applied science are integrally woven into the fabric of the practice of caring called nursing.

REFERENCES

1. What is nursing? Nurse Recruitment Magazine 1992;7(6):A2.
2. Donaldson SK. Nursing science for nursing practice. In: Omery A, Kasper CE, Page GG, eds. In search of nursing science. Thousands Oaks (CA): Sage, 1995:3–12.
3. Weiss SJ. Contemporary empiricism. In: Omery A, Kasper CE, Page GG, eds. In search of nursing science. Thousand Oaks (CA): Sage, 1995:13–26.
4. Kasper CE. Pragmatism: the problem with the bottom line. In: Omery A, Kasper CE, Page GG, eds. In search of nursing science. Thousand Oaks (CA): Sage, 1995:27–39.
5. Fry ST. Science as problem solving. In: Omery A, Kasper CE, Page GG, eds. In search of nursing science. Thousand Oaks (CA): Sage, 1995:72–80.
6. Johnson JL. The art of nursing. Image 1996;28:169–75.
7. Benner P. From novice to expert: excellence and power in clinical nursing practice. Menlo Park (CA): Addison-Wesley, 1984.
8. Gadamer HG, Lawrence FG, trans. Reason in the age of science. Cambridge (MA): MIT Press, 1991.
9. Bishop AH, Scudder JR Jr. The practical, moral, and personal sense of nursing: a phenomenological philosophy of practice. Albany (NY): State University of New York Press, 1990.
10. Bishop AH, Scudder JR Jr. Nursing: the practice of caring. New York: The National League for Nursing Press, 1991.
11. Bishop AH, Scudder JR Jr. Nursing ethics: therapeutic caring presence. Boston: Jones & Bartlett, 1996.
12. Benner P, Wrubel J. The primacy of caring: stress and coping in health and disease. Menlo Park (CA): Addison-Wesley, 1989.

The Authors Comment

Nursing as a Practice Rather Than an Art or a Science

Many nurses believe that nursing is often regarded as a mere collection of techniques and procedures for the care of the ill. Unfortunately, they have often tried to remedy this misconception by uncritically defining nursing as a science and an art. We believe this is the wrong approach because the worth of nursing should be found in nursing as practiced. We attempt to show that although nursing uses science and practices artfully, nursing is best conceived as a practice in the sense of the great philosopher Hans Georg Gadamer. Interpreting nursing as a practice shows the worth of nursing itself and suggests possibilities for future development of nursing out of its past achievements. (Please note that reference 11 in this article should read: Harder, I. [1993]. *The world of the hospital nurse: Nurse patient interactions—body nursing and health promotion. Illustrated by use of combined phenomenological/grounded theory approach.* Aarhus, Denmark: Sygeplejerskehojskole ved Aarhus Universitet, Skrift-serie fra Danmarks Sygeplejerskehojskole.)

—ANNE H. BISHOP
—JOHN R. SCUDDER

CHAPTER 66

What Is Nursing Science?

Elizabeth Ann Manhart Barrett

The enigma of defining nursing science is preceded by defining nursing, science, research, and nursing theory–guided practice. The context for exploring the meaning of nursing science is provided through examination of the totality and simultaneity paradigms. Differing views of nursing as a discipline are discussed. The position is taken that nursing is a basic science with various nursing schools of thought that constitute the substantive knowledge of the discipline. Finally, a definition of nursing science is presented that is broad enough to encompass all disciplinary knowledge. Despite current challenges, an optimistic vision is emerging. The nurse theorists and other nurse scholars who are furthering the development of this work are considered to be the cultural creatives of nursing and contributors to a larger movement toward wholeness in science and in society.

Definition of Nursing

What is nursing science? Although the term is quite familiar to many nurses, its definition remains an enigma. Trying to capture the meaning accurately is perhaps almost as difficult as trying to define love, because it is interpreted in many ways. At various times as I was pulling my thoughts together to answer what at first

About the Author

ELIZABETH ANN MANHART BARRETT was born in Hume, IL. She holds a PhD in nursing science from New York University, an MS in nursing, an MA, and a BS in nursing, summa cum laude, from the University of Evansville, IN. She has 5 children and 15 grandchildren. Dr. Barrett is Professor Emerita of Nursing, Hunter College, City University of New York. Currently, she maintains a private nursing practice of health patterning in New York City and is also a research consultant. The primary focus of Dr. Barrett's research and other scholarly activities is *Rogers' Science of Unitary Human Beings*. Reflecting Rogers' worldview, she developed a theory of power, an instrument to measure the power construct, and the practice methodology of Health Patterning.

seemed like such a simple question, I began to think this was an impossible mission.

Trying to define nursing is an age-old dilemma. Traditionally, *nursing* has been defined as a verb, meaning *to do*. Fawcett (2000a) defines the metaparadigm concept of nursing as "the actions taken by nurses on behalf of or in conjunction with the person, and the goals or outcomes of nursing actions" (p. 5). King (1981/1990) says nursing is "a process of action, reaction, and interaction" (p. 2). Orem (1997) views nursing as "a triad of interrelated action systems" (p. 28) that compose nursing agency (Fawcett, 2000a).

Rogers (1992), on the other hand, defines *nursing* as a noun meaning *to know*. She proposes that nursing is a basic science whose phenomenon of concern is unitary human beings in mutual process with their environments. She says, "The practice of nursing is not nursing. Rather, it is the use of nursing knowledge for human betterment" (Rogers, 1994, p. 34). Parse (1997) says "nursing is a discipline, the practice of which is a performing art" (p. 73). Most commonly, *nursing* is defined as both a noun and a verb. Orem also notes that in addition, *nursing* can be defined as a participle, as in *I am nursing* (Fawcett, 2000a).

I view nursing as a scientific art, which may seem like an oxymoron. However, I believe that the art cannot exist without the science. I define nursing as a basic science and the practice of nursing as the scientific art of using knowledge of unitary human beings who are in mutual process with their environments for the well-being of people. Personal definitions of nursing are quite varied, as they reflect our unique professional identities, as well as our philosophies of nursing and our paradigmatic propensities. This seems evident in the way nursing has been defined by the various nurse theorists as well as by other nurses. At this point, I need to make explicit what has been implicit, and that is that I speak through the bias of my own perspective.

Definition of Science

If these are some ways to look at defining nursing, what then is science? King (1997a) says *science* is *to know*. Parse (1997) defines *science* as "the theoretical explanation of the subject of inquiry and the methodological process of attaining knowledge in a discipline; thus, science is both product and process" (p. 74) and is arrived at through "creative conceptualization and formal inquiry" (p. 75). Others view science as product only, and propose that "science is a coherent body of knowledge composed of research findings and tested theories for a specific discipline" (Burns & Grove, 2000, p. 10). Science, as scientific knowledge, represents best efforts toward discovering truth. It is open-ended, evolving, and subject to revision and occasionally unfolds in dramatic shifts in thought.

Research is how we create science. *Research,* according to Parse (1997), is "the formal process of seeking knowledge and understanding through use of rigorous methodologies" (p. 74). Taking a narrower view, the National Institutes of Health propose that "research means a systematic investigation designed to develop or contribute to generalizable knowledge" (Daniel Vasgird, personal communication, November, 21, 2000).

What Is Nursing Science? Prelude

After this brief look at *What is nursing?* and *What is science?* we return to the question, *What is nursing science?* Although the term *nursing science* is used liberally throughout the literature, there are few definitions. Likewise, there are also few definitions of *nursing research.* It was amazing to discover this in computer searches and in a variety of books on nursing research and nursing theory. In other words, the majority of these authors do not differentiate nursing science from science produced by nurses, or nursing research from research conducted by nurses. This is the crux of the matter.

For most sources that do offer definitions, they may not be universally acceptable, nor can they be if they represent a particular philosophy, rather than the various philosophies that guide multiple schools of thought within the discipline. Failure to define key terms and failure to specify philosophical underpinnings are grave errors in building a unique body of disciplinary knowledge, which by definition reflects more than one paradigm (Parse, 1997). In addition, definitions need to be congruent with the philosophical underpinnings. To illustrate this point, in Fitzpatrick's (2000) *Encyclopedia of Nursing Research,* nursing science is not listed in the index, nor is nursing research. What is listed is *nursing care research,* and it is defined as "research directed to understanding the nursing care of individuals and groups and the biological, physiological, social, behavioral, and environmental mechanisms influencing health and disease that are relevant to nursing care" (p. 507). This reflects a particular worldview and does not reflect the discipline as a whole.

Context of Nursing Science

Munhall (1997) makes the important point that definitions require examination within their context and reflect assumptions as well as philosophical, political, and practical dimensions. Indeed, it is context that explains why different authors define and use the same nursing terms differently, and why many terms cannot be defined universally.

In attempting to rise above the bias of personal perceptions, it is indeed a formidable task to answer the question, What is nursing science? Nevertheless, this collegial journey is justified because, as Watson (1999) says so clearly, without a language, we are invisible. Nursing will remain invisible as a distinct discipline and be viewed as a subset of medical science or social science until we have clearly defined and embraced our unique identity. Yet, in many nursing circles, this conversation is dismissed as valueless.

Before nursing science can be defined, the point about context must be addressed. Fortunately, there are several ways to contextualize nursing science, including paradigmatic schemas developed by Fawcett in 1993, and Newman, Sime, and Corcoran-Perry in 1991. In 1984, Parse (as cited in Parse, 2000) designed the original, and most widely used, paradigmatic organization of nursing knowledge based on a conceptual differentiation of the totality and simultaneity paradigms (see Table 66-1). Each of these two paradigms is a worldview that expresses a philosophical perspective about the nursing discipline's unique phenomenon of concern; all nursing knowledge is connected with this phenomenon in some way (Parse, 1997). Nursing's phenomenon of concern focuses on the human as a whole being, the environment, and health. Some authors add other concepts, such as nursing and caring.

In general, there is agreement on nursing's phenomenon of concern, expressed by Parse (1997, 2000) as the human-universe-health process. However, the definitions of these terms differ according to paradigms, thereby serving to clarify rather than confuse, since the philosophical context is now explicated. The contrast between worldviews is often explained by the two paradigmatic views of the human as a whole person, although this is only one example of difference. The totality paradigm views the whole human as a biopsychosocioculturalspiritual being who can be understood by studying the parts, yet is more than the sum of parts. The person is separate from the changing environment, but interacts continuously with it. Health exists on a wellness-illness continuum. Most

Table 66-1
Comparison of Nursing Paradigms

| | Simultaneity | | |
	Human Becoming	Science of Unitary Human Beings	All Totality Theories
Human being	Open being cocreating meaning in multidimensional mutual process with the universe recognized by patterns of relating	Energy field in mutual process with environmental field	Biopsychosociospiritual organism interacting with environment
	Freely chooses in situation	Participates knowingly in change	Interacts by coping with or managing the environment
Health	Cocreated process of becoming as experienced and describedby the person, family, and community	A value	Physical, psychological, social, and spiritual well-being as defined by norms
Central phenomenon of nursing	Unitary human's becoming	Unitary human beings	Self-care, adaptation, goal attainment, or caring
Goal of the discipline of nursing	Quality of life	Well-being and optimal health	Promotion of health and prevention of disease
Mode of inquiry	Qualitative: Parse's research method: human becoming hermeneutic method	Quantitative and qualitative methods	Extant quantitative and qualitative methods
Mode of practice	True presence in all-at-once illuminating meaning through explicating, synchronizing rhythms through dwelling with, mobilizing transcendence through moving beyond	Patterns manifestation appraisal; pattern profile—perceptions, expression, experiences; deliberative mutual patterning	Nursing process with nursing diagnoses

NOTE: From *The Human Becoming School of Thought* (p. 11), by R. R. Parse, 1998. Thousand Oaks, CA: Sage. ©1998 by Sage. Reprinted with permission.

authors include King (1981/1990), Orem (1995), Roy (1997), Betty Neuman (1996), Peplau (1952), Leininger (1995), and others as totality paradigm theorists.

In the simultaneity paradigm *whole* means unitary, and the unitary human has characteristics that are different from the parts and cannot be understood by a knowledge of the parts. Moreover, the human cannot be separated from the entirety of the universe, as both change continuously in innovative, unpredictable ways, and together create health, a value defined by people for themselves (Parse, 1997,1998,2000; Rogers, 1992). The simultaneity theorists include Rogers (1994), Parse (1998), Margaret Newman (1990), and some, including myself, would say Watson (1999).

Although the two paradigms of nursing are different, neither is superior, and it is important to remember that a discipline requires more than one worldview of the phenomenon of concern (Parse, 1997). These differences give rise to different methods of inquiry and practice and provide sufficient scope to encompass all disciplinary activities.

Schools of Thought

Parse (1997) has advanced the conceptualization of schools of thought and proposes that each paradigm is composed of philosophically congruent schools of thought based on similar beliefs about the essential phenomenon of concern of nursing. She states, "Each

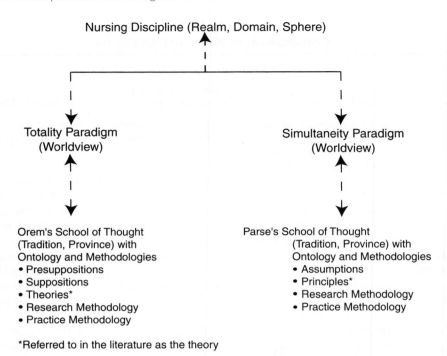

Figure 66-1   *From "The Language of Nursing Knowledge: Saying What We Mean," by R. R. Parse, in I. M. King and J. Fawcett (Eds.).* The Language of Nursing Theory and Metatheory *(p. 76), 1997, Indianapolis, IN: Sigma Theta Tau International Center Nursing Press. ©1997 by Sigma Theta Tau International Center Nursing Press. Reprinted with permission.*

school of thought is a knowledge tradition that includes a specific ontology (belief system) and congruent methodologies (approaches to research and practice)" (p. 74). In other words, schools of thought comprise the substantive knowledge of the discipline (Parse, 1997). Figure 66-1, developed by Parse, illustrates Orem's (1995) school of thought as one example from the totality paradigm and Parse's (1998) school of thought as one example from the simultaneity paradigm.

The ontology consists of the assumptions, postulates, and principles of the framework or theory. The epistemology flows from the ontology and gives rise to both research methods and practice methods that are congruent with the framework or theory.

Nursing frameworks and theories have birthed numerous research instruments to measure constructs operationally defined to provide consistency with the particular framework or theory. Such instrumentation is essential to advance nursing knowledge in some frameworks and theories, notably in the totality paradigm. Rogerian science may be the only framework or theory in the simultaneity paradigm that endorses quantitative as well as qualitative methods. At least 32 instruments have been developed specifically to measure constructs reflecting eight (King, 1981/ 1990; Neuman, 1996; Orem, 1995; Pender, 1996; Peplau, 1952; Rogers, 1994; Roy, 1997; Watson, 1999) nursing science frameworks and theories (Young, Taylor, & Renpenning, 2001).

Unique Research and Practice Methodologies

Of even greater significance is the development of unique research methodologies. Table 66-2 shows Fawcett's

Table 66-2
Nursing Discipline–Specific Research Methodologies

Conceptual Model or Theory	Research Methodology
Rogers' Science of Unitary Human Beings	Bultemeier's Photo-Disclosure Method
	Butcher's Unitary Field Portrait Research Method
	Cowling's Unitary Pattern Appreciation Case Method
Leininger's Theory of Culture Care Diversity and Universality	Ethnonursing Research Method
Newman's Theory of Health as Expanding Consciousness	Research as Praxis Method
Parse's Theory of Human Becoming	Parse's Method of Basic Research
	Cody's Human Becoming Hermeneutic Method of Basic Research
	Parse's Preproject-Process-Postproject Descriptive Qualitative Method of Applied Research

NOTE: From "The State of Nursing Science: Where Is the Nursing in the Science," by J. Fawcett, 2000b, *Theoria: Journal of Nursing Theory, 9*(3), p. 4. ©2000 by the Swedish Society for Nursing Theories in Practice, Research, and Education. Reprinted with permission.

(2000b) listing of those methods. They are all qualitative in nature. Fawcett insists that

> we must extricate ourselves from the research methods of other disciplines, such as the phenomenological methods that have their roots in psychology, the grounded theory method that comes from sociology, and the randomized, controlled trials methodology that originated in agriculture and now is frequently used by pharmacologists and physicians, (p. 5)

Fawcett does, however, endorse reformulation of a method within the parameters of a nursing framework or theory. For example, Leininger (1995) reformulated ethnography, a method from anthropology, within the view of her nursing theory, and thereby created the ethnonursing method (Fawcett, 2000b).

In 1998, I (Barrett) proposed that unique research methods are one direct route to moving nursing toward further disciplinary definition. These methods "facilitate creation of knowledge for colleagues who practice nursing in the new way" (Barrett, 1998, p. 95). Those who use them are on the cutting edge, experiencing the passion of blazing a new trail as they sing the diversity chant of pioneers on the nursing road less traveled (Barrett, 1998).

Nursing practice methodologies are another aspect of a school of thought and are essential for making the leap from the theoretical to the practical, and clearly demonstrating the practical nature of nursing theories. Fawcett (2000b) noted that Johnson (1992), King (1981/1990), Levine (1996), Margaret Newman (1990), Orem (1995), Rogers (1994), and Parse (1998), or scholars working with those frameworks and theories, have developed practice methodologies consistent with their work that can also form the basis for research methodologies. In other words, Fawcett (2000b), and earlier Newman (1990), proposed that information obtained during the practice of nursing can be regarded as research data.

Nursing Theory–Guided Practice

The American Academy of Nursing's Expert Panel on Nursing Theory–Guided Practice developed the following definition:

> Nursing theory–guided practice is a human health service to society based on the discipline-specific knowledge articulated in the nursing frameworks and theories. The discipline-specific knowledge reflects the philosophical perspectives embedded in the ontological, epistemological, and methodological processes that frame nursing's ethical approach to the human-universe-health process. (Parse et al., 2000, p. 177)

Nursing frameworks and theories provide two avenues to nursing practice by way of nursing theory–guided practice. The totality paradigm allows for adoption of evidence-based practice, defined differently in nursing than in medicine, particularly when it is nursing theory–guided. In medicine, the gold standard for evidence-based practice is outcomes of randomized controlled trials. Evidence-based nursing, linked with the current buzzword in medicine, refers to research usage, but Ingersoll (2000) proposes a definition of evidence-based nursing that, unlike medicine's definition, does include theory. Her definition states, "Evidence-based nursing practice is the conscientious, explicit and judicious use of theory-derived, research-based information in making decisions about care delivery to individuals or groups of patients and in consideration of individual needs and preferences" (p. 152).

Nursing theory–guided evidence-based nursing differs from evidence-based nursing in that the practice is guided by the discipline-specific knowledge reflected in the schools of thought within the totality paradigm. King (2000) has provided an example using her conceptual system. Her "theory of goal attainment within which a transaction process model was derived results in the following: Goals set lead to transactions which lead to goal attainment (outcomes) which is evidence-based practice" (p. 8).

Within the simultaneity paradigm, practice is simply nursing theory–guided or nursing science–guided. Evidence-based nursing is not compatible because it is philosophically incongruent. Its problem-oriented focus on diagnosis, interventions, and outcomes reflects the natural science approach, rather than the human science approach of the simultaneity paradigm.

Nursing as a Discipline

If nursing is a discipline, what then is a discipline? Parse (1997) describes a discipline as "a branch of knowledge ordered through the theories and methods evolving from more than one worldview of the phenomenon of concern" (p. 74). Her schema of worldviews in nursing, presented in Table 66-1, clarifies why the same words have different definitions and rather than serving to confuse, the different definitions serve to clarify when viewed within their appropriate place in the disciplinary domain.

To make matters more confusing, nursing is often called a practice discipline, or as Donaldson and Crowley described it in 1978, a professional discipline. Twenty-five years ago, many of us were still debating whether or not nursing was a profession, and we began to see these attributes on a continuum. Rather than asking if nursing was a profession, we started asking, "How professionalized is nursing?" But nursing has moved on and now the debate centers on the extent to which we are a discipline. Those who specify nursing as a professional discipline emphasize that nursing has a "social mandate to develop, disseminate, and use knowledge. In contrast, academic disciplines, such as physics, physiology, sociology, psychology, and philosophy, are mandated only to develop and disseminate knowledge" (Fawcett, 2000a, p. 692). The knowledge of academic disciplines can be practiced in a corresponding profession.

According to Newman et al. (1991), a discipline is

distinguished by a domain of inquiry that represents a shared belief among its members regarding its reason for being . . . . A professional discipline is defined by social relevance and value orientations. The focus is derived from a belief and value system about the profession's social commitment, the nature of its service, and an area of responsibility for knowledge development. (p. 1)

Fawcett's (2000a) description of the discipline, as she presented it in Figure 66-2, presents nursing science and the nursing profession as the two major dimensions. Nursing research is the means for developing the knowledge of nursing science, and the product of the research is all the knowledge that has been developed and disseminated. The nursing profession, in a reciprocal relationship to nursing science, is actualized in nursing practice, with the major activities being use and evaluation of the knowledge previously developed and disseminated (Fawcett, 2000a).

Fawcett (2000a) summarizes the thinking of several nurse scholars when she says that "the responsibility and

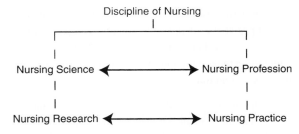

Figure 66-2 *From* Analysis and Evaluation of Contemporary Nursing Knowledge: Nursing Models and Theories *(p. 692), by J. Fawcett, 2000, Philadelphia: F. A. Davis. © F. A. Davis. Adapted with permission.*

goal of the professional discipline of nursing is to conduct discipline-specific research using discipline-specific methodologies and to engage in discipline-specific practice" (p. 693). She echoes Parse (1999), who notes that nothing less will establish nursing as an autonomous profession and define the unique gift that we contribute to the healthcare system. Leininger (1995) also argues that professional decisions and actions by nurses require substantive disciplinary knowledge.

What Nursing Science Is Not

Before proposing a working definition of nursing science, it seems important to ask, "What is it, then, that nursing science is not?" Rogers (1992), Parse (2000), and Fawcett (2000a) are all clear that research by nurses that generates or tests theories from other disciplines is not nursing research. Furthermore, findings of such research build the knowledge base of the other disciplines. Since most nursing research falls into this category, the premise is that we are using precious resources to build a knowledge base with strong roots in other disciplines. This is not to say this research should not be done. Scholars are free to pursue whatever route to knowledge that they choose. Yet, can we call it nursing knowledge if its origins are in other disciplines? One cannot help but wonder what progress could be made in developing the nursing discipline if all nursing research, by definition, was guided by the extant nursing frameworks and theories.

This is not to say that the knowledge of other disciplines is not valuable and is not used by nurses. Of course it is. It is simply knowledge required of a learned person. Likewise, nursing knowledge can be used by others. Knowledge, per se, does not belong to anyone. It is not a commodity to be bought and sold, even though in the not too distant past, access to medical knowledge, for example, was much more difficult to obtain. We simply need to be clear on what is nursing knowledge and what is not. However, there is a difference between access to information and the use of the discipline-specific knowledge to provide a professional service that constitutes the practice of a particular discipline. Furthermore, knowledge that is not nursing knowledge simply does not reflect the uniqueness of what nurses and nursing are about. In contrast, it is nursing knowledge from both paradigms that allows us to build our discipline so that nursing services reflect nursing's distinctive schools of thought.

Public's View of Nursing

Perhaps one reason the public is often unclear in defining what is unique about nursing is related to the fact that they may not have experienced the *real thing*. In other words, they may not have experienced being honored and cared for knowledgeably as humans who are whole and who are living life in an ever-changing and all-encompassing environment. Equally as important, they may not have experienced that their nurse caregivers are themselves humans who are aware of their wholeness and of living their life in an ever-changing and all-encompassing environment. The mutuality of the experience is what distinguishes this from the usual experience of clients who receive less than this standard of care. Instead, for the most part, the public views *nursing* as a verb that means doing, and nurses as those who carry out tasks of a certain nature. What nurses do is based on what nurses know. It is time to ask, "What is the foundational knowledge that drives the modus operandi of nursing practice?" Nursing theory–guided practice allows the discipline to escape from its low profile and create waves that demonstrate to the public why nursing services are essential to health and well-being.

Yes, those in the nursing theory movement are a minority on the road less traveled. Although the possibility cannot be ruled out that history will reveal that they are lone voices crying in the wilderness, I believe that will not be the case because this group is part of a larger movement in science, in society, in the universe. Nurse scholars who work within the new way of thinking about nursing are the cultural creatives of the discipline. You will be hearing more from them in the future. As the saying goes, *You haven't seen anything yet.* Those who walk down that road less traveled would do well to remember Margaret Mead's (as cited in Barrett, 1990) prophetic insight: "Never doubt that a small group of thoughtful, committed citizens can change the world; indeed it's the only thing that ever has" (p. xxi).

REFERENCES

Allison, S. E., & Renpenning, K. (1999). *Nursing administration in the 21st century.* Thousand Oaks, CA: Sage.

Anderson, C. A. (2000). The time is now. *Nursing Outlook, 48,* 257–258.

Barrett, E.A.M. (1990). Preface. In E.A.M. Barrett (Ed.), *Visions of Rogers' science-based nursing* (pp. xxi-xxiii). New York: National League for Nursing.

Barrett, E.A.M. (1998). Unique nursing research methods: The diversity chant of pioneers. *Nursing Science Quarterly, 11,* 94–96.

Burns, N., & Grove, S. K. (2000). *The practice of nursing research: Conduct, critique, & utilization* (4th ed.). Philadelphia: Saunders.

Daly, J., Mitchell, G. J., Toikkanen, T., Millar, B., Zanotti, R., Takahashi, T., et al. (1997). What is nursing science? An international dialogue. *Nursing Science Quarterly, 10,* 10–13.

Donaldson, S. K., & Crowley, D. M. (1978). The discipline of nursing. *Nursing Outlook, 26,* 113–120.

Fawcett, J. (1993). From a plethora of paradigms to parsimony in world views. *Nursing Science Quarterly, 6,* 56–58.

Fawcett, J. (2000a). *Analysis and evaluation of contemporary nursing knowledge: Nursing models and theories.* Philadelphia: F. A. Davis.

Fawcett, J. (2000b). The state of nursing science: Where is the nursing in the science? *Theoria: Journal of Nursing Theory, 9(3),* 3–10.

Fitzpatrick, J. J. (Ed.). (2000). *Encyclopedia of nursing research.* New York: Springer.

Frost, R. (1967). The road not taken. In R. Frost (Ed.), *Complete poems of Robert Frost* (p. 131). New York: Holt, Rinehart & Winston.

Gustafsson, B. (2000). The SAUC model for confirming nursing. *Theoria: Journal of Nursing Theory, 9(1),* 6–21.

Ingersoll, G. L. (2000). Evidence-based nursing: What it is and what it isn't. *Nursing Outlook, 48,* 151–152.

Johnson, D. E. (1992). The origins of the behavioral system model. In F. N. Nightingale (Ed.), *Notes on nursing: What it is, and what it is not* (Commemorative ed., pp. 23–27). Philadelphia: J. B. Lippincott.

King, I. M. (1990). *A theory for nursing: Systems, concepts, process.* Albany, NY: Delmar. (Original work published 1981)

King, I. M. (1997a). Knowledge development for nursing: A process. In I. M. King & J. Fawcett (Eds.), *The language of nursing theory and metatheory* (pp. 19–25). Indianapolis, IN: Center Nursing Press.

King, I. M. (1997b). Reflections on the past and a vision of the future. *Nursing Science Quarterly, 10,* 15–17.

King, I. M. (2000). Evidence-based nursing practice. *Theoria: Journal of Nursing Theory, 9(2),* 4–9.

Leininger, M. (1995). Culture care theory, research and practice. *Nursing Science Quarterly, 9,* 71–78.

Levine, M. E. (1996). The conservation principles: A retrospective. *Nursing Science Quarterly, 9,* 38–41.

Munhall, P. L. (1997). Deja vu, parroting, buyins, and an opening. In I. M. King & J. Fawcett (Eds.), *The language of nursing theory and metatheory* (pp. 79–87). Indianapolis, IN: Center Nursing Press.

Nagle, L. M. (1999). A matter of extinction or distinction. *Western Journal of Nursing Research, 21,* 71–82.

Neuman, B. M. (1996). *The Neuman systems model* (3rd ed.). Norwalk, CT: Appleton & Lange.

Newman, M. A. (1990). Newman's theory of health as praxis. *Nursing Science Quarterly, 3,* 37–41.

Newman, M. A., Sime, A. M., & Corcoran-Perry, S. A. (1991). The focus of the discipline of nursing. *Advances in Nursing Science, 14(1),* 1–6.

O'Neill, E. (2000, November). *Workplace Issues in Nursing.* Paper presented at the annual conference of the American Academy of Nursing, San Diego, CA.

Orem, D. E. (1995). *Nursing: Concepts of practice* (5th ed.). St. Louis, MO: Mosby.

Orem, D. E. (1997). Views of human beings specific to nursing. *Nursing Science Quarterly, 10,* 26–31.

Orlando, I. J. (1987). Nursing in the 21st century: Alternate paths. *Journal of Advanced Nursing, 12,* 405–412.

Parse, R. R. (1997). The language of nursing knowledge: Saying what we mean. In I. M. King & J. Fawcett (Eds.), *The language of nursing theory and metatheory* (pp. 73–77). Indianapolis, IN: Center Nursing Press.

Parse, R. R. (1998). *The human becoming school of thought: A perspective for nurses and other health professionals.* Thousand Oaks, CA: Sage.

Parse, R. R. (1999). The discipline and the profession. *Nursing Science Quarterly, 12,* 275.

Parse, R. R. (2000). Paradigms: A reprise. *Nursing Science Quarterly, 13,* 275–276.

Parse, R. R., Barrett, E., Bourgeois, M., Dee, V., Egan, E., Germain, C., et al. (2000). Nursing theory–guided practice: A definition. *Nursing Science Quarterly, 13, 177.*

Pender, N. J. (1996). *Health promotion in nursing practice* (3rd ed.). Stamford, CT: Appleton & Lange.

Peplau, H. (1952). *Interpersonal relations in nursing.* New York: Putnam.

Phillips, J. R. (2000). Rogerian nursing science and research: A healing process for nursing. *Nursing Science Quarterly, 13,* 196–203.

Ray, P. H., & Anderson, S. R. (2000). *The cultural creatives: How 50 million people are changing the world.* New York: Harmony Books.

Rogers, M. E. (1964). *Reveille in nursing.* Philadelphia: F. A. Davis.

Rogers, M. E. (1970). An *introduction to the theoretical basis of nursing.* Philadelphia: F. A. Davis.

Rogers, M. E. (1992). Nursing science and the space age. *Nursing Science Quarterly, 5,* 27–34.

Rogers, M. E. (1994). The science of unitary human beings. *Nursing Science Quarterly, 7,* 33–35.

Roper, N., Logan, W., & Tierney, A. J. (2000). *The Roper-Logan-Tierney model of nursing.* New York: Churchill Livingstone.

Roy, C. (1997). Future of the Roy model: Challenge to redefine adaptation. *Nursing Science Quarterly, 10,* 42–48.

Roy, C. (1999). *The Roy adaptation model-based research: 25 years of contributions to nursing science.* Indianapolis, IN: Center Nursing Press.

Watson, J. (1999). *Postmodern nursing and beyond.* New York: Churchill Livingston.

Wieck, K. L. (2000). A vision for nursing: The future revisited. *Nursing Outlook, 48,* 7–8.

Young, A., Taylor, S. G., & Renpenning, K. (2001). *Connections: Nursing theory, research, and practice.* St. Louis, MO: Mosby.

The Author Comments

What Is Nursing Science?

An Open Letter to Nurses of the 21st Century

In the second half of the 20th century, nurse theorists created a radical shift and developed discipline-specific knowledge that has boundless potential to radically change the face of nursing in the 21st century. I saw a need for a definition of nursing science that would encompass the work of theorists from the differing paradigms and guide the ongoing search for knowledge of nursing's unique phenomenon of concern, the human-universe-health process. Now, at a time when the world is moving so quickly that tomorrow is almost history, it is up to the students of today, who will soon be the nursing leaders of the future, to embrace, further develop, and use this knowledge for human betterment. Will you, the nurses of the 21st century, knowingly participate in continuing this revolution? You have power. Use it!

—ELIZABETH ANN MANHART BARRETT

Future Directions for Nursing Theory

This unit builds upon the writings presented in previous units, to extend and challenge the reader's developing perspectives on nursing theory. Traditional philosophic views about knowledge development, nursing science, practice, and technology are turned upside down. New philosophic views and paradigms are proposed. Although few of the ideas presented in these articles are actively practiced within nursing today, the ideas and the new thinking they will generate may find their way into mainstream nursing and transform how nurses do nursing theory.

Questions for Discussion

- Which ideas presented in these articles should find their way into mainstream nursing? Which should not?

- What might be your role, and those in your cohort, in challenging or extending existing perspectives on nursing theory?

A Treatise on Nursing Knowledge Development for the 21st Century: Beyond Postmodernism

Pamela G. Reed

This article explicates a framework for nursing knowledge development that incorporates both modernist and postmodernist philosophies. The framework derives from an "open philosophy" of science, which links science, philosophy, and practice in development of nursing knowledge. A neomodernist perspective is proposed that upholds modernist values for unified conceptualizations of nursing reality while recognizing the dynamic and value-laden nature of all levels of theory and metatheory. It is proposed that scientific inquiry extend beyond the postmodern critique to identify nursing metanarratives of nursing philosophy and nursing practice that serve as external correctives in the critique process. Philosophic positions related to the science, philosophy, and practice domains are put forth for continued dialogue about future directions for knowledge development in nursing.

Among the transitions currently facing nursing is the ending of what someday will be referred to as 20th-century nursing theorizing. For the past several years, nurses have been feeling the ground shift with the reforming of philosophic ideas that launched nursing as a science. Not since the advent of modernism and the birth of modern nursing at the end of the 19th century has nursing science been faced with such a wealth of possibilities for knowledge development. These possibilities have their roots in modernism to be sure, but they also are nurtured by the current dialogue postmodern thought has precipitated.

From P. G. Reed, A treatise on nursing knowledge development for the 21st century: Beyond postmodernism.
Advances in Nursing Science, *1995, 17(3), 70–84. Copyright © 1995. Reproduced with permission of Lippincott Williams & Wilkins.*

About the Author

PAMELA G. REED is Professor at the University of Arizona College of Nursing in Tucson, where she also served as Associate Dean for Academic Affairs for 7 years. She is a three-time graduate of Wayne State University in Detroit, receiving a BSN in 1974, an MSN in 1976 (with a double major in child–adolescent psychiatric mental health nursing and teaching), and her PhD with a major in nursing, (focused on life-span development and aging) in 1982. Dr. Reed pioneered research into spirituality and well-being with her doctoral research with terminally ill patients. She also developed a theory of self-transcendence and two widely used research instruments, the *Spiritual Perspective Scale* and the *Self-Transcendence Scale*. Her publications and funded research reflect a dual scholarly focus: spirituality and other facilitators of well-being and decision-making in end-of-life transitions, and nursing metatheory and knowledge development. Dr. Reed also enjoys time with her family, reading, classical music, swimming, and hiking in the mountains and canyons of Arizona.

Postmodernism has engaged nursing in a dialogue to reconcile a basic awareness about the uniqueness and differences in human beings and health, with basic beliefs in universals and values about human phenomena. It is a struggle, as a philosopher characterized that of feminism, to "modify the Enlightenment in the context of late modernity but not to capitulate to the postmodern condition."[1(p195)]

This article presents a framework that will help nursing science bridge modernist and postmodernist philosophies as nursing clarifies contemporary approaches to knowledge development. The framework builds on accomplishments of modernist nursing while exploiting opportunities of the postmodern context and, in this sense, is "neomodernist." The framework reaches beyond postmodern prescriptions for nursing science and proposes a neomodernist perspective on knowledge development that incorporates meta-narratives of nursing philosophy and nursing practice into scientific inquiry.

Historical Background: Modernism and Postmodernism

From premodern to postmodern times, paths to knowledge have crossed through the Age of Faith, the Age of Reason, to the Culture of Critique. The once dominant religious and metaphysical approach to reasoning about reality was transformed into avenues to truth that separated philosophic "beliefs" from empiric "knowing." Empiricism supplanted the Aristotelian emphasis on rationality that had inspired early modernists. Although modern science enlightened the world and enhanced everyday life, its approach failed to deliver the anticipated empirical base for ultimate meaning and truth about human beings and their world. Also, as philosopher Popper[2] helped scientists realize during the decline of positivism, knowledge development could not be purged of biases, contradictions, and values. Theories, like the fisherman's net, inevitably influenced what data were caught by the scientist. Postmodern thought helped move scientists toward the realization about the embeddedness of research data and the transitory nature of theory.

Postmodernism is a social movement and philosophy that originated among French literary theorists in the 1960s, although postmodern ideas were expressed prior to this time.[3] Postmodernism is a perspective or intellectual style of creating art, of theorizing, of doing science. And it is influencing nursing's approach to knowledge development.

Postmodernism challenges the modernist idea of a single, transcendent meaning of reality and the importance of the search for empirical patterns that correspond to and represent ultimate meaning. Metanarratives, grand or high theories, or other overarching discourses that identify essential truths and propose to re-present reality are not recognized as valid. The "postmodern condition"[4] is a "crisis of confidence in the narratives of truth, science and progress that epitomized modernity"[5(p98)]—a time of paradigms lost. Instead, there is focus on understanding multiple meanings, with the belief that every representation conceals and reveals meanings and that an inextricable link exists between meaning and power.[6] Whereas modernists fragmented the whole to study parts in the attempt to ultimately unify knowledge about the world, postmodernists fragment and dissolve unities, universals, and metanarratives believed to be entangled with values and beliefs that oppress people and fabricate reality. In postmodern thought, problems are not "solved," they are "deconstructed."

Postmodernists generally deny the existence of an essence of human beings, and they have incited ardent debate on the relevance of philosophy for science, given that a central purpose of philosophy is to examine questions about the intrinsic nature of human beings and the world, truth, and knowledge.[7] In postmodern thought, then, there is no autonomous subject to study; the subject is myth. What is studied is what the culture has inscribed on the object of study; in this sense, the focus of study is text. Meaning derives from the relationship between the text and the reader, and the content is not related to an external narrative. There is no transcendent referent for the knowledge builder and no source of meaning about human beings to be discovered and re-presented to others. So, in a phrase, the gods have fled. Any truths that appear to exist have come about not through historical teleologic progress, but as a product of time and chance, contingent on someone re-describing nature in a way that is temporarily useful to the current culture and context.[8,9] Thus, there is an epistemologic shift from concern over the truth of one's findings to concern over the practical significance of the findings.

Framework for Knowledge Development

Postmodernism's iconoclastic and pluralistic attitudes are dislodging nursing from cherished norms about knowledge development that tended to dichotomize essential units of inquiry: research and practice, inductive and deductive reasoning, qualitative and quantitative data. Twenty-first century approaches to developing knowledge will transcend these dichotomies.

Nursing's knowledge development activities have not been daunted by the shifts in philosophic thought, but instead are evolving out of both modernist and postmodernist influences. Nursing is embracing a broadened definition of scholarship that employs various key sources for development of nursing knowledge. These sources derive from the empirical, conceptual, and practice activities of nurses.[10–12] However, consistent with modern science, these domains have been regarded as independent throughout most of 20th-century nursing.

Science, philosophy, and practice have typically represented "orthogonal subspaces" of a discipline; each domain exists in its own dimension and has no image or projection in the plane of the other.[13] The schisms between these subspaces are a problem inherent in knowledge development. Yet despite the orthogonality and despite even the dominance of the scientific over the spiritual or philosophic modes of thought, none has been eliminated. It is as though each subspace represents some irreducible or essential basis of knowledge development. However, the independence between the domains, as enforced by modernists, proved to be an unsatisfactory approach to inquiry.

What instead may be needed for 21st-century nursing theory development is what Polis[13] labeled an "open philosophy," which deliberatively links phenomenon with noumenon and links empirical concepts that can be known through the senses with theoretical concepts of meaning and value that can be known through thought. The postmodern critique of modernism compels nursing to revisit the potential "openness" or linkages between scientific inquiry and the metanarratives of nursing philosophy and nursing practice as a means of both reforming and reaffirming nursing's approaches to knowledge development.

Nursing Science: Modern and Postmodern Influences

A nursing scientist uses valid and reliable systems of inquiry to gain understanding of phenomena of human health and healing processes. The scientist links empirical

is part of the culture being critiqued, complicity exists, as critics of postmodernism have explained.[1,28] And the critique cannot serve as its own external corrective; it describes a process but does not provide substance. Thus, it is suggested here that the nursing scientist's critique process be linked to a substantive overarching "ideal" or metanarrative. The metanarrative provides a base for examining knowledge as related to the context of a given discipline.[1] It functions as a "narrative foil"[28] against which scientists critique their work to form and reform knowledge.

Nursing knowledge development need not abandon completely modernist views about high theory or universal ideas. Rather than capitulate entirely to postmodernism, nurses can knowingly involve in their science the realm of perspectives and values, initially put forth by modernist nurses, that distinguish nursing knowledge and the caring application of that knowledge. In adopting a neomodernist view, nursing scientists would draw from the metanarratives of nursing for their critique. Metanarratives of nursing are found in nursing philosophy and nursing practice, as these two domains interface with nursing science in the development of knowledge.

Nursing Philosophy: Metanarratives for Knowledge Development

Philosophy, by definition, goes beyond analysis and critique by assigning values to human experiences.[29] In so doing, philosophy is a source for explicating the metanarratives of a discipline. Nursing philosophy is a statement of foundational and universal assumptions, beliefs, and principles about the nature of knowledge and truth (epistemology) and about the nature of the entities represented in the metaparadigm (ie, nursing practice and human healing processes [ontology]). A variety of philosophic schemes have been identified for understanding the nature of nursing phenomena.

One major scheme derives from philosopher Stephen Pepper's[30] widely recognized 1942 work in which he explicated what he conceived were the major

bases of truth about the world. Three of his six world-views, particularly as modified slightly by Lerner[31] and other developmental psychologists, predominantly have been used by scientists, including nursing scientists,[32] to frame philosophic assumptions of their discipline. Pepper's work predates philosophic schemes identified in nursing, and it likely provided a basis for conceptualizing the nursing worldviews and paradigms.[32–35] These extant nursing schemes, along with Pepper's original worldviews, are useful in organizing basic assumptions about nursing phenomena and in deriving a nursing metanarrative from philosophy for knowledge development. The three predominant worldviews are the mechanistic, organismic, and developmental–contextual, the latter previously labeled the "contextual–dialectic" worldview.[36]

Within the *mechanistic* worldview, the metaphor for human beings is the machine, composed of parts that can be measured, controlled, predicted, and added together to understand the whole. The whole is equal to the sum of the parts. Human beings are viewed as inherently at rest. Stability is assumed. Any change that occurs results from external forces and is deterministic and reversible, not developmental. The goal of change is to return to a state of equilibrium and balance. The individual's relationship with the environment is reactive. The unit of study is the part, devoid of context.

Within the *organismic* worldview, the metaphor for human beings is the biologic organism, composed of a complexity of interrelated parts. The parts are understood from the perspective of the whole, and the whole is represented in terms of the biologic organism itself. The environment assumes a more passive role, with the organism viewed as active on the environment. There is interactionism, primarily in the sense that the parts within the person interact and contribute to qualitative, developmental changes. Change is probabilistic and directed toward an end goal.

Within the *developmental–contextual* worldview, the metaphor for human beings is the historic event; that is, the individual is embedded in a context that is dynamic. Change, in both the human being and the environment, is ongoing and irreversible, innovative and developmental. Change occurs not as a result of the person's reaction to or action on the environment, but through a dialectic and interactive relationship with the environment. Change occurs in accord with Werner's[37] "orthogenetic principle" by which living systems develop through patterns of increasing complexity accompanied by increasing organization. Chaos and conflict can provide energy for progressive change. There is no one ideal goal for development that lasts a lifetime; each developmental phase (however defined) is qualitatively different and possesses its own ideals. The whole or basic unit of study is any living structure that manifests developmental patterns of change. Study of the person necessarily involves study of contextual factors.

Various philosophic systems have been put forth by nursing scholars, such as Hall's[33] change and persistence worldviews; Parse's[35] totality and simultaneity paradigms; Newman's[34] particulate–deterministic, interactive–integrative, and unitary–transformative worldviews; and Fawcett's[32] reaction, reciprocal interaction, and simultaneous action worldviews. These schemes reflect Pepper's[30] different depictions of reality and also extend his ideas by constructing worldviews that speak more directly to nursing and its phenomena of concern.

Some nursing scientists have appropriated worldviews from other disciplines, such as medicine and psychology. Medicine has advanced through three paradigms, namely the biomedical, biopsychosocial, and most recently the psychoneuroimmunologic paradigm.[38] Psychology's models of research and practice have evolved across behavioristic, psychodynamic, humanistic, and transpersonal schools of thought.[28,39]

The status quo in nursing seems to be that knowledge developers embrace the diversity of worldviews in critiquing knowledge and clarifying basic beliefs and assumptions about what are relevant and plausible issues of research and practice.[40] While this "plethora of paradigms"[41] available to nurses may be viewed in a positive way, it also may contribute to the potential for fragmentation within the discipline. This concern has been debated.[40,42] In the spirit of postmodernism,

nurses must question the status quo and continue to debate the logic of diversity in worldviews underlying nursing knowledge development. From a neomodernist perspective, this kind of diversity may not be entirely desirable.

Diversity or Fragmentation?

Diversity at the level of the worldview may inhibit clarification of a nursing philosophy[43] and nursing metanarrative for research and critique. The worldviews within each philosophic scheme define and interrelate the nursing metaparadigm concepts in radically different ways. Sanctioning all available worldviews for nursing in one sense reflects the postmodernist retreat from conceptualizing the whole and identifying unifying ideals. In attempting to achieve unity by preserving disparate worldviews, as some advocate,[40] nursing may be sacrificing coherence for diversity.

Does the diversity offer important distinctions in worldviews, each of which has a rightful role in guiding inquiry and critique within a discipline? Or might the diversity in philosophic schemes represent progress in knowledge about the nature of the world, such that some provide for fuller understanding than others? The former position seems less likely. Diversity does not mean that all points of view are equally valid and acceptable for a given context or discipline.[43] Moreover, preserving differences through compromise or coexistence rather than striving to resolve differences in ontology, values, and goals—a purpose of philosophy[44]—blocks dialogue and opportunities to further develop knowledge. Opposing beliefs about the nature of human health and nursing goals can perpetuate even more differences in nursing's epistemic and ethical claims and research funding priorities, "bringing about more confusion in our discipline rather than creating a sense of coherence necessary for its development."[45(p26)]

In addition to the question of the merits of diversity in worldviews for the discipline's progress, there is the more urgent question as to whether entertaining disparate worldviews best serves patients' well-being. Diplomacy and discourse aside, when choices available are between a mechanistic and developmental worldview, or between a paradigm in which the nurse and not the patient possesses the knowledge and authority and a paradigm in which patients are knowledgeable and knowing participants in their own healing process, is not one paradigm more emancipating (for patient and nurse) and more re-presentative of the nature of nursing than the other? The commitment for unity in diversity[42] may not be status quo but may be most appropriate in a postmodern world that tends to fragment focuses of inquiry, human beings, and their world.

To that end, then, the metanarrative of human developmental potential, transformational and self-transcendent capacity for health and healing, and recognition of the developmental histories of persons and their contexts is offered here as an external corrective of choice. It is a metanarrative originating in Lerner's[31] developmental–contextual worldview and congruent with the philosophic ideas expressed in Newman's[34] unitary–transformative paradigm and Parse's[35] simultaneity paradigm.

Given the alternatives, this metanarrative may be the best commitment to be made by the scientist and practitioner, at least at this point in the development of nursing knowledge. In proposing this metanarrative, however, one must acknowledge that inherent in this neomodernist framework is the realization that even metanarratives are temporary and "for the moment."[46] Although metanarratives by definition are more stable than lower levels of theory, their depictions of truth and reality are not fixed and must be open to developmental change themselves, subject in part to influences from the dynamic science and practice dimensions of nursing.

Nursing Practice: A Metanarrative for Knowledge Development

As if anticipating postmodernist values for the reality found in the culture and context of everyday life experiences, nurses have renewed focus on practice as connected to science. Nursing practice is regarded not only as a place of applying knowledge, but also as a place to generate and test ideas for developing knowledge. Early on, Peplau[47] identified practice as the context in which scientific knowledge was transformed into nursing knowledge. Linkages between science and practice help nursing move beyond grand theorizing and operationalize the metanarrative of "responsible participation and consideration of culture and context"[48(pviii)] and the emancipatory potential of nursing knowledge.

From a revisionist perspective of the early nursing theorists such as Peplau[47] and Paterson and Zderad,[49] it can be seen that nursing began moving beyond the reductionist and mechanistic approaches of modernism even before nursing recognition of postpositivism. As a result, nursing practice gave to nursing research a metanarrative that was patient oriented, context sensitive, pattern focused, and participatory. In her practice theory of interpersonal relations, for example, Peplau[47] incorporated practice and theory into her ideas of research. Resembling the hermeneutic circle, Peplau's research process began in practice, spiraled up, drawing in theories—or as she stated, "peeling out theories"—to explain the phenomenon, then returned to practice to examine the new knowledge in light of the experiences and reality of practice.

Paterson and Zderad[49] described a method of "nursology" as the study of nursing practice. They outlined five phases of phenomenologic nursology in which the practitioner role informed the research process: (1) preparing oneself to be an open window, (2) intuiting the rhythm of the other, (3) knowing the other scientifically, (4) synthesizing differences and similarities, and (5) arriving at a conception of the situation that has some universal meaning across many nursing practice situations.

More recently, Newman[50] described research as praxis, meaning an approach to research that takes the form of nursing practice in the researcher's relationship to the participant and in the enactment of values for human transformation through pattern recognition. Similarly, Parse[51] put forth a research methodology based on her "theory of human becoming." One essential step in the research process is "dialogical engagement," which involves establishing a therapeutic presence between researcher and participant.

These and other theorists' models of nursing depict ways in which doing science itself can be linked to the ideals and meta-narratives of practice. Guidelines for evaluating the emancipatory potential of the research process and product have been detailed.[52] Nursing practice frameworks are evolving scientific methods that are tailored not only to elicit desired data while protecting research participants' rights, but also to be therapeutic.

The Esthetic Order and Nursing Practice

Postmodernism has stimulated greater awareness among nurses of the culture of practice as a source of ultimate meaning about the object of that practice, human beings' health and healing. Concomitantly, there has been increased interest in research on nursing care processes ranging from nursing care systems to nursing caring behaviors, intuition, nursing presence, and the nurse-patient relationship. Rather than characterize this focus as a return to the mid-20th century focus of research on nurses, it may be more accurately viewed as a focus of inquiry influenced in part by the postmodern emphasis on context. In postmodernism, the ultimate locus of meaning is the culture or context of the object of inquiry.[2] Professional practice is a nursing context. And nursing practice increasingly is being viewed as a legitimate source of knowledge, in part because it is regarded as an esthetic order of nursing, imbued with meaning and beauty.[53]

Amidst the postmodern emphasis on culture and context as something external to the person, nursing must not lose sight of the other context of healing—the patient. The postmodern notion of context must be broadened in nursing to include, if not to emphasize, the patient as a context of health and healing. Human beings' inner healing nature cannot be dismissed, as postmodernists might have it.[38] Patient as environment was first conceptualized by several nurse theorists (eg, Levine,[54] Orem,[23] Paterson and Zderad,[49] and Neuman[55]) who wrote about the "internal environment" of the person as an inner reality and innate resource for health and development. The significance of an inner healing environment is supported by current worldviews about inner human potential and transformative

capacity.[28,30,34,35] A basic assumption of Nightingale was that the natural source of healing resided in the patient.[15] And Rogers[56] wrote emphatically about the coexistence of person and environment, regarding the two as one "person–environment mutual process."

Thus, it is proposed that the esthetic in nursing practice refers not only to the meaningful and beautiful experienced through nursing practice by the nurse, but also, and perhaps more appropriately, to that experienced through nursing practice by the patient. As Kim stated in describing one perspective of esthetics, "Certain aspects of nursing practice may be considered 'art' insofar as they communicate aesthetic ideas to perceivers, especially *clients.*"[57(p281)]

This perspective on the esthetics of nursing practice is contrary to the more commonly held view of the esthetic experience residing primarily in the nurse.[56] However, esthetic experience is not found primarily in the type of brushes the painter uses, or the way a musician holds an instrument, or the style of the conductor or poet. Rather, the esthetic is the beauty that is experienced in seeing the painting, hearing the music, and in reading or reciting the poem. Analogously, in nursing, the esthetic is not primarily that experienced by the practitioner; the esthetic is found in the beauty and meaning associated with the patient's experiences of health and healing—the phenomena of concern to nursing. The esthetic is what is desired, meaningful, beautiful—whether it is experienced through the art of a painter, a musician, or a nurse. Given the esthetic order underlying the nurse's art, then, nursing practice is recognized as possessing powerful metanarratives about health and the processes of healing.

Nursing Conceptual Models: Archetypes of Nursing Practice

The nursing conceptual models are a mechanism of translating the metanarrative of nursing practice for knowledge development. Nursing conceptual models broadly refer to extant conceptual and theoretical systems that describe the nature of nursing practice, patients as human beings, and health. Nursing conceptual models, their biases and preunderstandings notwithstanding,[58]

Development. Minneapolis, Minn: University of Minnesota Press; 1957.

38. Fox NJ. *Postmodernism, Sociology, and Health.* Toronto, Canada: University of Toronto Press; 1994.

39. Lundin RW. *Theories and Systems of Psychology,* 2nd ed. Lexington, Mass: Heath; 1979.

40. Barrett EAM. Response: disciplinary perspective: unified or diverse? Diversity reigns. *Nurs Sci Q.* 1992;5:155–157.

41. Fawcett J. From a plethora of paradigms to parsimony in world views. *Nurs Sci Q.* 1993;6:56–58.

42. Northrup DT. Commentary: disciplinary perspective: unified or diverse? A unified perspective within nursing. *Nurs Sci Q.* 1992;5:154–156.

43. Kikuchi JF, Simmons H, eds. *Developing a Philosophy of Nursing.* Thousand Oaks, Calif: Sage; 1994.

44. Moccia P. A critique of compromise: beyond the methods debate. *ANS.* 1988;10(4):1–9.

45. Laurin J. A philosophy of nursing: commentary. In: Kikuchi JF, Simmons H, eds. *Developing a Philosophy of Nursing.* Thousands Oaks, Calif: Sage; 1994.

46. Smith MC. Arriving at a philosophy of nursing: discovering? constructing? evolving? In: Kikuchi JF, Simmons H, eds. *Developing a Philosophy of Nursing.* Thousand Oaks, Calif: Sage; 1994.

47. Peplau HE. Interpersonal relations: a theoretical framework for application in nursing practice. *Nurs Sci Q.* 1992;5(1):13–18.

48. Chinn PL. A window of opportunity. *ANS.* 1994;16(4):viii.

49. Paterson JG, Zderad LT. *Humanistic Nursing.* New York, NY: Wiley; 1976.

50. Newman MA. Newman's theory of health as praxis. *Nurs Sci Q.* 1990;3:37–41.

51. Parse RR. Parse's research methodology with an illustration of the lived experience of hope. *Nurs Sci Q.* 1990;3:9–17.

52. DeMarco R, Campbell J, Wuest J. Feminist critique: searching for meaning in research. *ANS.* 1993;16(2):26–38.

53. Katims I. Nursing as aesthetic experience and the notion of practice. *Schol Inq Nurs Pract.* 1993;7:269–278.

54. Levine M. *Introduction to Clinical Nursing,* 2nd ed. Los Angeles, Calif: F. A. Davis; 1973.

55. Neuman B. *The Neuman Systems Model.* 3rd ed. Norwalk, Conn: Appleton-Lange; 1994.

56. Rogers ME. Nursing: a science of unitary man. In: Riehl JP, Roy C, eds. *Conceptual Models for Nursing Practice.* 2nd ed. New York, NY: Appleton-Century-Crofts; 1980.

57. Kim HS. Response to "Nursing as Aesthetic Experience and the Notion of Practice." *Schol Inq Nurs Pract.* 1993;7: 279–282.

58. Thompson JL. Practical discourse in nursing: going beyond empiricism and historicism. *ANS.* 1985;7(4):59–71.

59. Whall AL. Let's get rid of all that theory. *Nurs Sci Q.* 1993;6: 164–165.

The Author Comments

A Treatise on Nursing Knowledge Development for the 21st Century: Beyond Postmodernism

I wrote this article to articulate a philosophic position for reforming nursing's approach to knowledge development. I integrated the best of modernist and postmodernist thinking, without succumbing to the narrow view of reality that each alone conveys. The approach acknowledges the wealth of knowledge found in our canon of conceptual models and, at the same time, requires a critical perspective of any nursing metanarratives. I tried to extend the traditional views about science, nursing practice, and conceptual models in proposing a "neomodernist" stance for knowledge development. The "open philosophy" proposed in the article will hopefully encourage students to be innovative in thinking about how knowledge is developed in their discipline.

—Pamela G. Reed

The Unrecognized Paradigm Shift in Nursing: Implications, Problems, and Possibilities

Ann L. Whall
Frank D. Hicks

An important paradigm (or worldview) shift is occurring in science that affects the nature of nursing education, practice, and research. The shift from positivism to postmodernism and now to neomodernism has received little attention in US nursing and as such may forestall many opportunities related to such change. The nature of this paradigm shift and its effects on selected aspects of nursing education, practice, and research are described, and related implications, problems, and possibilities are explored. Neomodernism is discussed as one future for nursing that encompasses aspects of both positivism and postmodernism but yet goes beyond these to include important meta-narratives as traditional values and beliefs of nursing. The work of Laudan and Lakatos are explored as supportive of this neomodernist approach.

In the last decade of the 20th century, discussions of philosophic issues foundational to the discipline of nursing were infrequently published in nursing journals, although there were several noteworthy exceptions.[1-4] This seeming inattention was, for the most part, characteristic of the US nursing journals and became more apparent in the last decade because of the level of attention focused on other issues, such as nursing praxis, best practices, and evidenced-based practice. It appeared that topics garnering the most disciplinary attention in the United States were not seen as philosophically based and/or related to a worldview (or paradigm) shift affecting most disciplines, that is, a shift from positivism to postmodernism and increasingly to a neomodernist perspective. It is important that nursing not overlook the nature of the present paradigm shift,

Reprinted from Nursing Outlook, 50, A. L. Whall and F. D. Hicks, *The Unrecognized Paradigm Shift in Nursing: Implications, Problems, and Possibilities, 72–76. Copyright © 2002 with permission from Elsevier Ltd.*

totality claims of the positivists, as well as their claims regarding rationality and scientific truth.[8,23] Postmodernists often characterized positivists' research methods as "context stripping." This term denoted an inattention to the reciprocal relationships between individuals and their many environments and/or objectifying the observed and ignoring reciprocal relationships between the observer and the observed. The context could not, however, be ignored for clinical nursing research, because the clinical situation is often chaotic and characterized by multiple, diverse, and simultaneous interactions that, for the most part, are virtually uncontrollable. Because clinical nursing research was an early and continuing focus in nursing, the lack of control evident in clinical situations was problematic for those with positivistic views; postmodernism, however, allowed for more latitude for consideration of such contexts.

Several characteristics of the newer postmodernist paradigm were very congruent with traditional nursing values and experiences. Not only was the context important in research efforts for the postmodernist, but other freedoms were inherent within the new paradigm that were more consistent with the historical but often overlooked experiences of nursing. Nursing was a suspect entry into the hallowed halls of positivist researchers, often because nurse researchers deviated in both educational background and research training from that of other scientists. However, with a postmodernist view, expanded research training as well as newly accepted topics for research and expanded methods afforded nurse researchers possibilities not available in a positivistic world. In addition, nursing, under the influence of postmodernism, was free to explore the importance of cultural diversity for education, research, and patient care.

Postmodernism is not, however, without criticism. Certain characteristics of postmodernism, such as relativism; irrationalism, nihilism, and a deconstructionist methodology,[2,24] have been problematic for nursing. The tendency for postmodernists to overanalyze and deconstruct and yet provide little alternatives for reconstruction led some to nihilistic conclusions. One outcome of such a nihilistic attitude was the acceptance of all viewpoints as having equal merit/nonmerit. Someone once characterized the ultimate postmodern attitude as taking pleasure in the bottomless nature of a swamp of ever-inadequate knowledge.[6]

In nursing education, postmodernism was reflected by an era in which repeated analysis and evaluation of grand theories was addressed with use of truth criteria that may or may not have been appropriate. This repeated deconstruction of grand theories may have led to the nihilistic feelings inherent in the cry: "Let's get rid of all nursing theory."[25] Likewise, a tendency to eliminate "Philosophic Foundations of Nursing Theory" courses in master's and doctoral programs may be related to such nihilistic feelings and/or an era in which philosophic underpinnings of nursing education, practice, and research are unrecognized. Such outcries and movements in nursing rival the nihilism of the best postmodernists in any discipline.

Another example of the deconstructionist influence in nursing education is preference for a curricular structure that supports a "high wall" between specialties. At the master's level, in particular, faculty often cannot teach across divisional boundaries when a deconstructed view of knowledge prevails. An example of this, cited by the Bureau of Health Professions, is nurses with expertise in elder care (who are in short supply) who are not allowed to use this expertise across master's level specialties.[26]

Thus the influence of positivism and postmodernism remains variable both from discipline to discipline and within disciplinary segments, varying from almost total domination of either paradigm to a sometimes unrecognized allegiance to either of these approaches. In academia, unrecognized allegiance to either approach may have far-reaching and profound effects for nursing, with the selection of nursing faculty, as well as promotion and tenure decisions, riding on unspoken and often unrecognized paradigm assumptions.

Neomodernism as an Alternative Future

Exterior to nursing, the relative influence of and variable shift in the scientific paradigm (from positivism to postmodernism and to neomodernism) have been major topics of discussion for several years. These discussions range from the early views of Kuhn[27] to the more relevant views of Laudan[28] and Lakatos.[29] In an early but still influential view, Kuhn observed that the development of science was neither linear nor neat and that the process was not a smooth one from discovery to discovery, nor was scientific knowledge necessarily cumulative. Likewise, newer (or in his view, revolutionary) theses were not logically and systematically considered and were either not accepted or were discarded on the basis of the adequacy of scientific evidence. Rather, "phage groups" sought to interrupt the influence of new ideas, which might diminish their influence.

Revolutions in science, according to Kuhn, occurred because a particular worldview (or paradigm) delineating the theories and methods by which the discipline did its work was found to be no longer useful in addressing perplexing problems. When the accepted paradigm failed to sufficiently address phenomena relevant to the discipline, a revolution (ie, a gestalt switch) occurred that achieved a better way of viewing scientific problems. Ultimately, Kuhn[27] believed that the new paradigm supplanted the former in a radically different way. The switch was so drastic that the new view (as well its theories and methods) were incommensurable with the old view.

The incommensurability thesis was one of the most problematic aspects of Kuhn's theory,[10] because it suggested that a smooth transition and/or communication among scientists in different paradigms was impossible. Thus, in Kuhn's view, a neomodernist approach including both positivistic and postmodern views would be impossible, because these scientists could not communicate and essentially lived and worked in very different worlds.

Laudan[28] and Lakatos[29] challenged Kuhn's[27] views regarding this transition, including noncoherence of scientific bodies of knowledge and research traditions. Laudan[28] saw science as progressing along research traditions, with a collection of assumptions, tools, methods, and axioms guiding that science. Within these traditions, many theories resided that could change remarkably over time but commonalities remained that were sometimes grounded in the former research tradi-

tions. It is clear that Laudan's views are more descriptive of the state of the discipline of nursing, including that science is seen as a rational process used to solve problems. The hallmark of scientific progress in such a world would be the transformation of anomalous and unsolved problems into solved ones.

In nursing today, we see that the complete paradigm shift that Kuhn described has not occurred. There are nursing scientists (e.g., physiologists) still working within a positivist paradigm and other scientists (e.g., nurse anthropologists) who have never adopted a positivistic approach and essentially have always posited postmodernist views. These scientists manage to work side by side in a sometimes uneasy alliance, perhaps willing and able to let their views coexist because of some postmodern influence, such as tolerance for diversity.

Benner et al,[20] Reed,[2] and others have suggested several alternatives by which nursing may capitalize on the more useful aspects of both positivism and postmodernism but which go beyond both philosophic stances. Reed[2] has termed these "above and beyond efforts" *neomodernism* or an approach to nursing science in which a deliberative effort is made to use important traditional metanarratives to address current problems of nursing science. In Reed's view, this neomodernist approach includes the freedom to explore and propose alternative ways and methods for nursing science while taking into account important historic values and traditions. Neomodernism, therefore, offers an even more inclusive and seemingly a more liberated path than that of postmodernism.

Examples in nursing of cross-university research, wherein scientists from various philosophic backgrounds work to solve a specific scientific problem, are representative of a neomodernist perspective. In dementia research, bench scientists (who primarily use a positivist view) work with neomodernist nurse researchers to understand the nature of need-driven but dementia-compromised behavior in a cross-university effort.[30] There are many other examples of such interactive and integrative projects in nursing today. Nursing's scientific progress in the last two decades, therefore, appears more congruent with Laudan's perspective, which

CHAPTER 69

Philosophy of Technology and Nursing

Alan Barnard

This paper outlines the background and significance of philosophy of technology as a focus of inquiry emerging within nursing scholarship and research. The thesis of the paper is that philosophy of technology and nursing is fundamental to discipline development and our role in enhancing health care. It is argued that we must further our responsibility and interest in critiquing current and future health care systems through philosophical inquiry into the experience, meaning and implications of technology. This paper locates nurses as important contributors to the use and integration of health care technology and identifies nursing as a discipline that can provide specific insights into the health experience(s) of individuals, cultures and societies. Nurses are encouraged to undertake further examination of epistemological, ontological and ethical challenges to arise from technology as a focus of philosophical inquiry. The advancement of philosophy of technology and nursing will make a profound contribution to inquiry into the experience of technology, the needs of humanity and the development of appropriate health care.

Meaning in Technology

Technology embodies our desire to influence the world around us. At its most obvious, technology manifests itself as current, antiquated and failed objects and resources (e.g., stethoscopes, pharmaceuticals, machinery and devices) that are designed to enhance healthcare treatment through nursing and medical practice. In

About the Author

ALAN GORDON BARNARD was born in Australia and has qualifications in nursing, psychology, and education and holds a PhD. He has been involved in clinical practice and nurse education for more than 20 years and has extensive research and scholarly experience. Dr. Barnard has held positions in three Australian universities and has a professional commitment to qualitative method/methodology and furthering the theoretic basis of nursing. His research and scholarly interests relate to human experience of health care technology and the education of nurses, with particular emphasis on critical examination of beliefs and assumptions that inform the relations between technology and health care delivery. Dr. Barnard currently is currently the Course Coordinator for the Bachelor of Nursing Program, Queensland University of Technology, Australia.

addition, technology manifests as knowledge and skills associated with the use and application of resources and objects that nurses maintain and assess on a daily and ongoing basis. Finally, modern technology manifests increasingly within a technological system (technique) in which politics, organizations and humans are brought together with a primary aim of maximizing efficient and rational order. The relation of objects and resources to health-care practice is linked to the history of nursing practice and introduces patterns of activity that by their very nature influence patient care, values, knowledge, skills, political agendas, roles and responsibilities (Sandelowski, 1997; Barnard & Gerber, 1999b; Fairman & D'Antonio, 1999; Barnard, 2001c).

Technology is a word that engenders both confusion and meaning, and is used often to engender an aura of professionalism. The word is a commonplace descriptor for specialist and pseudo-specialist knowledge and skills (e.g., food technology, medical technology) that are influential in the ongoing development of specializations within healthcare and nursing. Its meaning is subject to historical and socio-cultural bias and is associated increasingly with sophisticated machinery, industrial objects, computerized or electronic automata, scientific knowledge and technical skills.

In recent years the dominant hierarchical model that treated technology as applied science has been replaced by a model that identifies science and technology as two separate bodies of knowledge and skills. It

has been recognized that technology often creates, develops and modifies existing technology using specific knowledge and skills and has a varied historical relation with science. In addition, numerous technological advances have originated from little or no understanding of science, and technological advances have preceded scientific knowledge and rationale. The development of the first aircraft and the steam engine are two commonly cited instances of technology developing separate from scientific explanation (Mumford, 1934; Ellul, 1964; Ihde, 1993).

Although science has provided technology with knowledge and insights for ongoing development, science should not be conceived of as essential for technological advancement from either an historical or a pre-conditional perspective (Barnard, 1996). Notwithstanding, throughout the last century science and technology combined increasingly to a point where both are interlinked in the process of discovery and development. Ihde (1993, p. 78) notes that technology and science now combine regularly to assist with modern research and development. Recent advancements are described best as techno-science because more than ever before, they rely on a fusion of scientific and technological knowledge and skills.

Technology has direct association with historical, scientific, philosophical and social precepts that are embodied in our lives, culture, politics, work, professions, language, values, education, knowledge and skills. Nurses are more than at any time before, required than a mere instrumental phenomenon. It is understood as *the* characteristic of modern society over and above political and economic ideology. In its extreme form it too fulfils the definition of being an essentialist perspective, because it is argued that technology is responsible for all the major challenges that afflict contemporary western societies (Feenberg, 1999).

Social constructivism focuses on social alliances that are important to technical choices. It is argued that different social groups (e.g., nurses, doctors, manufacturers, specialists) come together in one way or another in order to make choices and influence the use and development of technology. They influence the manifestation and/or experience(s) of technology through processes such as the supplying of resources, participation in its use, political support, financial support, etc., in the interests of differing groups, individuals and networks, who participate (or do not participate) in the process of accepting, rejecting and fostering technology. Technology is understood to be neither neutral nor autonomous. Technology reflects the outcome of a process of development that fixes the way it manifests and the social interests that may (not) accept a stake in its eventual form and influence (Feenberg, 1999).

Regardless of whether one assumes a substantivist, essentialist or social constructivist perspective (or a position somewhere in between), humanities philosophy of technology emphasizes critical examination of technology, and is positioned in opposition to the more hard-edged economic and technocratic view of the world that dominates much of current research and literature. It survives, somewhat tenuously, despite attempts to label it as anti-technology or unenlightened. The approach highlights nontechnical criteria in the interpretation of technology in order to develop a level of awareness that emphasizes human experience, values and understanding (i.e., the subject being dealt with, in addition to the object or agent of use). Contemporary humanities-orientated philosophers of technology such as Albert Borgmann, Andrew Feenberg, Don Ihde and Langdon Winner, confirm it is equally important to investigate the use and design of material artifacts as it is to understand machinery and equipment in terms of

human experience, gender, politics and culture. The perspective confirms that technology needs to be interpreted as more than material presence and/or instrumental action because technology embodies change, and is significant to interpreting gender, culture, traditions, action, values and praxis (Mitcham, 1994; Ihde, 1995; Feenberg, 1999).

Philosophy of Technology and Nursing

Bringing Forth Technology and Nursing Knowledge

The need to think about and find meaning in technology is evident increasingly in the practice development and future direction(s) of nursing. The task of understanding technology within nursing is both important and challenging due to its ubiquitous nature. Technology is everywhere we practice, yet we are not always aware of it. It seems at once to be both with us and yet not at the forefront of our experience. We use hundreds, if not thousands, of machines, pieces of equipment, tools, automata, policies and procedures in any one day, yet many of these things and activities go unnoticed as ordinary or commonplace. The technology of nursing is concealed often from our reflection, even though we have witnessed significant developments in technology and science. In fact, it is not until technology is revealed for its lack of utility and/or failure to respond in a desired manner that we notice it. In such cases, we may even award it a role in determining our life: 'the intravenous infusion pump will not work,' 'my watch has stopped' or 'the fridge is acting up.' Technology has seemingly a life of its own that we occasionally notice and engage with in a reflective way.

However, despite its quality of remaining hidden, it is important to recognize that nurses have always used tools and techniques in valued ways in order to achieve valued ends. Before the 20th century, nursing was a craft practised by individuals, of whom the vast majority were women who had gained experience in caregiving through religious orders and/or through families. Knowledge and skill developed by trial and error and were passed down through generations. Nursing practice relied on experience, intuition and faith, and was isolated to groups of individuals and geographical areas. Nurses relied less on scientific knowledge than on a personal and intuitive understanding and techniques developed and refined through practice (Abel-Smith, 1960; Reverby, 1987; Baly, 1995; Barnard, 2001b).

By the 1940s, nurses in developed countries were experiencing rapid expansion of knowledge and skills as a direct result of the development of medical science and technology. The rapid expansion led to the development of specialist wards/units/community services within environments that are noteworthy for their increasing patient acuity, changing values, computerization, unresolved ethical dilemmas, and changing economic, political, human and gender relations. In addition, nurses have accepted roles and responsibilities that have originated from the reassignment of medical and administrative duties (i.e., deputized to enact certain roles and responsibilities on their behalf). The deputation process (Barnard, 2001b) is ongoing and is characterized by an expansion of technical and administrative roles and responsibilities with varying degrees of nursing governorship (i.e., medicine often retains a supervisory and ownership role) (Reiser, 1978; Reverby, 1987; Brown, 1992; Walters, 1994; Fairman & Lynaugh, 1998; Barnard, 2001b).

The rapid growth of techno-science and the deputation of nurses has fostered the introduction of sophisticated technologies under the practice ambit of nurses. The process described has been central to our current position as a major contributor in the use of medical technology for health care delivery. Nurses accept a primary role for the use and integration of significant amounts of medical technology in health care in addition to the daily care of people in hospitals and the community. Therefore, nurses are positioned at an axis point between technology, individuals, clinical environments and communities and have a responsibility to take a primary role in interpreting and influencing the relationship(s) between technology, health care praxis and human experience.

Since the development of theories of nursing from the 1960s onwards, technology has become a focus of serious reflection. Nurse authors have focused on machinery and equipment use, alteration to skills and knowledge, nurse education, patient care outcomes and technology assessment as primary foci of concern (Carnevali, 1985; Jacox et al., 1990; McConnell, 1991; Calne, 1994; Locsin, 1995; McConnell, 1995; Pelletier, 1995; Hawthorne & Yurkovich, 1995; Bernardo, 1998). Nurse scholars have attempted to situate the outcomes of technological development and change within the contexts of nursing practice and care. They have stressed the need to develop technological intervention within various health care environments and in relation to changing health care practices.

In addition, there have been early advances in humanities-type perspectives that emphasize conceptual debate, historical analysis and critical inquiry. Literature has stressed the need for understanding of the relations between technology and the experience(s) of individuals and groups, nursing precepts, the future direction(s) for nursing practice, and conceptual/philosophical development (Ray, 1987; Allan & Hall, 1988; Fairman, 1992; Walters, 1995; Barnard, 1997; Sandelowski, 1997; Rudge, 1999; Purkis, 1999; Marck, 2000; Sandelowski, 2000; Barnard, 2001a, 2001c).

These developments represent a small yet growing collection of nursing research and scholarship that highlights technology as a principle focus of attention. Other developments important to furthering inquiry into technology and nursing have been, for example, the 1998 special edition of the journal *Holistic Nursing Practice 12*(4), the 1999 special edition of the Australian journal *Nursing Inquiry 6*(3), and the recently published books by Margarete Sandelowski (2000) entitled *Devices and Desires: Gender, Technology and American Nursing,* and Rozanno Locsin (2001) entitled *Advancing Technology, Caring, and Nursing.*

Technology: A Phenomenon Worthy of Philosophical Wonder

Technology is an important phenomenon and is worthy of significant philosophical reflection. Such worthiness demands a sustained focus on associated epistemological and refined analyses are required that rely less on generalizations about dehumanization, alienation or uncritical celebration of technology, than on considered critical reflection on specific relations between technology(ies), nursing care and healthcare practice(s). Broadening of interpretation is required that not only seeks macro examination of the relations between nursing and technology, but specific examination of discrete interventions and technology(ies). For example, there are domains of nursing practice that involve technologies that are subject commonly to cultural, gender and evolutionary alteration (e.g., care of the body, birthing practices). What was appropriate in the 1970s can bear little resemblance to our present time. In addition, technology manifests in certain social relations and is a reflection of cultural orientation, symbolism, technological systems and division of power. The use of technology can lead to 'positive' or 'negative' outcomes, but will most certainly not lead to outcomes that are neutral or do not require critical examination and reflection (Harding, 1980; Sandelowski, 2000; Marck, 2000; May et al., 2001; Barnard, 2001c; Barnard, 2001a).

Thirdly, philosophy of technology encourages us to reflect on technology from perspectives that are wider than the relation between technology and western culture. There are many countries that do not experience the same levels of techno-scientific development in healthcare services and nursing practices, although they are increasingly influenced by technical rationality. Therefore, for example, what are the implications of increasing technology in developing countries for current and future nursing practice and education? What lessons can be learned from contemporary nursing practice that may be instructive for healthcare provision and development?

Fourthly, it has been argued outside of nursing that issues related to cultural and global environments are of central and crucial concern, and the environmental movement is a potential source for the development of new healthcare perspectives (Ihde, 1993; Ferre, 1995). Foci specific to the environmental movement have potential for assisting with the development of nursing, partic-

ularly in relation to the use and disposal of health-related products and our role in the promotion of healthcare practices and lifestyles that are environmentally sensitive, appropriate and responsive to socio-cultural contexts. Ferre (1995) argues that the ecology movement has potential to provide assistance in 'postmodern' (alternative) interpretation(s) of technology. The movement has scope for greater synthesis of ideas and thinking that draws on the benefits of modern scientific analysis but is free to establish coherence in thinking that is not bound to the physics-based technological models of the pre- and current modern world. There is opportunity for scientific work that draws on the purposes and values of cultures, people, individuals and groups and emphasis on stability, durability, sustainability and satisfaction as dominant considerations rather than maximization of use, efficiency and rationalism. There is scope also to see nature and the human world as fundamentally intertwined with the objective world of technology and science. There are opportunities to make a significant contribution to thinking that seeks to correct what are according to Ferre (1995) the two great failures of modern technology: incoherence, or the failure to achieve synthesis for understanding, and inadequacy, or the failure to include subtle data in the powerful but ideally simplified concepts and models it uses.

Technology and Philosophical Reflection: Great Advance or Great Refusal

What is, and/or could be, the future for philosophy(ies) of technology and nursing? Can it assist nurses to interpret and engage with contemporary changes as they evolve rather than responding to them *post hoc?* Ihde (1993) notes that the use of philosophy/philosophers in applied ethics contexts such as medicine and healthcare comes too late. Philosophies are required to fix up or inquire into changes and developments that have occurred already in practice and contexts. Ihde (1993) emphasizes that even better assistance could be provided by philosophy through its inclusion in development processes. For example, it would be beneficial for nurses to be involved further in examining tele-medicine/nursing as approaches to the provision of healthcare services. May et al. (2001) note that although access to healthcare services is a primary reason for the development of tele-medicine, in the United Kingdom the reasons for its development are increasingly associated with economic/risk management. The technologies involved are seen increasingly as a political/technological fix to solving inequalities and the criteria used to assess the effectiveness of services are based commonly on objective measures such as efficiency, lowering costs, confidentiality and access to information. Whilst these measures are important, there are other measures of quality care that nurses would seek to include such as human-focused care, holistic treatment, the limitations of a lack of a physical presence in care, and the limitations of relying on digital information when undertaking healthcare assessment. These issues, and many more, require development and critique that arise from various philosophical perspectives.

The viewpoints expressed in this paper are predicated on the belief/assumption that the nursing discipline wants to progress understanding of technology that is based not only on dominant instrumentalist perspectives, but on critical analysis, reflection and evidence. To date, there has been a tendency within nursing and society(ies) to interpret technology based on inadequate and commonplace assumptions, and to foster a dominant agenda that has accepted technological development as a platform for professional advancement and prestige (Barnard, 1996, 1999b, 2000b, 2001c; Sandelowski, 1997; Purkis, 1999; Marck, 2000).

Professional advancement in association with technology is appropriate, but advancement must include active participation in seeking to optimize both health care intervention and understanding. The challenge is commonplace to society (and nursing) and was identified by Ellul (1997, p. 41) who noted that:

> People will ask, then, is a pure intellectual work what is needed? In a certain measure, yes. And it seems to me quite vain to want to dispense with intelligence in order to direct the action and to want to act right away and at any price, without knowing what one is going to do, without previously having

sat down to count the cost. Now this is very characteristic of the utopia and of technical solutions: one applies no serious intellectual method, and one seeks immediately to govern the action.

We need nursing practices that are culturally sensitive, individually aligned to specific needs, able to promote resistance and acceptance of technology(ies), and are reflective of adequate clinical reflection and judgement. If it is the case that we are not seeking to advance understanding of technology past instrumental action and application, then perhaps Marcuse (1964, p. 257) was correct when he argued that even if our thinking is judged by others to be incorrect or subversive, at minimum it is 'loyal to those who, without hope, have given there life to the great refusal.'

Conclusion: Technology and an Invitation to Inquiry

Philosophical and conceptual development that seeks to explain technology within the domain of nursing will assist to improve clinical practice, patient care and health care. Walters (1995, p. 339) highlighted its importance when he stated that:

> As nursing is practised in the midst of technology, acknowledging the material world of health care involves developing an understanding of technology used by nurses in their daily practice.

There is a need to (re)examine the relations between nursing and technology from not only an instrumental action but also from humanities-based perspectives that emphasize society, cultures and human experience. We require a type of technological thinking that seeks to examine our ambivalence towards technology with specific reference to its manifestation as 'both objective, material force and as a socially constructed and chameleon-like entity' (Barnard, 2001c, p. 372).

To these ends, there is need to critique rudimentary and popularized assumptions (popularized meaning: to make popular, especially by writing about (a subject) in a way that is understandable to most people) (Barnhart

The Author Comments

Philosophy of Technology and Nursing

Technology is significant to the history, contemporary practice, and future of nursing. Although nurses do an outstanding job at the delivery end of technology implementation, we have been less noteworthy in our critical examination of the relations between technology, nursing practice, and human experience. The article before the reader argues that theoretic/philosophic interpretation of technology is central to the future development of nursing as a profession. As we move forward into our new century, it is important that all nurses engage more with understanding the relations between technology and health care not only to provide care but also to determine appropriate care that is informed by debate and understanding. Philosophy of technology has the potential to assist us to raise our expectations and critically examine the many assumptions that inform clinical practice, research, and the education of nurses.

—ALAN GORDON BARNARD

CHAPTER 70

The Practice Turn in Nursing Epistemology

Pamela G. Reed

Nursing is a fascinating discipline. Nurses have the honor and expertise to participate closely in human healing processes of individuals, families, communities, and other systems of care. Yet, because the practitioner's expertise in healing is not fully understood, some account for it by relying on concepts (like intuition, tacit knowing, and gut feelings) that render nursing knowledge more mystical than professional. Admittedly, there are elements of mystery in nurses' patterns of knowing. However, contrary to philosophers of science Reichenbach and Popper, the *context of discovery* is not primarily mystical territory (Lamb & Easton, 1984), and this author believes it both possible and beneficial to obtain better explanations of how nursing knowledge is produced in the practice setting. Furthermore, trends in practice regarding evidence-based nursing, an intensified interest in advanced practice degrees, and the rise of the Doctorate of Nursing Practice degree all necessitate inquiry into nursing's epistemological infrastructure. In this column, the author proposes a rationale and a framework for thinking about knowledge production in nursing practice.

For too long, nursing has sustained the myth of the theory-practice gap and promulgated science as distinct from the discipline's art or practice. The researcher has been portrayed as the *producer* who hands down scientific knowledge to the clinician: as the *applier* of knowledge, sometimes *supplier* of ideas or researchable (aesthetic to technologic) to generate theories about healing processes that are facilitated by the caring acts of nursing practice.

Two basic assumptions underlie the model.

1. The practice setting is not only a place of knowledge application; it is a context wherein nurse-patient encounters generate important data for building nursing knowledge.
2. Knowledge production involves abstract thought and generation or refinement of nursing theory, at some level of theory.

Caveats and Conclusions

The characterizations of practitioner and researcher roles and other ideas put forth in the model admittedly are tentative and await further thought and dialogue. And the model begs for explanations about whether and how practitioners actually engage in the production of theory-based knowledge. Part of the answer lies in examining existing descriptions and theories about the various forms of human reasoning. Part of the answer will come from systematic study of practitioners in their daily work. And part of the answer resides in the goals and values nurses clarify concerning their science and practice.

Some may question the attention to nursing's epistemologic infrastructure in this column, given a general postmodern movement away from epistemology. But the concerns here shift from the classical normative epistemological stance to focus more on an empirical stance that seeks better explanation of the knowing process in nursing. Furthermore, this column, and Gary Rolfe's work that follows, provide evidence of a convergence of thought occurring independently across scholars, a phenomenon Lamb and Eastern (1984) called *multiple discoveries*. In other words, multiple people are sharing discoveries, in this instance regarding an intensifying interest in the untapped role of practice in nursing knowledge production, a questioning of traditional views of science that have perpetuated the subordination of clinicians, and pursuing what it means to know

and who are the legitimate knowers in nursing. It is hoped that more nurses will join the multiple discoveries unfolding concerning knowledge production in nursing practice.

REFERENCES

Abbott, A. (1988). *The system of professions.* Chicago: University of Chicago Press.

Alcoff, L. M. (1995). The problem of speaking for others. In J. Roof & R. Wiegman (Eds.), *Who can speak? Authority and critical identity* (pp. 97–119). Chicago: University of Illinois Press.

Baird, D. (2004). *Thing knowledge: A philosophy of scientific instruments.* Los Angeles: University of California Press.

Connor, M. J. (2004). The practical discourse in philosophy and nursing: An exploration of linkages and shifts in the evolution of praxis. *Nursing Philosophy, 5,* 54–66.

Diers, D. (1995). Clinical scholarship. *Journal of Professional Nursing, 11*(1), 24–30.

Doane, G. H., & Varcoe, C. (2005). Toward compassionate action: Pragmatism and the inseparability of theory/practice. *Advances in Nursing Science, 28*(1), 81–90.

Ellis, R. (1969). The practitioner as theorist. *American Journal of Nursing, 68,* 1434–1438.

Gibbons, M., Limoges, C., Nowotny, H., Schwartzman, S., Scott, P., & Trow, M. (1994). *The new production of knowledge: The dynamics of science and research in contemporary societies.* Thousand Oaks, CA: Sage.

Hess, D. J. (1997). *Science studies: An advanced introduction.* New York: New York University Press.

Lamb, D., & Easton, S. M. (1984). *Multiple discovery: The pattern of scientific progress.* Trowbridge, UK: Avebury.

Larsen, K., Adamsen, L., Bjerregaard, L., & Madsen, J. K. (2002). There is no gap 'per se' between theory and practice: Research knowledge and clinical knowledge are developed in different contexts and follow their own logic. *Nursing Outlook, 50,* 204–212.

Peplau, H. (1952). *Interpersonal relations in nursing.* New York: Putnam.

Peplau, H. (1992). Interpersonal relations: A theoretical framework for application in nursing practice. *Nursing Science Quarterly, 5,* 13–18.

Paterson, J., & Zderad, L. (1976). *Humanistic nursing.* New York: John Wiley & Sons.

Pickering, A. (1995). *The mangle of practice: Time, agency, and science.* Chicago: University of Chicago.

Pickstone, J. V. (2000). *Ways of knowing: A new history of science, technology and medicine.* Manchester, UK: Manchester University Press.

Reed, P. G. (1996). Transforming practice knowledge into nursing knowledge—A revisionist analysis of Peplau. *Image: Journal of Nursing Scholarship, 28*(1), 27–31.

Rolfe, G. (1996). *Closing the theory-practice gap: A new paradigm for nursing.* Oxford, UK: Butterworth-Heinemann.

Rolfe, G. (2000). *Nursing praxis and the reflexive practitioner: Collected papers 1993–1999.* London: NPI.

Rouse, J. (2002). *How scientific practices matter.* Chicago: University of Chicago Press.

Roy, C., & Obloy, M. (1978). The practitioner movement—toward a science of nursing. *American Journal of Nursing, 10,*1698–1702.

Shusterman, R. (1997). *Practicing philosophy: Pragmatism and the philosophical life.* New York: Routledge.

The Author Comments

The Practice Turn in Nursing Epistemology

This article was influenced by my interest in expanding nursing's knowledge-building capacity by more actively engaging practicing nurses in knowledge development. I see the move toward the practice doctorate as an opportunity to more deliberately integrate patients and practice experiences into theorizing. There are innovative approaches to theory development yet to be discovered in the 21st century. I hope educators can see their way to help develop nurses into scholars as well as practitioners of nursing. The ideas expressed in this chapter are summarized as five propositions in an article in the subsequent issue of *Nursing Science Quarterly,* Spring, 2007.

—Pamela G. Reed

CHAPTER 71

Nursing Praxis and the Science of the Unique

Gary Rolfe

Technical Rationality and the Theory-Practice Gap

The rise of research-based practice in the 1960s and 1970s and the growing influence of evidence-based practice over the past decade have served to establish technical rationality as the dominant discourse in nursing. The term *technical rationality* originated with Habermas (1970) and was employed by Schön (1983) to refer to the dominance of theory over practice (and hence of theorists over practitioners) and the one-way flow of information from research and researchers, through academic journals and textbooks, to nursing practice and practitioners. Under the rubric of technical rationality, new developments in nursing practice stem almost entirely from the findings of scientific (usually quantitative) research studies, and nurses are directed in their everyday practice by the writing of theorists.

However, the rise of theory (whether research-based *middle-range* theories or speculative *grand theories* and models) has also highlighted a gap or schism between theory and practice, in which the findings from research are not always smoothly translated or incorporated by nurses into their everyday practice. The most often cited resolution of the theory-practice gap was outlined by Hunt (1981) over two decades ago, and has been reiterated at regular intervals ever since. Hunt's explanations for the continued gap between theory and practice were the following: First, that nurses rarely read research reports; second, that when they do read them,

About the Author

GARY ROLFE was born in London and studied for a degree in philosophy at the University of Surrey, before training in Portsmouth as a psychiatric nurse. After working for several years in acute psychiatry, he took his master's degree and doctorate in the Department of Education at Southampton University. Gary lectured at the University of Portsmouth for many years before taking up a Chair in Nursing at Swansea University in Wales, where he currently lives with his wife and three children. Gary has published over 100 books, chapters, and journal articles, and has conducted research in the field of practice development and evidence-based practice. His current writing interests include postmodern philosophy, research methodology, and epistemology.

they rarely understand them; and third, even when they do read and understand research reports, they are reluctant or unable to apply the findings to practice for a number of personal and structural reasons. For supporters of technical rationality, the resolution of the theory-practice gap is thus for practitioners to make a greater effort to read and apply the findings of *gold standard* (usually quantitative) research to their practice.

Despite a variety of challenges to the dominance of positivist and/or quantitative research methodologies as the driving force of technical rationality, very few writers have questioned the paradigm of technical rationality itself. This is, perhaps, hardly surprising, since most of these writers are themselves theorists rather than practitioners, and any challenge to the dominance of theory over practice is also, to a greater or lesser extent, a challenge to the dominance of theorists over practitioners. Thus, while most theorists appear happy with Hunt's (1981) suggestion that the existence of the theory-practice gap is due largely to a reluctance or inability by nurses to apply research findings to their practice, very few writers have dared to suggest that perhaps the problem is one of inappropriate findings resulting from inappropriate research methodologies.

This suggestion is based on the suspicion that the social sciences might perhaps not provide us with the most appropriate research methodologies for nursing. These methodologies emerged from the desire of early social philosophers such as Auguste Comte and Emile Durkheim to replicate the huge technical advances made in the physical sciences during the 19th century,

and were therefore based on a similar model to physics and chemistry. Furthermore, since these early social scientists wished to study large social groups, they opted for statistical methodologies, which sought to generalize from carefully selected samples to the populations which those samples represented. Even when qualitative methodologies were later developed in the social sciences, many of them attempted to make similar generalizations from samples to populations. For example, while Husserlian phenomenology is not concerned with *statistical* generalizations, it nevertheless combines data from several respondents in order to make general statements about the lived experiences of members of particular social groups. Similarly, ethnographers usually attempt to generalize at the level of societies, rather than individuals.

Toward a Nursing Science of the Unique

When these methodologies were introduced to nursing by the first wave of nurse researchers (most of whom had taken doctorates in the social sciences), the aim was similarly to theorize at the macro level of social groups; to construct theories about nurses and patients *in general*. While theorizing at this macro level is entirely appropriate in the social sciences, where we wish to say something about how societies function, we run into difficulties in nursing, where we are (or should be) concerned with individual nurses and individual patients in which no two settings of clinical encounters

level? Can we still have a science of the unique in terms of communities?

GR: Yes, I think we can, so long as we then resist the temptation to generalize from the community to its individual members. I used the example of individual persons because I was curious that the noun *person* has two different plural forms, and I wished to make the point that it is possible to conceptualize and work with the concept of multiple individual persons as well as with the collective concept of people.

On Micro Theories and Clinical Theorizing

PR: Is your idea of theories about individual cases similar to what nursing introduced several years ago as micro level or practice theories, in contrast to theories of the mid-range or more abstract levels? Perhaps you and I are envisioning a clinical theorizing that requires more abstract thought than that for micro-level theories.

GR: The concept of micro theory was introduced by the sociologist Merton (1968) in the 1960s to refer to small-scale or specific theories that can usually be tested by a single empirical study. Some writers regard micro theories as more or less identical to research hypotheses, so that any midrange theory would generate a large number of micro theories, which could then be tested in a laboratory or practice setting. While such a concept bears similarities to my notion of informal clinical theories/hypotheses, there would appear to be a number of important differences. First, the purpose of micro theories is to test and refine midrange theories, whereas the primary purpose of my informal theories is to test and refine practice interventions. Second, micro theories are usually constructed and tested by researchers, rather than by practitioners as part of their praxis. And third, informal theories are just that, informal and disposable. An informal theory is formulated and tested, practice is modified, and the

practitioner/researcher casts it aside and moves on to the next informal theory. Informal theories are therefore largely instrumental and have little substantive knowledge-value in themselves.

On Scientific Knowledge and Patterns

PR: Doesn't scientific knowledge by definition describe *patterns* that apply to more than one case?

GR: While I agree that pattern description is one aim of science, I couldn't find a single definition of science that regards even description, far less *pattern* description, as a necessary condition. I would, in any case, be very cautious about asserting anything of science by definition, since there appears to be no single definition that even the majority of scientists agree upon. However, I suspect that this question is actually a restatement of your earlier one about whether it is possible to have a science that applies to single cases. As a supplement to my earlier response, I would add Ridley's (2001) point that the universe is the ultimate unique single case, and to reject a *science of the unique* as unscientific would be to accept that science has no role to play, for example, in a study of the origin of the universe.

On the Meaning of Praxis

PR: Do you have the source you used to define praxis in your book? Praxis has several different meanings. I usually think of praxis as the *enactment of one's values,* rather than enactment of theories, but I have seen the terms used in various ways.

GR: If you are referring to my book *Closing the Theory-Practice Gap* (Rolfe, 1996), then my main source was Carr and Kemmis' (1986) excellent book *Becoming Critical*, where praxis is defined as *doing action.* You are absolutely right to say that the term praxis is used in a variety of different ways. Its original Greek meaning is difficult to translate, but is often conceptualized as doing action in contrast to *theoria* (theory) and *poietike* (making-action). You are also quite right to point to its original moral component of *phronesis*, which is to say, of acting justly and truthfully. However, I am using the term in its modern Marxist/critical theorist meaning of mindful action.

On the Theory-Practice Gap as Attributable to Using the Wrong Kind of Theory

PR: What reactions have you received from your colleagues about your ideas on the practice-theory gap?

GR: My formulation of the theory-practice gap as being a function of the application of the wrong kind of theory resulted in a great deal of debate when I first published it (Rolfe, 1993). However, it appeared to capture the imagination of many practitioners and some theorists, who saw it as a way of validating and empowering nursing practice and practitioners. The introduction and growing popularity of evidence-based nursing has recently revived an interest in the importance of practitioners formulating and testing their own hypotheses, and the challenge now is to explore how nurses can legitimate their own informal sources of evidence.

Beyond Intuition

PR: I am interested in how one might view it as no less valid or scientific than researcher-based theorizing. I find the idea of the practitioners formulating and testing their own hypotheses exciting, particularly since it goes beyond mere intuition and preserves the link to science and theory in knowledge production.

GR: Part of my incentive for this work is precisely the desire, as you put it, to *go beyond mere intuition*,

since I always find it frustrating when practitioners claim that their mode of practice is tacit or based on gut feelings. While I appreciate that the intricacies of clinical practice might be difficult to put into words, I nevertheless share Schön's (1983) sentiment in his preface to *The Reflective Practitioner* that, "When people use terms such as 'art' and 'intuition', they usually intend to terminate discussion rather than to open up inquiry.... These attitudes have contributed to a widening rift between the universities and the professions, research and practice, thought and action" (pp. vii-viii). I hope that my comments in this column and the subsequent dialogue between us will be read as a simple and honest attempt to *open up inquiry* in the spirit of scholarly collegiality.

REFERENCES

Bacon, F. (1989). *The great instauration.* Arlington Heights, IL: Harlan Davidson.

Benner, P. (1984). *From novice to expert.* Menlo Park, CA: Addison-Wesley.

Carr, W., & Kemmis, S. (1986). *Becoming critical.* London: Palmer Press.

Dreyfus, H. L., & Dreyfus, S. E. (1986). *Mind over machine.* Oxford, United Kingdom: Basil Blackwell.

Gadamer, H. G. (1996). *The enigma of health.* Oxford, UK: Blackwell.

Habermas, J. (1970). *Toward a rational society* (J. Shapiro, Trans.). Boston: Beacon Press.

Hume, D. (1986). *A treatise of human nature.* New York: Penguin Classics.

Hunt, J. (1981). Indicators for nursing practice: The use of research findings. *Journal of Advanced Nursing, 6,* 189–194.

Merton, R. K. (1968). *Social theory and social structure.* New York: Free Press.

Popper, K. R. (1959). *The logic of scientific discovery.* London: Hutchinson.

Ridley, B. K. (2001). *On science.* London: Routledge

Rolfe, G. (1993). Closing the theory-practice gap: Model of nursing praxis. *Journal of Clinical Nursing, 2,* 173–177.

Rolfe, G. (1996). *Closing the theory-practice gap.* Oxford, UK: Butterworth Heinemann.

Sarvimaki, A. (1988). Nursing as a moral, practical, communicative- and creative activity. *Journal of Advanced Nursing, 13,* 462–467.

Schön, D. (1983). *The reflective practitioner.* London: Temple Smith.

Toulmin, S. (2003). *Return to reason.* Cambridge, MA: Harvard University Press.

The Author Comments

Nursing Praxis and the Science of the Unique

This article was the result of many years spent pondering the theory–practice gap in nursing and rejects the usually proposed solution of advocating that practice should more closely follow the directives of theory. In contrast, it suggests recasting theory to fit the demands of nursing practice as the concern with unique and individual therapeutic encounters rather than with general and generalizable prescriptions to respond in specific ways. In doing so, it resists the dichotomy between characterizing practice either in terms of a macro, rational nursing science or of a micro, intuitive nursing art. It does this by reformulating nursing as a science of the unique in which research and practice are brought together in the single unified action of nursing praxis. This view of nursing praxis challenges the hegemony of theory and theorists over practice and practitioners, and has profound implications for nursing in the 21st century.

—Gary Rolfe

CHAPTER 72

A Unitary Participatory Vision of Nursing Knowledge

W. Richard Cowling, III

This article responds to the calls by Margaret Newman for clarifying and expanding the nature of nursing knowledge. The unitary worldview proposed by Newman and the participatory worldview of action research are explicated, highlighting their respective major elements. A synthesis of unitary and participatory worldviews, grounded in a union of the elements of each, is proposed as a vision for the development of nursing knowledge. The unitary, participatory vision described offers the potential for inclusiveness and transcendence of previous perspectives of nursing knowledge.

This article poses a potential course for revisioning nursing knowledge based on a synthesis of unitary and participatory views of knowledge. The proposal is in response to calls by Newman[1-3] for clarifying and expanding the nature of nursing knowledge. Representations of nursing knowledge by Newman[1-3] and representations of action science by Reason and Bradbury[4,5] provide the foundation for the proposal.

Newman has argued for the necessity of clarifying the nature of nursing in general, and more specifically, for a transformation to a more inclusive realm of wholeness.[3] Hers is a call to "move to a realm of nursing that *includes and transcends* all of the realms that have gone before,"[2(p6)] using patterning as the dimension that brings everything together. Reason and Bradbury[4]

From W. R. Cowling, A unitary participatory vision of nursing knowledge. Advances in Nursing Science *2007, 30(1), 61–70. Copyright © 2007. Producedd with permission of Lippincott Williams & Wilkins.*

About the Author

WILLIAM RICHARD COWLING III was born at Clark Air Force Base, Manila, Philippines (where his mother and father were stationed after World War II), on December 10, 1948. He received a diploma in nursing (1969) and then a BS from the University of Virginia (1972), an MS in psychiatric mental health nursing from Virginia Commonwealth University (1979), and a PhD in nursing from New York University (1983). He is Professor and Director of the PhD Program in Nursing at the University of North Carolina Greensboro. Dr. Cowling is also the editor of the *Journal of Holistic Nursing*. The current focus of his scholarship is on a unitary, participatory, and appreciative understanding of the lives of women who have survived child abuse. Key contributions made to the discipline are creating scholarship that provokes new and deepened understandings of the wholeness of women's lives, developing methods of inquiry specific to unitary research and practice, developing approaches to inquiry that integrate healing, and supporting the development of students and others in learning about and using the unitary perspective in their work. His hobbies and interests are focused on gardening, feeding birds, reading, and watching movies that are unique in their presentation of life, and on his partner, his daughter, two granddaughters, and his animal companions Sammy, Paulo, and Atticus.

assert that the purpose of knowledge making, consistent with action research, is liberation of the human body, mind, and spirit and the making of a better world for everyone—also a purpose of nursing. Referring to Skolimowski's[6] work, they suggest that a style of inquiry that supports such knowledge making requires "the courage to imagine and reach for our fullest human capabilities."[4(p11)]

A Unitary View of Nursing Knowledge

Newman[2] identifies the focal points of nursing knowledge evolution as physical and environmental factors, actions to stabilize and assist patients, interpersonal processes of the nurse-patient relationship, behavioral correlates of health (defined as absence from disease), nursing diagnosis, nursing paradigms and conceptual models, and integration. Newman represents the evolution of nursing knowledge against the backdrop of evolving epistemologies of knowledge, including a science of observables and valid observations. She portrays an evolution in nursing knowledge toward inclusiveness, with each realm of nursing knowledge incorporating prior realms of knowledge. Furthermore, she views

these prior realms as special cases of the "patterning of the whole," which she saw as the realm bringing all aspects together.

Newman's[1-3] views are associated with the science of unitary human beings, the conceptual system from which she developed her theory of health as expanding consciousness. This conceptual system portrays human beings as fields of energy, entirely whole—not becoming whole, in mutual process with the environment. Each human field has a unique identity or individuation that expresses itself in the form of a pattern. Patterns are not directly observable, but their manifestations are conveyed in objective and subjective ways in a variety of human phenomena—physical/material, emotional/mental, social/cultural, and spiritual/mystical. These manifestations are facets of the wholeness and pattern of human beings or groups of human beings. Wholeness cannot be reduced to any one of these manifestations, but each provides a clue to wholeness and pattern. Newman emphasizes meaning as a critical expression of wholeness and pattern.

Newman[2] cites Wilber's[7] description of the evolution of theory as support for her perspective. Wilber proposed a vision of the evolution of theory as moving "from *matter* to *body* to *mind* to *spirit* with each subsequent realm of knowledge *transcending and including* the realm that preceded it."[2(p3)] His view has been described as a holarchy, rather than a hierarchy, with each of the realms being at once whole and a part of a larger whole. *Hierarchy* implies levels of evolution that are distinct, whereas *holarchy* implies levels of wholeness embedded in previous levels of wholeness. Newman characterizes nursing knowledge as a holarchical progression that "has moved from emphasis on *physical* care to *interpersonal* process to an *integrative* approach to a *unitary* perspective" in which "each succeeding level *transcends and includes* the previous ones."[2(p3)] In Newman's view, the unitary perspective does not discard physical, interpersonal, and integrative knowledge but accounts for it in the patterning of the whole, which is its primary focus. The unitary perspective accomplishes a current task of nursing, according to Newman, which is "to reconcile the seemingly contradictory points of view"[2(p3)] existing within nursing's knowledge domain.

Newman[3] has built the case for a unified perspective on the discipline. She also calls attention to the tendency of scientists within and outside of nursing to dichotomize things. Wilber,[8] influenced by Eastern philosophical thinking, described a typical manifestation of solving the problem of opposites as eradicating one, for instance, disease. Newman[3] uses the example of fluctuating body temperature as a manifestation of unitary patterning and the process of health *and* disease in one. She argues that there are no boundaries between art and science and between research and practice. In addition, she notes the convergence of various nursing theories, such as caring and health as expanding consciousness, as an indication of movement away from distinct boundaries in conceptualizing nursing knowledge. Newman has suggested further development in this direction, asking, "What is the transcendent unity of theories of nursing?"[3(p241)]

To answer this question, Newman argues that "the process of emerging nursing knowledge is one of including and transcending that which has gone before."[3(p243)] She grounds her point of view in the work of Wilber,[8] who suggested that schools of thought in science are complementary approaches to the various levels of individuals and opposites are complementary aspects of the same reality. Newman emphasizes that literature supports "the synthesis of caring and health with the underlying concepts of wholeness, pattern, mutual process, consciousness, transcendence, and transformation."[3(p243)] She has compiled a comprehensive statement from authors holding a variety of theoretical convictions to illustrate the transcendent unity of theories of nursing.

Newman[1–3] advocates a coherent message to society about nursing that flows from a clear disciplinary perspective. She argues for breaking with a paradigm that focuses on the other as object, fixing things, and hierarchical 1-way interventions. A unitary transformative perspective directs nursing toward the we in relationship, the meaning of the whole, and mutual process partnering, revealing a transforming world in process.[1]

The picture of nursing knowledge that represents Newman's view is emergent and evolving. It can be characterized as follows:

- nursing knowledge grounded in wholeness;
- nursing knowledge focused on patterning;
- nursing knowledge aimed at inclusiveness and transcendence; and
- nursing knowledge open to reconciliation with no boundaries.

Nursing Knowledge Grounded in Wholeness

Newman emphasizes the importance of grounding nursing knowledge in wholeness.[2,3] She describes her own theoretical and methodological journey in seeking to understand wholeness as the basic concept of the discipline of nursing, consistent with the unitary-transformative paradigm of the discipline.[9] Newman's perspective is clearly ontological. "Unbroken wholeness is what is real—not the fragments we devise with our way of describing things."[1(p37)] Cody has insisted that "we are compelled to apprehend, describe, and explain the full breadth of human diversity"[10(p98)] guided by discipline-wide emphasis on the wholeness of the human being.

sculpture, movement, and dance, drawing on aesthetic imagery. *Propositional knowing* draws on concepts and ideas, and *practical knowing* consummates the other forms of knowing in action in the world."[5(pp207–208)] Several other forms of knowing have been linked to the participatory worldview, including relational, reflective, representational, and feminist.[4] All of these extended epistemologies subscribe to multiple ways of knowing that arise from a relationship between self and other, involve participation and intuition, and assert the centrality of sensitivity and attunement at the moment of relationship.

Relational Ecological Form

The participatory worldview is more than a theory of knowledge—it is a political statement. This worldview implies democratic peer relationships affirming "people's right and ability to have a say in decisions that affect them and that claim to generate knowledge about them."[5(p208)] The participatory agenda includes liberating voices that are muted because of social restrictions resulting from poverty, sexism, racism, homophobia, class structures, and neocolonialism. In the generation of knowledge, connections between power and knowledge are illuminated. Relationships considered important in a participatory worldview extend beyond human to what is termed "more-than-human." For instance, as pointed out by Bradbury and Reason,[5] the systemic character of the planet's ecosystem and humanity's role in natural processes are emblematic of participatory concerns.

Purpose and Meaning: Spirit and Beauty

The development of knowledge is centered on the flourishing of life, including the life of persons, communities, and the "more-than-human."[5] The participatory worldview asks us "to inquire into what we mean by 'flourishing' and into the meaning and purpose of our endeavors."[5(p208)] The participatory worldview also encompasses the spiritual, enhancing consciousness toward a resacrilization or reenchantment of the world.[6,18,19] Ferrer[20] considers the participatory vision as a cornerstone for revisioning *transpersonal theory,* a developmental psychological theory having to do with transcending the

sphere of the individual, in relation to human spirituality. "Sacred experience is based in reverence, in awe and love for creation, valuing it for its own sake, in its own right as a living presence."[5(p209)] In the participatory worldview, the practical response to human problems is placed in a wider spiritual context—"Human practice inquiry is a spiritual expression, a celebration of the flowering of humanity and of the cocreating cosmos, and as a part of sacred science, it is an expression of the beauty and joy of the cosmos."[5(p209)] Reason and Bradbury[4] propose that the purpose of human inquiry is to heal the alienation that characterizes modern experience.

A Synthesis of Unitary and Participatory Views of Knowledge

The unitary view of nursing knowledge and the participatory view of knowledge provide complementary perspectives that offer insights and a potential vision to clarify and expand nursing knowledge.[2] Newman has noted the complementary nature of the unitary and participatory worldviews, acknowledging that "research in a paradigm characterized by pattern and process is participatory research."[1(p38)] She suggests that knowing a reality of wholeness and pattern requires experiencing it and engaging with it through the process of practice. Participation in research aids participants in understanding their situations and the potential for action.

Newman's[1] views concerning participatory research are consistent with the major philosophical assumption of most participatory research, which emphasizes the shortcomings of attempting to study something from the outside. However, Newman's conceptualization of participatory research methods is grounded in the ideal of seeking to understand the meaning of the whole through its pattern—a pattern that is constantly unfolding. For Newman, participatory research is a requisite of unitary science and the development of nursing knowledge because it provides the means for "entering into" the pattern as it is unfolding, rather than attempting to understand it from the outside.

The perspective on nursing knowledge that synthesizes unitary and participatory worldviews is characterized by the following elements:

- the nature of the cosmos as participatory, wholeness;
- patterning as the focus of practical being and acting;
- unitary knowing encompassing extended participatory epistemologies;
- a unitary, relational ecological form of inclusiveness and transcendence; and
- purpose and meaning opening to reconciliation with no boundaries.

The Nature of the Cosmos as Participatory, Wholeness

The proposed unitary, participatory view of nursing knowledge would be grounded in an ontology of the cosmos as participatory, wholeness. Laszlo has put forward a provocative image of the cosmos as a "whispering pond" with scientists, wherever they look, seeing nature "acting and evolving not as a collection of interdependent parts, but as an integrated, interacting, self-consistent, and self-creative whole."[4(p7),21] Ferrer[20] considers a participatory vision a way of explaining transpersonal, spiritual events, and argues that participatory refers to the "ontological predicament" of human beings. "Human beings are—whether they know or not—always participating in the self-disclosure of Spirit by virtue of their existence."[20(p121)] In the unitary, participatory version of ontology, this given participatory worldview is extended to all phenomena. Ferrer[20] proposes that the participatory predicament he describes is also the ontological foundation of other forms of participation, implying that all phenomena are participatory in nature.

Patterning as the Focus of Practical Being and Acting

The practical being and acting associated with participatory action research would be broadened to encompass a patterning focus. The referent point for the practical would be the unitary patterning of individuals and communities or any groups of individuals in concert with the environment. Theories could be generated that would illuminate patterning-based action, guide it, and provide it with meaning. This would assist the nursing community in articulating further the nature of knowing and a body of knowledge associated with wholeness and patterning—one that has practical consequences. The focus on practical being and acting based on patterning amplifies nursing's longstanding value concerns—our relationship with others and the environment, our questions about what is worthwhile for the human condition, and our pursuit of purpose and meaning.

Unitary Knowing Encompassing Extended Participatory Epistemologies

A unitary, participatory ontological view requires extended epistemologies, which have been developed and continue to be developed in the field of participatory inquiry. A multiplicity of modes of knowing is drawn upon to reveal participatory, wholeness in its varied patterning forms. Potential extended epistemologies that would support inquiry into phenomena of concern to nursing from a unitary, participatory perspective would include the representational, relational, and reflective forms of knowing described by Park.[22] These forms of knowledge are viewed by participatory researchers as extending beyond objective knowledge. They address the need for broadening "existing epistemological horizons to include forms of knowledge associated with various human concerns"[22(p83)]—and not dealt with through objective forms.

Representational knowledge can be either functional or interpretive. *Functional knowledge* is the portrayal of one entity or experience as a variable related to another; for example, "powerlessness is a function of proverty."[22(p82)] *Interpretive knowledge* "manifests itself as understanding of meaning and requires that the knower come as close to the to-be-known as possible.[22(p83)] "This involves taking into account backgrounds, intentions, and feelings in seeking to understand human affairs and creations. *Relational knowledge* is a kind of knowing that comes from knowing another human being affectively. This type of knowing is infused with relational meaning that can bring people together. "It resides in the act of relating and shows itself in words, expressions, and other forms of doing relationship."[22(p85)] *Reflective knowledge* is associated with the critical tradition incorporating the notion that human knowledge must move beyond understanding to changing the world. This form of knowledge involves change-producing activity through conscious reflection. It embraces the dignity of human beings as autonomous beings capable of acting on their own behalf.

The core forms of knowing associated with participatory research would be a starting point.[4] *Experiential knowing* would serve as a primary mode of entering into the field of wholeness and appreciating the nature of patterning from the standpoint of direct encounter with the person, place, or thing. *Empathy and resonance* would be skills developed to facilitate in-depth knowing. *Presentational knowing* offers a way of creatively and meaningfully expressing wholeness and patterning through story, picture, sculpture, movement, dance, and other types of aesthetic imagery. *Propositional knowing* would be based upon previous forms of knowing and would provide theoretical understandings of wholeness and patterning. *Practical knowing* would consummate the other forms of knowing, providing for the development of skills of inquiry and ways of living that are grounded in wholeness and focus on patterning through knowing participation in change.

A Unitary, Relational, Ecological Form of Inclusiveness and Transcendence

The unitary perspective has an implied political agenda that accompanies a theory of knowledge. The unitary, participatory view, as with any worldview, will find its expression in political structures and organizational forms. The relational and ecological form of the participatory worldview will find expression in political structures and organizational forms that integrate the unitary values of inclusiveness and transcendence. The political dimension of participatory wholeness asserts the primacy of people's right and ability to be involved in generating knowledge about them that is not fragmenting, alienating, and restricting in the manifestation of their

human existence and experience. The notion of participatory, wholeness extends to groups and communities as well as individuals, implying the need to include muted voices and respect the richness and infiniteness of human patterning. From this perspective flows the potential for the fullest exercise of the power of people to produce their own knowledge that serves their purposes.

Newman, in a world of no boundaries, characterizes a liberated person as transcending "opposites, like good and evil . . . moving to unity consciousness."[3(p241)] Furthermore, she advocates release of rights and wrongs as a basic dichotomy pervasive in our society. While these statements may appear to stand in counter distinction to the emancipatory aims of participatory research, Newman's overarching value of nursing as a transformative enterprise supports human liberation and advancement. For instance, she advocates that nurses take several actions to release themselves from boundaries in constructing nursing knowledge and practice. These include (1) fulfilling one's purpose in society by "letting go of imposed, external values and allowing one's inner voice to emerge"[3(p244)]; (2) "reaching out to others who hold values contrary to one's own and support their action potential"[3(p244)]; and (3) creating caring communities exemplified by transformation.

Purpose and Meaning Opening to Reconciliation With no Boundaries

According to the participatory worldview, the purpose of human inquiry is the flourishing of human life.[4] This worldview calls for a participative consciousness that embraces sacred experience and recognizes the mystery that entails seeing the world as a sacred place. Beyond searching for truth, there is a desire to heal alienation in the human experience and condition. Rather than the notion of healing to make whole, the participative, wholeness perspective accepts wholeness as inherent in all beings. Thus, a conceptualization of healing that would serve the purpose and meaning of the participatory, wholeness worldview is one that appreciates wholeness.[11] This appreciation occurs from being open to the ideals of reconciliation and envisioning a world with no boundaries. Ferrer[20] described participatory knowing in a way that suggests congruence with unitary knowing. His description demonstrates reconciliation with no boundaries. This knowing "refers to a multidimensional access to reality that includes not only the intellectual knowing of the mind, but also the emotional and empathic knowing of the heart, the sensual and somatic knowing of the body, the visionary and intuitive knowing of the soul, as well as any other way of knowing available to human beings."[20(p121)]

Summary

Newman,[2] using Bernstein[23] as a source of support, argues for integration of knowledge to frame nursing science—one that would assimilate empirical, interpretive, and critical dimensions to create a theoretical orientation aimed at practical activity. This view might be held as impossible, or at least highly flawed by empiricists. In addition, the overwhelming hegemony of empiricism in nursing and medical science that such an integrative approach might face in competing for funding could prevent significant advancement of unitary, participatory research programs. Yet, the unitary participatory vision of nursing knowledge, with its participatory approaches aimed at capturing the patterning of wholeness that underlies human life and relationships, clearly adds to the repertoire of methods that can address societal concerns. Just as community-based participatory research has gained prominence in scientific funding, approaches grounded in the unitary, participatory perspective will be valued as extensions of research.

In the conclusion of her essay on a world with no boundaries, Newman portrays her work as an "effort to open our hearts and minds to the boundaryless nature of nursing knowledge."[2(p244)] She depicts the profession of nursing as positioned to facilitate the transformation of the world—attributing to it a ripeness that is even more prominent today. "We must cease the binding conflict that exists in a struggle to protect false boundaries. As we explore a world of no boundaries, we will experience the compassion of and creativity of unity consciousness."[2(p244)]

Reason and Bradbury[4] call attention to the paucity of debate about the purpose of knowledge making. They note the primary value placed by academia and institutions of science on the knowledge-making process of pure research unburdened by practical concerns. They view action research as lacking interest in the production of academic theories based on action, theories about action, and theoretical or empirical knowledge applied in action; rather, its primary purpose is "to liberate the human body, mind, and spirit in the search for a better, freer world."[4(p2)]

Ferrer calls for a participatory vision of human spirituality that positions scientists and practitioners to talk about knowledge of a more liberated self and world, a central purpose of nursing, "not so much in terms of 'things as they really are,' but of 'things as they can be' or even 'things as they should be.'"[20(p177)] In line with a world that can be or should be, Bradbury and Reason[5] call researchers to both search for and develop a world worthy of human aspiration. The unitary, participatory view of nursing knowledge represents the vision of such a world.

REFERENCES

1. Newman MA. Experiencing the whole. *ANS Adv Nur Sci.* 1997;20(1):34–39.
2. Newman MA. The pattern that connects. *ANS Adv Nur Sci.* 2002;24(3):1–7.
3. Newman MA. A world of no boundaries. *ANS Adv Nur Sci.* 2003;26(4):240–245.
4. Reason P, Bradbury H. Introduction: inquiry and participation in search of a world worthy of aspiration. In: Reason P, Bradbury H, eds. *Handbook of Action Research: Participative Inquiry and Practice.* Thousand Oaks, Calif: Sage; 2001:1–14.
5. Bradbury H, Reason P. Issues and choice points for improving the quality of action research. In: Minkler M, Wallerstein N, eds. *Community-based Participatory Research for Health.* San Francisco: Josey-Bass; 2003:201–220.
6. Skolimowski H. *A Sacred Place to Dwell: Living With Reverence Upon the Earth.* Rockport, Mass: Element; 1993.
7. Wilber K. *The Marriage of Sense and Soul: Integrating Science and Religion.* New York: Random House; 1998.
8. Wilber K. *No Boundary: Eastern and Western Approaches to Personal Growth.* Boulder, Colo: Shambhala; 1981.
9. Newman MA, Sime AM, Corcoran-Perry SA. The focus of the discipline of nursing. *ANS Adv Nur Sci.* 1991:14:1–6.

10. Cody WK. Lyrical language and nursing discourse: can science be the tool of love? *Nurs Sci Q.* 2002;15(2):98–106.

11. Cowling WR. Healing as appreciating wholeness. *ANS Adv Nurs Sci.* 2000;22(3):16–32.

12. Heron J. *Co-operative Inquiry: Research Into the Human Condition.* London: Sage; 1996.

13. Heron J, Reason P. A participatory inquiry paradigm. *Qual Inq.* 1997;3(3):274–294.

14. Skolimowski H. *The Participatory Mind.* London: Arkana; 1994.

15. Heron J. Quality as primacy of the practical. *Qual Inq.* 1996;2(1):41–56.

16. Macmurray J. *The Self as Agent.* London: Faber & Faber; 1957.

17. Heron J, Reason P. The practice of co-operative inquiry: research "with" rather than "on" people. In: Reason P, Bradbury H, eds. *Handbook of Action Research: Participative Inquiry and Practice.* Thousand Oaks, Calif: Sage; 2001: 179–188.

18. Berman M. *The Reenchantment of the World.* Ithaca, NY: Cornell University Press; 1981.

19. Berry T. *The Dream of the Earth.* San Francisco: Sierra Club; 1988.

20. Ferrer J. *Revisioning Transpersonal Theory: A Participatory Vision of Human Spirituality.* Albany: State University of New York Press; 2002.

21. Laszlo E. *Holos: The Fabulous World of the New Sciences: Exploring the Emerging Vision of Quantum, Cosmos, Life and Consciousness* [unpublished work]. Cited by: Reason P, Bradbury H. Introduction: inquiry and participation in search of a world worthy of aspiration. In: Reason P, Bradbury H, eds. *Handbook of Action Research: Participative Inquiry and Practice.* Thousand Oaks, Calif: Sage; 2001:1–14.

22. Park P. Knowledge and participatory research. In: Reason P, Bradbury H, eds. *Handbook of Action Research: Participative Inquiry and Practice.* Thousand Oaks, Calif: Sage; 2001: 81–90.

23. Bernstein R. *Beyond Objectivism and Relativism: Science, Hermeneutics, and Praxis.* Philadelphia: University of Pennsylvania; 1983.

The Author Comments

A Unitary Participatory Vision of Nursing Knowledge

I was inspired to write this article because there was a convergence of the unitary perspective and the participatory perspective in my work in seeking to understand the life patterning, healing, and health of people. In particular, I was motivated by the calls by Margaret Newman for clarifying and expanding the nature of nursing knowledge. Both the unitary and participatory views had guided my theoretical understandings and my methodological choices in exploring the lives of women in despair. I sought to explicate the distinctive features of each perspective and to articulate a unification of the elements that could guide a vision of nursing knowledge—one that would include and transcend previous perspectives and offer a more liberated view of nursing knowledge worthy of human aspiration.

—WILLIAM RICHARD COWLING, III

Author Index